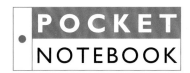

POCKET
NOTEBOOK

Pocket
OBSTETRICS
AND GYNECOLOGY

Second Edition

Edited by

K. JOSEPH HURT, MD, PhD

Assistant Professor
Department of Obstetrics and Gynecology
University of Colorado School of Medicine

T0200319

Wolters Kluwer

Philadelphia · Baltimore · New York · London
Buenos Aires · Hong Kong · Sydney · Tokyo

Acquisitions Editor: Chris Teja
Development Editor: Ashley Fischer
Editorial Coordinator: Lindsay Ries
Marketing Manager: Rachel Mante-Leung
Production Project Manager: Bridgett Dougherty
Design Coordinator: Teresa Mallon
Manufacturing Coordinator: Beth Welsh
Prepress Vendor: Aptara, Inc.

2nd edition

9 8 7 6

Printed in China

Library of Congress Cataloging-in-Publication Data

Names: Hurt, K. Joseph, editor.
Title: Pocket obstetrics and gynecology / edited by K. Joseph Hurt.
Other titles: Pocket notebook.
Description: 2nd. | Philadelphia : Wolters Kluwer, [2019] | Series: Pocket notebook | Includes index.
Identifiers: LCCN 2018040264 | ISBN 9781496366993 (spiral bound)
Subjects: | MESH: Genital Diseases, Female | Gynecologic Surgical Procedures | Pregnancy Complications | Obstetric Surgical Procedures | Handbooks
Classification: LCC RG107 | NLM WP 39 | DDC 618.1/075—dc23
LC record available at https://lccn.loc.gov/2018040264

CONTENTS

Contributors	x
Foreword	xiv
Preface	xv

WELL-WOMAN VISIT AND PRIMARY CARE
Elizabeth Patberg, Reeva Makhijani, Leo Han, and Sharon T. Phelan

Well-Woman (Annual) Exam	1-1
Benign Breast Disease	1-3
Breast Cancer	1-5
Cervical Cancer Screening	1-7
Lipids and Cholesterol	1-10
Obesity	1-11
Osteoporosis	1-12
Skin Cancer Screening	1-13
Domestic Violence	1-15
Substance Abuse	1-16
Depression and Psychiatric Disease Screening	1-16
Contraception and Sterilization	1-16
Emergency Contraception (EC)	1-18
Vaccinations	1-19
Women's Health Epidemiology and Research	1-20

EMERGENCY ROOM
Eduardo Hariton and Roxanne A. Vrees

Imaging in OBGYN	2-1
Ultrasound in Early Pregnancy	2-2
Acute Pelvic Pain	2-2
Ectopic Pregnancy	2-3
Early Pregnancy Failure	2-5
Ovarian Cysts	2-7
Adnexal Torsion	2-7
Pelvic Inflammatory Disease (PID)	2-8
Acute Uterine Bleeding	2-9
Trauma in Pregnancy	2-11
Sexual Assault	2-12

OPERATIVE OB-GYN
K. Lauren Barnes, David I. Shalowitz, and Leigh A. Cantrell

Perioperative Patient Management	3-1
Postoperative Ileus	3-5
Postoperative Fever	3-6
Surgical Site Infections (SSI)	3-6
Perioperative DVT/PE	3-7
Sepsis	3-8
Perioperative Oliguria	3-9
Bowel Obstruction	3-10
Complications of Laparoscopy	3-11
Complications of Hysteroscopy	3-12

OB-GYN ANESTHESIA

Ross Harrison and Lisa Gill

Gynecologic Anesthesia	4-1
Parenteral Analgesia in Obstetrics	4-1
Neuraxial Anesthesia in Obstetrics	4-2
Local Anesthetics in Obstetrics	4-5
Nonpharmacologic Analgesia in Obstetrics	4-6
General Anesthesia in Obstetrics	4-6
Postoperative Pain Management	4-7
Inhalational Analgesia in Obstetrics	4-7

GENERAL GYNECOLOGY

Polina Rovner, Dana Marie Scott, Jessica Opoku-Anane, and Teresa M. Walsh

Vulvovaginitis	5-1
Bartholin Gland Cyst and Abscess	5-2
Uterine Fibroids	5-3
Adenomyosis	5-5
Endometriosis	5-5
Abnormal Uterine Bleeding (AUB)	5-8
Postmenopausal Bleeding	5-10
Dysmenorrhea	5-11
Premenstrual Syndrome (PMS) and Premenstrual Dysphoric Disorder (PMDD)	5-12
Chronic Pelvic Pain	5-13
Vulvar Pain/Vulvodynia	5-14
Female Sexual Dysfunction	5-15
Menopause	5-16
Hormone Therapy	5-17
Pregnancy Termination	5-18
Adnexal Masses	5-19

PEDIATRIC AND ADOLESCENT GYNECOLOGY

Evelyn Hall and Kavita Shah Arora

Puberty	6-1
Precocious Puberty	6-2
Delayed Puberty	6-4
Amenorrhea	6-6
Androgen Insensitivity Syndrome	6-9
Congenital Adrenal Hyperplasia (CAH)	6-11

PELVIC SURGERY AND UROGYNECOLOGY

William D. Winkelman and Sherif El-Nashar

Physiology and Mechanisms of Micturition	7-1
Physiology and Mechanisms of Defecation	7-1
Pelvic Organ Prolapse (POP)	7-1
Urinary Incontinence	7-4
Overactive Bladder and Urge Incontinence	7-5
Stress Incontinence	7-6
Overflow Incontinence	7-7
Bypass Incontinence and Urogenital Fistulae	7-7

Interstitial Cystitis	7-8
Anal Incontinence	7-9

INFERTILITY
Pietro Bortoletto and Christine Conageski
Infertility Evaluation	8-1
Premature Ovarian Insufficiency (POI)	8-2
Polycystic Ovarian Syndrome (PCOS)	8-2
Tubal Factor Infertility	8-3
Recurrent Pregnancy Loss (RPL)	8-4
Müllerian Anomalies	8-4
Male Factor Infertility	8-8
Ovulation Induction and Assisted Reproduction	8-9
Fertility Preservation	8-10
Preimplantation Genetic Testing	8-11
Ovarian Hyperstimulation Syndrome (OHSS)	8-11

PRENATAL CARE
Meghan Klavans, Amy Nacht, and Todd J. Stanhope
Routine Prenatal Visits	9-1
Nutrition in Pregnancy	9-3
Clinical Pelvimetry	9-4
Common Prenatal Complaints	9-5
Fetal Ultrasound: Anatomy and Echocardiography	9-8
Congenital Anomalies	9-9
Genetic Screening	9-12
Amniocentesis and Chorionic Villus Sampling (CVS)	9-13

NORMAL LABOR AND DELIVERY
Benjamin S. Harris and Jessica C. Ehrig
Antenatal Fetal Testing	10-1
Fetal Lung Maturity Testing by Amniocentesis	10-2
Newborn Respiratory Distress	10-2
Group B Streptococcal Disease	10-3
Spontaneous Labor and Delivery	10-4
Induction of Labor (IOL)	10-6
Intrapartum Fetal Monitoring	10-7
Operative Vaginal Delivery	10-12
Vaginal Birth After Cesarean	10-13
Fetal Cord Blood Gas Analysis	10-14
Routine Postpartum Care	10-15
Breastfeeding	10-15
Affiliated Obstetrical Providers	10-16

COMPLICATED PREGNANCY AND DELIVERY
Tana Kim, Neggin B. Mokhtari, and Shane Reeves
Gestational Hypertensive Disorders	11-1
Hydrops Fetalis	11-2
Intrauterine Growth Restriction	11-3
Multiple Gestation	11-4
Cervical Insufficiency & Short Cervix	11-5
Preterm Premature Rupture of Membranes	11-6

Preterm Labor   11-8
Postpartum Hemorrhage (PPH)   11-9
Placental Abruption   11-12
Placenta Previa   11-13
Vasa Previa   11-14
Placenta Accreta   11-14
Uterine Inversion   11-15
Amniotic Fluid Embolism   11-15
Malpresentation   11-16
Fetal Meconium   11-16
Intraamniotic Infection   11-17
Endomyometritis   11-18

CARDIOLOGY AND CARDIOVASCULAR DISEASE
Lauren Carlos and Sarah Rae Easter
Cardiovascular Disease in Pregnancy   12-1
Cardiovascular Changes in Pregnancy   12-2
Chronic Hypertension (CHTN)   12-3
Hypertensive Crisis   12-5
Pregnancy-Related Hypertension   12-6
Coronary Artery Disease/Acute Coronary Syndrome   12-10
Pulmonary Hypertension   12-11
Valvular Heart Disease   12-12
Peripartum Cardiomyopathy   12-15

PULMONARY
Anne Holland Mardy and David I. Shalowitz
Pulmonary Function Testing   13-1
Respiratory Changes in Pregnancy   13-2
Arterial Blood Gas (ABG) Analysis   13-3
Pneumonia   13-4
Pulmonary Edema   13-5
Influenza in Pregnancy   13-6
Asthma and Pregnancy   13-6
Anaphylaxis   13-7

NEPHROLOGY AND URINARY TRACT
Shriddha Nayak and Catherine Hudson
Urinary System Changes in Pregnancy   14-1
Acute Kidney Injury (AKI)   14-1
Chronic Kidney Disease   14-3
Urinary Tract Infection (UTI)   14-4
Pyelonephritis   14-6
Nephrolithiasis   14-7
Fluids and Electrolytes   14-8

GASTROENTEROLOGY
Jennifer R. McKinney, Melissa Teitelman, and Chad A. Grotegut
Gastrointestinal Changes in Pregnancy   15-1
Cholelithiasis   15-1
Cholecystitis   15-1
Pancreatitis   15-1

Appendicitis	15-3
Irritable Bowel Syndrome (IBS)	15-4
Inflammatory Bowel Disease	15-5
Viral Hepatitis	15-7
Intrahepatic Cholestasis of Pregnancy (ICP)	15-9
HELLP Syndrome	15-10
Acute Fatty Liver of Pregnancy (AFLP)	15-11
Total Parenteral Nutrition (TPN)	15-12

HEMATOLOGY

Ashley E. Benson, Chelsea K. Chandler, Sarah Rae Easter, and Todd J. Stanhope

Hematologic Changes of Pregnancy	16-1
Anemia	16-1
Hemoglobinopathies	16-3
Thrombocytopenia (Plt <150000/μL)	16-4
Venous Thromboembolic Disease	16-6
Thrombophilia Evaluation	16-10
Coagulopathies	16-11
Antiphospholipid Antibody Syndrome (APS)	16-12
Alloimmunization	16-13
Neonatal Alloimmune Thrombocytopenia (NAIT)	16-15
Blood Products for Hemorrhage and Critical Care	16-15

ENDOCRINOLOGY

Maeve Hopkins, Pietro Bortoletto, Megan R. Barrett, and Jon G. Steller

Hormonal Regulation	17-1
Type I Diabetes Mellitus	17-2
Diabetic Ketoacidosis (DKA)	17-3
Type II Diabetes Mellitus	17-4
Hyperosmolar Hyperglycemic State	17-4
Diabetes in Pregnancy	17-5
Gestational Diabetes (GDM)	17-7
Hypothyroidism	17-8
Hyperthyroidism	17-9
Adrenal Disorders	17-10
Hyperandrogenism	17-12
Hirsutism	17-13
Parathyroid Disorders	17-14
Pituitary Disorders	17-16

NEUROLOGY

Ashish Premkumar and Irina Burd

Headache (HA)	18-1
Migraine	18-2
Seizure Disorders	18-3
Eclampsia	18-5
Stroke in Pregnancy	18-6
Cerebral Venous Thrombosis	18-7
Multiple Sclerosis in Pregnancy	18-8
Neuropathies in Pregnancy	18-8

PSYCHIATRY
Emily Fay and M. Camille Hoffman

Substance Abuse	19-1
Depression	19-3
Anxiety Disorders	19-4
Bipolar Disorder	19-5
Psychosis	19-5
Schizophrenia	19-6

DERMATOLOGY
Said S. Saab and Misha D. Miller

Dermatologic Changes in Pregnancy	20-1
Lichen Sclerosus	20-2
Lichen Simplex Chronicus	20-3
Lichen Planus	20-3
Psoriasis	20-4
Hidradenitis Suppurativa	20-5
Apocrine Miliaria	20-5
Gyn-Derm Cysts	20-6
Common Dermatologic Manifestations of Systemic Disease	20-6

INFECTIOUS DISEASE
Christina Megli and Catherine Albright

HIV/AIDS in Women	21-1
TORCH Infections	21-2
Other Infections in Pregnancy	21-4
Human Papilloma Virus (HPV)	21-6
Syphilis	21-7
Molluscum Contagiosum	21-9
Chancroid	21-9
Pubic Lice	21-10
Genital Ulcers	21-10

GYNECOLOGIC ONCOLOGY
Erin Blake, Allison Gockley, and Ritu Salani

Types of Hysterectomy	22-1
Cervical Cancer	22-2
Uterine Cancer	22-4
Epithelial Ovarian Cancer (EOC)	22-7
Germ Cell Tumors	22-8
Sex Cord-Stromal Tumors	22-10
Vaginal Cancer	22-11
Vulvar Cancer	22-12
Gestational Trophoblastic Neoplasia	22-14
Chemotherapy	22-16
Radiation Therapy	22-18

APPENDIX 1: OB-GYN ANATOMY PRIMER
OB-Gyn Anatomy Primer   23-1

APPENDIX 2: COMMON PROCEDURES AND SURGERIES
Misha Pangasa and Brittney D. Bastow
Intrauterine Device Insertion (IUD)   24-1
Subdermal Device Insertion   24-1
Bartholin Abscess Incision and Drainage   24-2
Loop Electrosurgical Excision Procedure (LEEP)   24-4
Endometrial Biopsy   24-5
Amniocentesis   24-5
Dilatation and Curettage (Evacuation)   24-5
Cold Knife Conization (CKC)   24-5
Operative Hysteroscopy   24-6
Endometrial Ablation   24-6
Hysteroscopic Tubal Ligation   24-7
Operative Laparoscopy   24-7
Total Abdominal Hysterectomy   24-7
Vaginal Hysterectomy   24-8
Cesarean Section   24-8
Postpartum Tubal Ligation   24-9
Cervical Cerclage   24-10
Repair of Obstetrical Laceration   24-10
Pudendal Nerve Block   24-10
Male Circumcision   24-11
Common Surgical Instruments   24-11

APPENDIX 3: DRUG REFERENCE
Kevin W. McCool and Allison Faucett
Medications in Obstetrics & Gynecology   25-1

APPENDIX 4: ACLS ALGORITHMS
ACLS Algorithms   26-1

APPENDIX 5: NRP ALGORITHM
Neonatal Resuscitation Program Algorithm   27-1

ABBREVIATIONS   28-1

INDEX   I-1

CONTRIBUTORS

Catherine Albright, MD, MS
Assistant Professor
Maternal Fetal Medicine
Obstetrics & Gynecology
University of Washington
Seattle, Washington

Kavita Shah Arora, MD, MBE
Assistant Professor
Obstetrics & Gynecology and
  Bioethics
Case Western Reserve University
Cleveland, Ohio

K. Lauren Barnes, MD
Resident, Obstetrics & Gynecology
Harvard Medical School
Boston, Massachusetts

Megan R. Barrett, MD
Assistant Professor
Obstetrics & Gynecology
Duke University School of
  Medicine
Durham, North Carolina

Brittney D. Bastow, MD
Senior Instructor
Obstetrics & Gynecology
University of Colorado
Aurora, Colorado

Ashley E. Benson, MD
Resident, Obstetrics &
  Gynecology
University of Utah
Sale Lake City, Utah

Erin Blake, MD, MSc
Resident, Obstetrics &
  Gynecology
University of Colorado
Aurora, Colorado

Pietro Bortoletto, MD
Resident, Obstetrics & Gynecology
Harvard Medical School
Boston, Massachusetts

Irina Burd, MD, PhD
Associate Professor
Maternal Fetal Medicine
Gynecology & Obstetrics
Johns Hopkins School of
  Medicine
Baltimore, Maryland

Leigh A. Cantrell, MD, MSPH
Associate Professor
Gynecologic Oncology
Obstetrics & Gynecology
University of Virginia School of
  Medicine
Charlottesville, Virginia

Lauren Carlos, MD
Resident, Obstetrics & Gynecology
Yale School of Medicine
New Haven, Connecticut

Chelsea K. Chandler, MD
Resident, Obstetrics &
  Gynecology
Magee-Womens Hospital
University of Pittsburgh
Pittsburgh, Pennsylvania

Christine Conageski, MD
Assistant Professor
Obstetrics & Gynecology
University of Colorado
Aurora, Colorado

Sarah Rae Easter, MD
Fellow
Maternal Fetal Medicine and
  Anesthesia
Obstetrics & Gynecology
Harvard Medical School
Boston, Massachusetts

Jessica C. Ehrig, MD
Fellow
Maternal Fetal Medicine
Obstetrics & Gynecology
University of Colorado
Aurora, Colorado

Sherif El-Nashar, MD, PhD
Associate Professor
Female Pelvic Medicine &
    Reconstructive Surgery
Obstetrics & Gynecology
Case Western Reserve University
Cleveland, Ohio

Allison Faucett, MD
Assistant Professor
Maternal Fetal Medicine
Obstetrics & Gynecology
University of Colorado
Aurora, Colorado

Emily Fay, MD
Fellow
Maternal Fetal Medicine
Obstetrics & Gynecology
University of Washington
Seattle, Washington

Lisa Gill, MD
Assistant Professor
Maternal Fetal Medicine
Obstetrics & Gynecology
University of Minnesota
Minneapolis, Minnesota

Allison Gockley, MD
Fellow
Gynecologic Oncology
Obstetrics & Gynecology
Harvard Medical School
Boston, Massachusetts

Chad A. Grotegut, MD
Associate Professor
Maternal Fetal Medicine
Obstetrics & Gynecology
Duke University
Durham, North Carolina

Evelyn Hall, MD
Resident, Obstetrics &
    Gynecology
Northwestern University
Chicago, Illinois

Leo Han, MD, MPH
Assistant Professor
Family Planning
Obstetrics & Gynecology
Oregon Health and Science
    University
Portland, Oregon

Eduardo Hariton, MD, MBA
Resident, Obstetrics &
    Gynecology
Harvard Medical School
Boston, Massachusetts

Benjamin S. Harris, MD, MPH
Resident, Obstetrics &
    Gynecology
Duke University
Durham, North Carolina

Ross Harrison, MD
Resident, Obstetrics &
    Gynecology
University of Wisconsin
Madison, Wisconsin

**M. Camille Hoffman, MD,
    MSCS**
Associate Professor
Maternal Fetal Medicine
Obstetrics & Gynecology, and
    Psychiatry
University of Colorado
Aurora, Colorado

Maeve Hopkins, MD, MA
Resident, Obstetrics &
    Gynecology
Duke University
Durham, North Carolina

Catherine Hudson, MD
Assistant Professor
Female Pelvic Medicine and
    Reconstructive Surgery
Obstetrics & Gynecology
The Ohio State University
Columbus, Ohio

Tana Kim, MD
Resident, Obstetrics & Gynecology
University of Minnesota
Minneapolis, Minnesota

Meghan Klavans, MD, MBA
Resident, Obstetrics & Gynecology
University of Virginia
Charlottesville, Virginia

Reeva Makhijani, MD
Resident, Obstetrics & Gynecology
Brown University
Providence, Rhode Island

Anne Holland Mardy, MD
Resident, Obstetrics & Gynecology
Columbia University
New York, New York

Kevin W. McCool, MD, PhD
Resident, Obstetrics & Gynecology
University of Wisconsin
Madison, Wisconsin

Jennifer R. McKinney, MD, MPH
Resident, Obstetrics & Gynecology
University of Colorado
Aurora, Colorado

Christina Megli, MD, PhD
Resident, Obstetrics & Gynecology
Oregon Health and Science University
Portland, Oregon

Misha D. Miller, MD
Assistant Professor
Mohs Surgery and Cutaneous Oncology
Dermatology
University of Colorado
Aurora, Colorado

Neggin B. Mokhtari, MD
Resident, Obstetrics & Gynecology
Magee-Womens Hospital
Pittsburgh, Pennsylvania

Amy Nacht, DNP, CNM, MPH
Assistant Professor
Women, Children, & Family Health
College of Nursing
University of Colorado
Aurora, Colorado

Shriddha Nayak, MD
Resident, Obstetrics & Gynecology
Johns Hopkins School of Medicine
Baltimore, Maryland

Jessica Opoku-Anane, MD, MS
Assistant Professor
Minimally Invasive Gynecologic Surgery
University of California San Francisco
San Francisco, California

Misha Pangasa, MD
Resident, Obstetrics & Gynecology
Magee-Womens Hospital
Pittsburgh, Pennsylvania

Elizabeth Patberg, MD
Resident, Obstetrics & Gynecology
Emory University
Atlanta, Georgia

Sharon T. Phelan, MD
Professor Emeritus
Obstetrics & Gynecology
University of New Mexico
Albuquerque, New Mexico

Ashish Premkumar, MD
Resident, Obstetrics & Gynecology
University of California San Francisco
San Francisco, California

Shane Reeves, MD
Associate Professor
Maternal Fetal Medicine
Obstetrics & Gynecology
University of Colorado
Aurora, Colorado

Polina Rovner, MD
Resident, Obstetrics & Gynecology
University of Colorado
Aurora, Colorado

Said S. Saab, MD, MPhil
Resident, Obstetrics & Gynecology
University of Pennsylvania
Philadelphia, Pennsylvania

Ritu Salani, MD, MBA
Associate Professor
Gynecologic Oncology
The Ohio State University
Columbus, Ohio

Dana Marie Scott, MD
Resident, Obstetrics & Gynecology
University of Minnesota
Minneapolis, Minnesota

David I. Shalowitz, MD, MSHP
Assistant Professor
Gynecologic Oncology
Obstetrics & Gynecology
Wake Forest Baptist Health
Winston-Salem, North Carolina

Todd J. Stanhope, MD
Obstetrics & Gynecology
North Memorial Health Care
Robbinsdale, Minnesota

Jon G. Steller, MD
Fellow
Maternal Fetal Medicine
Obstetrics & Gynecology
University of Colorado
Aurora, Colorado

Melissa Teitelman, MD, MSCE
Associate Professor
Gastroenterology
Department of Medicine
Duke University
Durham, North Carolina

Roxanne A. Vrees, MD
Assistant Professor
Obstetrics & Gynecology
Brown University
Providence, Rhode Island

Teresa M. Walsh, MD
Assistant Professor
Obstetrics & Gynecology
University of Texas Southwestern
    Medical Center
Dallas, Texas

William D. Winkelman, MD
Resident, Obstetrics &
    Gynecology
University of California San
    Francisco
San Francisco, California

FOREWORD

It is my pleasure to introduce the completely updated second edition of *Pocket Obstetrics & Gynecology*. This indispensable reference combines all the virtues of a handbook with many of the values of the millenials who will use it.

Merriam-Webster defines a handbook as "a book capable of being conveniently carried as a ready reference." Clearly, *Pocket OB-Gyn* meets this criterion fully. The well-organized information covers almost any situation a provider will encounter in general (or more complicated) OB-Gyn practice, and *Pocket OB-Gyn* accomplishes this in minimum space, allowing busy clinicians to carry it everywhere.

In addition to providing the most relevant diagnostic and management algorithms, each topic reviews the knowledge supporting those guidelines. Often, you will be rushed to find appropriate treatments, plans, drug doses, and other considerations in a matter of seconds. *Pocket OB-Gyn* meets learners' needs in this regard because it was written by busy trainees who have compiled efficient condensed bullet lists, tables, and graphics. When you have more time, though, you can return to the same sections and review the physiology, basic science, and original references in more depth. I highly encourage you to do this frequently – to germinate ideas on particularly difficult cases that propel you to investigate more. Those are the times that "great questions" are born, and the scientific discoveries supporting tomorrow's newest cures emerge. I hope each of you will think about the clinical problem(s) you will pursue in your lifetime, and seek opportunities to develop and expand the knowledge that the authors will include in the *next* revision of *Pocket OB-Gyn*.

All of the authors from across the country should be highly commended for creating such an efficient resource and for tending to our women's health clinical compendium with such intelligence and care.

NANETTE SANTORO, MD
Professor and E Stewart Taylor Chair of Obstetrics and Gynecology
University of Colorado School of Medicine
Aurora, Colorado

PREFACE

We are proud to present the completely revised second edition of *Pocket Obstetrics & Gynecology*. The enthusiastic response to the first edition confirmed the need for a quick Pocket Medicine style reference for women's care. For this revised edition, we have again recruited resident, fellow, and attending authors from the top OB-Gyn training programs across the country. The materials are thoroughly updated, as always accompanied by current references and best practice recommendations.

Each chapter contains the brief physiology, differential diagnoses, clinical algorithms, and key references that will be most useful for initial evaluation and management. Where possible we strive to link the latest understanding of pathophysiology with clinical science, bridging early basic medical training and clinical clerkships. The format is consistent with the other books in the series, so we group problems by organ system. Because OB-Gyn involves so much interdisciplinary learning and training, you may find that some closely related topics are spread among different chapters (e.g., preeclampsia and eclampsia are found in the cardiovascular and neurology chapters). Appendices on pelvic anatomy, typical OB-Gyn procedures, and common medications keep useful data right at your fingertips for quick review before a case or presentation. We added a chapter on psychiatric disorders and expanded the index, on the suggestion of our readers. We hope that *Pocket Obstetrics & Gynecology* will continue to be your go-to rapid reference.

Of course medicine is rapidly and constantly evolving, and this book is *not* comprehensive – nor can it take the place of years of training and clinical experience. We encourage you to be aware of updates in the field and changes in standard of care. Please let us know of any suggestions or feedback, and once again we will incorporate those in the next edition. Email me directly at *LWW.PocketOBGYN.Editor@gmail.com* to share your thoughts.

We hope that you find here the core knowledge and practice guidelines that will facilitate excellent patient care, and also make your work a little more efficient. From students to midlevel providers to senior attendings, on L&D and in the OR, we hope you will find *Pocket Obstetrics & Gynecology* an indispensable aid.

K. Joseph Hurt, MD, PhD
Aurora, Colorado

WELL-WOMAN (ANNUAL) EXAM

Well-Woman Visit *(Obstet Gynecol 2012;120:421)*

- **Purpose:** Promote healthy lifestyle, minimize health risks. Screen, evaluate, counsel, & immunize. Identify reproductive concerns. Address age-specific risks. Offer contraception & preconception planning. Optimize primary care health.

Age-stratified well-woman exam components				
Age group	**Screening**	**Labs & tests**	**Health/risk assessment**	**Immunizations**
13–18	Complete H&P inc. sexual and gyn hx. Physical w/ tanner staging, pelvic exam if indicated	GC/CT, HIV testing if sexually active	Sexuality: development, high-risk behaviors, contraception, preventing STDs, internet/ phone safety Fitness/Nutrition: screen for eating disorders, obesity, MV + folate, calcium Psychosocial: screen for suicide/depressive sx, gender identity & sexual orientation, emotion/ physical/sexual abuse	TDAP: booster ages 11–18 with Td booster q10y; Hep B series, HPV vaccines ages 9–26, Influenza qyearly, Meningococcal vax ages 13–18, MMR and VZV if not previously given
19–39	Complete H&P inc OB, GYN, sexual hx. Physical w/ clinical breast exam, pelvic exam >21, earlier if indicated	Pap: 21–29: Cytology + HPV reflex q3y; >30: cytology + HPV co-testing q5y; GC/C, HIV >24; earlier if indicated	Sexuality: contraception, reproductive health plan, high-risk behaviors, preconception/genetic counseling, sexual function, STDs Fitness/Nutrition: Folate supplement, Ca Psychosocial: IPV CV risk factors Health/Risk assessment: Breast self-awareness	TDAP x1 followed by Td q10y; HPV series, influenza qyearly, MMR and VZV if not previously given
40–64	Complete H&P + OB/GYN/ Sexual hx, screen for pelvic organ prolapse, menopausal sx, urinary/ fecal incontinence; Physical w/ breast and pelvic exam	Pap with co-testing q5y, colonoscopy @ age 50, screen for diabetes age 45, lipids q5y at 45, Hep C screening x1 if born b/w 1945–1965, yearly mammogram	Sexuality: contraception, sexual function Fitness/Nutrition Psychosocial: Intimate Partner Violence CV risk factors including h/o PEC, GDM, PIH Health/Risk Assessment: ASA for stroke prevention ages 55–79, breast self-awareness, HRT	TDAP x1, Td q10y, herpes zoster vax x1 at age 60, influenza qyearly, MMR and VZV if not previously immunized

	Age group 65+	Screening	Labs & tests	Health/risk assessment	Immunizations
		Complete History & Physical w/ screening for pelvic organ prolapse, menopausal sx, urinary/ fecal incontinence, when woman's age or health issues are such that she would want intervention, can defer pelvic exam	Bone Mineral density q2y, can d/c pap smears at age 66 if adequate prior screening, colonoscopy q10y, mammogram yearly, lipids q5y, diabetes q3y, TSH q5y, UA, Hep C screening x1	Sexuality: sexual function, barrier protection, high-risk behaviors Fitness/Nutrition Psychosocial Health/Risk Assessment	Zoster x1, Influenza yearly, Pneumococcal vaccine x1, Td q10y, VZV if not previously immunized/ nonimmune

For complete guide of age-stratified well-woman exam components, visit http://www.acog.org/About-ACOG/ACOG-Departments/Annual-Womens-Health-Care/Well-Woman-Recommendations

- **Screening:** Diet/nutrition/exercise, safety/seat belts, IPV, STD/sexual health screening, diabetes, obesity, metabolic syn, osteoporosis, thyroid dz, breast cancer, cervical dysplasia, colon cancer, and skin cancer
- **Timing:** 1st Ob/Gyn visit at 13–15 yo
- **Hx for well-woman visit:**
  Chief complaint/HPI w/review of systems/PMH/PSH
  Ob hx: Including dates, outcomes, gestational age, infant wt, deliv mode, complications, anesthesia
  Gyn hx: LMP – certain/regular
    Menstrual hx: Age at menarche? Regular cycles? Cycle length (days)? Days of flow? Degree of flow (light, mod, heavy)? Dysmenorrhea? Assoc sx?
    STIs: Gonorrhea, chlamydia, herpes, syphilis, HIV, other? Rx?
    # lifetime sexual partners? Current sexual partners (men, women, or both)?
    Cervical ca screening: Abn pap ever? If h/o abnl screening – any colpo/LEEPs/ CKCs? Date of last pap smear
    Contraception: Past & current forms of birth control?
    Domestic Violence: H/o physical, sexual, or emotional abuse?
    Incontinence: Urinary or fecal?
    Sexual: Desire? Pain? Other concerns?
  Meds: Current meds w/dose, route, schedule, indication
  Allergies: Including nondrug & environmental allergens, w/rxn & severity
  Soc hx: Including tobacco, EtOH, & illicit drug use. THC use (in legal states)?
  FHx: Specifically address Gyn cancers including cervical, endometrial, ovarian, breast. Also colon cancer, bleeding/clotting disorders, fetal anomalies/birth defects.
- **Physical exam for well-woman visit:**
  VS, ht, wt, BMI, general appearance, general physical exam, breast, thyroid, cardiovascular, pulmonary, abdominal, rectal, & pelvic (speculum/bimanual)
  Pelvic exam: Annual pelvic exam for ≥21 yo (expert opinion). Not req before OCP start in otherwise healthy, asymptomatic women. External only <21 yo unless indicated; exam under anesthesia for very young. Include external and internal (urethral meatus, vaginal introitus, perianal, speculum exam of vagina and cervix, bimanual uterus, cervix, adnexa ± rectovaginal exam).

Leading causes of death among females of all races in the United States (2015)						
Age 15–19	**Age 20–24**	**Age 25–34**	**Age 35–44**	**Age 45–54**	**Age 55–64**	**Age 65+**
Unintentional injury	Unintentional injury	Unintentional injury	Cancer	Cancer	Cancer	Heart dz
Suicide	Suicide	Cancer	Unintentional injury	Heart dz	Heart dz	Cancer
Cancer	Homicide	Suicide	Heart dz	Unintentional injury	Chronic respiratory dz	Alzheimer's disease
Homicide	Cancer	Heart dz	Suicide	Chronic liver dz	Unintentional injury	Stroke
Heart dz	Heart dz	Homicide	Chronic liver dz	Stroke	Diabetes mellitus	Chronic respirator dz
Birth defects	Pregnancy complications	Pregnancy complications	Stroke	Chronic respiratory dz	Stroke	Diabetes
Pregnancy complications	Birth defects	Diabetes	Diabetes	Suicide	Chronic liver disease	Influenza & pneumonia

From CDC Leading Causes of Death in Females at www.cdc.gov/women/lcod/2015/all-females. Accessed April 1, 2018.

Cancer Screening Guidelines
- **Cervical dysplasia:** See section below on Cervical Cancer Screening.
- **Breast cancer:** See section below on Breast Cancer.
- **Colorectal cancer:** Begin age 50 yo. Consider 45 yo if AA. Younger if FHx. Prefer colonoscopy q10y; other acceptable methods:
  Fecal occult bld or fecal immunochemistry testing q1y w/ 3 collected samples
  Flexible sigmoidoscopy q5y
  Combination of fecal occult bld & flexible sigmoidoscopy
  Double contrast barium enema q5y
- **Skin cancer:** Counsel regarding ultraviolet exposure. Consider annual skin exam & referral for high risk. Use asymmetry/border/color/diameter/enlargement criteria.
- There are no recommended guidelines for routine screening for **ovarian, endometrial,** or **lung** cancer. H&P guide investigation.

BENIGN BREAST DISEASE

Likely benign mass: Mobile, soft, smooth, <2 cm
Concerning mass: Hard, fixed, single, irreg margins, >2 cm, adenopathy, bloody nipple discharge, overlying skin changes, nonsymmetric breast appearance

Abnormal Radiology Findings
- Poorly defined soft tissue density, irreg borders – sometimes in a "star" appearance
- Clustered microcalcifications in 1 area
- Calcification in a soft tissue mass/density
- Asym in the breast, or skewing of breast tissue
- New abnormality not previously seen
- **Worrisome findings:** Soft tissue mass, clustered microcalcifications
- Most common breast mass in <25 yo, gradual growth, "lumpy" on exam, low risk for cancer → if increasing in size, consider bx

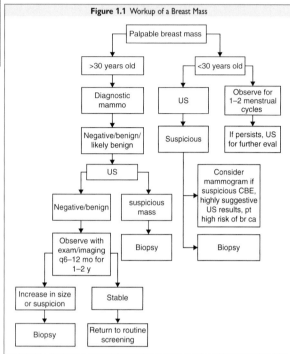

Figure 1.1 Workup of a Breast Mass

Mammography, BIRADS (Breast Imaging Reporting and Data System) score			
Score	Description	Risk of cancer	F/u
0	Incomplete	NA	Need to rpt mammogram or breast US
1	Negative	Minimal	Continue routine screening
2	Benign finding	Minimal	Continue routine screening
3	Probably benign findings	2%	F/u mammogram in 6 mo to reassess
4	Suspicious abnormality	25–30%	May need bx
5	Highly suggestive of malig	95%	Core or excisional bx of mass
6	Biopsy-confirmed breast cancer known	100% (known)	Excision, chemo, or radiation

Benign breast disease	
Mastalgia	**Definition:** Breast pain, can be cyclic or noncyclic *Cyclic:* Usually most painful before menses, relieved w/menses, usually bilateral. Due to hormonal changes that cause proliferation of breast tissue. Can also be associated with HRT or OCPs. *Noncyclic:* More likely to be unilateral and variable in its location in the breast. Etiologies inc stretching of Cooper's ligaments, diet/lifestyle, HRT, ductal dysplasia, chest wall pain. **Tx:** Reassurance, most self-resolves. **Danazol** only FDA-approved tx, but has severe androgenic effects; tamoxifen for severe mastalgia, but has menopausal side-effects. Some can be helped w/NSAIDs, acetaminophen, supportive bras, warm compresses, low fat/high complex carb diet, OCPs, recommend decreasing caffeine & chocolate intake, minimal data for evening primrose oil and vit E
Mastitis	**Definition:** Acute cellulitis that can progress to an abscess, typically seen in breast-feeding women; presents often in a wedge distribution of ducts w/ warmth, erythema, tenderness, fevers, & malaise made by clinical dx **Tx:** Dicloxacillin 500 mg QID ×10 d, or cephalexin 500 mg QID ×10 d, warm compresses, pt must continue pumping to help provide an outlet for drainage. Infants are safe to breast-feed as bacteria originated from infant's mouth flora (*Staph* and *Strep* species).
Breast cysts	**Definition:** Classified by US appearance. Fluid-filled cyst is usually simple from terminal duct, common in 35–50 yo, causes localized breast pain, usually resolves. Microcysts and cysts with thin septa usually benign. **W/u:** Expectant mgmt for 6 w or breast US → if simple cyst, no further intervention required; consider aspiration if severe pain or obstruction of adjacent breast tissue → if recurs or concerning on radiology, refer for further imaging, breast bx/excision
Fat necrosis	**Definition:** Hard or indurated areas usually after trauma (seat belt, bx, radiation, infxn). Common in subareolar region. **W/u:** Can assess w/mammography or breast US
Fibroadenoma	**Definition:** Most common breast mass in <25 yo, gradual growth, "lumpy" & mobile on exam, low risk for cancer **W/u:** If increasing in size, consider bx

Nipple Discharge
- Very common complaint, usually benign
- **Nml discharge:** Common with stimulation, bilateral, serous
- **Galactorrhea:** Typically bilateral, milky discharge unrelated to Preg, bilateral.
  Causes: Unknown, endocrine abnormalities a/w amenorrhea or hypothalamic dysfxn from endocrine abnormalities or pituitary mass, many psychiatric meds (dopamine inhibitors)
  W/u: HPI asking about visual changes, HAs, menses, thyroid sx, current meds; PE looking at visual field defects (tunnel vision)
  Labs: Prolactin, TSH, free T4, CT head looking for a pituitary adenoma if elevated prolactin
- **Nonbenign discharge:** Unilateral, bloody (guaiac test if not visible), serous, or colored discharge can be a/w breast mass or overlying skin changes. Caused by carcinoma, intraductal papilloma, duct ectasia, fibrocystic changes.
  W/u: Send discharge for cytology, mammogram if >35 yo or breast US if <35 yo. Cytology is of little value & has a low sens.

BREAST CANCER

Epidemiology
- Breast cancer is the most common cancer among women. 2nd most common cause of cancer death in women (after lung cancer) in USA. From 1998–2007 the incid & mortality rates have decreased. Developed nations have a higher incid than developing. Lifetime risk of breast cancer is 12% (1 in 8 women).
- AA women have a lower incid rate, higher mortality rate, & higher stage at dx

Risk Factors
- **Age >40 yo:** 95% of breast cancers occur in women >40 yo
- **FHx of breast cancer:** 1st-degree relatives, premenopausal breast cancer, BRCA1 and BRCA2 mutations (tumor suppressor genes, autosomal dominant, account for 2–7% dx, but confer 40–70% lifetime breast cancer risk). General population risk 1/400, Ashkenazi Jews 1/40 chance of having mutation.
  - **BRCA1/2:** 45–65% risk breast cancer, 10–15% risk ovarian cancer → risk reducing mastectomy decreases risk by >90%. Prophylactic BSO reduces br ca risk by 50% and ovarian ca risk by 80–95%. BRCA testing recommended for 1st-degree relative w/breast cancer, relative w/breast cancer <50 yo, 3+ 1st- or 2nd-degree relatives w/breast cancer, breast/ovarian cancer in 1st- or 2nd-degree relative, 2+ 1st- or 2nd-degree relatives w/ovarian cancer, male breast cancer. Recommend annual MRI/mammogram starting at age 25 and q6mo pelvis US and CA-125 if declines RR BSO. Can use tamoxifen for chemoprevention (*Obstet Gynecol* 2017;130:e110).
- **Increased hormonal exposure:** Early menarche (<12 yo), late menopause (>55 yo), older age w/1st Preg, fewer pregnancies (all these → increased lifetime estrogen exposure)
- **Personal h/o breast cancer:** 0.5–1% risk of developing breast cancer in contralateral breast, majority of recurrences are w/i the 1st 5 y
- **Radiation exposure:** 35% lifetime risk
- **Diet & exercise:** Physical activity & wt control are protective

Breast cancer screening modalities		
Screening	**Performance**	**Guidelines**
Breast self-awareness (awareness of normal look & feel of one's breasts)	Difficult to assess	ACOG: Recommended ACS: Recommended NCCN: Recommended
Self-breast exam (monthly exam, day 7–10 of cycle)	Difficult to assess	Breast awareness education, all ages. ACOG: Consider for high-risk pts USPSTF: Not recommended ACS: Optional for >20 yo NCCN: 20–39 yo q1–3 y; >40 yo annually 50–70% of breast cancer found on self-exam
Clinical breast exam (5+ min/breast by health professional)	Sens 54% Spec 94% PPV 3–4% (*JAMA* 1999;282:1270)	ACOG: 20–39 yo every 1–3 y; >40 yo annually USPSTF: Insuff data to assess ACS: Not recommended for avg risk women NCCN: 25–39 yo q1–3 y; >40 yo annually
Ultrasound	Sens 80–85% Spec 60–70% (*Int J Clin Pract* 2009; 63:1589)	Adjunct to mammography, esp in young women w/dense breast tissue. Can help further eval inconclusive findings, guide bx, differentiate cyst vs. solid mass. Not 1st line.
Mammogram	Sens 85% Spec 90% (bcsc-research.org/)	ACOG: >40 yo annual screening, or 10 y younger than 1st-degree affected relative. Stop at age 75. USPSTF: 50–74 yo q2y ACS: >45–54 yo annual screening, >55 yo q1–2 y NCI: >40 yo, screen every 1–2 y NCCN: 20–39 yo q1–3 y; >40 yo annually
Breast MRI	Sens 77% Spec 86% (*Ann Int Med* 2008;9:671)	For >20% lifetime risk, or known BRCA1 or BRCA2, 1st-degree relative w/BRCA & no personal testing, h/o chest radiation btw 10 & 30 yo, genetic syndromes (eg, Li-Fraumeni, Cowden). Not recommended for personal h/o breast cancer or dysplasia, & not for avg risk women.

Data from *Obstet Gynecol* 2017;130;e1. *JAMA* 2015;314:1599. *JNCCN* 2009;10:1060. *Ann Int Med* 2009;151:716.

Premalignant Lesions
- **Atypical hyperplasia:** Ductal or lobular, proliferative lesion similar to carcinoma in situ; includes intraductal papilloma, ductal epithelial hyperplasia, sclerosing adenosis → excision and counseling on risk reduction strategies

- **DCIS:** Precancerous lesion with 30% risk of developing into cancer in 10 y. Most common noninvasive breast cancer (1 of 5 new cases), usually dx by mammogram alone, can have breast conserving rx ± tamoxifen ± XRT
- **LCIS:** More common in premenopausal women, risk factor for invasive ca, may also be precursor lesion. Recommend excision ± tamoxifen.

Invasive Cancer
- **Infiltrating ductal:** 60–70% breast cancer; includes mucinous, tubular, & medullary carcinomas, classified by cell type, architecture of mass, & pattern of spread
- **Infiltrating lobular:** 10–15% breast cancer, arising in lobules, multifocal, higher incid of cancer in contralateral breast
- **Inflamm:** 6% of breast cancer, p/w skin changes, rapid onset in a few weeks, causes diffuse induration & swelling. Dx w/punch bx of skin & mammogram, tx w/ chemo
- **Phyllodes tumor:** Similar to fibroadenoma, epithelial lined spaces surrounded by monoclonal & neoplastic stromal cells. Classified as benign, intermediate, or malignant based on atypia, mitosis, abundance of stromal cells, median age of dx 40 yo, can metastasize to distant organs w/lung as primary site; tx w/wide local incision.
- **Paget dz:** Presents as focal skin changes, assoc mass identified in 60% of cases. Underlying DCIS in 2/3 of cases & invasive cancer in 1/3.

Breast Cancer Staging/Prognosis
- Tumor size, differentiation, & nodal metastasis strongly correlated w/prog
- High expression of estrogen or progesterone a/w better prog
- Overexpression of HER2 (human epidermal growth factor receptor) a/w worse prog
- ER/PR status a/w improved survival rates b/c of targeted therapy of SERMs & aromatase inhibitors (reduce circulating estrogens).

TNM staging for breast cancer		
T (tumor)	**N (lymph node)**	**M (metastasis)**
Tx: Tumor cannot be assessed	Nx: LN cannot be assessed	M0: No metastasis
T0: No evid of primary tumor	N0: No LN metastasis	M1: Distant clinical, radio-logic, or histo-logic lesions >0.2 mm. *All M1 dx stage 4 prior to neo-adjuvant chemo
TIS: Carcinoma in situ (DCIS, LCIS, Paget's)	N1: Mets to movable ipsilateral level I, II axillary LNs	
T1 (mi, a, b, c): Tumor <20 mm in greatest dimension	N2 (a, b): Mets in ipsilateral level I, II axillary LNs fixed or matted to one another or other structures; or ipsilateral internal mammary nodes in the *absence* of axillary LN mets	
T2: Tumor >20 mm, <50 mm	N3 (a, b, c): Mets in ipsilateral infraclavicular (level III axillary) LN w/or w/o level I, II axillary LN involvement; or clinically detected ipsilateral internal mammary LN w/clinically evident level I, II axillary LN mets; or mets in ipsilateral supraclavicular LN w/or w/o axillary or internal mammary LN	
T3: Tumor >50 mm		
T4 (a, b, c, d): Tumor of any size, direct extension to the chest wall and/or skin (ulceration/nodules)		

Used with the permission of the American College of Surgeons. Amin, MB, Edge, SB, Greene, FL, et al. (Eds.) *AJCC Cancer Staging Manual.* 8th ed. Springer New York, 2017.

Treatment
Depends on stage and location of cancer. Includes surgery, radiation, chemo. #1 lawsuit reason for gynecologist (apart from OB): Failure to diagnose or adequately/quickly refer breast cancer (*Med Law* 2005;24:1).

> **Surg:** Std of care is breast conserving surg = wide local excision (aka lumpectomy) w/ sentinel lymph node biopsy followed by radiation and hormonal therapy General Ob/Gyns refer to breast specialist or general surgeon for eval & excision

CERVICAL CANCER SCREENING

Epidemiology and Definitions (*Obstet Gynecol* 2016;128:e111)
- 2nd most common cancer in women worldwide. Mean age at dx: 40–59 y; bimodal distribution peaks 35–39 y & 60–64 y. Cervical cancer and related mortality ↓ 50%

from 1975 to 6.7/100000 women in 2011 due to pap smear screen. ~50% women dx w/ cervical ca now had no screening; 10% not screened in 5 y of dx.

Pathophysiology

- Caused by HPV infxn. An effective immune system clears HPV infxn; cervical cancer thought to be from long-term HPV infxn. >90% young healthy women clear cervical HPV w/i 1–3 y, esp if <21 yo. Most clear in 8 months or reduce to undetectable levels in 8–24 mo.
- **HPV:** E (early) & L (late) E6, E7 proteins expressed in malignant cells. E6 → degradation of tumor suppressor p53 → ↑ cell proliferation. E7 binds tumor suppressor pRb (retinoblastoma gene product) → release E2F transcription factors → ↑ replication & cell division. Unchecked cell cycle → ↑ malig.
  High-risk HPV strains: 16, 18, 31, 33, 35, 45, 58 are carcinogenic; HPV 16 in ~60% of all cases, HPV 18 in ~15% of cases
  Low-risk HPV strains: 39, 51, 52, 56, 59, 68, 73, 82 (6, 11 cause genital warts)
- **Risk factors:** Increased sexual contacts, smokers, new sexual partner, HIV+ or immunosuppression (→ decreased viral clearance)

Pap Smear Guidelines (J Low Genit Tract Dis 2012;16:175)

- Pap smear adequate if transformation zone (junction of squamous & columnar cells) is present for cytologic eval. Sens 51%; spec 98%. HPV typing from pap smear cells can also be performed. Pap + HPV cotesting (Sens 100%, Spec 92.5%)
- Start screening ≥21 yo regardless of sexual Hx. Do NOT screen ≤21 yo, except HIV+ pts. Recent ↓ in testing frequency retains benefits but minimizes unnec procedures. Regardless of pap screening, annual Gyn exam recommended for all. If abn pap, consult current ASCCP guidelines (www.asccp.org).

Pap smear screening schedules			
	USPSTF	ASCCP	ACOG
When to start screening	21 yo	21 yo	21 yo
How frequently should you test?			
Age 21–29 yo (pap smear alone if nml)	Every 3 y	Every 3 y	Every 3 y
Age 30 & older			
Pap smear alone if nml	Every 3 y	Every 3 y	Every 3 y
Pap smear w/HPV cotesting	Every 5 y	Recommended, but no more frequently than every 5 y	Every 5 y as recommended strategy
Age to stop	65 yo if adequate screening	65 yo w/adequate screening & no h/o CIN 2+ in last 20 y	65 yo if adequate screening & no h/o CIN 2, CIN 3, or adenoCa in situ or cervical cancer in last 20 y
After hysterectomy including cervical removal w/no h/o CIN 2–3, adenoCa in situ, or prior cervical cancer in last 20 y	No pap screening needed, but annual exam for vaginal & vulvar dz should continue		
HPV vaccinated	No change in screening		
HIV+ women, immunocomp, or in utero DES exposure	1st pap w/l 1st year of sexual activity OR diagnosis but no later than 21 yo, then annually. If 3 consecutive nl paps, can do q3y. Cont paps throughout lifetime, do not stop at 65 yo (Obstet Gynecol 2016;128:920)		

- Pap (cytology) results reported as:
  ASCUS: Atypical cells of undetermined significance
  LSIL: Low-grade squamous intraepithelial lesion ~ corresponds to CIN 1
  HSIL: High-grade squamous intraepithelial lesion ~ corresponds to CIN 2–3
  AGC: Atypical glandular cells (means columnar cells, has association with CIN 2–3)
- **Management:**
  ASCUS → reflex high-risk HPV testing; if HPV positive refer to colposcopy; if HPV negative rpt according to age appropriate guidelines (www.asccp.org) – OR → rpt

pap in 6 mo → if rpt = ASCUS or more refer to colposcopy, if negative return to annual screening

Pts w/negative cytology & positive HPV cotesting should either be referred directly to colposcopy or perform high-risk HPV typing. If high-risk type then referral to colposcopy should be made. If no high-risk type (16 or 18) then rpt w/ coscreening in 1 y.

LSIL/HSIL/AGC: Refer to colposcopy, AGC needs colpo + ECC

Special cases	
Cervical cancer screening in pregnancy (ASCCP)	
ASCUS and positive HPV	Refer to colposcopy during preg or 6 w postpartum, no ECC during preg. If neg HPV, rpt cytology in 12 mo
LSIL	Refer to colposcopy during preg or 6 w postpartum, no ECC during preg
HSIL/AIS/AGS	Refer to colposcopy during preg, no ECC during preg
Adols should not be screened before 21 yo, but if they have been:	
Past ASCUS, LSIL, CIN 1	Rpt annually for 2 y & then further screening delayed until 21 yo; refer to colposcopy if persists
Past HSIL, AGC, ASC cannot exclude HSIL, CIN 2–3	Refer to colposcopy w/ECC
Adols w/HIV	1st pap w/l 1st year of sexual activity or 1st year of diagnosis but no later than 21 yo. Annually until 3 neg consecutive paps, then q3y (Obstet Gynecol 2016;128:920)

Primary HPV screening is an acceptable alternative to cytology – growing evidence of improved detection of high-risk lesions and negative more reassuring than negative cytology. If positive HR HPV → colpo, if +other HPV strain → cytology and then colpo if ≥ ASC-US (Obstet Gynecol 2016;127:185).

Colposcopy
- **Definition:** Direct visualization of the cervix, vagina, & vulva w/a mobile lighted binocular microscope to identify, map, & bx cervical lesions. Deemed adequate if transformation zone is visualized on all sides since this is the region in which abn changes occur. Visualization is aided by:
  Acetic acid: Dehydrates cells → lighter appearance in dysplastic cells w/↑ n/c ratio/↑ chromatin = "acetowhite changes."
  Lugol iodine: Stains nml cervicovaginal epithelial cells dark due to high glycogen content, while dysplastic cells are lighter; used in place of or in addition to acetic acid
- Abn colposcopic findings include:
  Punctation: Small bld vessels visible as small dots
  Mosaicism: An interspersing of white & nml epithelial cells
  Acetowhite changes: A range of white-hued epithelium w/diffuse or sharp borders
  Atypical vessels: Larger vessels w/i lesions may indicate a more advanced lesion
- Any abn lesions are biopsied to evaluate for preinvasive cancer; colposcopy does not always mean bx; only abn lesions & endocervical canal are sampled.
- **Endocervical curettage:** Curetting the endocervical canal to obtain glandular cells or nonvisualized lesions.
- **Bx results:** Reported as:
  CIN 1: Mild cellular atypia confined to lower 1/3 of squamous epithelium
  CIN 2: Moderate cellular atypia confined to basal 2/3 of epithelium
  CIN 3: Severe cellular atypia encompassing >2/3 and includes full thickness lesions w/o invasion of basement membrane (formerly known as carcinoma in situ)
  AIS: Premalignant glandular condition, only precursor to cervical adenocarcinoma vs. SCC

Cervical Dysplasia Management (Obstet Gynecol 2013;121:829)
- CIN 1 → Can follow conservatively w/surveillance; consider conization if persists >2 y
- CIN 2 → Consider conization or follow w/rpt pap/colposcopy, esp if young (21–24 yo)
- CIN 3 → Conization/LEEP (30% of untx CIN 3 will progress to cancer in 30 y) vs. hysterectomy if completed child-bearing
- AIS → Hysterectomy recommended vs. conservative mgmt. with LEEP if future fertility desired
- Invasive cancer → Refer to GYN/ONC (see Chap. 22)
- See ASCCP for most up-to-date recommendations (www.asccp.org)

LIPIDS AND CHOLESTEROL

Screening and Treatment
- Cardiovascular dz is the leading cause of death (all ages) in women (22%)
- ACOG Screening Recs: Assess lipid profile every 5 y starting at age 45 unless high risk
  Risk factors warranting earlier screening (18–44 y): FHx of familial hyperlipidemia, DM, PVD, premature CVD (<50 for M/<60 for F); personal h/o obesity, CHD or risk equivalents, DM, more than 1 CHD risk factors (ie HTN and cig smoking)

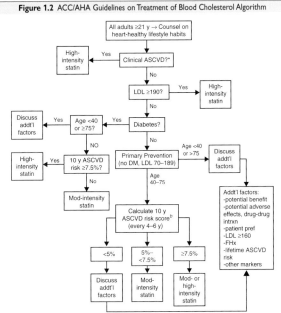

Figure 1.2 ACC/AHA Guidelines on Treatment of Blood Cholesterol Algorithm

a Clinical ASCVD (atherosclerotic cardiovascular disease) = coronary heart disease, acute coronary syndrome, h/o myocardial infarction, angina (stable or unstable), coronary revascularization, stroke, TIA, peripheral arterial disease
b 10-y ASCVD risk score is based on age, race, gender, total cholesterol, HDL, smoking status, diabetes diagnosis, and blood pressure. Updated calculator at: http://my.americanheart.org/cvriskcalculator.
(Adapted from Am Fam Physician 2014;90(4):260–5.)

Cholesterol treatment guidelines			
Therapy	Effect	Examples	Population
High-intensity statin	≥50% ↓ LDL	Atorvastatin (Lipitor) 40–80 mg Rosuvastatin (Crestor) 20–40 mg	• Clinical ASCVD • DM and ≥7.5% 10-y risk score • LDL ≥190
Moderate-intensity statin	30–50% ↓ LDL	Atorvastatin 10–20 mg Rosuvastatin 5–10 mg Simvastatin 20–40 mg Pravastatin 40 mg Lovastatin 40 mg	• DM and <7.5% 10-y risk score • Age 40–75 and 5–7.5% 10-y risk score

Therapy	Effect	Examples	Population
Low-intensity statin	<30% ↓ LDL	Simvastatin 10 mg Pravastatin 10–20 mg Lovastatin 20 mg	• Consider in pts. Age <40 or >75 with DM or 10-y risk score >7.5% after discussion of risks/benefits • Pts who cannot tolerate higher doses
Life-style modification	Various	Diet and exercise – includes decreased saturated fat (<7% total calories) total daily cholesterol intake <200 mg (NCEP diet), decreased salt intake, exercise 40 min 3–4×/wk	All adults
Bile acid sequestrants	15–30% ↓ in LDL	Cholestyramine, colestipol	• 2nd-line agents • For use in those who cannot tolerate statins • Consider adding as a 2nd agent in high-risk pt who has had inadequate response to statins • Insuff evid to rec use of nonstatin meds in addt to statins to further reduce risk of ASCVD events
Cholesterol absorp inhibitor	20% ↓ in LDL	Ezetimibe	
Nicotinic acid	10–15% ↓ in LDL 15–30% ↑ in HDL 40% ↓ in triglyc	Niacin	
Fibrates	5–15% ↓ in LDL 10–20% ↑ in HDL 30–50% ↓ in triglyc.	Fenofibrate	

There is insufficient evidence to recommend for or against treating to specific target cholesterol levels.
Adapted from *Circulation* 2014;129(25 suppl2):S13.

- Hormone effects on lipids:
  Estrogen: ↓ LDL, ↑ HDL, & ↑ TG
  Progestin: Antagonizes estrogen changes → ↑ LDL, ↓ HDL, & ↓ TG
- Contraception: If multiple ASCVD risk factors (including dyslipidemia, smoking, DM), avoid CHCs (MEC Cat 3/4). POPs, LNG IUD, and implants MEC 2
- Postmenopausal women on HRT (estrogen &/or progestin) → 29% ↑ in CHD events; no indication for HRT to prevent CHD. Women on HRT had a 41% ↑ in stroke events (*JAMA* 2002;288:321). Newer data since the WHI trial sugg younger postmenopausal women (<60 yo) on HRT do not have ↑ CHD. (See Chap. 5.)

OBESITY

	Definitions for obesity	
WHO wt category	**BMI for adults (>21 yo)**	**Recommended wt gain in preg**
Underweight	<18.5	28–40 lb
Normal weight	18.5–24.9	25–25 lb
Overweight	25–29.9	15–25 lb
Obese	≥30	11–20 lb
Class 1 obesity	30–34.9	
Class 2 obesity	35–39.9	
Class 3 obesity	≥40	

BMI = weight (lb)/[height (in)]^2 × 703 = weight (kg)/[height (m)]^2

Epidemiology (CDCNHANES 2011–2014)
- 37% of all US adults (34% ♀ age 20–39) are obese, a dramatic ↑ in the past 20 y; disparities by race w/ 57% of AA women obese
- 17% of all US children & adols are obese → increased heart dz, diabetes, & metabolic syn

Obesity and Gynecology

- **Infertility:** Oligo-ovulation & anovulation, ↓ gonadotropin resp, initial rx is wt loss/lifestyle modification followed by ovulation induction with clomid/letrozole
- **Contraception:** ↓ Levels of circulating progestins, but epidemiologic/clinical correlate still unclear, may still use patch/COCs/implants
- **Anesthesia/surgical risk:** ↑ Difficulty w/spinal/epidural anesthesia, ↑ intubation risk w/higher Mallampati score, consider preoperative anesthesia consult, ↑ wound breakdown w/laparotomy. ↑ DVT risk, consider prophylaxis, ambulation, SCDs, compression stockings.
- **Endometrial cancer risk:** Unopposed estrogen (androstenedione → estrogen by adipose tissue aromatase) → endometrial hyperplasia

Obesity and Obstetrics (Obstet Gynecol 2015;126(6):e112–26)

- **Fetal anomalies:** ↑ Anomalies such as cleft lip/palate, neural tube, cardiac defects
- **Antepartum complications:** 20%↑ risk miscarriage, 40%↑ risk stillbirth (5–13× ↑ if Class III at term), 46% of time wt gain is higher than recommended (11–20 lb for obese); ↑ fetal macrosomia; ↑ gestational diabetes, gestational HTN/preeclampsia, cardiac dz
- **Labor & deliv:** Difficult to follow fetal HR w/tocometry → ↑ interventions such as fetal scalp electrode placement. Protracted labor curve & ↑ labor dystocia → ↑ cesarean deliv. ↓ VBAC success rate. ↑ Shoulder dystocia.
- **Postpartum complications:** ↑ Endometritis, wound dehiscence, VTE, depression, anemia; ↓ breastfeeding

Treatment

- **Nonsurgical:** Nutrition & exercise programs, goal setting w/provider, close f/u appointments, some limited pharmacotherapy; initial goal of 10% reduction in weight, then repeat to ultimate goal BMI <25
- **Surgical:** Bariatric Surg for BMI >40 or >35 w/other comorbidities w/gastric banding, sleeve gastrectomy, or gastric bypass. Attention to contraception should be paid to women who get bariatric surg as their fertility may ↑.

OSTEOPOROSIS

Definition (Obstet Gynecol 2012;120:718)

- Low bone mass, microarchitectural deterioration, increased bone fragility. Defined by WHO based on DEXA T-scores:
    - **T-score:** Std deviation from mean BMD of a healthy young (30 yo) adult
        - **Nml:** T-score ≥ −1
        - **Osteopenia:** T-score < −1 but > −2.5
        - **Osteoporosis:** T-score ≤ −2.5
    - **Z-score:** Std deviation from mean BMD of age-matched pop, informative in cases of sev osteoporosis

Epidemiology (AJOG 2006;194:S3)

- 8–17% US postmenopausal women have osteoporosis
- Incid increases w/age → 48–70% affected by age 80
- By age 70, Caucasian women in US have a 40% risk of hip, spine, or forearm fracture

Etiology

Osteoporosis risk factors	
Etiologies	**Risk factors**
Age-dependent bone loss	Age
Low bone mass	Thin, small frame, Caucasian, Asian, Prev personal fracture, FHx of fracture
Estrogen deficiency (hypogonadal states)	Postmenopausal, amenorrhea, anorexia nervosa
Endocrine disorders	Hyperparathyroidism, hyperthyroidism, DM
GI disorders	Celiac dz & malabsorption, pancreatic dz, gastric bypass or GI surg
Nutrition	Calcium, vit D, protein deficiency
Meds	Depo-Provera, glucocorticoids, gonadotropin-releasing hormone agonists, heparin & anticonvulsants, tamoxifen, cancer chemotherapeutics
Lifestyle	Cigarette smoking, excessive EtOH use Sedentary

Clinical Manifestations

- Clinically silent until fracture. Hip fracture, esp trochanteric vs. intracapsular, is the most serious complication. Vertebral fracture often p/w back pain, kyphosis, & loss of ht. Forearm fracture also possible.

Screening

- **FRAX risk assessment tool** (www.shef.ac.uk/FRAX/) calculates 10-y fracture risk
- **DEXA** (gold std) at 65 yo, earlier if postmenopausal w/fracture, risk factors (h/o fragility fracture, body wt <127 lb, medical causes of accelerated bone loss, smoker, alcoholism, rheumatoid arthritis, FHx of hip fracture in parent). FRAX 10-y risk >9.3% (65 yo risk) → early screening.

DEXA screening guidelines	
Organization	Criteria
National Osteoporosis Foundation	All women over age 65
	Personal h/o bone fracture after 50
	<65 & postmenopausal w/risk factors
USPSTF	All women over age 65
	All women whose FRAX fracture risk is >9.3% due to risk factors
ACOG	All women over age 65
	<65 postmenopausal w/ risk factor or FRAX 9.3% risk of fracture

- **Other screening modalities** (US, CT, x-ray, photon absorptiometry) are available but are less cost-effective, accurate, & available
- **Biochemical markers** of bone turnover include:
  Bone resorption markers: Hydroxyproline, pyridinium cross-links
  Bone formation markers: Alk phos, osteocalcin, procollagen 1 propeptides
  Fasting urinary calcium/Cr ratio indicates balance btw resorption & formation

Treatment and Medications

- **Prevention and nonpharmacologic:** Regular weight-bearing exercise + 800 IU Vit D daily + 1200 mg calcium daily + avoid cigarette smoking & excessive EtOH intake. Fall precautions for older or unsteady pts. ACOG calcium/Vit D recommendations:
  Age 9–18: Calcium 1300 U QD, Vit D 600 U QD
  Age 19–50: Calcium 1000 U QD, Vit D 600 U QD
  Age 51–70: Calcium 1200 U QD, Vit D 600 U QD
  Age ≥70: Calcium 1200 U QD, Vit D 800 U QD
- **Pharmacologic:** Initiate rx for >50 yo & vertebral/hip fracture or T-score ≤−2.5 at the femoral neck or spine or T-score −1 to −2.5 at the femoral neck or spine & 10-y fracture risk ≥3% or 10-y osteoporosis fracture risk ≥20% or low trauma fracture (esp vertebral/hip)
  Bisphosphonates: 1st line, oral, or IV administration (alendronate, risedronate, ibandronate, etidronate). Side effects – esophagitis, myalgias, gastric ulcers, osteonecrosis of the jaw (rare), subtrochanteric fx (rare)
  SERM: Oral (raloxifene). Side effects – vasomotor sx, DVT, leg cramps
  Calcitonin: Last line. Subcutaneous or nasal administration. Side effects – nausea, rhinitis
  Parathyroid hormone: Subcutaneous administration. For pts who have failed or are intolerant of other tx. Side effects – HyperCa, nausea, leg cramps.
  Estrogen: Oral, transdermal administration. WHI demonstrated ↓ osteoporosis for both estrogen alone & estrogen–progestin therapy. Side effects – ↑ VTE, cardiovascular dz, breast cancer. Risks much less in women w/i 10 y of menopause.
- **Monitoring resp to therapy:** F/u DEXA 1–2 y after beginning of therapy, decreased frequency thereafter if adequate resp

SKIN CANCER SCREENING

Basal Cell Carcinoma (*J Natl Compr Canc Netw* 2010;8:836; *BMJ* 2012;345:37s)
- **Definition:** Arises from epidermal basalis, locally invasive
- **Epidemiology:** Most common skin cancer. Account for 75% of nonmelanoma skin ca. Likely 1–3 million BCC/y in US. 15–28% lifetime risk in women.
- **Risks:** Age, race, male sex, *UV light exposure esp intermittent & intense*, chronic arsenic exposure, ionizing radiation, immunosuppression, & PUVA therapy for psoriasis

- **Pathophysiology:** Sun exposure/inflammation. Genetics – PTCH1, chromo 9, tumor suppressor gene, two-hit hypothesis.
- **Clinical manifestations:** 85% on face and neck, 15% on trunk
  - **Nodular:** 60% of cases, flesh-colored papule, pearly or translucent, telangiectatic vessel, may have ulceration
  - **Superficial:** 30% of cases, mostly on trunk, scaly plaque, rimmed w/translucent micropapules
  - **Morpheaform:** Smooth, flesh-colored plaques, atrophic, ill-defined borders, aggressive
  - **Basal cell nevus syn:** Autosomal dominant inheritance, PTCH1 mutation, p/w multi BCCs at a young age, macrocephaly, bifid ribs, bone cysts, palmar pitting, & medulloblastoma
- **Tx: Low-risk BCC** (<10 mm on head/neck, <20 mm all other areas; nodular or superficial histopathology, no perineural invasion; primary lesion, defined borders, immunocompetent, no prior radiation) → electrodessication & curettage, surgical excision. High-risk BCC → Mohs Surg, surgical excision, XRT.
- **Prog:** Excellent, metastasis rate 0.55%; however, deep invasion and recurrence can cause morbidity. 40% of pts → 2nd BCC ≤5 y

Squamous Cell Carcinoma (NEJM 2001;344:975)
- **Definition:** Arises from epidermal keratinocytes, locally invasive
- **Epidemiology:** 2nd most common skin cancer, 25% of nonmelanoma skin ca. 4–9% lifetime risk for US women
- **Risks:** Same as BCC, see above
- **Pathophysiology:** UV light, esp >30000 cumulative h →leading to p53 gene mutation. Prevention: Protection from sun exposure, retinoids.
  - **Actinic keratoses:** Precursor lesion, scaly erythematous macules, 1% progress to SCC, 60% of SCC arise from actinic keratoses
- **Clinical manifestations:** Typically occur on sun damaged skin
  - **SCC in situ** (Bowen dz): Well-defined borders, scaly plaque, erythematous
  - **Invasive SCC:** Hyperkeratotic papules or nodules, firm, may have ulcerations
  - **Verrucous carcinoma:** Well-defined, cauliflower-like growths
  - **Xeroderma pigmentosum:** Multigenic, autosomal recessive, sev sun sens, degeneration of skin & eyes
  - **Epidermolysis bullosa:** Blister formation w/no prev trauma, increased risk of aggressive SCC
- **Tx:** Staging based on TNM criteria full physical exam → if low risk (same criteria as BCC) then electrodessication & curettage, surgical excision, radiation. If high risk → Mohs Surg, surgical excision, radiation. (See www.NCCN.org for most recent detailed guidelines for treatment)
- **Prog:** 5-y cure rate 0–>90%, 5-y recurrence rate 8%, 5-y metastasis rate 5% (cure rate, recurrence rate, and metastasis rate depends on tumor stage)

Melanoma (NEJM 2006;355:51)
- **Definition:** Arises from epidermal melanocytes, most fatal form of skin cancer
- **Epidemiology:** 4% of all skin cancers, but responsible for 80% skin cancer deaths
- **Risks:** Age, race, UV light exposure & intermittent, atypical nevi, high nevus count, FHx. MRAT: www.cancer.gov/melanomarisktool/
- **Prevention:** Insuff evid to recommend universal screening by USPSTF, but remain alert. High-risk pts → yearly screening from a dermatologist
- **Clinical manifestations:**
  - **Superficial spreading melanoma:** 70% of all melanomas, variably pigmented macules, irreg borders
  - **Nodular melanoma:** 15–30% of all melanomas, darkly pigmented, pedunculated nodules
  - **Lentigo maligna melanoma:** Begins as brown macule that grows to be darker, asym, & have raised areas
  - **Acral lentiginous melanoma:** <5% of all melanomas, most common form of melanoma in darker-skinned people, most commonly on palms of hands & soles of feet
  - **ABCDE:** Asymmetry, border irregularities, color variegation, diameter >5 mm, evolving lesion (Dermatology 1998;197:11). Sens 97% if single criterion met, 43% if all 5 criteria met. Spec 36% if single criterion met, 100% if all 5 criteria nml.
  - **Glasgow criteria:** Referral if 1 major criterion, presence of minor criteria reinforces need for referral
    - **Major:** Change in size or new lesion, change in shape, change in color
    - **Minor:** Diameter >6 mm, inflammation, crusting or bleeding, sensory change
  - **Ugly duckling sign:** Used to observe a pt w/multi nevi, refer if a pigmented lesion appears different from the surrounding lesions

- **Tx:** Staging based on tumor thickness, mitotic rate, & ulceration → wide local excision, LN excision, & adjuvant immunotherapy
- **Prognosis:** Based on tumor thickness (*J Clin Oncol* 2009;27:6199); 14% 5-y survival with metastatic melanoma

Melanoma prognosis by tumor thickness		
Tumor stage	Invasion thickness	10-y survival rate
T1	<1 mm	92%
T2	1.01–2 mm	80%
T3	2.01–4 mm	63%
T4	>4 mm	50%

From *J Clin Oncol* 2009;27:6199.

DOMESTIC VIOLENCE

Definitions
- Intentional controlling or violent behavior by someone in a relationship w/the victim. Includes emotional/psychological abuse and economic deprivation
- **Intimate partner violence:** Physical/sexual violence, stalking or psychological aggression (including coercive acts) by a current/former intimate partner (CDC)
- **Common couple violence:** Not connected to general control behavior, arises in a single argument where one/both partners are injured
- **Intimate terrorism:** General pattern of abuser control, emotional & psychological abuse, not mutual, more likely to escalate over time, more likely to involve serious injury
- **Violent resistance:** Self-defense, violence by victim against abuser
- **Phases of abuse:** Tension-building: Poor communication, fear, victim tries to pacify the abuser. Acting-out: Outburst of violent, abusive behavior. Honeymoon: End of violence → affection & apology.

Epidemiology (CDC *National Intimate Partner and Sexual Violence Survey* 2010, see www.cdc.gov/ViolencePrevention/pdf/NISVS_Report2010-a.pdf)
- 1 in 3 (35.6%) ♀ experience IPV, ~1 in 5 (18.3%) ♀ have been raped
- Higher prevalence if under age 35, single, divorced/separated, EtOH or drug abuse, smoking, pregnant, lower socioeconomic class, h/o childhood abuse
- **Elder abuse:** 10% of women over 65 report physical, sexual, or verbal abuse or neglect. Risks: Advanced age, AA, disability in self-care, dementia, depression, h/o hip fracture, h/o stroke, social isolation, low socioeconomic status, and institutional staffing shortages.
- **Pregnancy:** IPV affects 7–20% of pregnancies, 3-fold higher risk if preg is unintended. Preg can result from reproductive coercion (forced preg by contraception sabotage). Victims more likely to deliver preterm & via C-section. 3-fold ↑ risk of attempted/completed homicide. Highest risk of IPV in 3rd trimester & postpartum.
- No typical abuser or victim; IPV affects all ages, races, & socioeconomic classes

Clinical Manifestations
- Inconsistent explan of injuries or delay in seeking tx. Somatic complaints (HAs, abdominal/pelvic pain, fatigue). Depression, anxiety, eating disorders.
- Presenting late to PNC. Frequent ED visits. Noncompliance w/rx. Skin tears, bruises, bone fractures, malnutrition, dehyd, & pressure ulcers common in victims of elder abuse.
- Most injuries on breasts, abd, & genitals, esp in preg. Defensive wounds on hands, arms. Bruises of different ages.

Diagnostic Workup/Studies
- Screen routinely in all pregnant pts, for well-woman/preventive visits. ACOG recommends screening annually but does not endorse any particular screening tool. No strong evid that routine screening decreases harm (USPSTF).
- **SAFE questions** (*JAMA* 1993;269:2367)
  "Do you feel safe in your relationship?"
  "Have you ever been in a relationship where you have been threatened, hurt, or afraid?"
  "Are your family/friends aware that you have been hurt? Could you tell them and would they be able to give you support?"
  "Do you have a safe place to go and resources you need in an emergency?"

- Example screening questions from ACOG Committee Opinion (Number 518, Feb 2012)
    - "Has your current partner ever threatened you or made you feel afraid?"
    - "Has your partner ever hit, choked, or physically hurt you?"
    - "Has your partner ever forced you to do something sexually that you did not want to do, or refused your request to use condoms?"
- **BASE** & the **CTS** can be used to screen for elder abuse (*JAGS* 2004;52:297)

Treatment and Medications

- **RADAR:** Routinely screen, Ask direct questions, Document your findings, Assess safety, Review options. Provide supportive counseling & validation of a pt's fear.
- **Assess risk for escalation:** Presence of weapons in the home, increasing violence frequency/severity, partner's knowledge that victim is planning to leave, threats of homicide
- Refer to social workers, safe houses, ER. 1-800-799-SAFE provides information regarding local resources in every state
- Specific, detailed, accurate, & nonjudgmental documentation is essential in case the victim seeks legal redress, and is required by law in some states
- Reporting: Mandatory reporting of child abuse in all states and of elder abuse in most states (napsa-now.org). Required reporting of IPV-related injuries (definitions vary) in all US states *except* AL, WY, and NM. Must report any case of IPV in KY (w/ or w/o injury). State specific policies: acf.hhs.gov/sites/default/files/fysb/state_compendium.pdf

SUBSTANCE ABUSE

- Substance abuse screening is part of well woman and primary care OB-Gyn. See Chapter 19 (page 19-1).

DEPRESSION AND PSYCHIATRIC DISEASE SCREENING

- Depression and psychiatric screening is part of well woman and primary care OB-Gyn. See Chapter 19 (page 19-3).
- **Screening** (2-item tool): "During the last month, have you felt down, depressed, or hopeless?" & "During the last month, have you felt little interest or pleasure in doing things?" PHQ-9: Assesses 9 sx of DSM-IV-TR definition of depression.

CONTRACEPTION AND STERILIZATION

Epidemiology (*Contraception* 2011;83:397)

- ~50% of pregnancies in US are unintended
- **PRAMS:** 33% of ♀ w/unintended preg did not think they could get pregnant at the time of conception; 22% stated their partner did not want to use contraception; 16% cited side effects; 10% cited access
- Contraceptive efficacy should be compared to 85% unprotected preg rate in 1 y. Assessed by *perfect use* (failure rate if used exactly according to guidelines) & *typical use* (failure rate for the usual compliance).

Contraceptive methods (*see also below)			
Method	Perfect use	Typical use	Primary mech of action
Sterilization			
Female*	<1%	<1%	Mechanical obstruction
Male Outpt procedure (urology)	<1%	<1%	Mechanical obstruction
Long-acting reversible contraception (LARC)			
Etonogestrel implant* (Implanon/Nexplanon)	<1%	<1%	Inhibition of ovulation
Levonorgestrel IUD* (Mirena)	<1%	<1%	Cervical mucus thickening, sterile inflamm rxn
Copper T IUD* (PARAGARD)	<1%	<1%	Sterile inflamm rxn, interferes w/sperm fxn

Method	Perfect use	Typical use	Primary mech of action
Combined hormonal			
Pills, patch, vaginal ring*	<1%	9%	Inhibition of ovulation
Progestin only			
Depo-provera	<1%	6%	Inhibition of ovulation
POPs	<1%	9%	Cervical mucus thickening
Barrier			
Male condom ↓ STI/HIV infxns	2%	18%	Mechanical obstruction for sperm
Female condom ↓ STI/HIV less than male condom	5%	21%	Mechanical obstruction for sperm
Diaphragm + spermicide*	6%	12%	Mechanical & chemical obstruction for sperm

*Special Considerations for Contraceptive Methods
- WHO or CDC criteria for contraceptive considerations w/medical problems; see www.cdc.gov/reproductivehealth/unintendedpregnancy/usmchm
- **Female sterilization** ("CREST Study" *Am J Obstet Gynecol* 1996;174:1161):
  Postpartum salpingectomy: Most effective method of female sterilization (10-y cumulative failure rate = 7.5/1000 BTL; performed up to 2 d after deliv.
  Interval sterilization: Sterilization at other than postpartum period. Varying LSC approaches.
  Hysteroscopic sterilization (Essure): Was not available for the CREST study, but is highly effective, outpt. Minimally invasive method w/o limitations by BMI, adhesive dz. Requires confirmation of tubal occlusion with HSG at 3 mo.
- **Combined hormonal methods (= estrogen + progestin):**
  Side effects – Breakthrough bleeding, breast tenderness, HA, nausea/vomiting
  OCPs: Both estrogen & progestin or progestin-only pills. Can interact w/other meds (antiretrovirals, antiepileptics) → potential ↓ efficacy of either or both meds. Useful for menorrhagia, dysmenorrhea, hirsutism, & acne. ↓ Risk of endometrial & ovarian cancer. Different dosing and hormonal preparations are available. Monthly vs. continuous dosing is acceptable, continuous dosing may be preferable for endometriosis, PMS/PMDD, lifestyle reasons.
  Contraceptive patch: Replaced weekly × 3 w then removed for 1 w (menses). Less effective in women >90 kg.
  Vaginal ring: Placed intravaginally × 3 w then removed for 1 w (menses). Small ↑ in vaginitis, vaginal discharge, & leukorrhea compared to OCPs.
- **Progestin-only methods:**
  Mech of action: Thickened cervical mucus, thinned endometrium, ovulation inhib
  Side effects: Breakthrough bleeding, acne, follicular cysts, wt gain, mood changes
  POP: Preg rate <1% perfect use, 9% typical use. Must be taken around same time every day. Shorter half-life, therefore missed doses more likely.
  DMPA: Preg rate <1% perfect use, 6% typical use. One intramuscular or subcutaneous injection every 90 d (12 w). Side effects: Wt gain 3–6 lb/y, esp in obese adols ↓ BMD, but reversible after discontinuation (DEXA scan not recommended).
  Etonogestrel implant (Implanon/Nexplanon): Placed in upper arm, in-office, effective for 3 y, possibly longer. Side effects: Breakthrough bleeding common → major reason for early discontinuation, no ↓ BMD like DMPA, risks of insertion include pain, bleeding, infxn, & difficult removal.
  Levonorgestrel IUD (Mirena/Liletta): Inserted in-office, lasts for 5 y. Effective for menorrhagia, dysmenorrhea, endometriosis, endometrial hyperplasia, & possibly Grade 1 Stage I endometrial cancer. Adolescence, nulliparity, prev STI, & prev ectopic Preg are **not** contraindications to IUD placement. ↑ Ectopic preg w/IUD, but overall rate of ectopic ↓ due to decreased Preg.
- **Nonhormonal methods**
  Copper IUD: Inserted in-office. Effective for 10 y. Does not impact menstrual regularity, but may cause slightly heavier menses. Adolescence, nulliparity, prev STI, & prev ectopic preg are not contraindications to IUD placement.
  Diaphragm with spermicide: Requires fitting, not common in US. Refit if recent Preg or change in wt. Increases risk of urinary tract infxn. Insert up to 6 h prior to intercourse, remove 6–24 h after intercourse.
  Withdrawal: Preg rate: 4% perfect use, 22% typical use. Used by up to 56% of women using contraception, usually secondary in conjunction w/condoms.

Lactational amenorrhea: Preg rate: 2% perfect use, 5% typical use. Effective for 1st 6 mo postpartum *only if* exclusive breast-feeding (only nutrition for infant), breast-feeding every 4 h during the day & at least every 6 h at night, no menses if ≥56 d postpartum.

Rhythm method: Preg rate: 0.4–5% perfect use, 12–23% typical use. Relies on regular menstrual cycles & the limited viability of ova/sperm w/o fertilization. Can use menstrual calendars, cervical mucus changes, basal body temperature, or ovulation kits to avoid intercourse during midcycle fertile days.

EMERGENCY CONTRACEPTION (EC)

Definition (Obstet Gynecol 2015;126(3):e1–11)
- Use of oral pills or an IUD as an emergency measure to prevent preg
- Intended for occasional or backup use, not as a primary contraceptive method
- **Indications:** No contraception use, or contraceptive failure/misuse, during sexual intercourse w/i the prev 120 h

Mechanism of Action
- For EC pills: inhibition or delay of ovulation. For copper IUD: Interference w/tubal transport or fertilization. Prevention of implantation.
- EC does *not* interrupt preg & is ineffective after preg has been established
- Since oral EC only delays ovulation, patients must be counseled that unprotected intercourse after taking EC will NOT be protected

Treatment and Medications (Obstet Gynecol 2015;126(3):e1–11)
- Physical exam & lab tests not req prior to EC. Exclude preg esp before IUD. No contraindications based on medical conditions according to CDC MEC.
- **Levonorgestrel** (Plan B): 1.5 mg PO in a single dose. Effective up to 120 h from unprotected intercourse, though most effective w/i 1st 72 h. 98% of pts menstruate w/i 21 d (mean 7–9 d). Administer preg test if no menses w/i 28 d. Side effects – irreg bleeding, nausea/vomiting (give antiemetics). Redose if vomiting w/i 2 h of administration.
- **Ulipristal** (Ella): 30 mg PO in a single dose. Selective progesterone receptor modulator. Effective up to 120 h from unprotected intercourse. More effective than levonorgestrel from 72–120 h after unprotected intercourse.
- **Copper IUD** (ParaGard): Must be inserted w/i 120 h from unprotected intercourse. Most effective form of EC. Provides long-term, effective contraception along w/EC
- **Yuzpe method:** 2–5 combined OCPs q12h ×2 within 72 h of unprotected intercourse. Less effective than other EC but may be more accessible. Dosing by pill formulation available at bedsider.org

Methods of emergency contraception					
Method	Dosing	Timing	Access	Efficacy	Side effects
Selective progesterone receptor modulator (Ella)	30 mg PO ulipristal acetate ×1	Up to 5 d after intercourse	Prescription only	1.4% pregnancy rate	HA (19%) Nausea (12%) Irr bleeding (16%)
Progestin only (Plan B)	Levonorgestrel 1.5 mg PO ×1 OR Levonorgestrel 0.75 mg PO ×12h ×2	Up to 3 d after intercourse	Available OTC w/o age restriction Available OTC if >17 yo	2.2% pregnancy rate (60–94% pregnancy prevention rate) Less effective if obese	Similar to ulipristal
Combined progestin-estrogen pills (CHCs)	Various formulations[a]	Up to 5 d after intercourse	Prescription needed	59–89% pregnancy prevention rate ~50% higher RR of pregnancy than Plan B	Nausea (more than others methods)

Method	Dosing	Timing	Access	Efficacy	Side effects
Copper IUD (Paragard)	n/a	Up to 5 d after intercourse	Requires office visit and insertion by clinician	0–2% pregnancy rate	<1% uterine perf ↑ duration menses dysmenorrhea

Formulations of OC's used for EC available at http://ec.princeton.edu/questions/dose.html
Adapted from *Obstet Gynecol* 2015;126(3):e1–11.

VACCINATIONS

Figure 1.3 Recommended United States Adult Immunization Schedule 2016

	Age group (yrs)		
Vaccine	**19–26 years**	**27–64 years**	**≥65 years**
Influenza	1 dose annually		
Tetanus, diphtheria, pertussis (Td/Tdap)	Substitute Tdap for Td once, then Td booster every 10 yrs		
Varicella	2 doses, if non-immune		
Human papillomavirus (HPV) Male or Female	3 doses		
Zoster			1 dose
Measles, mumps, rubella (MMR)	1 or 2 doses depending on indication		
Pneumococcal 23-valent polysaccharide	1 or 2 doses depending on indication		1 dose
Hepatitis A	2 doses		
Hepatitis B	3 doses		
Meningococcal	1 or more doses depending on vaccine and indication		
Haemophilus influenzae type b (Hib)	1 or 3 doses depending on indication		

☐ Recommended for all persons who meet the age requirement, lack documentation of vaccination, or lack evidence of past infection; zoster vaccine is recommended regardless of past episode of zoster ☐ Recommended for persons with a risk factor (medical, occupational, lifestyle, or other indication) ☐ No recommendation

From Advisory Committee on Immunization Practices, Department of Health and Human Services, Centers for Disease Control and Prevention. More information and complete recommendations and notes: http://www.cdc.gov/vaccines/schedules/downloads/adult/adult-schedule.pdf. Accessed January 2018.

Figure 1.4 Adult vaccines by medical indication 2016

	Indication					
Vaccine	**Pregnancy**	**Immuno-compromising conditions (excluding HIV infection)**	**HIV infection CD4+ count (cells/μL) < 200**	**HIV infection CD4+ count (cells/μL) ≥ 200**	**Diabetes**	**Healthcare personnel**
Influenza	1 dose annually					
Tetanus, diphtheria, pertussis (Td/Tdap)	1 dose each pregnancy	Substitute Tdap for Td once, then Td booster every 10 yrs				
Varicella	Contraindicated			2 doses		
Human papillomavirus (HPV) Female	3 doses through age 26 yrs					
Zoster	Contraindicated			1 dose for all ≥60 yo		
Measles, mumps, rubella (MMR)	Contraindicated			1 or 2 doses depending on indication		
Pneumococcal polysaccharide (PPSV23)	1 to 3 doses depending on indication					
Hepatitis A	2 or 3 doses depending on vaccine					
Hepatitis B	3 doses					
Meningococcal	1 or more doses depending on vaccine and indication					
Haemophilus influenzae type b (Hib)	Post bone marrow transplant only	1 dose				

☐ Recommended for all persons who meet the age requirement, lack documentation of vaccination, or lack evidence of past infection; zoster vaccine is recommended regardless of past episode of zoster ☐ Recommended for persons with a risk factor (medical, occupational, lifestyle, or other indication) ☐ No recommendation

From Advisory Committee on Immunization Practices, Department of Health and Human Services, Centers for Disease Control and Prevention. More information and complete recommendations and notes: http://www.cdc.gov/vaccines/schedules/downloads/adult/adult-schedule.pdf. Accessed January 2018.

US women's mortality: Top causes for all females, all ages, 2015

1. Heart dz, 22.3%
2. Cancer, 21.1%
3. Chronic lower respiratory dzs, 6.2%
4. Stroke, 6.1%
5. Alzheimer dz, 5.7%
6. Unintentional injuries, 4.0%
7. Diabetes, 2.7%
8. Influenza & pneumonia, 2.3%
9. Kidney dz, 1.8%
10. Septicemia, 1.6%

From CDC "Leading Causes of Death in Females." 2015 data. https://www.cdc.gov/women/lcod/2015/index.htm. Accessed April 1, 2018.

Annual US Gyn new cancer diagnoses and deaths, 2016

Cause	Cases (% all new ca dx)	Deaths (% all ca deaths)
Endometrial	60050 (3.6)	10470 (1.8)
Ovarian	222280 (1.8)	14240 (2.4)
Cervical	12990 (0.8)	4120 (0.7)
Vulvar	5950 (0.4)	1110 (0.2)
Vaginal	4620 (0.3)	376 (<0.1)

From NIH SEER Program, Cancer Fact Sheets, 2016. http://seer.cancer.gov/statfacts/. Accessed 10/11/2016.

Epidemiology terms

Sens	% w/dz w/positive result on a test
Spec	% w/o dz w/negative result on a test
PPV	% w/a positive test who *actually have* condition
NPV	% w/a negative test who do not have the condition; PPV & NPV change w/prevalence
Incid	Number of new events in a specific time period per pop at risk at the start of the time interval
Prevalence	Number of people w/a dz at a *point* in time per pop at risk at that time
OR	Odds of an exposure w/dz over odds in a control group; common for case-control studies
RR	Proportion of exposed who develop a condition over proportion of unexposed who develop a condition (I_{exp}/I_{unexp}); for cohort studies
AR	Probability of a medical event (as a % of all who could have the event). ARR = difference of ARs btw 2 groups
NNT	1/the ARR in %; number of pts to treat for 1 prevented case (=1 avoided risk outcome)
CI	If exp repeated 100×, truth is in this range 95× (w/i the 95% CI). If CI crosses 1, the finding is not signif (=no effect)
Intention to treat analysis	Based on how subjects were originally randomized & includes all of them; no dropouts or problem pts subtracted from the groups
Type 1 error (α)	Rejecting the null hypothesis when it is actually true, causes you to believe there was an effect when there was not; usually set at $p < 5\%$
Type 2 error (β)	Accepting the null hypothesis, when it is actually false; causes you to believe there was no effect when there actually was
Power	Ability of your study to detect a true difference ($1 - \beta$); often set at 80%

Calculating sensitivity, specificity, PPV, NPV

	Dz+	Dz–	
Test pos	a (true pos)	b (false pos)	PPV = $[a/(a + b)] \times 100$
Test neg	c (false neg)	d (true neg)	NPV = $[d/(c + d)] \times 100$
	Sens = $[a/(a + c)] \times 100$	Spec = $[d/(b + d)] \times 100$	

Types of studies	
Case series	**What:** Summary of cases & outcomes for an unusual event **Pro:** Good for rare, interesting, or new conditions or rxs **Con:** Only descriptive, not controlled, no causality
Cohort	**What:** Follow exposed & control group for specific outcomes (in real time or after the outcome has already occurred). Looks forward for outcome. Define by exposure → eval outcome. **Pro:** Can be retrospective ("historical cohort") or prospective **Con:** No causality; prospective is expensive & lengthy
Case control	**What:** Search for prior exposure in cases (w/condition) compared w/ controls (w/o condition). Looks backward. **Pro:** Can be run quickly w/existing databases. Good for rare conditions. **Con:** No causality; matching cases & controls can be difficult
RCT	**What:** Follow randomized groups of pts w/rx or placebo to assess outcomes/complications. A "true experiment." **Pro:** Level 1 evid; gold std for clinical research **Con:** Often difficult to recruit & expensive. May not be feasible or ethical for certain clinical questions (eg, many obstetrical concerns).

Phases of Clinical Trials (Understanding Clinical Trials, NIH, clinicaltrials.gov)
- **Phase 1:** Tests an experimental drug or rx in a small group of people (10–80) to evaluate safety, determine a dosage, & identify side effects
- **Phase 2:** The experimental study drug or rx is given to a larger group of people (100–300) to see if it is effective & to further evaluate safety
- **Phase 3:** The experimental study drug or rx is given to large groups (1000–3000) to confirm effectiveness, monit side effects, & collect safety data
- **Phase 4:** Postmarketing review of risk/benefit & unexpected events

Ultrasound (US)

- **Transabdominal US:** 4–5 mHz curvilinear transducer, better if pt's bladder is full; Common indications – FAST scan, fetal presentation
- **Transvaginal US (TVUS):** 5–10 mHz transducer, better visualization of pelvic organs, pt's bladder should be empty
  Common indications – pregnancy location, evaluation of adnexa
- **Doppler:** Change in frequency of reflected US shows blood flow. Useful to assess flow. In acute setting, can help evaluate for flow to the ovaries, evaluation of retained products of conception, assessment of FHT, etc. In early pregnancy, M-mode is preferred for documenting fetal FH overpulsed Doppler.
- **Normal measurements:**
  Uterus is $8 \times 5 \times 4$ cm (smaller in prepubertal or postmenopausal women). Normal AP diameter 3–5 cm & length 6–10 cm.
  EMS is <15 mm (premenopausal) & <8 mm (postmenopausal). In screening for postmenopausal vaginal bleeding, use nml <5 mm (PPV 9% & NPV 99% for endometrial cancer). EMS measured from echogenic interfaces of the anter & post basalis layers.
  Ovary vol is 9.8 ± 5.8 cm^3. Ovarian follicles up to 2.5 cm diameter. Avg nml ovary is $3.5 \times 2.5 \times 1.5$ cm $\rightarrow 2 \times 1.5 \times 1$ cm postmenopausal.
  Fallopian tubes are not normally visible unless there is pathology (eg hydrosalpinx). Small amount of fluid in the posterior cul-de-sac may be physiologic.

Radiography (XR)

- Common indications: Fractures, displaced IUDs, cardiopulmonary evaluation, trauma, other nonpregnant conditions. Abdominal shielding used.

Computed Tomography (CT)

- Common indications: Acute abdomen, postoperative symptoms, intracranial evaluation, suspected gyn malignancy IV contrast ok in Preg
- **Noncontrast CT:** Nephrolithiasis, neuropathology (hemorrhagic stroke, head trauma, intracranial hemorrhage, intracranial lesions/masses, skull fracture)
- **Contrast CT:** Vascular pathology (aneurysm, dissection, ischemic stroke), trauma, bowel pathology (diverticulitis, appendicitis), abscesses, pulmonary embolism

Magnetic Resonance Imaging (MRI)

- Can help evaluate pregnant patients for acute appendicitis or sinus venous thrombosis

Imaging During Pregnancy (Obstet Gynecol 2016;127:75; Am J Obstet Gynecol 2012;206:456)

- No reports of adverse fetal affects w/ US or MRI
- With few exceptions, ionizing radiation from CT or XR is lower dose than a/w fetal harm and should not be withheld if indicated → risks depending on exposure & GA
  Extremely high-dose ionizing radiation → "All or nothing" effect w/ early Preg loss. At <18 w, 500 rad is the estimated threshold for embryonic demise

Fetal radiation exposure during imaging	
Procedure	Estimated fetal radiation exposure (mrad)
CXR (2 views)	0.02–0.07
Abdominal film (single view)	100
Hip film (single view)	200
CT scan of head or chest	<1000
CT scan of abd & lumbar spine	3500
CT pelvimetry	250

At term, 2000 rad is the threshold & fetal risks same as maternal risks.
Risk of anomalies, growth restriction, or SAB not increased w/ radiation exposure of <5 rad. True threshold dose is likely >20 rad.
Risk of CNS effects (eg, microcephaly, mental retardation) highest at 8–15 w. There is no established risk at <8 or >25 w.
The threshold dose of ionizing radiation → mental retardation at <16 w is 35–50 rad. After 16 w, the threshold is 150 rad.
1–2 rad fetal exposure may ↑ leukemia risk by 1.5–2, but baseline childhood cancer risk is 0.2–0.3%; therefore, overall risk is still low.

No single diagnostic procedure provides radiation doses significant enough for adverse embryonic/fetal effect, especially mid to late Preg.
- **Nuclear medicine:** Radioactive iodine contraindicated in Preg. Tc-99m usually results in fetal exposure of <0.5 rad.
- **Contrast agents:** Iodine-based contrast safe for use in Preg. Gadolinium contraindicated in Preg – assess risks/benefits of contrast & obtain consent. Gadolinium crosses placenta → excreted into amniotic fluid. Unk exposure duration & effect on fetus.

ULTRASOUND IN EARLY PREGNANCY

Ultrasound in Pregnancy (Obstet Gynecol 2009;113:451; NEJM 2013;369:1443)
- **1st trimester US:** TVUS best in early Preg to confirm IUP, evaluate ectopic Preg, determine GA, evaluate Preg chorionicity, confirm cardiac activity, evaluate adnexal masses. Also obtain nuchal translucency, nasal bone for prenatal screening.
    GS: Visible by ~4 w GA, eccentrically implanted in the mid-upper fundus w/ a bright decidual rxn (double-ring sign), visible in 2 planes. Not used to determine final GA. Mean sac diameter (the avg of 3 measurements in mm) + 30 = GA (days) ± 3 d
    Yolk sac: Visible at 5 w GA, should be seen when the mean GS diameter is >13 mm
    Embryo: Visible at 6 w GA, or when mean GS diameter is ≥20 mm.
    1st trimester CRL is most accurate dating. If ≤9.5 w GA, CRL in mm + 42 = GA (days) ± 3 d.
    FHM: Observed when the embryo is ≥5 mm CRL. FHR = 100 bpm at 5–6 w GA, & → peak 175 bpm at 9 w GA. If FHM is seen, SAB rate is 2–3% in asymptomatic low-risk women. Women <35 yo who p/w VB = 5% SAB rate if the US is nml & shows FHM.
    To quickly estimate EDD from LMP, use Naegele's rule: Add 1 y, subtract 3 mo, & add 7 d (= 280 d from LMP)
    US Dx criteria of failed preg: Crown–rump ≥7 mm and no HR, mean sac diam ≥25 mm and no embryo, absence of HR 2 w after scan with gest sac but no yolk sac, or absence of HR 11 d after scan with gest sac and yolk sac
- **2nd & 3rd trimester US** – see Fetal Ultrasound in Chap. 9 (page 9-8)
- **US for determination of GA:** US dating takes preference over menstrual dating when the discrep is >7 d in the 1st trimester; >10 d in the 2nd trimester. In the 3rd trimester, accuracy of a US is w/i 3–4 w.

ACUTE PELVIC PAIN

Definitions and Epidemiology (Natl Health Stat Report 2010;6:1)
- Lower abdominal or pelvic pain present for <7 d. Most common presenting complaint & primary dx for women of ages 15–64 who are seen in the ER.

Causes of pelvic pain	
OBGYN causes of acute pelvic pain	**Other causes of acute pelvic pain**
Dysmenorrhea	Gastroenteritis
Ectopic Preg	Appendicitis
Spont miscarriage	Small bowel obst
Ovarian tumor or cyst	Severe constipation
Ovarian torsion	Hernia
PID	Diverticulitis
TOA	Nephrolithiasis
Degenerating leiomyoma	Pyelonephritis
Herpes simplex virus, chancroid	Cystitis
Bartholin duct cyst or abscess	

From Flasar MH, Cross R, Goldberg E. Acute abdominal pain. Prim Care 2006;33(3):659.

Pathophysiology and Clinical Manifestations (Prim Care 2006;33:659)
- **Visceral pain:** Stretch, distention, torsion, or contraction of abdominal organs is detected by autonomic, afferent nociceptors → "slow", C-fibers relay the signal to the CNS → pain is usually midline or bilateral, poorly localized, dull, achy, or cramping

- **Parietal pain:** Direct irritation of the peritoneal lining is detected by somatic, afferent nociceptors → "fast," A-delta fibers relay the signal → pain is unilateral, localized, sharp
- **Referred pain:** Visceral nerve afferents carrying stimuli from a diseased organ enter the spinal cord at the same level as somatic afferents from a remote anatomic location (eg, free fluid in the abd can irritate the diaphragm causing referred pain in the shoulder).

Physical Exam
- Fever, tachy, hypotension → expedite w/u, concern for sepsis/infxn, intra-abdominal bleeding (eg, ruptured ectopic Preg, hemorrhagic ovarian cyst), ovarian torsion, appendicitis.
- **Abdominal exam:** Note prior surgical scars, distention, bowel sounds (hyperactive/high pitched vs. hypoactive), rebound, guarding, rigidity. Palpate 4 quadrants.
- **Pelvic exam:** Note swelling, erythema, lesions, bleeding, discharge, masses, nodularity, cervical motion tenderness, or pain

Diagnostic Workup and Studies
- **Labs:** Urine or serum bhCG (on every reproductive age woman in the ER), CBC, urinalysis +/- culture, vaginal wet prep, gonorrhea, & chlamydia PCR
- **Imaging:** FAST scan, transabdominal or transvaginal US
- **Culdocentesis:** Rarely used. Aspiration of fluid from the post cul-de-sac. Considered in limited resource settings.
- **Diagnostic laparoscopy:** Consider for the unstable pt w/ abdominal pain, esp if +hCG
- Rx & medications depend on dx (see other sections, below)

ECTOPIC PREGNANCY

Definitions & Epidemiology *(Obstet Gynecol 2008;111:1479; NEJM 2009;361:379)*
- Preg outside of the endometrial cavity. 2% of 1st trimester pregnancies
- 3–4% of all pregnancy-related deaths (leading cause of death in the 1st trimester)
- Ectopic Preg increasing (4.5/1000 pregnancies in 1970 → 19.7/1000 in 1992)
- Rate of rupture w/ ectopic Preg is 20–35%

Etiology
- Blastocyst implants & invades improperly at nonendometrial site. 97% in fallopian tubes, most frequently in the ampullary region. Other implantation sites include the isthmic portion of the tube, fimbria, uterine cornua, cervix, ovary, prior C/S scar, or abd.
- Heterotopic Preg → 2 or more implantation sites (ie, an IUP & ectopic Preg). Extremely rare, only 1:4000 nml pregnancies. Increased to 1/100 in IVF pts.
- **Risk factors:** Prior ectopic Preg, prior tubal Surg, tobacco smoking, prior PID, *Chlamydia trachomatis* infxn, 3 or more prior spont miscarriages, age >40 y, prior medical or surgical abortion, infertility >1 y, lifelong sexual partners >5, current IUD use, IVF/ART. However, 50% of women with ectopic pregnancies have NO risk factors.

Clinical Manifestations and Physical Exam
- Lower abdominal pain on the affected side. Vaginal bleeding.
- Clinical findings are often unremarkable w/ unruptured ectopic Preg. Only 75% develop marked abdominal tenderness. May p/w shoulder pain, dizziness, syncope. Hx & risk factors are useful to assess index of suspicion.
- VS & clinical assessment to look for signs of hemodynamic stability.
- **Pelvic exam:** Adnexal mass. Abdominal exam: Tenderness to palpation. Evaluate for surgical abd: Rebound, guarding, rigidity.

Diagnostic Workup and Studies
- **Labs:** CBC (sometimes serial Hgb), bld type (RhoGAM if Rh-negative), CMP for BUN/Cr, & AST/ALT (if considering MTX)
- **Serum (quantitative) hCG:**
    If hCG above "discriminatory zone" (DZ) of 1500–2000 mIU/mL, nml IUP can be seen on TVUS.
    If hCG >1500–2000 mIU/mL & no IUP on TVUS → likely abnl Preg (eg, ectopic Preg, incomplete AB, resolving completed AB) unless twins/multiples
    If hCG <DZ & no IUP → rpt hCG in 48 h (at SAME lab as values differ by lab).
    In 85% of women w/ a nml IUP, the hCG will ↑ ≥63% in 48 h
    In 99% of women w/ a nml IUP, the hCG will ↑ ≥53% in 48 h
    An ↑ in serum hCG of <53% in 48 h → abn Preg. Of note, 21% of ectopic pregnancies have normal rise in hCG

- **TVUS:** Sensitivity of TVUS for dx of ectopic Preg ranges from 73–93%, depending on GA and sonographer. Extrauterine GS or embryo seen in only 15–30% of cases. Most common US finding is an adnexal mass btw the ovary & uterus.
  Adnexal mass (other than a simple ovarian cyst) is 84% sensitive & 99% specific for ectopic Preg
  Trilaminar endometrial stripe (only) is 38% sensitive & 94% specific for an ectopic Preg
  Pseudosac (intrauterine midline fluid collection) is neither sensitive nor specific for the dx of ectopic Preg. Do not confuse pseudosac for IUP.
- **Serum progesterone:** Often not definitive. Levels from 5–20 ng/mL are equivocal
  Serum progesterone <5 ng/mL sugg abn Preg (100% specific, 60% sensitive)
  Serum progesterone >20 ng/mL sugg nml IUP (40% specific, 95% sensitive)
- **Endometrial curettage:** For "Preg of unk location," Uterine curettage with D&C or Manual vacuum aspiration (MVA) can evaluate POCs (float villi), & assist in decision for medical vs. surgical management vs. dx of abnl intrauterine Preg

Management Options
- **Expectant mgmt:** 68% → successful resolution *(Lancet 1998;351:1115)*
  If initial hCG is <200 mIU/mL, 88% resolve w/o rx
  Recheck hCG 48 h after initial lab tests to ensure declining serum hCG
- **Medical mgmt:** MTX inhibits dihydrofolate reductase → decreased tetrahydrofolate → ↓ purine nucleotide synthesis → ↓ DNA/RNA in S-phase of cell cycle → prevent proliferation (in active tissues like trophoblast, bone marrow, buccal/intestinal mucosa). 2 commonly used protocols (see below). Multidose regimen more effective for advanced GA, high initial bhCG levels (>5000) & +fetal cardiac activity.
  Side effects: Usually self-limited. Most common are nausea, vomiting, stomatitis, conjunctivitis, worsening abdominal pain 2–3 d after MTX dose due to expansion of the affected gestational tissue, transient liver dysfxn, & uncommonly myelosuppression, alopecia, pulmonary damage, anaphylaxis.
  Pt education: Stop taking prenatal vitamins & folate supplements, avoid sun exposure, refrain from EtOH consump, intercourse, & vigorous physical activity
  Absolute contraindications to MTX: Tubal rupture or hemodynamic instability, breast-feeding, alcoholism, alcoholic liver dz, or chronic liver dz, immunodeficiency, pre-existing bld dyscrasias (bone marrow hypoplasia, leukopenia, thrombocytopenia, signif anemia), active pulmonary dz, peptic ulcer dz, hepatic, renal, or hematologic dysfxn, Cr >1.3 mg/dL, AST or ALT >50 IU/L, sensitivity to methotrexate, inability to comply with required follow-up
  Relative contraindications to MTX:
  GS >3.5–4.0 cm. Single-dose MTX 93% effective when the GS is <3.5 cm. Decreases to 87–90% efficacy when >3.5 cm. Large GS → ↓ success.
  Embryonic cardiac activity. Single-dose MTX is 87% effective if + fetal heart motion
  Serum hCG level >5000 mIU/mL. Failure w/ single-dose MTX is 14.3% if hCG >5000 mIU/mL (compared to 3.7% failure if hCG <5000 mIU/mL). Consider multidose regimen or surgical mgmt.

Single-dose MTX regimen
89% success rate, MTX dose: 50 mg/m^2 Day 1: Check hCG (& other labs above), administer MTX Days 4 & 7: Check bhCG ↓ In hCG of ≥15% from day 4–day 7 → continue to monitor weekly serum hCG levels until undetectable (Note: hCG may ↑ from day 1–day 4) If hCG does not fall appropriately from day 4–day 7 → consider rpt US, then rpt MTX dose or perform laparoscopy

Multidose MTX regimen
93% success rate MTX dose: 1 mg/kg + Leucovorin (folinic acid) dose: 0.1 mg/kg 　Day 1: Check hCG, administer MTX 　Day 2: Administer Leucovorin 　Day 3: Check hCG. If hCG has NOT decreased by 15% from day 1, then administer MTX 　Day 4: Administer Leucovorin 　Day 5: Check hCG. If hCG has NOT decreased by 15% from day 3, then administer MTX 　Day 6: Administer Leucovorin 　Day 7: Check hCG. If hCG has NOT decreased by 15% from day 5, then administer MTX 　Day 8: Administer Leucovorin If 4 doses of MTX are given w/o a 15% decline in hCG over 48 h → proceed w/ laparoscopy If there is a ≥15% decline in hCG over 48 h → follow weekly serum hCG levels until undetectable

Two-dose MTX regimen
87% success rate

MTX dose: 50 mg/m² IM

Day 0: Administer MTX

Day 4: Check bhCG and repeat MTX 50 mg/m² IM

Day 7: Check bhCG. If the decrease is >15%, monitor weekly serum hCG levels until undetectable. If <15% decrease in hCG levels, readminister MTX 50 mg/m2 on days 7 and 11, measuring hCG levels.

Day 11: Administer MTX 50 mg/m². If hCG levels decrease 15% between days 7 and 11, continue to monitor weekly until nonpregnant hCG levels are reached.

If the decrease is <15% between days 7 and 11, consider surgical treatment.

- **Surgical mgmt:** Appropriate when patient does not meet criteria for medical mgmt. If surgical mgmt. is indicated, laparoscopy preferred over laparotomy. If the pt is HDS → shorter operative times, less bld loss, less analgesic requirements, shorter hospital stay, no difference in tubal patency rates, similar rates of subseq IUP.
    Salpingostomy: Gold std Surg for ectopic. Open affected tube & evacuate ectopic POCs. Esp useful for pt w/ abn contralateral tube who desires future fertility. Persistent ectopic Preg in 4–15% of cases. Consider empiric dose of MTX postoperatively if not contraindicated. Follow weekly serum hCG levels until they are undetectable. Check pathology to confirm POCs.
    Salpingectomy: Removal of entire affected fallopian tube. Appropriate for pts w/ a nml appearing contralateral tube who desire future fertility, or pts who do not desire future fertility. Eliminates risk of persistent ectopic Preg, or recurrent, ipsilateral ectopic Preg. If confident that all trophoblast removed, no need for serial hCGs.

EARLY PREGNANCY FAILURE

Definition and Epidemiology (Fertil Steril 2003;79:577; Obstet Gynecol 2005;105:333)

- Completely dependent on how we define a clinical pregnancy
- SAB (miscarriage) occurs before 20 w 0 d & <500 g
- 10–20% of clinically recognized pregnancies end in spontaneous abortion
- Early Preg failure complicates 12–15% of known pregnancies & 17–22% of all pregnancies; 80% occur in the 1st 12 w of gest; fertilization → 30% implantation failure → 30% early loss (= 60% loss before recognized clinical Preg) → 12–15% clinical Preg SAB → 25% live birth.
- Vaginal bleeding in 20–40% known 1st trimester pregnancies → ~50% of those = SABs
- Once fetal cardiac activity is noted, 90–96% have ongoing Preg
- **Risk factors:** ↑ Mat age, prev SAB, heavy smoking, EtOH, cocaine, NSAIDs, fevers, caffeine >200 mg daily may be a/w SAB, chronic mat dz (DM, autoimmune, APLA syn), short interpregnancy interval, uterine anomalies

Types of spontaneous abortions (<20 w 0 d)					
Name	Sx	Bleeding?	Internal cervical os?	Tissue passed?	Notes
Missed	No sx; +/− fetal pole no cardiac activity. No cramping.	± (may be scant)	Closed	None	Includes "anembryonic" & "blighted ovum"
Threatened	Any bleeding gives dx, ± pain	Yes	Closed	No	Increases loss & PTB rate
Inevitable	Imminent miscarriage, usually w/ painful cramps	Yes	Open	No	
Incomplete	Bleeding & passage of some POCs	Yes	Open	Partial	Treat medically or surgically

Name	Sx	Bleeding?	Internal cervical os?	Tissue passed?	Notes
Complete	After passage of POCs, ± cramping	Yes or resolving	Closed	All POCs passed	Usually no medical intervention
Septic AB	Usually cramping/uterine tenderness, ± fever/chills/malaise/discharge	±	±	No or partial; infected POCs are retained	May be VERY ill
Recurrent	2–3 consecutive early losses	Any of the above	Any of the above	Any of the above	Refer for RPL w/u

Etiologies

- Chromosomal abnormalities (50%); congen anomalies; trauma (early GA uterus generally protected from blunt trauma); host factors (eg, uterine abnormalities [septum]), maternal endocrinopathies, infection, inherited or acquired thrombophilias, corpus luteum dysfxn; unexplained
- **Diff:** Cervical, vaginal or uterine pathology (polyp, malig, trauma), ectopic Preg, infxn, molar Preg, SAB (see above), subchorionic hemorrhage, vaginal trauma

Clinical Manifestations and Physical Exam

- Amenorrhea, vaginal bleeding, &/or pelvic pain/cramping
- Cessation of nml sx of Preg (eg, nausea, breast tenderness)
- Speculum/digital exam to assess cervical dilation, POCs
- Evaluate extent of bleeding (eg, hemorrhage) & maternal stability

Diagnostic Workup (Obstet Gynecol 1992;80:670; Ultrasound Obstet Gynecol 1994;3:63)

- **Passed tissue:** "Float villi" in saline to evaluate frond-like chorionic villi; send to pathology
- **Transvaginal US:** Distinguishes IUP vs. extrauterine Preg, viable vs. nonviable, presence of gestational trophoblastic dz, retained POCs, ectopic
- **Missed AB:** No fetal cardiac activity + CRL >7 mm OR mean sac diameter >25 mm and no embryo OR absence of embryo with HR >2 w after scan that showed GS w/o yolk sac OR absence of embryo with HR >11 d after scan that showed GS w/ yolk sac
- **Findings suggestive of early Preg failure:** Grossly distorted sac, absence of yolk sac w/ MSD >13 mm; absence of embryonic pole w/ MSD >20 mm; enlarged yolk sac (>6 mm); irreg or low lying sac; slow FHT (<100 bpm at 5–7 w); small GS (difference btw MSD & CRL <5 mm); subchorionic hematoma >25% vol of the GS
- Quantitative bhCG: Low yield once IUP confirmed. If no IUP, serial hCGs q48h to rule out ectopic → ↓ hCG = nonviable IUP or spontaneously resolving ectopic

Management of First Trimester Abortions

Management of first trimester abortions	
Spontaneous	If evidence of complete passage & no excessive bleeding, no further mgmt needed. If highly desired, no infxn/bleeding, & esp if unsure dating, may manage expectantly.
Missed, incomplete, or inevitable	Expectant mgmt if <13 w w/ stable VS & no e/o infxn. ~40% will ultimately need uterine evacuation; ~80% success w/ expect mgmt for incomplete. **Medical:** Misoprostol (PGE1 analog) in 1st trimester; contraindications: Allergy, unlocated pregnancy, ectopic Preg or pelvic infxn, hemodynamic instability **Missed AB:** 800 µg vaginally q24h up to 3 doses OR 400 µg per vagina q4h ×4 OR 600 µg sublingually q3h ×2 if needed (71% success by 3 d, 84% success by 8 d; 12% need D&C) **Incomplete AB:** 600 µg PO OR 400 µg sublingually ×1 (82% success by 5 d, 95% success by 7 d; 3% need for D&C) **Surgical:** Suction D&C or manual vacuum aspiration. Risks include uterine perforation, intrauterine adhesions, cervical trauma, & infxn Recommended: Doxycycline 100 mg PO preop & 200 mg PO postop (97% success rate)

Threatened	**Expectant mgmt:** Bleeding precautions, pelvic rest. No effect of proges-terone for threatened AB, but may ↓ recurrent AB *(Cochrane Database Syst Rev 2013;10:CD003511)*

If Rh(D)-negative & unsensitized, give RhoGAM 50–300 μg IM (prevent alloimmunization) Offer chromosomes/pathology. Grief counseling. Pain meds (NSAID, ± narcotics). Bleeding warnings. Antiemetic for nausea. F/u US in some circumstances (varies with clinical presentation).

Data from *NEJM 2005;353:761; Am J Obstet Gynecol 2005;193:1338; Obstet Gynecol 2014;123:676.*

OVARIAN CYSTS

Definitions *(Obstet Gynecol 2011;117:1413; Am Fam Physician 2009;80:815)*
- **Functional ovarian cysts:** Follicular cysts form when an unruptured ovarian follicle fills w/ serous fluid → capsule distention/pain. Corpus luteum cysts, normally present in early Preg; can bleed → distention or active hemorrhage.
- **Benign & neoplastic ovarian cysts** (see also Chap. 22): Dermoid, stromal & germ cell tumors, fibroma, epithelial neoplasm, cystadenoma, endometrioma

Epidemiology and Etiology
- Incidence of ovarian cysts = 5–15%. Lifetime risk 5–10% surgery for adnexal mass
- **Diff dx:** Leiomyomata, TOA, hydrosalpinx, ectopic Preg, paratubal cysts, diverticular abscess, appendiceal abscess, nerve sheath tumors, ureteral diverticulum, pelvic kidney, bladder diverticulum, peritoneal inclusion cysts, malignancy

Clinical Manifestations
- Most are asymptomatic, but may p/w pain, pressure, dyspareunia
- Intermittent pain may indicate ovarian torsion. Acute, sev pain may represent ovarian torsion or cyst rupture. Increased abdominal girth, bloating, wt loss, & early satiety raise concern for malig

Physical Exam & Diagnostic Workup
- **Pelvic exam:** 45% sens & 90% spec. ↓ detection w/ BMI >30
- **Labs:** hCG, CBC, urinalysis, other labs depending on presentation & Hx
- **Imaging:** Ultrasound is the imaging test of choice for evaluating the ovaries; TVUS sens 82–91% & spec 68–81% for distinguishing benign from malignant dz. Classic US appearance of a simple cyst is anechoic, well circumscribed, echolucent w/ postacoustic enhancement.
- See Chap. 22 for w/u for malig, tumor markers, & referral to gyn oncology

Treatment and Medications
- **Observation:** Most simple ovarian cysts spontaneously regress in 6 mo. ↑ adnexal/ ovarian torsion at 6–10 cm mass. 0–1% risk of malig if cyst is unilocular, thin walled, sonolucent, <10 cm in diameter, & has smooth, regular borders.
  Premenopausal women w/ cyst <3 cm do not require f/u
  Premenopausal women w/ cyst 4–10 cm who desire expectant mgmt → rpt US for resolution in 12 w (4–12 w depending on concern)
  Postmenopausal women w/ cysts 4–10 cm & CA-125 <35 U/mL who desire expectant mgmt → serial USs every 4–6 w
- **Surgery:** Provides definitive treatment and pathologic dx. Indicated for hemodynamic instability, cyst >6–10 cm, concern for malig, concern for torsion, or persistent sx
  Laparoscopy: ↓ Operative morbidity, postoperative pain, analgesics, recovery time, & cost
  Laparotomy: Usually for malig (w/ appropriate staging), hemodynamic instability, or failed laparoscopy
  Cystectomy vs. oophorectomy: Consider the pt's age, reproductive desires, menopausal status, & preoperative dx (If a corpus luteum cyst is removed during Preg at <12 WGA → progesterone supplementation)

ADNEXAL TORSION

Definition and Epidemiology *(Am J Obstet Gynecol 1985;152:456)*
- Twisting of adnexal components (most commonly ovary ± fallopian tube) on their ligamentous supports → venous, arterial, & lymphatic obst
- 5th most common gyn emergency; 2.7% of female surgical emergencies

- Females of all ages (fetal/neonat to elderly); however, 70% are of ages 20–39
- Increased risk w/ Preg (20–25% of all cases) & ovarian hyperstimulation

Etiology (Clin Exp Obstet Gynecol 2004;31:34; Am J Obstet Gynecol 1991;164:577)
- 86–95% a/w adnexal mass (48% cysts, 46% neoplasms). ↑ w/ masses 6–10 cm
- Congenitally long ovarian ligaments
- ↑ w/ strenuous exercise, intercourse or sudden ↑ in abdominal pressure
- Right ovarian torsion more common than left (protection from sigmoid colon)

Pathophysiology
- Compromise of vascular pedicles impedes arterial inflow & lymphatic & venous outflow →
  Venous drainage interrupted before arterial due to less compressibility of arterial walls →
  Marked ovarian enlargement can develop w/ continued perfusion & blocked outflow

Clinical Manifestations and Physical Exam (Ann Emerg Med 2001;38:1506)
- **Acute pelvic pain** (83%): Sudden/sharp pain (59%) radiating to back/flank/groin (51%) w/ peritoneal signs (3%)
- **Nausea &/or vomiting** (70%): Colicky or sporadic sx from intermittent torsion
- **Neonates:** Usually in 1st 3 mo of life w/ feeding intolerance, vomiting, abdominal distention, & fussiness/irritability – usually ovarian cysts have already been identified w/ prenatal US (Arch Pediatr Adolesc Med 1998;152:1245).
- Resolution of sx seen after ~24 h due to ischemic death of involved structures. Functionality can be preserved w/ immediate intervention.
- **Bimanual exam:** Adnexal mass (72%), tenderness on affected side
- **Fever** (<2%): May be a marker of necrosis, particularly in the setting of increased WBC

Diagnostic Workup/Studies
- Adnexal torsion is largely a clinical diagnosis
- Dx confirmed at Surg. ~40% correct preop dx (J Reprod Med 2000;45:831)
- **Clinical dx:** (1) Lower abdominal pain, (2) ovarian torsion, & (3) diminished or absent bld flow in the ovarian vessels on color Doppler flow imaging. Rule out ectopic Preg, PID, appendicitis, diverticulitis, nephrolithiasis, & leiomyoma-related sx.
- **Lab studies:** hCG to rule out Preg; CBC, BMP, may see anemia, leukocytosis, or electrolyte abnormalities from vomiting
- **US:** Cystic or solid mass (70%), free fluid in post cul-de-sac (>50%), enlarged heterogeneous appearing ovary (J Ultrasound Med 2001;20:1083). Nml ovary on US does *not* rule out torsion, but abnl is suggestive of torsion.
  Doppler: Controversial; some studies w/ sens & spec of 100% & 97%, others w/ 43% & 92% (Eur J Obstet Gynecol Reprod Biol 2002;104:64); color Doppler flow ↑ dx of torsion when absent but not reliable when flow is present.
  Whirlpool sign: Doppler finding in vascular pedicle (J Ultrasound Med 2009;28:657)
  MRI/CT: Limited value, can detect ovarian edema; diagnostic criteria not well defined or validated, and costly/time consuming. CT potentially useful in excluding alternative diagnoses on differential.

Treatment (NEJM 1989;321:546; Obstet Gynecol Surv 1999;54:601)
- **Swift operative eval:** Preserve ovarian fxn & prevent infxn from necrosis
- **Laparoscopic detorsion** w/ cystectomy is preferred in in premenopausal pts, majority regain full function, even if ischemic appearing intraoperatively. No ↑ risk of clot dislodgement/PE with detorsion. Consider oophoropexy for prevention esp w/ recurrent ovarian torsion.

PELVIC INFLAMMATORY DISEASE (PID)

Definition and Epidemiology (Obstet Gynecol 2010;116:419)
- **PID:** Clinical spectrum of inflamm disorders of the female upper genital tract including endometritis, salpingitis, TOA, & pelvic peritonitis
- >800,000 cases/y in US; true magnitude unk due to difficult dx
- **Risk factors:** Age <25, young age at 1st intercourse, nonbarrier contraception, multiple sexual partners, oral contraception, cervical ectopy, IUD insertion w/i prev 3 w

Etiology and Microbiology (NEJM 1975;293:166; Ann Intern Med 1981;95:685)
- **Neisseria gonorrhoeae:** 1/3 of cases; 15% w/ endocervical gonorrhea develop PID
- **C. trachomatis:** 1/3 of cases; 15% w/ endocervical chlamydia develop PID
- **Other pathogens:** Vaginal flora (eg, anaerobes, Gardnerella vaginalis, Haemophilus influenzae, enteric gram-negative rods, & Streptococcus agalactiae)

Clinical Manifestations
- Lower abdominal pain (90%). Mucopurulent discharge (75%).
- **Long-term sequelae:** Infertility (18%), ectopic Preg, chronic pelvic pain, dyspareunia

Diagnosis of PID	
CDC diagnostic criteria (Dx is imprecise. Maintain low threshold for rx due to long-term sequelae)	1. Pelvic or lower abdominal pain 2. No cause other than PID can be identified 3. One or more minimum criteria are present on physical exam: (a) cervical motion tenderness, (b) uterine tenderness, or (c) adnexal tenderness
Additional criteria (enhance spec)	1. Oral temp. >101°F (>38.3°C) 2. Abn cervical or vaginal mucopurulent discharge 3. Presence of abundant # of WBCs on wet mount 4. Elevated ESR 5. Elevated CRP 6. +GC/CT 7. Lab-proven chlamydia or gonorrhea infxn
Specific criteria (if needed)	Endometrial bx w/ endometritis TVUS or MRI w/ hydrosalpinx or free pelvic fluid Laparoscopic confirmation of pelvic infxn

From CDC. Sexually Transmitted Diseases Treatment Guidelines, 2015. http://www.cdc.gov/std/tg2015/pid.htm

Treatment
- **Indications for hospitalization:** Preg, outpt therapy failure after 72 h, noncompliance, sev illness (eg, N/V, high fever), or TOA
- **IUD:** Do not need to remove IUD, close clinical f/u if remains in place
- Screen for additional STIs. F/u in clinic in 3 d
- Expedited partner therapy (EPT) is indicated to prevent reinfection in all cases of confirmed infection: See state-specific legislation: http://www.cdc.gov/std/ept/legal/default.htm

CDC 2015 treatment guidelines		
Inpt	Cefotetan 2 g IV q12h OR Cefoxitin 2 g IV q6h + Doxycycline 100 mg PO or IV q12h × 14 d	D/c IV abx 24–48 h after clinical improv & afebrile
	Clindamycin 900 mg IV q8h + Gentamicin IV or IM (2 mg/kg) ×1, then 1.5 mg/kg q8h or 3–5 mg/kg QD	
Outpt	Ceftriaxone 250 mg IM* ×1 OR Cefoxitin 2 g IM ×1 & Probenecid 1 g PO ×1 OR 3rd gen cephalosporin (ceftizoxime/cefotaxime) + Doxycycline 100 mg PO q12h × 14 d & ± Metronidazole 500 mg PO q12h × 14 d *If allergic to 3rd gen cephalos, can consider levofloxacin 500 mg PO QD OR ofloxacin 400 mg q12h OR moxifloxacin 400 mg QD + metronidazole 500 mg PO QD ×14 d	

*Note: Oral cephalosporins no longer recommended to treat gonorrhea due to growing resistance (as high as 6%) in some states. CDC. MMWR. 2012;61(31):590.
From CDC Sexually Transmitted Diseases Treatment Guidelines, 2015. http://www.cdc.gov/std/tg2015/pid.htm.

ACUTE UTERINE BLEEDING

Definition and Epidemiology (Fertil Steril 2011;95:2204; Obstet Gynecol 2002;99:1100)
- Abnormal uterine bleeding: Any alteration in the volume or pattern of menstrual blood flow

- **Acute abnormal uterine bleeding:** An episode of bleeding sufficient to require immediate intervention to prevent further blood loss. May or may not occur in the setting of Chronic Abnormal Uterine Bleeding. See Chap. 5 (pp. 5-8 to 5-9), Abnormal Uterine Bleeding.
- Affects 10–30% of women. 12% of gyn visits in ER. Also, see SABs above.
- **Diff dx:** Ruptured ectopic preg, placental abruption, placenta previa, PPH, acute severe menorrhagia, genital trauma, SAB, invasive malignancy, drugs, coagulopathy

Physical Exam
- **Rapidly determine acuity:** General appearance & stability. Tachycardia, hypotension, orthostatic VS.
- Targeted history: LMP, timing, duration, quantity, s/sxs of hypovolemia
- **Speculum exam:** Rule out nonuterine causes (eg, rectal bleeding, genitourinary, vaginal lacerations, cervical lesions), quantify bleeding, cervix dilated? Check for obvious lesions,
- **Bimanual exam:** Evaluate for structural abnormalities, such as a prolapsing fibroid, focal tenderness

Diagnostic Workup/Studies
- Always rule out Preg – qualitative hCG. Labs: CBC, coags including fibrinogen, type, & screen. Imaging: Consider TVUS if clinically indicated

Treatment and Medications
- If unstable: 2 large bore IVs, crystalloid fluid resusc
- Consider transfusion of 2 U packed RBCs if Hgb <7.5
- If anemic, start PO ferrous sulfate at discharge from hospital
- Initiate goal-directed therapy

Medical management of acute uterine bleeding			
Category	**Agent**	**Dose**	**Comments**
Estrogen	Premarin (consider rx for antiemetic)	25 mg IV q4–6h up to 24 h	Avoid in smokers >35 yo, uncontrolled HTN, CAD, Hx VTE, stroke, liver dz
COCs	EE/norethindrone (consider rx for antiemetic)	35 µg/1 mg TID × 1 w, then QD × 3 w	Avoid in smokers >35 yo, uncontrolled HTN, CAD, h/o VTE, stroke, liver dz; Consider antiemetics to minimize side effects
Progestin	Aygestin (norethindrone acetate)	5 mg TID × 1 w, then BID × 3 w	Use w/ caution in pts w/ Hx VTE, stroke or MI, liver dz
	Provera (Medroxyprogesterone)	20 mg TID × 1 w, then BID × 3 w	
Nonhormonal	Tranexamic acid	1.6 g PO TID × 5 d OR 10 mg/kg IV q8h up to 5 d	Avoid in pts w/ active renal disease, thromboembolic dz or intrinsic risk of thrombosis

Data from *Obstet Gynecol* 2006;108:924; J *Obstet Gynecol* 1997;37:228; Am J *Obstet Gynecol* 1982;59:285.

Surgical management of acute uterine bleeding	
Intracavitary tamponade	Foley balloon (30–50 cc); Bakri balloon (not to exceed 500 cc)
D&C; hysteroscopy	Reserve for emergent cases; may help w/ acute episode, subseq menses unchanged
UAE	Reserve for emergent cases; particularly w/ leiomyoma or suspected AVM
Hysterectomy	Reserve for emergent life threatening cases; definitive

Based on the Clinical Guideline for Heavy Menstrual Bleeding, National Institute for Health and Clinical Excellence, Updated March 2018.

TRAUMA IN PREGNANCY

Epidemiology (Int J Gynaecol Obstet 1999;64:87; Obstet Gynecol 2009;114:147)
- Complicates 3–8% of pregnancies; 2/3 from motor vehicle collisions. Leading cause of nonobstetric maternal death during Preg (Am J Obstet Gynecol 2013;209:1).
- Incidence of trauma increases as pregnancy progresses
- Up to 20% of pregnant women are victims of DV. Preg alone is an independent risk factor for DV (Am J Obstet Gynecol 1991;164:1491).
- Outcomes directly related to GA & severity/mechanism of injury
- 40–50% fetal loss rate w/ life-threatening maternal trauma (eg, shock, head injury leading to coma, emergency laparotomy for maternal indications) (Obstet Gynecol Clin North Am 1991;18:371)
- 1–5% fetal loss w/ non–life-threatening injuries, but b/c more common, >50% of fetal losses occur w/ minor trauma
- **Blunt trauma:** Placental abruption (40% sev cases, 3% nonsevere cases), direct fetal injury (<1%), uterine rupture (<1%), mat shock, mat death
- **Penetrating trauma:** Gunshot wounds or stab wounds; fetal prog generally worse than mat prog
- **Pelvic fractures:** Fetal mortality rate 35%; may result in signif retroperitoneal bleeding. Not an absolute contraindication for vaginal delivery.
- **Burns/electrical injury:** Can range from unpleasant sensation to fetal/maternal death. Evaluate for spontaneous abortion, placental abruption, cardiac arrhythmias, fetal burn and intrauterine fetal death

Clinical Manifestations and Physical Exam (Obstet Gynecol 2009;114:147)
- **Placental abruption:** Vaginal bleeding, uterine tenderness, abdominal pain, back pain, fetal distress, high-frequency uterine contractions, uterine hypertonus, decreased fetal movement, or even fetal death
- **Primary survey:** Note that pregnant women can lose a significant amt of bld before manifesting vital sign abnormalities due to their increased intravascular vol; determination of uterine size/gestational age is critical
- **Abd:** Ecchymoses (new & old), seat belt injury, penetrating abdominal injuries, palpate for contractions or tenderness
- **Speculum:** Bleeding, rupture of membranes, vaginal lacerations, pelvic bone fragments

Diagnostic Workup/Studies (Obstet Gynecol 2009;114:147)
- **US:** Fetal cardiac activity, fetal GA & presentation, free peritoneal fluid or mat hemorrhage. Consider FAST to assess for free fluid in perihepatic, perisplenic, pelvic, & pericardial areas
- **Radiologic eval:** Should not be deferred if required for maternal assessment regardless of modality or concern for radiation exposure

Initial Management (ACOG 1998)
- **Maternal:** Main goal is to establish maternal cardiopulmonary stability. Supplemental O_2; 2 large-bore IVs; early IV fluid resusc in ratio 3:1 based on bld loss; left lateral uterine displacement after 20 w (if spinal injury suspected, manual displacement or a wedge under a backboard ok); labs – CBC, type & screen, coags, & hold tube. Kleihauer–Betke & RhoGAM for Rh-negative patients.
- Once mother stabilized, proceed w/ **fetal assessment**
  Viability 23–24 w GA, depending on institution
  <Viable: Document FHR by Doppler or real time US; tocometer if high concern for abruption by Hx or physical exam
  >Viable: 4–6 h continuous fetal monitoring (includes FHR & tocodynamometry). If >6 contractions in an hour, high risk mechanism or severe injury → prolonged monitoring for 24 h. Nonreactive NST → further eval (BPP or prolonged fetal monitoring).
- In setting of maternal **cardiopulmonary arrest**, delivery by emergent C/S (resuscitative hysterotomy) if >4 min has elapsed or nonshockable rhythm. Improves mat resusc by decreasing uterine compression of venous return.

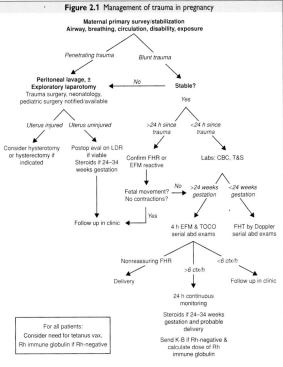

Figure 2.1 Management of trauma in pregnancy

Maternal primary survey/stabilization
Airway, breathing, circulation, disability, exposure

Penetrating trauma — *Blunt trauma*

Peritoneal lavage, ±
Exploratory laparotomy ← *No* — Stable?
Trauma surgery, neonatology,
pediatric surgery notified/available
Yes

Uterus injured — *Uterus uninjured* — *>24 h since trauma* — *<24 h since trauma*

Consider hysterotomy
or hysterectomy if
indicated

Postop eval on LDR
if viable
Steroids if 24–34
weeks gestation

Confirm FHR or
EFM reactive

Labs: CBC, T&S

Fetal movement?
No contractions?

No — *>24 weeks gestation* — *<24 weeks gestation*

Yes

Follow up in clinic

4 h EFM & TOCO
serial abd exams

FHT by Doppler
serial abd exams

Nonreassuring FHR — *>6 ctx/h* — *<6 ctx/h*

Delivery

24 h continuous
monitoring

Steroids if 24–34 weeks
gestation and probable
delivery

Send K-B if Rh-negative &
calculate dose of Rh
immune globulin

Follow up in clinic

For all patients:
Consider need for tetanus vax,
Rh immune globulin if Rh-negative

Data from *Am J Obstet Gynecol* 1990;162:1502; *Am J Obstet Gynecol* 2004;190:1661; *Am J Obstet Gynecol* 2004;190:1461; *Am J Obstet Gynecol* 2013;209:1 UNC SOM OB Algorithms 2004; ATLS Course Manual 2012.

SEXUAL ASSAULT

Epidemiology
- Defined as a wide range of behaviors that involve unwanted sexual contact
- Lifetime prevalence of 18–19% in US women. Varies in other countries.
- All patients seen should be screened for intimate partner violence or sexual abuse.
  Risk factors: Female gender, age <25 y, prior assault, college women, military status,
  institutionalized or developmentally delayed.

Initial Evaluation
- Acute medical needs: Assessment and treatment of physical injuries, pregnancy
  assessment and emergency contraception, STI/HIV prophylaxis as indicated,
  psychological assessment and support
- Forensic evaluation: Should be completed as soon as possible and up to 96 h
  following an assault. A Sexual Assault Nurse Examiner (SANE) or other qualified
  provider is recommended whenever possible as it will facilitate prosecution of
  perpetrator if trained professional completes evidentiary collection
- Screening for STIs is not required if prophylaxis is given.
- HIV PEP (postexposure prophylaxis) should be discussed with all sexual assault
  survivors with exposure of vagina, rectum, mouth or any mucous membrane to
  blood, semen, or vaginal/rectal secretions AND who present for care within 72 h of
  exposure

Treatment

- Empiric STI therapy should include 250 mg ceftriaxone IM, 1 g azithromycin PO, and 2 g metronidazole PO to treat for gonorrhea, chlamydia, and trichomonas. Flagyl should be avoided for 24 h following alcohol use
- HIV PEP should include Tenofovir 300 mg + Emtricitabine 200 mg po daily (Truvada) × 1 dose plus Raltegravir 400 mg po bid × 1 dose followed by 28-d course. (Provide 4-d supply to patient) and follow up with a provider experienced with managing PEP (eg PCP, ID specialist)
- Tetanus/diphtheria/pertussis (Tdap) 0.5 mL, IM injection × 1 dose if there was penetration of a foreign object by the perpetrator and the last tetanus toxoid booster is unknown or more than 10 y ago
- HPV vaccination is recommended for female survivors aged 9–26
- Mandatory reporting is required for vulnerable populations, minors, elderly, and if weapons were involved (eg gun/knife)
- All survivors should be offered law enforcement and local advocacy/support resources

PREOPERATIVE EVALUATION

- Preop eval is needed for all pts before all procedures, w/ complete **medical/surgical Hx & periop risk assessment**

American Society of Anesthesiologists' (ASA) physical status classification system	
ASA-I	Normal, healthy
ASA-II	Mild systemic disease
ASA-III	Severe systemic disease
ASA-IV	Severe systemic disease that is constant threat to life
ASA-V	Moribund pt not expected to survive

Based on American Society of Anesthesiologists Physical Status Classification System. https://www.asahq.org/resources/clinical-information/asa-physical-status-classification-system. Updated October 15, 2014. Accessed May 6, 2018.

- **Review of current meds & allergies:** Discuss holding NSAIDs, antiplatelet agents, anticoagulant supplements (eg, fish oil); consider bridging long-acting anticoagulants to shorter-acting meds (eg, warfarin to heparin). Review herbal medications.
- Review relevant prior **operative reports**
- Most healthy women w/ no identifiable RFs require no further **testing or consultation**
- Consider ECG in women >50 y. Depending on invasiveness & urgency of the procedure, periop eval by PCP ± anesthesia or other specialist is recommended. Additional testing based on identified risk.
- **Informed consent,** w/ balanced discussion of:
  Risks, benefits, alternatives (incl nontreatment & poss additional procedures), & complications
  Healthcare team & their roles including trainees & supportive teams
  Permission to take photos or videos for documentation or teaching
  Possibility of bld or bld product use
- Identify existing advance directive & healthcare proxy/power of attorney. Consider creating an advance directive if one does not already exist.
- Discuss expected postop course (hospital stay, recovery, change in fxn, etc.)
- Identify special needs for OR (eg, interpreter services, special equipment)

PERIOPERATIVE OPTIMIZATION

- New or uncontrolled medical conditions → consultation/optimization w/ appropriate specialist + primary care input
- **Pulm dz:**
  RFs = older age, current smoking, obesity, obstructive sleep apnea, low serum albumin (<3 g/dL) & BUN >30 mg/dL, higher ASA scores are a/w higher risk for postop pulm complications (Ann Surg 2000;232:242; Ann Intern Med 2006;144(8):581)
  Well-controlled asthma not a/w pulm postop complications
  Advise smoking cessation >8 w before elective Surg (if <8 w, no dec in pulm complications)
  Preop PFTs/CXR/ABG if unexplained dyspnea or respiratory sx; consider if COPD of unclear severity
  Postoperatively: Deep breathing exercise, incentive spirometry, early ambulation, upright position, & adequate pain control are effective in preventing postop pulm complications
- **Cardiovascular dz:**
  Most abdominal/pelvic surg is considered intermediate risk regarding cardiac morbidity
  Selected procedures may be of low risk (eg, D&C) or high risk (major debulking surg)
  Nonemergent surg should be delayed or canceled if pt has (1) unstable coronary syns, (2) decompensated heart failure, (3) signif arrhythmia, or (4) sev valvular dz

Revised Cardiac Risk Index (RCRI)

Presence of any of the following puts pt at higher risk for major periop cardiac morbidity:

1. High-risk surgery – eg open abd procedure
2. Ischemic heart dz (h/o MI, angina, use of nitrate therapy, positive stress test, Q wave on ECG)
3. Heart failure
4. Cerebrovascular dz
5. Insulin-requiring diabetes (DM)
6. Renal insufficiency w/ Cr >2 mg/dL

From Circulation 1999;100(10):1043.

Testing by RCRI factors		
Low risk	No RCRI factors	No testing Consider ECG for >50 yo
Intermediate risk (1–2 RCRI factors)	Good functional status, no h/o angina or PVD	No testing
	Poor/indeterminate functional status, h/o angina or PVD	Consider noninvasive stress test: If negative: No further intervention indicated If positive: Discuss cardiac cath & revascularization w/ cardiology No beta blockade in pts w/ RCRI scores ≤2. Dec risk of MI, but inc risk of nonfatal stroke (*Lancet* 2008;372:1962)
High risk (3+ RCRI factors)	Primary sx are related to failure, arrhythmia, or valve	Medical optimization
	Pts w/ >2 cardiac RFs who ALSO have extensive stress-induced ischemia on noninvasive testing	Revascularization (*Eur Heart J* 2009;30:2769)

Beta-blockers & statins should be initiated only if indication for long-term use. Start rx weeks prior to surgery. Target HR 60–80 bpm.
Data from 2009 ACCF/AHA; *J Am Coll Cardiol* 2009;54:2102.

- **Hematology:**
    Anemia: Investigate if unexplained; correct anemia w/ iron suppl if there is time before Surg or transfuse if Hgb <7 g/dL, symptomatic, or for high anticipated bld loss. Consider menstrual suppression if menorrhagia is a contributing factor. Consider erythropoiesis-stimulating agents or iron suppl if transfusion refused.
    Thrombocytopenia: Goal is generally Plt >50k for open surgery; consider hematology consult if concern that plt function is impaired, regardless of plt count
    Pt on anticoagulation:
    Determine risk of stopping anticoagulation perioperatively. Stop warfarin 5 d prior to procedure, goal INR <1.5. Consider heparin bridge if at high risk of thrombosis.
    Avoid elective Surg w/i 1 mo of acute venous or arterial thrombosis
    Consider IVC filter if recent thrombosis & high risk of bleeding w/ anticoag
- **Endocrine:**
    DM (*Diabetes Care* 2017;40(Suppl 1):S120–7):
    Periop gluc problems: (1) Surgical stress, (2) preop NPO, (3) decreased PO postop, (4) type of anesthesia (general > neuraxial)
    Critical considerations: (1) Type 1, type 2, or gestational diabetes; (2) timing, length, & invasiveness of procedure; (3) current med regimen
    Poor periop gluc control a/w (1) increased risk of infxn, (2) poor wound healing, (3) neuro/cardiac sequelae of hypoglycemia
    Postop goals: Maintain euglycemia (80–180 mg/dL) & prevent ketoacidosis & nonketotic hyperosmolar state
    In critically ill patients, liberal glucose management is recommended as intensive control increases mortality (*NEJM* 2009;360:1283–97)
    Metformin contraindicated w/ renal insufficiency or poor tissue perfusion; thiazolidinediones may exacerb edema or precipitate CHF

Perioperative DM management		
PREOP	Type 2 DM, diet controlled	Fingerstick gluc pre- & postop
	Type 2 DM, PO med controlled	Hold meds morning of Surg
	Insulin-controlled DM (type 1 or type 2)	Continue basal/long-acting insulin, consider dose-reduction. Reduce preop intermediate-acting PM dose 50% (eg, NPH). D5 in IVF. Consider IV insulin for long, complex cases.

POSTOP	Noninsulin-requiring DM	SS inferior to basal/bolus regimen, use only if needed & NPO (Diabetes Care 2011;34:256) Resume home meds if no contraindication, as soon as taking PO well
	Insulin-requiring DM	**Continue basal insulin to prevent ketogenesis in Type 1 DM.** Consider dose reduction. NPO: Home basal insulin + regular SS q6h, D5 in IVF W/ PO diet: Home basal/bolus regimen OR 0.5 U/kg divided btw basal & preprandial short-acting (AC) insulin at meals

- **Thyroid dz:**
  Hyperthyroid: If new dx or uncontrolled, postpone Surg, consult endocrinology, continue chronic meds
  Hypothyroid: Consider endocrinology consult if new dx. Otherwise, continue meds. No need for IV/IM thyroid replacement if NPO for <7 d.
  For hypo- & hyperparathyroidism: Follow for calcium imbalance
- **Adrenal insufficiency:**
  Higher risk for periop adrenal crisis (HoTN, HoNa)
  Minimal suppression of the HPA axis in pts w/ <5 mg prednisone (or equiv) daily; <10 mg prednisone every other day; or ANY dose of glucocorticoid for <3 w. These pts do not require supplemental steroids (N Engl J Med 2003;348:727).
  Replacement based on type of Surg (JAMA 2002;287:236):
    Minor Surg (outpt Surg or minimally invasive): → Consider 25 mg hydrocortisone on day of procedure vs. usual dose → pt returns to regular dose
    Obstetric cases & all gynecologic Surg: → 50 mg hydrocortisone just before procedure → followed by 25 mg IV q8 h for 24 h → back to maint dose
    For sev surgical stress (consider in extensive debulking surgeries): 100–150 mg hydrocortisone on day of procedure → rapid taper to usual dose over 1–2 d
    Critically ill pts (septic shock): → 50–100 mg hydrocortisone IV q6–8h until shock is resolved → taper slowly (monit sodium)
- **Elderly pts:**
  Polypharmacy: Carefully review meds & potential interactions
  Avoid bowel prep due to higher risk of dehyd/electrolyte derangement
  Higher risk for the following postoperatively (Am J Obstet Gynecol 2003;189:1584)
    Delirium & mental status changes; ensure sleep hygiene, orientation to environment & careful dosing of psychoactive meds. W/u medical causes of delirium.
    Pulm edema w/ heart failure due to fluid overload; monit fluid balance
    MI & stroke
    Slow return of bowel fxn
- **Obese pts:**
  Higher risk for the following postoperatively (Am J Obstet Gynecol 2010;202:306):
    SSI; plan incision & dose Abx appropriately based on weight
    Pulm complications/OSA; encourage early ambulation & pulm toilet; CO_2 monitor
    Thromboembolic complication; consider weight-based anticoagulant dosing

---

PREOPERATIVE MEASURES

- **Preg test:** For ALL women of reproductive age
- **Bld type & Ab screen:** Consider T&S/cross-match for intermediate/high-risk surgeries
- **Antibiotic ppx for prevention of SSI:** See below
- **Antibiotic ppx for prevention of SBE:**
  Not routinely recommended for GU procedures. Used in women w/ highest potential risk (prosthetic valve, prev infective endocarditis, pt w/ unrepaired cyanotic heart dz, repaired heart dz w/i 6 mo of procedure, or repaired dz w/ residual defects near prosthetic material, cardiac xplant w/ signif valvular dysfxn) (JACC 2014;63:22).
- **Venous thromboembolism ppx:** See below
- **Bowel prep:** Mechanical bowel preparation (eg, magnesium citrate, polyethylene glycol) not recommended for most gynecologic or colorectal Surg (Am J Obstet Gynecol 2011;205:309).
- **Fasting:** Preop NPO reduces aspiration risk. Milk or fried/fatty food: 8 h; light meal not including milk: 6 h; clear fluids: 2 h (Anesthesiology 2011;114:495). See ERAS
- **Skin prep:** SSI, see below
- **Positioning & incision selection:** Neurologically neutral positioning & padding of all jnts. Avoid prolonged lithotomy (>4 h) or steep Trendelenburg. Select incision for appropriate exposure & to avoid excessive retraction.

Common nerve injury in gynecologic surgery

Nerve and deficit	Presentation	Mechanism and risk factors	Prevention
Femoral nerve (L2–4)	• Weakened hip flexion, leg extension • Difficulty climbing stairs • Sensory changes to anterior and medial leg	Femoral nerve pierces the psoas muscle to pass under the inguinal ligament. Common neuropathy after gynecologic Surg, esp abd hysterectomy (~11%). RFs: Use of self-retaining retractors, wide Pfannenstiel or Maylard incision, BMI <20 kg/m², operation >4 h, poorly developed rectus muscle, Narrow pelvis, hip hyperflexion, or external rotation in lithotomy	Avoid compression of the psoas muscle by self-retaining retractors Avoid extending Pfannenstiel incision beyond the lateral border of rectus abdominis Avoid hyperflexion & external rotation of the hip within footrests
Ilioinguinal (T12–L1) & iliohypogastric (T12–L1) nerves	• Mons and lateral labia pain	Ilioinguinal nerve & iliohypogastric nerve course ~3 cm inferomedially to ASIS. Risk of entrapment or transection at the lateral edge of Pfannenstiel incision. Prone to neuroma formation after injury.	If need to extend incision lateral to rectus muscle body, curve fascial incision cephalad Avoid lateral placement of sutures when closing fascia (<1.5 cm lateral to the edge)
Genitofemoral (L1–2) & lateral–femoral cutaneous (L2–3) nerves	• Labial and thigh pain/paresthesia	These nerves lie on the belly of the psoas muscle lateral to the external iliac artery Excessive lateral retraction Transection during pelvic LND	Avoid lateral excessive lateral traction on the psoas muscle Isolate the nerves during pelvic LN
Obturator nerve (L2–4)	• Weakness in hip adduction	Obturator nerve lies post to the psoas muscle & passes through the obturator canal Direct injury during pelvic LND Passing of the TOT sling	Careful dissection in the obturator fossa to identify nerve Careful passing of the trocar during TOT sling
Pudendal nerve (S2–4)	• Perineal pain	Exits pelvis through the greater sciatic foramen & enters again through the lesser foramen around the ischial spine (lateral 1/3 of the sacrospinous ligament) Injury during sacrospinous fixation Entrapment w/ vaginal mesh	Avoid the lateral 1/3 of sacrospinous ligament during fixation
Peroneal nerve (L4–5, S1–2)	• Weakness in dorsiflexion of the foot. Foot drop	Wraps around the lateral fibular head Excessive compression on the lateral aspect of the knee	Good padding of the lateral aspect of the knee during Surg in candycane stirrups Early ambulation after Surg

Nerve and deficit	Presentation	Mechanism and risk factors	Prevention
Brachial plexus (C5–8, T1)	• Weakness/ tingling in arm or hand • Severe: Erb's or Klumpke's palsy	Wraps around the lateral aspect of the neck & upper shoulder Hyperabduction of the shoulder Compression w/ shoulder braces Prolonged steep Trendelenburg Morbid obesity	Avoid use of shoulder braces (preferred antislip devices include egg-crate foam or vacuum-beanbag mattresses) Avoid abduction of shoulder >90°

Adapted from *Obstet Gynecol* 2004;103:374.

ENHANCED RECOVERY AFTER SURGERY (ERAS)

Definition (*Obstet Gynecol* 2016;128(3):457–66): Protocols to improve patient education and expectations for surgery, decrease fasting periods, optimize multimodal pain control, decrease opioid use and infections, and encourage rapid return to normal diet and activity

Preoperative:
• Multimodal pain control with opioid sparing agents (acetaminophen, gabapentin, NSAIDs/celecoxib) and regional anesthesia if indicated
• Allow clear liquids until 2 h preop ± carb rich drink 2 h prior to surgery
• Appropriate preop antibiotics and VTE prophylaxis

Intraoperative:
• Restrictive or goal-directed fluid admin, regulate body temperature
• Minimize long-acting opioids and paralytics, use local anesthetics around incision
• Anesthetic agents chosen to decrease postop nausea

Postoperative:
• Early feeding, mobilization, and discharge based on criteria
• Scheduled bowel regimen and minimization of opioids to dec risk of ileus

POSTOPERATIVE ILEUS

Definition
• Obstipation w/ intolerance to oral intake due to postop intestinal dysmotility
• Physiologic ileus can last 1–3 d postop depending on procedure. Longer duration may be abnl.

Etiology
• Inhibition of nml motility by postop inflammation, inhibition of spinal reflexes, opioids, vasoactive intestinal polypeptide, substance P, nitric oxide

Clinical Manifestations
• Inability to tolerate PO diet, abdominal pain, distention, tympany on exam, decreased bowel sounds, delayed/decreased flatus

Diagnosis
• Generally clinical, though should rule out small bowel obst (see below)
• Intestinal dilation w/o evid of transition point on CT, XR imaging of abd

Treatment
• Bowel rest, NG tube if necessary. Vol resusc, repletion of electrolytes PRN, ambulation.
• Reduce/eliminate aggravating med (eg, opioids, ondansetron)
• Serial abdominal exams until abdominal decomp
• Advance diet with return of flatus/bowel sounds

Prevention
• Epidural + local anesthesia instead of systemic or epidural opioids (*Cochrane Database Syst Rev* 2000;(4):CD001893)
• Alvimopan (selective opioid receptor antag) postop. FDA has limited access to med as may inc risk MI in some pts.
• Gum chewing immediately postop (*World J Surg* 2009;33(12):2557)
• **Scheduled** bowel regimen after hysterectomy (*Am J Obstet Gynecol* 2007;196(4):311.e1)
• Minimize manipulation of bowel intraop
• Routine NG tube placement is NOT indicated (*Cochrane Database Syst Rev* 2007;18(3):CD004929)

POSTOPERATIVE FEVER

Definitions
- Nml temperature ranges from 36.5–37.5°C
- Fever is as temperature >38.0°C or >100.4°F

Workup
- **Hx:** Review records for preop infxn, intraop complications, xfusion, med list, allergies, urinary catheter, vascular access sites. Ask about diarrhea, skin rash, new onset pain, sputum production, preop illness
- **Physical exam:** Temperature (& trends), pulse, bld pres, & respiratory rate. Examine skin (rash), lungs (decreased breath sounds, rales, brhonchi), heart (new murmurs), abd (tenderness or peritoneal signs), operative site (including vaginal cuff, poss), catheter/drain/IV sites, & lower extremities (DVT).
- **Lab:** Based on Hx, exam, & diff. May include urinalysis & culture, CBC w/ diff, bld culture ×2 before Abx (1 set from indwelling central line if present), sputum culture (generally low yield), wound culture (low yield), CXR, lower limb US for DVT, & PE protocol CT scan. W/u for other medical conditions as appropriate.

	Common causes of postoperative fever by onset/timing
Immediate (1st 24 h)	• Primarily noninfectious: Med effect, xfusion rxn, preop infxn, malig hyperthermia (rarely); atelectasis
Acute (1–7 d)	• Infectious: Nosocomial infxn (most commonly PNA; in critical pts may be VAP, aspiration PNA) & UTI, *Clostridium difficile*; community-acquired infxns; SSI & vascular catheter–related infxns, endometritis • Noninfectious: Surgical site inflammation – common after uterine Surg (eg, myomectomy); med rxn; thromboembolism (DVT, PE); CVA; pancreatitis; EtOH withdrawal; rheumatologic conditions; hyperthyroidism
Subacute (1–4 w)	• Primarily infectious: SSI (including abscess); central venous catheter–related; UTI; sinusitis (esp if NG tube in place); PNA; *C. difficile*. • Noninfectious: Med rxns; thromboembolism (DVT, PE). Consider septic pelvic thrombophlebitis
Delayed (>1 mo)	• Primarily infectious: Community-acquired or nosocomial infxns; SBE; *C. difficile*; FB infxn; osteomyelitis; unrelated infxns

- **Mgmt:** Based on etiology, if Abx indicated, target to suspected sources; tailor to culture results when available

SURGICAL SITE INFECTIONS (SSI)

Definition, Microbiology, and Epidemiology
- SSI introduced at time of Surg by endogenous flora
- **Common organisms:** *Staphylococcus aureus*, enterococcus, *Escherichia coli*, coagulase-negative staphylococci. Gyn SSI more likely caused by gram-negative bacilli, enterococci, group B streptococcus, anaerobes
- **RFs:** Obesity, existing infxn, diabetes, smoking, corticosteroids, immunosuppression, poor nutrition, long duration of Surg, active bact vaginosis or cervicitis

Surgical wound classification		
Case type	**Examples**	**Infection rate**
I. Clean: Uninfected, closed primarily, does not enter bowel/vagina	Dx Lsc, BSO, lsc tubal, hsc	2.6%
II. Clean Contaminated: GU or GI tracts entered, controlled	Hysterectomy, vag surg	3.6%
III/IV. Contaminated/dirty: Gross spillage from GI tract, open wounds, infected	Debridement of infected wound, perforated bowel	10.5%

Data from *Arch Surg* 1999;134:1041.

Prophylaxis *(Infect Control Hosp Epidemiol 2008;29:S51)*
- **Skin prep:** Chlorhexidine-alcohol superior to povidone-iodine in lsc and open surgery, but benefit not seen in Cesarean delivery (*NEJM* 2010;362:18; *J Matern Fetal Neonatal Med* 2017;30:1–8)

- Sterile technique, avoid razor hair removal (trim/clip instead), avoid hyperglycemia
- **Antimicrobial ppx** (Am J Obstet Gynecol 2008;199:301.e1, Obstet Gynecol 2009;113:1180; Am J Heal Pharm 2013;70(3):195–283):
  Administer <30 min before Surg (Ann Surg 2009;250:10), or at time of anesthesia
  Redosing required for longer surg (ie Cefazolin redosed q4h, Clinda q6h) and for EBL >1500 (excl Vanc/Gent for either indication)
  Obese patients require increased dose based on weight

Antibiotic prophylaxis for ob-gyn surgery	
Procedure	**Antibiotic options (single dose)**
Hysterectomy & urogynecologic procedures	Cefazolin* 2 g IV (3 g IV if wt >120 kg) Clindamycin 600 mg IV + gentamicin 1.5 mg/kg IV or ciprofloxacin 400 mg IV or aztreonam 1 g IV Metronidazole 500 mg IV + gentamicin 1.5 mg/kg IV or ciprofloxacin 400 mg IV
Surgical abortion	Doxycycline 100 mg PO/IV 1 h before, 200 mg PO after proc Metronidazole 500 mg PO BID ×5 d
HSG with PID or hydrosalpinx	Doxycycline 100 mg PO BID ×5 d
Cesarean	A 1st-generation cephalosporin (eg, cefazolin 1 g IV) + Azithromycin 500 mg IV if during labor or 4 h after ROM Clindamycin 600 mg IV + gentamicin 5 mg/kg IV
No ppx for laparoscopic or open clean cases, hysteroscopy, IUD placement, endometrial bx, or urodynamics	

*Acceptable alternatives: Cefotetan, cefoxitin, cefuroxime, or ampicillin–sulbactam.
Data from Obstet Gynecol 2009;113:1180; and Obstet Gynecol 2011;117:1472; and N Engl J Med 2016; 375: 1231–41.

Clinical Manifestations (Infect Control Hosp Epidemiol 1992;13:606; Infect Dis Obstet Gynecol 2003;11:65)
- **Incision cellulitis:** Warmth, swelling, erythema, pain w/o fluid collection
- **Superficial incisional SSI** (skin, subcutaneous tissue): Positive cx, purulent drainage
- **Deep incisional SSI** (fascia, muscle): Spont dehiscence, abscess
- **Vaginal cuff cellulitis:** Edema, induration, & erythema of the vaginal cuff
- **Organ space:** Pelvic abscess, vaginal cuff abscess
- **Nec fasciitis:** Erythema, swelling/edema, pain disproportionate to exam (followed by analgesia), crepitus, gray-colored discharge

Workup
- CBC (leukocytosis ± bandemia), gram stain + cx of incision or abscess fluid, bld culture
- **US:** Inexpensive, sens 56–93%, spec 86–98% for pelvic abscess (J Emerg Med 2011;40:170)
- **CT:** Abscess characterized by multilocular (89%), thick enhancing wall (95%) (J Reprod Med 2005;50(3):203)

Treatment
- **Incisional cellulitis:** Antimicrobial rx w/ gram-positive coverage, consider MRSA coverage
- **For more complicated SSI:** Parenteral antibiotic therapy ± abscess drainage
- **Nec fasciitis:** Emergent wide local debridement + beta-lactam/beta-lactamase inhib + **clindamycin** (antitoxin effect) + MRSA coverage

PERIOPERATIVE DVT/PE

Definition and Epidemiology
- **VTE:** DVT & PE are common periop complications. See Chap. 16 for full details on diagnosis and management.
- **Rates of postsurgical VTE w/o rx:** 29% for benign Gyn & 38% for Gyn oncology (Br Med J 1978;1:272; Aust N Z J Obstet Gynecol 1983;23:216)

VTE perioperative risk stratification

Points	Risk factors (point given for each factor present)
1	Age 41–60; minor Surg; BMI >25; swollen legs; varicose veins; Preg/postpartum; h/o recurrent SAB; OCPs/HRT; sepsis <1 mo; lung dz (ie, PNA) <1 mo; abn pulm fxn; acute MI; CHF <1 mo; h/o IBD; bed rest
2	Age 61–74; open Surg >45 min; laparoscopy >45 min; cancer; >72 h bed rest; central venous access
3	Age ≥75; h/o VTE; family h/o VTE; FVL; G20210A; lupus anticoagulant; anticardiolipin Ab; ↑ homocysteine; HIT; thrombophilia
5	Stroke <1 mo; hip/pelvis/leg fx, spinal cord injury

Thromboprophylaxis

Points (Risk VTE)	Average-risk bleed	High-risk bleed
0 (<0.5%)	Early ambulation	
1–2 (~1.5%)	Mechanical ppx, preferably intermittent pneumatic compression (IPC)	
3–4 (~3%)	LDUH or LMWH or IPC	Mechanical ppx, prefer IPC
≥5 (~6%)	LDUH or LMHW + ES or IPC	IPC alone until bleeding risk gone, then add LDUH or LMWH
Cancer	LDUH or LMWH + ES or IPC + LMWH for 4 w after discharge	IPC alone until bleeding risk gone, then add LDUH or LMWH
Contraindication to heparin	Fondaparinux or low-dose ASA (160 mg) + IPC	IPC until bleeding risk gone → add ASA or fondaparinux
Dosing	LDUH = UFH 5000 U SQ q12h or q8h LMWH = Enoxaparin 40 mg SQ daily; dalteparin 5000 U SQ daily Fondaparinux = 2.5 mg SQ daily	

From *Chest* 2012;141:e227S.

Perioperative prevention of DVT and PE

Risk	Pt & Surg	Suggested ppx
Low	Minor (<30 min) in pts <40 w/ no additional RF	• Early mobilization
Mod	Surg <30 min w/ RF, Surg >30 min in pts of age 40–60 w/o RF; major Surg in pts <40 w/o RF	• UFH 5000 units q12h or • LMWH: Dalteparin 2500 units QD or enoxaparin 40 mg QD or • IPCDs or stockings
High	Surg <30 min in pts of age >60 w/ RF; major Surg in pts >40 w/ RF	• UFH 5000 units q8h or • LMWH: Dalteparin 5000 units QD or enoxaparin 40 mg QD &/or • IPCD or stockings
Highest	Major Surg in pts >60 yo w/ cancer or prior VTE or hypercoagulable state	• UFH 5000 units q8h or • LMWH: Dalteparin 5000 units QD or enoxaparin 40 mg QD & • IPCDs or stockings & • LMWH for 4 w after ca surgery

Data from *Obstet Gynecol* 2007;110:429; *Chest* 2008;133: 381S; *Obstet Gynecol* 2012;119:155. *N Engl J Med* 2002; 346:975–80.

SEPSIS

Definitions (*JAMA* 2016;315(8):801–10)
- **Sepsis** is a life-threatening organ dysfunction caused by a dysregulated host response to infection causing an amplified, uncontrolled, self-sustaining intravascular inflamm response. Hospital mortality rate >10%.
- **Septic shock:** Subset of sepsis in which circulatory, cellular, and metabolic abnormalities are associated with a greater risk of mortality than sepsis alone. Signs incl elevated lactate >2 mmol/L and vasopressors to maintain MAP>65. Hospital mortality rate >40%.

Epidemiology (*NEJM* 2003;348:16)
- **Incid:** 240 cases per 100,000, 9% annual ↑ from 1979–2000

Clinical Manifestations

- Bact wall components (endotoxin, LPS) & products (exotoxins) activate host defense, w/ initial excessive resp of inflamm mediators (TNFα & IL-1) activating coagulation cascade & formation of microvascular thrombi, impaired tissue oxygenation & tissue damage
- HoTN, initial ↑ cardiac output, but eventual systolic & diastolic failure
- **AMS (encephalopathy):** Agitation, confusion, obtundation
- **Acute renal failure due to hypoperfusion/hypoxia:** Oliguria, electrolyte abnormalities
- Pulm edema → V/Q mismatch → hypoxemia → ARDS

Workup

- Obtain appropriate cx (eg, bld, urine, wound, catheter tip)
- CXR to assess acute lung injury & ARDS (diffuse bilateral infiltrates)
- Imaging studies (eg, CT) to confirm infxn site & sample poss source
- **SOFA Score:** Score based on PaO_2/FiO_2, plt count, bilirubin, MAP, GCS, Cr, and UOP used to stratify risk. With score ≥2 abnormal = overall mortality risk 10%
- **qSOFA (quick SOFA):** RR >22, altered mentation, SBP ≤100 mmHg used to triage
- Monitor lactate level as marker for tissue perfusion

Management (Crit Care Med 2008:36:296; JAMA 2017;317(8):847–8)

- **IV Abx:** Obtain cultures and give broad spectrum abx directed at most likely pathogens **w/i 1 h of sepsis recognition.** De-escalate based on cultures or clinical improvement.
- **Adequate access:** CVC if septic shock or shock and large-bore IVs
- **Aggressive fluid resusc:** Administer 30 mL/kg of IV crystalloid within 3 h. Additional fluid given based on frequent reassessment necessary to prevent organ dysfxn
  Goals: CVP ≥8 mmHg (12 mmHg if ventilated), MAP ≥65 mmHg, UOP ≥0.5 mL/kg/h
- **Vasopressors:** If BP not responsive to IV fluid (septic shock), use vasopressors to maintain MAP >65 mmHg (norepinephrine 1st line, alternatives include phenylephrine, epinephrine, vasopressin, dopamine)
- **Early respiratory stabilization:** Pulse oximetry, mechanical vent as needed for resp fail
- **Corticosteroids:** Consider hydrocortisone IV (for adrenal insufficiency) only if BPs unresponsive to fluid resusc

PERIOPERATIVE OLIGURIA

Definitions

- Generally, urine output of <30 mL/h for 2–3 h or <500 mL/d
- According to RIFLE criteria for AKI (Crit Care 2007;11:R31)
  Risk: UOP <0.5 mL/kg/h for 6–12 h; or Cr ↑ >50%
  Injury: UOP <0.5 mL/kg/h for >12 h; or Cr ↑ >100%
  Failure: UOP <0.3 mL/kg/h for >24 h or anuria for 12 h; or Cr ↑ >200%, or Cr >4 w/ acute rise >0.5 mg/dL. Or institution of renal repl tx (RRT).
  Loss: RRT >4 w
  End stage: RRT >3 mo

Common causes of perioperative oliguria	
Prerenal	• *True vol depletion* – gastrointestinal dz (vomiting, diarrhea), renal losses (diuretics, osmotic diuresis, DI), skin or respiratory losses (insensible losses, sweat, burns), & 3rd space sequestration (edema, crush injury, skeletal fracture, preeclampsia) • *HoTN (septic or cardiac shock); heart failure, cirrhosis, & nephrotic syn; selective renal ischemia*
Renal	• *Tubular* – acute tubular necrosis from prolonged intraop HoTN, nephrotoxic agents (NSAIDs, ACE inhibs, or angiotensin II blockers) • *Glomerular* – vasculitides • *Interstitial* – acute interstitial nephritis from nephrotoxic agents
Postrenal	• *Ureteral injury/blockade* • *Reflex spasm of the voluntary sphincter* b/c of pain or anxiety; use of meds such as antichol & narcotics; detrusor atony as a result of Surg manipulation or anesthesia • *Mechanical obst* from an expanding hematoma or fluid collection or an occluded Foley catheter

Workup

- History & physical exam
- Check the Foley catheter & irrigate as a 1st step
- Bladder scan if concern for obstruction
- Check meds & hold/replace NSAIDs & other nephrotoxic meds. Renally dosing other meds as needed.
- Review operative report & anesthesia record: Intraop I/Os & BP
- **Labs**
  Urinalysis w/ review of sediment for muddy brown, granular casts (ATN) & eos (interstitial nephritis)
  CBC, Cr, serum electrolytes & urinary electrolytes/Cr
  Serum BUN/Cr: Ratio >20 generally sugg prerenal dz
  FE_{Na}: <1% in prerenal dz & >2% in intrinsic renal dz. **Note FE_{Na} not useful if not oliguric.** Consider FE_{urea} if recent use of diuretics.
- **Renal US:** Postrenal obst, chronic renal dz

Management

- **Prerenal:** Fluid challenge of 500–1000 cc of crystalloid. Cr resolves in 1–3 d.
- **Renal:** Identification & tx of underlying cause
- **Postrenal:**
  Acute retention: Transurethral or suprapubic catheter
  Ureteric/bladder injuries: Consider percutaneous nephrostomy tube, trial of stenting (antegrade or retrograde) followed by delayed repair. Drain if urinoma.

BOWEL OBSTRUCTION

Definition

- Failure of intestinal contents to progress normally through either the small bowel or the large bowel. Small bowel obstruction (SBO) more common following surgery

SMALL BOWEL OBSTRUCTION

Etiology

- Adhesive dz, malig, hernia most likely. Up to 42% of women w/ ovarian cancer (*Ann Oncol* 1993;4(1):15)
- Stricture (eg, postradiation or from inflamm bowel dz), intussusception, volvulus, gallstone ileus less likely

Clinical Manifestations

- Nausea, vomiting (± feculent), crampy abdominal pain, inability to tolerate PO
- Extent of abdominal distention may depend on site of obst
- Generally no flatus or BM
- May be clinically hypovolemic
- Peritoneal signs may indicate ischemic bowel or perforation (suspect if Lactate elev)

Diagnosis

- Radiographic evid (XR, CT) of "transition point" w/ prox dilation & distal decomp of bowel
- CT more sensitive for signs of bowel ischemia/strangulation, perforation, closed loop (prox + distal) obst, hernia, additional intra-abdominal pathology
- Consider lactate for biochemical evid of ischemia a/w SBO

Treatment

- Conservative measures include bowel rest, NG tube to low suction for decomp, vol resusc & electrolyte repletion PRN. TPN if indicated.
- Consider therapeutic use of Gastrografin (water-soluble contrast) (*World J Surg* 2008;32(10):2293)
- Consider medical rx w/ octreotide for pts w/ advanced ovarian cancer to dec secretions (*Cochrane Database Syst Rev* 2010;7:CD007792)
- Exploratory laparotomy if concern for strangulation/ischemia, perforation, early SBO after laparoscopic Surg w/ concern for port site hernia, failure of conservative mgmt
- NGT may be removed if (1) passage of flatus or stool, (2) residual vol of gastric contents <100 cc after 4 h clamped

- In gynecologic Surg, most often related to malig
- Unlikely to respond to conservative mgmt
- Rx options include colostomy creation or endoscopic stent, depending on location & clinical situation

COMPLICATIONS OF LAPAROSCOPY

Incidence (*Clin Obstet Gynecol 2002;45(2):469*)
- Occur in 0.2–10.3% of all laparoscopic cases
- Over 50% during entry into the abdominal cavity

Complications of Laparoscopy (*J Minimally Invasive Gynecol 2006;13:352*)
- **Extraperitoneal insufflation:** Misplacement of Veress needle → peritoneal tenting
    Signs: Immediate insufflation pres >15 mmHg, abdominal wall fullness/crepitus, hypercarbia, respiratory compromise if large volume
    Prevention: Monitor insufflation pres, reposition Veress needle as appropriate
    Mgmt: Alert anesthesiologist; should resolve w/ supportive measures
- **Nerve injury:** See table with summary above
- **Vascular injury:** During entry (Veress needle or port placement) or intraop
    Common vessels injured: Inferior/superior epigastric artery, aorta, vena cava, iliac vessels
    Signs: Port site bleeding, intra-abdominal bleeding on entry, tachy, HoTN
    Prevention: Correct needle placement & direct visualization of trocar sites
    Open (Hasson) entry may minimize vascular injury risk (*Aust N Z J Obstet Gynecol 2002;42:246*)
    Manage: Small vessels → tamponade or ligation, large vessels → laparotomy, abdominal packing, & fluids if vascular surgeon not immediately available (*J Min Invas Gynecol 2010;17:692*)
- **GI injury:** Incid 13/1000, occurs during entry or intraop (*Br J Surg 2004;91:1253*)
    Signs: If not recognized intraop, worsening abdominal pain, tachy, fever
    Intraperitoneal air not reliable sign, occurs in 38.5% laparoscopy (*J Reprod Med 1976;16(3):119*)
    RFs: Prior Surg, intra-abdominal pathology (endometriosis, PID, adhesions)
    Prevention: NG or OG tube decomp of stomach. In high-risk pts consider nonumbilical entry point (**Palmer's point** – 3 cm below costal margin in left midclavicular line).
    Mgmt: Surgical repair (oversewing or resxn), Abx
- **Postop bleeding:**
    Signs: Tachy, >expected Hgb/Hct drop, HoTN, oliguria, AMS, increased abdominal pain, bleeding from incision or vagina
        Abd compartment syn: Bleeding/ascites → ↑ intra-abdominal pres → ↓ lung compliance, ↓ venous return, ↓ kidney fxn → hypoxemia, oliguria, renal failure.
        Requires surgical decompression.
    Manage: Fluid resusc, monit UOP, NPO, trend CBC, poss surgical exploration
- **Urinary tract injury:** Incid in TLH 0.3% for ureter and 0.8% for bladder injury (*Obstet Gynecol 2015;126(6):1161–9*)
    Only 18% of ureter injuries and 79% of bladder injuries recognized during operation
    Signs: Abdominal/flank pain, peritonitis, hematuria, oliguria/anuria, fever, leakage of urine from incision or vagina, elevated Cr. Consider CT ± urogram, sampling free fluid in abd if suspect urinoma; send fluid for BUN/Cr. If close to serum, then transudate (ascites); if higher, suspect urine leak.
    Prevention: Decomp of bladder w/ Foley, direct visualization during trocar placement, dissection, & visualization of ureters (peristalsis), routine stenting not recommended
    Mgmt: Closure for large cystotomy, postop bladder decomp, ureter repair
- **Trocar site hernia:** Incid 0.5% (*Br J Surg 2012;99:315*)
    Signs: Bulging, small-bowel obst
    RFs: Pyramidal trocars, size ≥12-mm trocars (3% vs. <1%) (*AJOG 1993;168:1493*)
    Prevention: Close port defects ≥10 mm (*Arch Surg 2004;139:1246*)
    Mgmt: Surgical vs. expectant depending on severity
- **Shoulder pain:** Common, referred pain from diaphragmatic irritation (CO_2, bld, fluid)
- **Air/CO_2 embolization** (rare) → circulatory collapse (sudden ↓ O_2 sat, ↓ BP, dysrhythmia).
    Place pt in left lateral decubitus w/ head tilted down, cardiopulmonary support.

COMPLICATIONS OF HYSTEROSCOPY

Complications and Management (Obstet Gynecol 2011;117:1486; Best Pract Res Clin Obstet Gynaecol 2009;23:619)

- **Fluid overload (5–6%):** Excessive intrauterine Absorp of distending media
  - **Main types of distending fluid:**
    - **Nonelectrolyte** (glycine, mannitol, sorbitol): For use w/ monopolar instruments
    - **Electrolyte** (saline, LR): For diagnostic hysteroscopy & w/ bipolar or mechanical instruments
  - **Pathophysiology:** Vol overload: CHF, pulm edema; metabolic imbalance: HypoNa, ↓ serum osm, ↑ ammonemia, hyperglycemia, acidosis; ↓serum Na by ~10 mmol/L/ 1000 mL glycine deficit (Lancet 1994;344:1187); neurologic sequelae: Cerebral edema, nausea, visual changes, sz, coma. Prevent overload: Select distending media that minimizes risk of overload (isotonic, electrolyte-containing solutions), monit fluid deficit frequently, use automated fluid monitoring system.
  - **Manage:** D/c infusion (J Am Assoc Gynecol Laparosc 2000;7:167)
    - Nonelectrolyte solution >1000–1500 mL
    - Electrolyte solution >2500 mL
    - OR serum Na <130 mmol/L
    - If severely hyponatremic → hypertonic saline. Loop diuretics are not indicated unless there is clinical evid for vol overload; may exacerb electrolyte abnormalities. Low threshold for xfer to ICU for intensive monitoring.
- **Hemorrhage (2–3%):** From resection, cervical lacerations, tenaculum site, perforation
  - **Manage:** Electrocautery, inject vasopressin, suturing tenaculum site, balloon tamponade (AJOG 1983;147:869), laparoscopic suturing, hysterectomy, UAE
- **Uterine perforation (1–1.5%)** → Retroperitoneal hematoma, bowel/bladder injury, or signs of acute bld loss
  - **Prevention:** Careful sounding, adequate cervical dilation, operate resectoscope toward user (not toward uterine wall)
  - **Mgmt:**
    - Hemodynamically stable → monit for bleeding, pain, infxn
    - Large perforation, unstable or perforation w/ electrocautery → surgical exploration w/ repair
- **Infxn:** Rare complication of hysteroscopy (<1%)
- **Air/CO$_2$ embolization** (gas rarely used as distention medium) → circulatory collapse (sudden ↓ O$_2$ sat, ↓ BP, dysrhythmia). Place pt in left lateral decubitus w/ head tilted down, cardiopulmonary support.

GYNECOLOGIC ANESTHESIA

- Many office procedures & selected transvaginal operations may be performed under local anesthesia, w/ or w/o sedation/analgesia
  Examples: Loop electrosurgical excision procedures, 1st trimester dilation & curettage, hysteroscopy, endometrial ablation
  Technique: Paracervical block or intracervical block
- Local anesthetic toxicity
  Usually occurs following inadvertent intravascular injection
  CNS effects typically precede CV effects
    CNS: Prodrome of excitation, metallic taste, tinnitus, perioral numbness, confusion, agitation → brief seizures → coma
    CV: Initial HTN, tachy; followed by hypotension, arrhythmias, cardiac arrest
    Exception: Bupivacaine-cardiotoxicity predominates; prolonged Na⁺ channel blockage
    Treatment: Call for help, stop injection, assess airway, BNZs for seizure suppression, manage arrhythmia per ACLS guidelines, lipid emulsion (1.5 mg/kg IV)
  Epinephrine may be added to ↓ overall uptake, allow increased local effect, and to indicate vascular uptake; most effective when using shorter-acting agent; less useful for long-acting/lipophilic anesthetic (eg, bupivacaine)
  Contraindications to use of epi. Absolute: Untreated/severe HTN, CHF, arrhythmias, CAD, hyperthyroidism, ergot alkaloid use. Relative: Tricyclic antidepressant use, MAOI use, beta blockade, cocaine use, asthma, diabetes, phenothiazine use.

Common local anesthetics					
Mech: Block voltage-gated Na channels, prevent nerve depolarization/action potential					
High lipid solubility = favors entry into cells = more potent, longer duration					
Anesthetic	**Type**	**Lipid solubility**	**Concentration**	**Max dose w/o epi**	**Max dose w/ epi**
Lidocaine	Amide	++	1% 10 mg/mL	4 mg/kg	7 mg/kg
Bupivacaine	Amide	++++	0.25% 2.5 mg/mL	2.5 mg/kg	3 mg/kg
2-chloropro-caine	Ester	+	2% 20 mg/mL	11 mg/kg	14 mg/kg
Ropivacaine	Amide	+++	1% 10 mg/mL	3 mg/kg	N/A
Mepivacaine	Amide	++	1% 10 mg/mL	4 mg/kg	7 mg/kg

From Hawkins JL, Bucklin BA. Obstetrical anesthesia. In: Gabbe SG, ed. *Normal and Problem Pregnancies.* 6th ed. Philadelphia, PA: Saunders, Elsevier; 2012:362.

- Laparoscopic & prolonged gynecologic surgeries usually performed under GA
  Laparoscopic procedures require paralysis
  Standard anesthesia techniques & precautions apply
  Many laparoscopic procedures require prolonged Trendelenburg positioning for access to pelvis – ventilation may be difficult
- Physiologic change w/ pneumoperitoneum:
  Cardiac: ↑ SVR, MAP; rarely profound bradycardia from vagal response to peritoneal stretch
  Pulmonary: ↓ Lung volume, functional residual capacity & compliance; ↑ PCO_2
- Transvaginal procedures & many abdominal procedures may be performed under neuraxial anesthesia/sedation, particularly if pt not candidate for GA due to medical comorbidities (precludes use of paralytics)
  Examples: Dilation & curettage/evacuation, operative hysteroscopy, vaginal hysterectomy or abdominal hysterectomy in pts not candidates for GA
- Both minilaparotomies & some laparoscopic procedures (most commonly sterilization) may be performed under sedation w/ local anesthesia only

PARENTERAL ANALGESIA IN OBSTETRICS

- All nonneuraxial methods provide only partial relief of labor pain
  May help laboring women cope w/ pain
  Useful in cases of absolute contraindication, pt refusal of neuraxial anesthesia, or situation where neonatal concerns wouldn't limit opioid use (eg, IUFD)
- Opioids act as opioid receptor agonists: Mu, kappa, delta

- Transfer across the placenta is rapid & signif; fetal effects may limit use
  - Drug transfer affected by prot binding capacity, size, ionization
  - In general, all local anesthetics & opioids transfuse freely across the placenta
  - Fetal acidosis results in ion trapping → fetal drug accum
- Side effects of systemic opioids
  - **Maternal:** Sedation, respiratory depression, N/V, pruritus, somnolence
  - **Fetal:** Decreased fetal HR variability during labor; pseudosinusoidal HR pattern, respiratory depression at birth. Use short-acting opioid w/ no active metabolites, if poss. Monit fetus continuously during administration of systemic opioids. Avoid administration shortly before deliv.
- **Sedatives:** Do not provide analgesia; typical use is for sleep/relaxation in latent labor

Parenteral opioids			
Opioid	Onset	Neonat half-life	Disadvantages
Fentanyl Remifentanil – also fast acting	1 min IV	5.3 h	Short duration; may not control labor pain well; remifentanil is potent resp depressant
Morphine	5 min IV 40 min IM		Longer duration can result in prolonged sedation
Nalbuphine	2–3 min IV 15 min IM	4.1 h	Partial agonist/antag: Antag properties limit side effects but may also limit relief
Meperidine Historic 1st choice in labor, *no longer widely used*	5 min IV 30–45 min IM	13–22 h, 63 h for active metabolite	Both drug & active metabolite normeperidine cross placenta: Prolonged fetal sedation; risk of lethal serotonin syn in pts taking MAOIs limits use

From *Obstet Gynecol* 2002;100:177.

Methods of administration of parenteral opioids		
Method	Advantages	Disadvantages
Intermittent administration Administered by nurse Short- to medium-acting opioids	No pump req, no staff needed to set up apparatus RN oversight of fetal status for administrations	Less autonomy, more delays, more total opioid used
Patient-controlled analgesia (PCA) Programmed to deliver on-demand boluses Short-acting (eg, Fentanyl)	Pt autonomy, less delay in administration; results in less total opioid used	Requires pump apparatus, anesthesia staff for setup Risk of self-administration during period of fetal distress

NEURAXIAL ANESTHESIA IN OBSTETRICS

Mechanisms of pain in labor			
Pain	Mech	Pathways	Neuraxial anesthesia
Visceral	a. Contractions → ischemia → release of pain mediators b. Stretch/distention	Sensory nerves follow symp nerve pathways, enter spinal cord at T10–L1	Block T10–L1 afferents
Somatic	Fetal head distends vagina/ perineum Pain from lacerations	Pudendal nerves enter spinal cord at S2–4	Extend block to S4 Or: Pudendal block, local infiltration

- Most effective method for labor pain; standard for C/S, postpartum tubal ligations, urgent postpartum procedures whenever poss
- Indications for neuraxial anesthesia in labor: Maternal request; anticipation of operative vaginal deliv or shoulder dystocia; breech extraction; twin delivery; high risk of C/S; risk of hemorrhage; difficult intubation; maternal condition where signif

pain or stress would create medical risk (eg, sev respiratory or cardiac dz); maternal condition which could worsen & potentially limit use of neuraxial anesthesia later in labor course (eg, worsening thrombocytopenia or coagulopathy)
- Contraindications to neuraxial anesthesia in labor:
    Absolute: Maternal refusal, uncooperative pt; soft tissue infxn of site; uncorrected hypovolemia; uncorrected therapeutic anticoagulation; Lovenox w/i 24 h; certain spinal conditions (eg, ependymoma); severe thrombocytopenia (<50 K), increased intracranial pressure
    Relative: Certain spinal conditions (eg, discectomy, rod fusion); mod thrombocytopenia (<75 K); LP shunt, some neurologic dzs (ie, multiple sclerosis); fixed cardiac output conditions (ie, AS)
- Types of neuraxial blocks: Spinal, epidural, & CSE
    Spinal: Anesthetic/opioid delivered directly into spinal fluid w/ needle through dural puncture
    Benefits: Rapid onset (2 min); 1/20 epidural dose used so less risk tox; sacral blockade
    Disadvantages: Limited duration (1–1.5 h)
    Epidural:
    Anesthetic/opioid delivered into epidural space via continuous infusion through catheter
    Benefits: Ability to continuously infuse & adjust dosage as needed; pt controlled
    Disadvantages: Slower onset (20 min), larger doses used (20× spinal doses)
    Combined spinal–epidural (CSE):
    Meds delivered directly into spinal fluid, then catheter placed in epidural space
    Benefit: Combination of rapid onset & ability to continuously infuse
    Disadvantages: More technically challenging than epidural or spinal alone; increased risk of PDPH compared to spinal alone

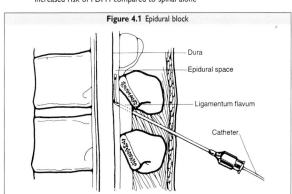

Figure 4.1 Epidural block

Dura
Epidural space
Ligamentum flavum
Catheter

Modified from Mulroy MF. *Regional Anesthesia: An Illustrated Procedural Guide.* Philadelphia: PA, Lippincott Williams & Wilkins; 2002:104.

Complications of neuraxial anesthesia			
Complication	Incidence	Mechanism	Treatment
Hypotension	28–31% Prehydration = slightly less	Local anesthetic causes sympathetic blockade	Prehydration decreases to some degree Epi/phenylephrine Avoid aortocaval compression
Fever >100.4°F (incid above that in women w/ parenteral opioids)	15–33% nullips 1–5% multiples	Not well understood; noninfectious, inflamm resp, altered thermoregulation	Conservative measures Acetaminophen does not reliably treat epidural fever

Complication	Incidence	Mechanism	Treatment
Fetal HR decelerations (transient)	8%	Maternal hypotension, decreased uterine perfusion, ↓ maternal epinephrine release	Maternal positioning, hydration, oxygen, epi
Postdural puncture headache ("spinal HA")	1.5–3% spinal 1–2% epidural overall; 60–80% w/ epidural "wet tap"	Leakage of CSF through dural puncture	Supine position, oral analgesics, caffeine Blood patch very effective; indicated if HA lasts 24+ h
Pruritus (w/ opioid in spinals/ epidurals)	1.3–26% epidural 41–85% spinal	Periph morphine agonist effects	Nalbuphine 2.5–5 mg IV; naloxone 40 μg IV
Inadq blockade	9–15% epidural		

Rare complications: Epidural hematoma, abscess, total spinal blockade (high spinal; caused by intrathecal injection of local anesthetic), local anesthetic tox

From *Obstet Gynecol* 2002;100:177.

- Combination of local anesthetic & opioid typical. The local anesthetic provides the best anesthetic effect, but also causes motor blockade & potential tox (0.02% after epidural) (*Int J Obstet Anesth* 2004;14:37; *Am J Obstet Gynecol* 2001;185:128). The opioid has a synergistic effect w/ the local anesthetic, allowing for lower dose (20–30% less local anesthetic) & has no intrinsic motor blockade.

Neuraxial anesthetics		
Local anesthetic	Advantages	Disadvantages
Bupivacaine (most common choice) Ropivacaine (very similar to bupivacaine)	Good motor/sensory differentiation Long duration Good safety, no tachyphylaxis (acute ↓ in resp to drug after its administration)	Cardiotoxicity, prolonged Na$^+$ channel block Slower onset: 20 min
Lidocaine	Rapid onset: Used for test dose, rapid bolus for perineal repairs, instrumental deliv	Poor sensory–motor differentiation More tachyphylaxis
Chloroprocaine	Very rapid onset: Used for test dose, rapid bolus for perineal repairs, instrumental deliv	Poor sensory–motor differentiation Very short duration

Neuraxial anesthetics		
Opioid	Advantages	Disadvantages
Fentanyl (most common choice) Sufentanil: Similar SE profile, more potent	Less side effects than morphine More rapid onset	Pruritus (occurs w/ all opioids)
Morphine		Pruritus, N/V Slower onset
Hydromorphone	Superior analgesia to fentanyl in some studies; similar crossing of bld–brain barrier as fentanyl but longer half-life	Similar SE profile to morphine limits use

Effect of neuraxial anesthesia on labor course and outcome	
1st stage of labor	No significant effect on the duration of the first stage of labor
2nd stage of labor	Avg ~14 min longer likely due to decreased sensation/urge to push
Labor augmentation	Increased rates of labor augmentation (RR 1.19)
Operative vaginal deliveries	Slightly increased rates of operative vaginal deliveries (RR 1.38)
C/S rate	No ↑ cesarean delivery rate overall; small increased risk for cesarean for fetal distress (RR 1.43)
Reference:	*Cochrane Database Syst Rev* 2005;4:CD000331.

LOCAL ANESTHETICS IN OBSTETRICS

- Indications for local anesthetics:
  - Skin infiltration for episiotomies/assisted deliveries (nonemergent settings), perineal laceration repair (w/ or w/o other analgesia)
  - **Nerve blocks:** Pudendal, paracervical (close proximity to large vessels → higher potential for tox)
  - Placement of spinal & epidural anesthesia
- In an emergent setting where access to general anesthesia will be delayed, local anesthetics may be administered in large amts to perform C/S, followed by general anesthesia when available

Figure 4.2 Neuraxial and Regional Anesthesia placement

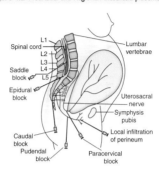

Adapted from Cheek TG, Gutsche BB, Gaiser RR: The pain of childbirth and its effect on the mother and fetus. In Chestnut DH, ed. *Obstetric Anesthesia: Principles and Practice.* 2nd ed. St Louis, MO: Mosby; 1999:323.

Figure 4.3 Pudendal and cervical anesthetic blocks

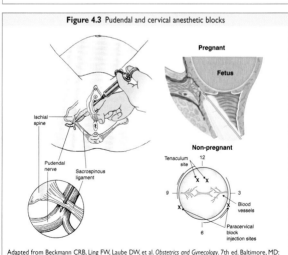

Adapted from Beckmann CRB, Ling FW, Laube DW, et al. *Obstetrics and Gynecology.* 7th ed. Baltimore, MD: Lippincott Williams & Wilkins; 2013 and Vidaeff AC. Pudendal and paracervical block. Eckler K, ed. UpToDate. Waltham, MA: UpToDate Inc. http://www.uptodate.com (Accessed on June 12, 2018) and Jain S, Inamdar DB, Majumdar A, Jain DK. Effectiveness of paracervical block for pain relief in women undergoing hysterosalpingography. *J Hum Reprod Sci.* 2016;9(4):230.

NONPHARMACOLOGIC ANALGESIA IN OBSTETRICS

- **Advantages:** Empowering, few side effects, may improve overall satisfaction w/ labor experience
- **Disadvantages:** Incomplete relief; pts may perceive eventual pharm rx as failure
- **Evid:** Poor study quality; heterogeneity in techniques used and outcomes measured

Nonpharmacologic analgesia methods	
Method	**Effect**
Labor support	Decreased analgesic, shorter labor; more likely to have vaginal delivery; greater satisfaction. Should be continuous, one-to-one nursing (*Cochrane Database Syst Rev 2011;2:C003766*)
Breathing	Lack of evid for pain control, but may be calming
Touch, massage	Massage & casual touch ↓ anxiety, perception of pain (*J Nurse Midwifery 1986;31:270*)
Music	Improves satisfaction, decreases distress, may ↓ need for analgesia (*Pain Manag Nurs 2003;4:54*)

Nonpharmacologic analgesia methods	
Method	**Effect**
Water immersion	Decreased use of neuraxial anesthesia; ~30 min shorter first stage. (*Cochrane 2009;2:CD000111*). No increased maternal/neonatal infection, even w/ ROM. ACOG: Water birth "experimental" and should only be done w/ informed consent in clinical trials.
Hypnosis	Women using self-hypnosis may have significantly decreased use of epidural anesthesia; better satisfaction. Very limited evid; not all women can successfully use hypnosis (*BR J Anaesth 2004;93:505*)
Acupuncture	Does not provide adequate analgesia. No standard; few trials
TENS	Not effective pain relief during labor when compared to placebo
Sterile water injections	Rationale of counter-irritation: Irritate nerves in dermatome of pain. May be useful for back pain a/w labor; however, no change in labor outcomes or use rescue analgesia. Disadvantage of acute somatic pain during injection (*Cochrane Database Syst Review 2012*)

GENERAL ANESTHESIA IN OBSTETRICS

- Rarely indicated for vaginal deliv except for emergent, unanticipated procedures (eg, breech extraction, internal version, shoulder dystocia)
- In US, 10% of C/S are performed under general anesthesia (*Anesthesiology 2005;103:645*)
  Emergent ("crash") C/Ss are the most common setting for general anesthesia
  Other situations include nonemergent C/S in a pt w/ absolute contraindications to neuraxial anesthesia
    Advantages: Rapid, complete anesthesia; ability to administer 100% oxygen
    Disadvantages: Risk of difficult intubation; risk of aspiration; risk of infant respiratory depression; anesthetics cause uterine atony, leading to more bld loss; pregnant women have low tolerance for apnea during intubation
- **Other uses:**
    Uterine inversion: Obstetric emergency where body of uterus inverts following deliv resulting in massive hemorrhage
    Nitric oxide or halogenated anesthetics relax uterus & facilitate replacement. Nitroglycerine may be given IV/sublingually if delay in general anesthesia is anticipated.
    Can be considered in cases of retained placenta due to Bandl's ring or head entrapment for breech extraction; must balance w/ risk of uterine atony

POSTOPERATIVE PAIN MANAGEMENT

- Post C/S pain include visceral (uterus) & somatic pain (abdominal wall)
- Multimodal medication regimens:
- **Goals:** (1) Adequate pain control (2) ↓↓ opioids to ↓ assoc side effects such as ileus, sedation, & effects on infant via secretion of active compounds into breast milk
  Oral pain meds – preferred mgmt once pt is tolerating PO; scheduled dosing of nonopioids may be beneficial to reduce opioid exposure
  Opioids – carry above side effects
  NSAIDs – very effective for visceral pain from uterine involution
  Acetaminophen – good maternal/neonatal safety profile
  Breast-feeding: Opioids, acetaminophen, & NSAIDs considered generally compatible w/ breast-feeding
  Exception: Meperidine – prolonged infant sedation by active metabolite normeperidine

Postoperative pain management after cesarean section		
Method	**Advantages**	**Disadvantages**
Epidural/spinal: Single dose long-acting opioid Morphine, morphine XR Fentanyl Sufentanil Hydromorphone	Better pain relief than PCA, less systemic side effects Long acting Can remove catheter after dose	Pruritus N/V Respiratory depression potential – need extended monitoring
PCEA	Same pain relief as above Decreased side effects Pt control → less total drug used	Pruritus N/V Catheter must remain in place
Epidural/spinal: Addition of local anesthetic	↓ Dose of opioid side effects	More motor blockade
Patient-controlled IV analgesia: PCA	Superior to IM opioid; less total drug used	Sedation – less w/ demand-only dosing
Wound infiltration Single injection or catheter left in wound	Decreased systemic effects Decreased total dose of analgesic used Decreased opioid use postpartum	No effect unless catheter left in wound for continued infiltration
Transversus abdominis plane block T6–L1 nerve root block w/ local anesthetic	Improves pain control in women who do not receive intrathecal morphine; less side effects (Can J Anesth 2012;59:766)	Requires postop procedure

- **Postpartum bilateral tubal ligation:**
  Avoid long-acting intrathecal/epidural opioid/local anesthetic if goal is discharge soon after procedure. Infiltration of skin, fallopian tubes w/ local anesthetic shown to ↓ total analgesic use, ↑ time to analgesic use postoperatively. Sufentanil, bupivacaine, lidocaine all effective.
- **Postdischarge pain control:**
  Acetaminophen + NSAIDs typically adequate following vaginal delivery; opioids commonly prescribed after cesarean delivery but amount of opiate taken is usually less than what is prescribed

INHALATIONAL ANALGESIA IN OBSTETRICS

- **Nitrous oxide:** Most common inhalational agent used; use in US limited (~1%) but more common in UK & Canada; patient self-administers N_2O in anticipation of contractions; mechanism of action poorly understood – possibly by release of endogenous opioids
  Benefits: High satisfaction, rapid elimination; no evidence of neonatal risks due to rapid metabolism (half-life <3 min)
  Side effects: N/V (common), paresthesias, dizziness, somnolence

Definition *(Obstet Gynecol 2006;107:1195)*
- Vulvovaginal sx such as itching, burning, irritation, & abn discharge. BV (most common), vulvovaginal candidiasis, & trichomoniasis.
- **Nml vaginal flora:** ↑ Estrogen → ↑ vaginal epithelial glycogen → ↑ glucose source → ↑ lactobacilli → ↑ lactic acid → ↓ vaginal pH @ 3.8–4.5 *(NEJM 2006;355:1244)*

Pathophysiology and Risk Factors

Pathophysiology & risk factors			
Type of vaginitis	**Pathogenesis**	**Risk factors**	**Sequelae**
Bacterial vaginosis (BV)	2° shift in vaginal flora from lacto-bacilli to mixed flora (ie *Gard-nerella vaginalis*)	>1 partner, change in partners (last 30 d), same-sex partner, douching	↑ risk of STIs, ↑ complications after surg, PTD, PPROM, SGA (unclear benefit to treat asx in pregnancy)
Candidiasis	Mostly 2° *Candida albicans*. Rarely by nonalbicans species (*glabrata*).	Preg, luteal phase, nulliparity, spermi-cides, ↓ age, broad-spectrum abx use, immunosup-pressed	Adverse preg out-comes (PPROM, PTD, SGA)
Trichomonas	Common vaginal parasite	New partner, sex ≥2×/w, 3+ partners/mo, presence of other STI	Adverse preg out-comes (PTD, PPROM)

Data from *NEJM* 2006;355:1244; *MMWR* 2010;59:NO.RR-12.

Clinical Manifestations *(NEJM 2006;355:1244; JAMA 2004;291:1368; Obstet Gynecol 2006;107(5):1195)*
- **BV:** Copious, thin, whitish-gray, fishy smelling discharge. Less likely pruritus.
- **Candidiasis:** Thick, white, curdy ("cottage cheese") discharge. + Pruritus, dysuria, vaginal erythema. Dx should not be made based on H&P alone.
- **Trichomonas:** Copious yellow to greenish, frothy discharge. Often foul odor. ± Pruritus, postcoital bleeding, dysuria, postcoital bleeding. ± Vaginal or cervical erythema ("strawberry cervix").
- **DIV:** Abnormal yellow or green discharge, burning, dyspareunia. Rare form of vaginitis, generally found in peri/postmenopausal patients. Diagnosis of exclusion.

Diagnostic Studies *(NEJM 2006;355:1244)*
- **BV:** Nugent score = gold std, Gram stain w/ scored bacteria & clue cells. Amsel criteria = common, simple diagnostic criteria

Amsel clinical criteria for BV requires presence of 3 out of 4 clinical findings	
1. Vaginal pH >4.5	Touch swab to midportion of vaginal sidewall, then to pH paper. Cervical mucus, semen, or blood can alter pH
2. Thin, gray watery discharge	Visualize/assess on speculum exam
3. >20% clue cells on wet mount	Clue cells = epithelial cells w/ borders obscured by bacteria
4. "Amine" odor test	Add 10% KOH on slide → + if distinctive (fishy) odor

Data from *Am J Med* 1983;74:14; *Obstet Gynecol* 2006;107:1195.

- **Candidiasis:** Presence of hyphae or spores on KOH or saline wet mount OR yeast cx (useful if pt c/o sx but negative wet mount or if recurrent infections).
- **Trichomonas:** Presence of mobile trichomonads on wet mount; ↑ PMNCs often present.
- **Result on Pap:** Candidiasis, BV, or Trichomonas on Pap is NOT confirmatory and requires additional testing. If patient asx for BV or Candidiasis, do not need to test/treat.

Treatment of vulvovaginitis	
BV	[b]Metronidazole 500 mg PO BID × 7 d[d] OR gel 0.75% 1 applicator PV QD × 5 d OR Clindamycin cream 2% 5 g, 1 applicator PV QHS × 7 d OR Clindamycin 300 mg PO BID × 7 d[d] OR 100 mg ovules PV QD × 3 d OR (alternative regimen) [b]Tinidazole 2 g PO QD × 2 d OR 1 g PO QD × 5 d (alternative regimen)
Candida	**Rx PO** Fluconazole 150 mg PO × 1 dose
	OTC PV Butoconazole 2% cream 5 g PV × 3 d Clotrimazole 1% cream 5 g PV × 7 d or 2% cream 5 g PV × 3 d[d] Miconazole 2% cream 5 g PV × 7 d[d], or 4% cream 5 g PV × 3 d, or 100 mg vaginal suppository-1 tab PV × 7 d, OR 200 mg vaginal suppository-1 tab PV × 3 d, OR 1200 mg vaginal suppository1 tab PV QD × 1 d OR Tioconazole 6.5% ointment 5 g PV × 1 application
	Rx PV Butoconazole 2% cream, 5 g PV × 1 OR Nystatin 100,000-U vaginal tab, 1 tab QD × 14 d OR Terconazole 0.4% cream 5 g PV × 7 d, or 0.8% cream 5 g PV × 3 d OR 80 mg vaginal suppository-1 tab PV × 3 d
	Recurrent (4+/y) 7–14 d of topical azole therapy AND Fluconazole 100 mg, 150 mg, or 200 mg PO q72h × 3 doses → weekly × 6 mo
	Severe infxn 7–14 d of topical azole OR Fluconazole 150 mg PO q72h × 2 doses
	Nonalbicans) 7–14 d of topical or oral azole therapy If recurs – Boric acid 600 mg PV × 14 d
Trich	[b]Metronidazole 2 g PO × 1 dose[d] or 500 mg PO BID × 7 d (alternative regimen) OR [b]Tinidazole 2 g PO × 1 dose Treat sex partners. EPT (expedited partner tx) not routinely recommended
DIV	Clindamycin 2% cream PV QD × 14 d (ACOG Obstet Gynecol 2015)

[a]Safe/preferred in Preg
[b]Avoid ETOH use during treatment
From MMWR Recomm Rep 2015;64.

BARTHOLIN GLAND CYST AND ABSCESS

Definition (J Obstet Gynaecol 2007;27:241)
- Bartholin glands secrete mucous for vaginal lubrication. Located at ~4 and 8-o'clock on labia minora bilaterally, behind hymenal ring. Not palpable unless pathologic. Usually women b/w 20–30 yo.

Etiology and Pathophysiology
- Blockage of gland outflow → accumulation of mucous → Bartholin duct cyst
- Infection of a Bartholin cyst → Bartholin duct abscess. Polymicrobial. Most common bacteria are anaerobic & facultative aerobes.
- Bartholin cyst & abscess uncommon >40 yo. Consider biopsies of cyst wall to r/o cancer.

Clinical Manifestations and Physical Exam
- Small cysts are asx. Larger may c/o vaginal pressure or dyspareunia. Typically unilateral, round, & tense.
- Abscess = severe pain, difficulty walking, sitting, engaging in sex. May be tender w/ erythema/induration, fluctuance, purulent drainage.
- **DDx:** Epidermal inclusion cysts, mucous cyst of vestibule, cyst of canal of Nuck, Skene duct cyst (J Obstet Gynaecol 2007;27:241)

Treatment (See also Appendix of Common Procedures)
- Small, asx cyst requires No rx. OTC analgesics, warm compresses, & sitz baths may provide sx relief and aid in drainage in some cases.
- Abscess may drain spontaneously. Immediate pain relief will occur w/ drainage.

- Surgical mgmt reserved for recurrences, abscesses, or large symptomatic cyst.
    - (1) **I&D:** Relief but incision can reseal → reaccumulation of fluid. High recurrence rates after I&D. Word catheter (or pediatric Foley) allows continued drainage & tract epithelialization. Leave catheter 4–6 w but often drains fall out before that time.
    - (2) **Marsupialization:** Create new drainage site. Incise roof of cyst → sew edges of cyst wall to skin edges. Requires anesthesia, time, & placement of sutures. Lower recurrence after marsupialization.
    - (3) **Bartholin gland excision:** Reserved for repeated recurrences. ↑ Risk of bleeding. Not performed if active infxn.
- Antibiotics
- Antibiotics should be empirically provided after surgical management of abscess. Cx rarely changes mgmt (*Am Fam Physician 2003;68:135*).
    Obtain culture if concern for MRSA or in high risk patients (immunocompromised, pregnant)
    Use broad spectrum abx

UTERINE FIBROIDS

Definition
- Benign smooth muscle tumors, originating from myometrial tissue (leiomyoma)
- Uterine fibroids can be classified based on their anatomical location

Type	Location
0	Pedunculated submucosal
I	<50% intramural
II	>50% intramural
III	Contacts endometrium
IV	Intramural
V	Subserosal >50% intramural
VI	Subserosal <50% intramural
VII	Pedunculated subserosal
VIII	Other

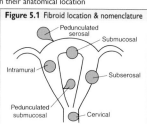

Figure 5.1 Fibroid location & nomenclature

Epidemiology (*Obstet Gynecol Clin N Am 2011;38:703*)
- By 50 yo, fibroids are found in ~70% of Caucasians & >80% of African Americans. Indication for 30–40% of hysterectomies.
- Risks: >40 yo, African American, FHx, nulliparity, obesity

Pathology
- **Gross:** Pearly, round, well circumscribed. Size & location vary. Relatively avascular but surrounded by rich vasculature system.
- **Histology:** Smooth muscle cells aggregated in bundles
- **Leiomyoma types:** Hyaline (65%), myxomatous (15%), calcific (10%, mainly older women), cystic (4%, hyalinized areas) → liquefaction, fatty (rare), carneous (red) necrosis (esp *pregnant* pts, acute d/t outgrowing blood supply → acute muscle infarction → severe pain & local peritoneal irritation)
- Leiomyomas do not transform into leiomyosarcoma. Likely a de novo neoplasm.

Pathophysiology
- Fibroids are estrogen- & progesterone-sensitive tumors. Fibroids create ↑ estrogen environment → ↑ growth & size maint. ↑ Estrogen conditions (obesity, early menarche, PCOS, pregnancy) → ↑ fibroid risk.

Clinical Manifestations
- Mostly asx. Sx depend on size, location, & number. In general, the larger the fibroid, the larger the chance of sx.
- Abnormal uterine bleeding (AUB) = most common symptom; can result in anemia
- **Other sx:** Pelvic pain, pressure, urinary frequency, dyspareunia, incontinence, constipation, infertility and for large tumors, hydronephrosis or DVT (compression of ureters, IVC)
- Evid sugg that myomas are the primary cause of infertility in only a small # of women. Myomas that distort the uterine cavity & larger intramural myomas may have adverse effects on fertility (*Fertil Steril 2008;90:S125*).

Physical Exam and Diagnostic Studies

- **Findings:** Uterine enlargement, irreg uterine contour
- Must r/o other causes of abn bleeding. Postmenopausal bleeding w/ fibroids should be evaluated the same way as women w/o fibroids.
- **Imaging:**

  US: Defines pelvic anatomy & effective in locating fibroids (*J Ultrasound Med* 2003;22:601)

  SIS: Allows eval of uterine cavity, particularly if infertility or AUB is a concern. Good for submucosal type.

  MRI: Very accurate but expensive. Useful to map out location of fibroids or to differentiate from adenomyosis.

  Hysteroscopy: Gold stnd for submucosal fibroid

Treatment and Medications

- **Observation:** Asx fibroids do not require intervention, no matter their size or the patient's age
- **Medical mgmt** (*Obstet Gynecol Clin N Am* 2011;38:703): Tailored to alleviating sx. Cost & s/e of rx may limit long-term use.

  NSAIDs: No data to support use as sole agent for therapy. Good for dysmenorrhea based on role of PGs as pain mediators.

  OC: 1st line. OC useful in those with AUB and pain, but not effective in decreasing bulk symptoms

  Levonorgestrel IUD: Beneficial for AUB sx (FDA approved). May decrease uterine volume. Those using LARC for AUB-L have higher continuation rates than those on OC (*BJOG* 2017;124(2):302)

  GnRH agonist (Leuprolide 3.75 mg IM QM or 11.25 mg IM q3mo): GnRH desensitization → ↓ FSH & LH. Reversible amenorrhea, 35–65% ↓ in fibroid size w/i 3 mo. Use preop ↓ uterine size if it will change surgical approach (ie, minimally invasive approach vs. open approach), OR ↑ Hgb prior to surgery. Softens fibroids & makes planes harder to see → avoid prior to myomectomy. Induces menopause sx & ↓ bone density. Consider add-back therapy, can be started right away.

  GnRH antagonists (cetrorelix, ganirelix): Avoid initial flare of GnRH agonists, rapid onset of action. Cons: Daily injections.

  Aromatase inhibitors (eg, Letrozole): Block ovarian & peripheral estrogen production, ↓ estradiol level after 1 d of rx. ↓ S/e compared to GnRH w/ rapid results. Not FDA approved.

  Antiprogestins (Mifepristone 5 or 10 mg/d × 6 mo): 26–74% ↓ in volume & slower recurrent growth after cessation. S/e: Endometrial hyperplasia (dose-dependent). Not FDA approved

- **Nonsurgical mgmt:**

  UAE: IR injects polyvinyl EtoH particles into bilateral uterine arteries → ischemia & necrosis → ↓ size and sx. *Postembolization syn* may require hospitalization postop for pain control. Successful pregnancies occur after UAE though may have abnormal placentation, but long-term data limited.

  High-Intensity Focused Ultrasound (HIFU) or Magnetic Resonance-Guided Focused Ultrasound (MRgFUS): Under MRI guidance. US waves directed at fibroid → protein denaturation, cell damage, necrosis. Modest ↓ volume but may provide sx control. Long-term studies needed.

- **Surgical Mgmt:**

  Hysteroscopic myomectomy: 1st line for symptomatic submucosal fibroids (type 0, I, II). Risks: Fluid overload, perforation.

  Ultrasound-guided radiofrequency thermal ablation (RFA): Electrode directed into myoma via US guidance, then ablated → reabsorption. Fertility preserving. Re-intervention rate similar to myomectomy or UAE. TRUST study: Randomized RFA vs. myomectomy vs. UAE (*Curr Obstet Gynecol* 2016;5(4):318)

  Myomectomy: For those desiring fertility or declining hysterectomy. Goal to remove visible & accessible fibroids & reconstruct uterus. Via laparoscopically, robotic-assisted, or laparotomy. Incidence of recurrence ↑ with number of fibroid. Risks: Unexpected hyst (<1%), blood loss or transfusion. CS delivery @ 37–38 w gest may be required depending on size and location of myomectomy (*Obstet Gynecol* 2011;118:323).

  Hysterectomy: Definitive surgical rx. Satisfaction rate >90%.

ADENOMYOSIS

Definition
- Presence of endometrial glands & stroma w/i myometrium
- Amt & degree of invasion vary. Diffuse (adenomyosis) or circumscribed focal (adenomyoma) glandular deposits.

Epidemiology
- 70–80% of cases seen in 4th & 5th decades. Only 5–25% of adenomyosis seen <39 yo.

Pathology
- **Gross:** Globally enlarged uterus, red myometrial discoloration, spongy with focal areas of hemorrhage
- **Histology:** Ectopic foci of glands and stroma in myometrium
- Often coexist with other uterine diseases (fibroids, endometriosis)

Pathophysiology
- Unclear etiology, but several theories: Invagination of endometrium into myometrium or misplaced stem cells of Müllerian remnants
- Estrogen & progesterone likely play role in dev & maint. Often develops during reproductive years & regresses after menopause. Risk factors: Parity, ↑ age

Clinical Manifestations and Physical Exam Findings
- AUB, dysmenorrhea. CPP, many asx. Severity correlates w/↑ ectopic foci & extent of invasion. Other complaints: Dyspareunia infertility.
- Ectopic endometrial tissue proliferates → enlarged globular uterus on exam

Diagnostic Workup (J Minim Invasive Gynecol 2011;18:428)
- Definitive dx by histology
- TVUS preferred imaging technique = ill-defined myometrial heterogeneity, myometrial cysts (round anechoic areas), asymmetry in anterior and posterior wall, projections of endometrium extending into myometrium
- MRI may be complementary = large asym uterus, thickened junctional zone (innermost myometrial layer), no fibroids

Treatment and Medications
- No medical therapy exists at this time to treat sx while allowing pts to conceive
- Conservative, medical mgmt for symptomatic adenomyosis similar to AUB or dysmenorrhea. Goal: Symptom relief of primary complaint.
- NSAIDs often given. May consider: Continuous oral contraceptives, progestins, Mirena IUD, & GnRH agonist.
- **Surgical Mgmt** (J Minim Invasive Gynecol 2011;18:428):
  UAE: Improvement in 83%, decreased uterine volume by 3 mo (J Vasc Interv Radiol 2017;28(12):1629). Less successful if fibroids also present.
  Endometrial ablation = Treats AUB sx only. Injury to lining can activate invagination and *cause* adenomyosis
  Nonexcisional techniques: Uterine sparing including electrocoagulation of myometrium, ablation with high frequency US (HIFU), radiofrequency ablation. Described in literature in several small studies (Fertil Steril 2014;101(2):472–87).
  Focal excision: Must be able to identify area, margins, & extent of dz. Low efficacy (50%). May have fertility & delivery implications.
  Hysterectomy = Treatment of choice for those done w/ childbearing

ENDOMETRIOSIS

Definition and Epidemiology (Obstet Gynecol 2011;118:69)
- Defined as viable, estrogen-sensitive, endometrial glands, and stroma associated with an inflammatory response outside the uterus
- Prevalence: Reproductive age: 6–10%, Infertile: 20–50%, CPP: 71–87%
- If 1st-degree relative affected, 7–10 fold ↑ risk of developing endometriosis
- **Risk factors:** Early menarche (<11 yo), menstrual cycles <27 d, heavy & prolonged menses
- **Protective factors:** ↑ Parity, ↑ lactation periods, regular exercise (>4 h/w)

Etiology
- Classic theories of spread: Retrograde menstruation or direct implantation, coelomic metaplasia, lymphatic/hematogenous spread. Newer theories: Hormone receptor abnormalities, altered immunity.

Clinical Manifestations (Obstet Gynecol 2011;118:69)

- Often asymptomatic
- Classic triad dysmenorrhea, deep dyspareunia, subfertility. Other sx − chronic pelvic pain, dyschezia.
- Pelvic pain described as cyclic pain before onset of menses (2° dysmenorrhea), deep dyspareunia (worse during menses). Atypical endometriosis pain can also be continuous
- Can involve bowel or bladder; pain usually cyclic: Dyschezia, hematuria, dysuria

Diagnostic Workup/Studies (N Engl J Med 2010;362:2389)

- **Physical exam findings:** Uterosacral ligament nodularity, adnexal mass
- Laparoscopy w/ or w/o bx for histology (gold std). Path: Endometrial glands/stroma w/ varying amts of inflammation/fibrosis. Blood or hemosiderin-laden macrophages. Bx not req, but definitive.
- **Visual appearance:** Classical lesions = black powder burn. Nonclassical = red or white.
- No correlation b/w severity of visual dz & degree of pain or prog w/ rx but some association with depth of infiltration
- No serum markers or imaging studies useful in dx
- Sensitivity of imaging (MRI, US) is dependent on the type of endometriosis present. Peritoneal and ovarian implants are unlikely to be seen, vs. pelvic/adnexal masses are readily identified
- **US:** Ovarian endometriomas appear as cyst w/ low-level, homogenous internal echoes from old blood. TVUS = imaging of choice to detect deeply infiltrating endometriosis of rectum or rectovaginal septum.

Classification

- Numerous schemes proposed. ASRM classification most common. Value = uniform recording of OR findings & comparing therapeutic interventions.
- **ASRM criteria:** Stage I (minimal) → Stage IV (severe). Based on extent, size, & location of endometriosis lesions seen during operative procedure. Not good predictor of pregnancy after treatment and does not correlate with pain, dyspareunia, or infertility

Treatment and Medications

- No medical therapy exists at this time to treat sx while allowing pts to conceive
- Should always begin with medical therapy

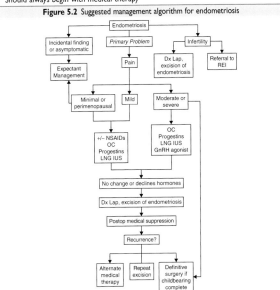

Figure 5.2 Suggested management algorithm for endometriosis

Modified from Hoffman BL, Schorge JO, Schaffer JI, et al., eds. *Williams Gynecology.* 2nd ed. New York, NY: McGraw-Hill; 2012.

- Best treated with long-term medical mgmt w/ surgical backup
- **Medical therapy** (Fertil Steril 2008;90:S260): Medical suppressive therapies are ineffective for infertility (Int J Gynaecol Obstet 2001;72:263)
    - **NSAIDs:** Inconclusive evidence as to NSAIDs efficacy for treatment of endometriosis pain (Cochrane Database Syst Rev 2017;23:1)
    - **OCs:** Traditional first line. Continuous more effective than cyclic. Not helpful in dyspareunia and atypical endo.
    - **Progestins:** New first line. Antagonize estrogenic effects on endometrium → eventual endometrial atrophy of endometriosis foci.
        Medroxyprogesterone acetate (MPA) 20+ mg PO QD or 150 mg IM q3mo (depot) or 104 mg SQ q3mo: No max dose of progesterone. Similar effectiveness as GnRH agonist to ↓ pain. Safe for long-term use
        Norethindrone 2.5–5 mg QD, Effective in dysmenorrhea, deep dyspareunia, atypical endometriosis pain, dyschezia. ↑ Patient satisfaction. Good control of bleeding
        LNG-IUS q5y: Improves pain in stage I–IV
        Etonogestrel q3y: Limited data. Similar pain and patient satisfaction scores to MPA
    - **GnRH agonists:** ↓ Signaling of HPA-axis → ↓ estrogen → amenorrhea & endometrial atrophy. Nasal spray (nafarelin acetate) or depot formulation (leuprolide acetate) q1–3mo. S/e = menopause sx + ↓ bone density. Not useful in post-menopausal endometriosis. **Add-back therapy** w/ progesterone or combo (estrogen/progesterone) to ↓ s/e can be initiated immediately, and required in long-term use. Theory = amt necessary to prevent menopause sx < amt to stimulate endometriosis. Does not diminish efficacy. Norethindrone acetate (only hormone FDA approved for add-back therapy) 5 mg PO QD w/ or w/o low-dose estrogen 0.625 mg QD × 12 mo. Also start on daily Ca 1000 mg. GnRH agonist FDA approved 12 mo.
    - **Danazol** (600–800 mg QD): Inhibit LH surge → chronic anovulatory state. Substantial androgenic & hypoestrogenic s/e profile make it unacceptable. S/e = acne, hirsutism, bloating, voice changes, hot flashes, muscle cramps.
    - **Aromatase inhibitors:** Primarily in research setting. Literature suggest use in postmenopausal endometriosis. Insufficient data to recommend routine use.
    Cochrane review concluded that for pain, suppression of menses with GnRH agonist, LNG-IUD, and danazol was beneficial (Cochrane Database Syst Rev. 2014 Mar 10;(3): CD009590).
- **Surgical therapy** (Fertil Steril 2008;90:S260): Relief of pain after surgical rx = 50–95%. Laparoscopic resection of visible lesions improves pain. All visible lesions should be treated. ↑ Risk of recurrence if no postop suppression and ovaries left in situ and younger patients have higher risk of reoperation.
    - **Conservative Surg** (diagnostic laparoscopy, lysis of adhesions, ablation/excision of visible implants, normalization of anatomy) = 1° approach for symptomatic or large endometriomas b/c medical therapy will not lead to complete resolution. Cyst excision in endometriomas has improved outcomes over cyst drainage.
    - **Uterosacral nerve ablation:** Previously believed to disrupt efferent nerve fibers in the uterosacral ligaments → ↓ uterine pain for intractable dysmenorrhea. No benefit over conservative surgery alone.
    - **Presacral neurectomy:** Interrupts symp innervation to uterus @ level of superior hypogastric plexus. Benefit in midline pain only. Technically challenging w/ risk of bleeding. S/e: Constip, urinary dysfxn.
    - **Hysterectomy + BSO:** For those w/ debilitating sx, completed childbearing, & failed other therapies. If ovaries look normal, ovarian conservation should be considered. Even with BSO, there is a 10–15% risk of persistent pain usually due to deep infiltrating endometriosis. Consider leaving ovaries in situ and counseling about possible need for additional surgery if persistent symptoms (5–20% chance of reop). If oophorectomy performed, long-term adherence w/ HRT req to prevent ↑ risk of mortality a/w BSO prior to menopause (Obstet Gynecol 2010;116:733; Obstet Gynecol Clin North Am 2014;41:371–83). Use estrogen/progesterone therapy d/t risk of unopposed estrogen may stimulate growth of endometrial implants.
- Surg, followed by medical therapy offers longer sx relief than surg alone. OC, progestins, GnRH analogs, have been shown to ↓ pain & ↑ time until recurrence (Fertil Steril 2008;90:S260; Hum Reprod 2011;26:3).

ABNORMAL UTERINE BLEEDING (AUB)

Definition and Etiology
AUB: Menstrual flow outside of nml vol, duration, regularity, or frequency. Excessive blood loss is based on pts' perception.

PALM-COEIN classification	
Structural causes of AUB	
P	Polyp
A	Adenomyosis
L	Leiomyoma (submucosal, other)
M	Malignancy, hyperplasia
Nonstructural causes of AUB	
C	Coagulopathy (Warfarin, heparin, LMWH, and 20% with HMB have underlying bleeding d/o)
O	Ovulatory dysfunction
E	Endometrial
I	Iatrogenic (eg, breakthrough bleeding associated with contraception, TCAs)
N	Not yet classified
Pair AUB with terms to describe bleeding pattern to indicate etiology (eg, AUB-P, AUB-A, AUB-L). Data from *Int J Gynecol Obstet* 2011;113(1):3.	

Pathophysiology
- See PALM-COEIN table
- Anovulation → unopposed estrogen → ↑ risk of endometrial hyperplasia & malignancy

Differential Diagnosis
- Always consider Preg or related complications (SAB, ectopic)
- **Teens:** MCC d/t persistent anovulation d/t dysregulation of HPA, coagulopathy, contraception, infxn, tumor
- **Reproductive age (19–39 y):** Structural abnormalities (PALM), anovulatory cycles, contraception, endometrial hyperplasia. Cancer less common but may occur.
- **Perimenopause:** Endometrial hyperplasia, cancer, anovulatory bleeding d/t declining ovarian fxn, PALM

Diagnostic Workup (*BMJ* 2007;334:1110; *Obstet Gynecol Clin N Am* 2008;35:219)
- Detailed history & physical exam, including bimanual exam to evaluate uterus & speculum exam to evaluate cervix & vagina. Complete menstrual Hx & can provide dx w/ sufficient confidence that rx can begin empirically
- History: C/o hirsutism, heat intolerance; HMB since menarche OR PPH, bleeding with dental work OR (two of the following) bruising 1–2×/mo, epistaxis 1–2×/mo, gum bleeding, FH of bleeding sx (*Fertil Steril* 2005;84:1345)
- Physical: Hirsutism, enlarged thyroid, acanthosis nigricans, petechiae
- Fibroids, adenomyosis: Regular, heavy menses
- Polyps: Intermenstrual spotting, heavy menses
- **Lab tests:** Preg test, CBC, TSH, PRL. Consider Pap test & chlamydia testing. R/o bleeding disorders (particularly in teens)
- An EMB is not always req, except for >45 yo OR younger with risk factors (eg, if long-term unopposed estrogen exposure, failed medical management, persistent AUB)
- Imaging including ultrasound and SIS reserved to evaluate findings on physical, when sx persist despite rx, or suspicious for intrauterine pathology (AUB-P, AUB-L). SIS superior to TVUS for diagnosing intracavitary lesions (polyps, submucosal fibroids) though hysteroscopy with biopsy is gold standard (*J Obstet Gynaecol* 2011;31(1):54–8).

Treatment and Medications (*Obstet Gynecol Clin N Am* 2008;35:219; *Menopause* 2011;18:453)
- Treat underlying etiology, start empiric medical rx with progestin-only therapies or COCPs. Expect improv in 3 mo. Failure to improve → need to r/o other etiologies before changing mgmt. See also Chap. 2 for acute bleeding.
- **Medical management (acute):**
  CEE: 25 mg IV q4–6h; shown to stop bleeding within 8 h of administration (*Obstet Gynecol* 1982;59:285–91)
  COCPs: Monophasic with 35 μg PO, TID × 7 d
  Medroxyprogesterone: 20 mg PO, TID × 7 d
  Tranexamic acid: 1.3 g PO or 10 mg/kg IV (max 600 mg/dose), q8h × 5 d

- **Medical management (chronic)**
- For long-term treatment for AUB-A, AUB-O, AUB-L, options include LNG-IUD, COCPs (continuous), MPA, norethindrone, NSAIDs, TXA. DPMA or Etonogestrel implant can be offered but SE include irregular bleeding, so may not be best options depending on etiology of AUB
- For those with EIN and poor surgical candidate or fertility desire:
  MPA 10–20 mg/d or 12–14 d/mo (cyclic)
  DPMA 150 mg IM q3mo
  Micronized vaginal progesterone 100–200 mg/d or 12–14 d/mo (cyclic) × 3 mo
  Megestrol acetate 40–200 mg/d
  LNG-IUD 52 mg/5 y
  → Follow-up with serial EMB × q3–6mo to look for regression (though appropriate freq not clearly known)
- **Rx goals:** (1) Reverse abnormalities of endometrium d/t chronic anovulation, (2) induce or restore cyclic menses of nml vol & duration
- Surgical management:
  Acute surgical mgmt: If hemodynamic unstable, bleeding refractory to 2 doses of IV estrogen, or blood loss that cannot be replaced w/ transfusion, OR mgmt (D&C) req. Should continue medical therapy after D&C. Informed consent should include hysterectomy. Uterine artery embolization may be considered as alternative, if available.

  Operative hysteroscopy: AUB-P and submucosal AUB-L

  Endometrial ablation: High success rate. 25–50% are amenorrheic, & 80–90% have ↓ bleeding. Effective alternative to hysterectomy. ↑ Success if pretreated w/ progestins or GnRH agonists. R/o cancer prior to Surg. Up to 1/3 will eventually elect for hysterectomy. NOT first line.

  Hysterectomy: High satisfaction, more morbidity & riskier for pts w/ multiple medical conditions

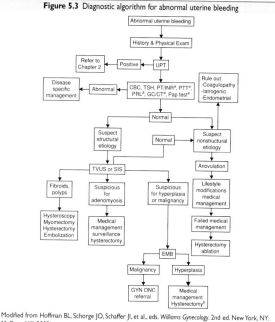

Figure 5.3 Diagnostic algorithm for abnormal uterine bleeding

Modified from Hoffman BL, Schorge JO, Schaffer JI, et al., eds. *Williams Gynecology.* 2nd ed. New York, NY: McGraw-Hill; 2012.
[a]Study obtained as indicated from patient history.
[b]GYN ONC referral for complex atypical hyperplasia, per provider discretion.

POSTMENOPAUSAL BLEEDING

Definition, Epidemiology, and Etiology (Obstet Gynecol 2010;116:168)
- **PMB:** Vaginal bleeding occurring after ≥12 mo of amenorrhea
- PMB "is endometrial cancer until proven otherwise." Malig w/ PMB = 1–14%. Predictive value depends on age & risks: Obesity, HTN, diabetes, low parity.
- Differential diagnosis: Cancer, atrophy (most common), endometrial hyperplasia, HRT, polyps

Diagnostic Workup (Obstet Gynecol 2010;116:168)
- **Comprehensive H&P:** Pelvic exam to evaluate rectal, vulvar, vaginal, or cervical origin
- **Goal of endometrial eval:** (1) Exclude malignancy, (2) rx based on proper etiology (anatomic vs. nonanatomic pathology)
- **Endometrial eval:**
  Transvaginal US: Transvaginal ultrasound with EMS ≤4 reliable excludes endometrial cancer (Obstet Gynecol 2009;114:409–11). Limitations: EMS not always visible. Incidental found EMS >4 mm in an asx pt does NOT require intervention. If EMS ≤4 mm but bleeding persists, warrants further w/u.
  EMB: Accurate for excluding cancer, but only samples 4–12% of endometrium. Sens 99%, Spec 98%. High rate of insufficient or failed sampling (0–54%) → further eval via D&C ± hysteroscopy (Maturitas 2011;68:155)
  Sonohysterography: Imaging w/ saline infusion (SIS) overcomes some TVUS limitations
  D&C: Useful when unable to obtain EMB (cervical stenosis, pt intolerance, etc.). Risks: 1–2% complication rate. May miss 10% of endometrial lesions.
  Hysteroscopy: Helpful for focal lesions that could be missed on EMB

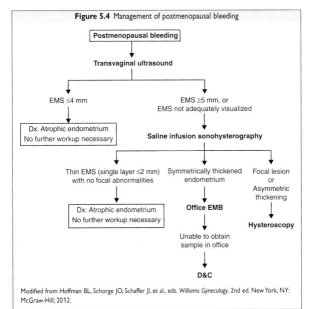

Figure 5.4 Management of postmenopausal bleeding

Postmenopausal bleeding
↓
Transvaginal ultrasound

EMS ≤4 mm → Dx: Atrophic endometrium / No further workup necessary

EMS ≥5 mm, or EMS not adequately visualized
↓
Saline infusion sonohysterography

Thin EMS (single layer ≤2 mm) with no focal abnormalities → Dx: Atrophic endometrium / No further workup necessary

Symmetrically thickened endometrium → Office EMB → Unable to obtain sample in office → D&C

Focal lesion or Asymmetric thickening → Hysteroscopy

Modified from Hoffman BL, Schorge JO, Schaffer JI, et al., eds. *Williams Gynecology*. 2nd ed. New York, NY: McGraw-Hill; 2012.

DYSMENORRHEA

Definitions and Epidemiology
- Dysmenorrhea = painful menstruation. One of the most common gyn complaints.
- Primary dysmenorrhea (PD) = Painful menses without underlying pelvic pathology. Affects 43–91% of young women; severity varies. Most prevalent in ages 20–24; prevalence ↓'s thereafter. Risks: Early menarche, smoking. No association with parity, exercise (Contraception 2010;81:185; Obstet Gynecol 2006;108:428).
- Secondary dysmenorrhea (SD) = Painful menses d/t underlying pelvic pathology. Risks: BMI <20, nulliparity, early menarche, short cycles (<27 d), heavy/long menses, family hx, depression, PID, h/o sexual assault, & heavy smoking (Obstet Gynecol 2010;116:223).

Pathophysiology and Etiology
- PD: Premenstrual ↓ in progesterone → ↑ PGF2 → ↑ uterine contractility → pain/cramps (Contraception 2010;81:185)
- SD: Most common cause = endometriosis
    Gyn causes: Adenomyosis, fibroids, IUD, PID, adhesions, Müllerian anomalies
    Nongyn etiology: IBD, IBS, UTI, nephrolithiasis, interstitial cystitis, chronic pelvic pain, psychosomatic (BMJ 2006;332:1134; Am Fam Phy 2014;89:341)

Clinical Manifestations
- **PD:** Onset shortly after menarche. Midline, cramping pain, beginning w/ onset of menses. Resolves over 12–72 h. May be a/w HA, N/V, backache, & diarrhea.
- **SD:** Onset any time after menarche. Timing during menstrual cycle variable. May be a/w dyspareunia (Contraception 2010;81:185; BMJ 2006;332:1134)

Diagnosis
- Diagnose PD by history & normal. Consider SD if abnormal exam, no response to empiric TX, or if sx follow years of painless menses (Contraception 2010;81:185)
- Pelvic ultrasound: Evaluate for structural etiologies (eg noncommunicating uterine horn)

Treatment and Medications (Obstet Gynecol 2006;108:428; Obstet Gynecol 2010;115:206)
- **PD:**
    NSAIDs: *1st-line therapy.* Efficacy ~90%. Start day *prior to* or *at onset* of menses; continue regular dosing throughout. Specific COX-2 inhibs (celecoxib) also shown to be effective (not FDA approved for PD).
    COCs: Efficacy 70–80%. Suppress ovulation & endometrial thickening → ↓ PG → ↓ pain. OCs w/ medium-dose estrogen. Continuous OC ↓ pain longer than monthly but ↑ breakthrough bleeding. Intravaginal ring also effective
    Progestin-only medications:
    Progestin-only pills: Good for women with contraindication to estrogen. Do not consistently inhibit ovulation, but thin the endometrium to decrease dysmenorrhea
    Depot medroxyprogesterone(150 mg IM q3mo): Limited data for PD. ↓ Bleeding → ↓ pain.
    Levonorgestrel-releasing IUS: Meta-analysis & RCT data show LNG-IUS is as effective as GnRH analogue in controlling dysmenorrhea (Contraception 2007;75:S134; Hum Reprod 2005;20:1993)
    Etonogestrel subdermal implant: 81–82% reduction in PD
    Nifedipine (20–40 mg QD): ↓ Uterine contractility → ↓ pain. S/E: Flushing, tachy, & HAs.
    Narcotics: Use as sparingly as possible due to risk of dependence
- **SD:** Treat underlying disorder

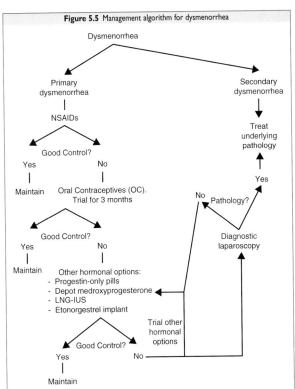

Figure 5.5 Management algorithm for dysmenorrhea

Dysmenorrhea

Primary dysmenorrhea → NSAIDs

Secondary dysmenorrhea → Treat underlying pathology

Good Control?
- Yes → Maintain
- No → Oral Contraceptives (OC). Trial for 3 months

Good Control?
- Yes → Maintain
- No → Other hormonal options:
  - Progestin-only pills
  - Depot medroxyprogesterone
  - LNG-IUS
  - Etonogestrel implant

Good Control?
- Yes → Maintain
- No → Trial other hormonal options

Pathology?
- No
- Yes → Diagnostic laparoscopy

Modified from Hoffman BL, Schorge JO, Schaffer JI, et al., eds. Williams Gynecology. 2nd ed. New York, NY: McGraw-Hill; 2012.

PREMENSTRUAL SYNDROME (PMS) AND PREMENSTRUAL DYSPHORIC DISORDER (PMDD)

Definition and Epidemiology (Am J Psych 2012;169:465; Obstet Gynecol 2010;115:206; Maturitas 2015;82:436–40)

- **PMS:** Presence of at least one symptom (bloating, breast tenderness, peripheral swelling, mild mood changes, sleep disturbance) during luteal phase that impairs functioning
- **PMDD (DSM-5 Diagnostic Criteria):** Severe form of PMS. 5 or more of the following during the week prior to menses, resolving within a few days after the onset of menses. At least 1 of the 5 sx must be a core symptom (bolded below). Symptoms must cause significant distress/interference with work/school/relationships
  Symptoms: **Marked affective lability, marked irritability/anger, markedly depressed mood, marked anxiety,** decreased interest in usual activities, difficulty concentrating, lethargy/decreased energy, marked change in, hypersomnia/insomnia, feeling overwhelmed, physical sx
  Dx of exclusion: Not due to other mood d/o, substance use, medical condition
- PMS: 30% of menstruating women. PMDD: Affects 3–8% of reproductive-age women.
- Important impact on lifestyle. Affected women have ↑ rates of work absences, ↑ medical expenses, ↓ health-related quality of life

Etiology

- Multifactorial: Triggered by changes in ovarian steroids during luteal phase in susceptible women → cause changes in the opioid, GABA, & serotonin systems. Women w/ PMS/PMDD have normal estrogen & progesterone levels, but have an abnormal response to these hormonal fluctuations

Diagnostic Workup/Studies

- Menstrual/general hx, physical, CMP, CBC, serum TSH
- 2–3-mo prospective menstrual calendar: Document sx & time correlation with menses
- **DDx:** Mood & personality disorders, domestic abuse, thyroid disorders, perimenopause, anemia, endometriosis, chronic fatigue syndrome, IBS, fibromyalgia

Treatment and Medications

- Goal to ↑ unaffected days & ↓ symptom severity → ↑ psychosocial functioning
- Lifestyle modifications: Exercise, decreased stress, dietary modification (↑ complex carbs)
- **Dietary Supplements/Herbal Meds:** Calcium carbonate 1200 mg QD (48% reduction in symptoms compared to placebo). Vitamin B6 (pyridoxine) 80 mg QD (more effective at treating mood sx than placebo, not physical sx). Vitex agnus-castus (Chasteberry) – Only herb proven to control PMS-associated mood swings and PMDD, 40 drops/d.
- **COCs:** Multiple studies w/ favorable results. For PMDD – Drospirenone-containing COCs w/ 24 active d have improved symptoms (compared to 21 active d). For PMS, COCs beneficial, but efficacy differences between COC types are not clear
- **SSRIs:** *1st line for severe PMS & PMDD w/ primarily emotional sx.* Meta-analysis of RCT – 60% resp rate. Daily dosing has better effect than luteal phase-only dosing. Fluoxetine 20 mg/d, paroxetine 20–30 mg/d, citalopram 20–30 mg/d, sertraline 50–150 mg/d.
- **Other psychotropic medications:** Clomipramine (TCA) – effective for PMS at low doses. Benzodiazepines – helpful if irritability is dominant symptom. Neither as effective as SSRI
- **GnRH agonists** (Leuprolide 3.75 mg IM qmo, 11.25 mg IM q3mo): Meta-analysis – Improved PMS/PMDD symptoms (OR 8.66), more effective for physical than psychological sx. Side effects (amenorrhea, bone loss, vasomotor, flushing) limit its long-term use. If used for >6 mo, "add-back" tx (estrogen/progestin) recommended, but this can increase PMS/PMDD symptoms.
- **Oophorectomy:** Last-resort treatment for patients that have failed other options, but have had success w/ trial of GnRH agonists. Hormonal add-back is required.

CHRONIC PELVIC PAIN

Definitions, Epidemiology, and Etiology (Clin Obstet Gynecol 1990;33:130; Br J Obstet Gynaecol 1999;106:1149)

- Noncyclic pain, lasting ≥3–6 mo, located in the pelvis (below the umbilicus), causes functional disability or request for medical care
- Prevalence of CPP 4–16%. Only ~1/3 of women seek medical care.
- **Differential Diagnosis (Wide):**
  Gynecologic (20%): Endometriosis, leiomyoma, adenomyosis, recurrent ovarian cysts, hydrosalpinx, ovarian remnant syndrome, pelvic inflammatory disease, pelvic adhesive disease, post-tubal ligation pain syndrome
  Urologic (30%): Interstitial cystitis/painful bladder syndrome, radiation cystitis, bladder cancer, urethral syndrome, recurrent cystitis
  Gastrointestinal (38%): Irritable bowel syndrome, inflammatory bowel disease, chronic constipation, colorectal carcinoma, celiac disease, abdominal/pelvic hernias
  Musculoskeletal: Abdominal wall myofascial pain, pelvic floor dysfunction, fibromyalgia, coccygodynia, piriformis syndrome
  Neurologic: Abdominal wall cutaneous nerve entrapment (ilioinguinal/iliohypogastric), pudendal neuralgia, central sensitization of pain
  Vascular: Pelvic congestion syndrome
  High prevalence of concurrent psychiatric disorder, history of abuse

Diagnostic Workup/Studies

- **History:** Detailed history including urinary, gastrointestinal, gynecologic, musculoskeletal, sexual, and psychosocial symptoms

- Consider standardized form (International Pelvic Pain Society "Pelvic Pain Assessment")
- Pain characteristics and location (associated, provocative/palliative, quality, radiation, setting, temporal aspects)
- **Physical exam:** Systematic complete exam, including back, abdomen, and extremities
- **Pelvic Exam: Visual inspection of external genitalia, Cotton swab test** (light palpation with moistened cotton swab starting on thighs and moving medial to vestibule), **examination of pelvic floor** (palpation of levator ani, internal transverse perineal, obturator internus for tenderness or contraction), **bimanual exam, speculum exam** (use smallest speculum possible)
- **Labs:** CPP itself causes no lab changes. Labs used to exclude other etiologies: Pregnancy test, Urinalysis/culture, Gonorrhea, Chlamydia, Trichomonas, wet prep, trich.
- **Imaging:** Pelvic US to evaluate pelvis, particularly if enlarged uterus/adnexal mass on exam, h/o abnormal bleeding. Consider MRI if deep infiltrating endometriosis suspected
- If symptoms/exam indicate alternate source of pain, consider referral to appropriate provider, ie, Urology, GI, psych, pelvic physical therapy *(Obstet Gynecol 2002;100:337)*

Treatment and Medications *(Barbieri RL, Treatment of Chronic Pelvic Pain in Women, UpToDate)*
- Target treatment to suspected underlying causes. Often requires long-term care.
- Multifactorial etiology often requires multidisciplinary approach
- **Pain management:** NSAIDs are first line. Avoid opiates if possible.
- **Lifestyle modifications/nonmedical therapy:** Exercise, heat packs, acupuncture, massage, PT
- **Empiric Management:**
  Endometriosis: OCs/NSAIDs. If no improvement in 2–3 mo, trial continuous progestin (Medroxyprogesterone acetate 10–50 mg/d, norethindrone 2.5–30 mg/d, Depo Medroxyprogesterone acetate 150 mg IM q3mo, LNG-IUS) or GnRH agonist
  Irritable Bowel Syndrome: Diet/behavioral modifications
  Interstitial Cystitis: Behavior modification (avoid bladder irritants [caffeine, artificial sweeteners, hot pepper, vitamin C, alcohol], fluid management), pelvic floor PT, Amitriptyline, Pentosan polysulfate sodium
  Myofascial pain syndrome: Physical therapy, trigger point injections, muscle relaxants
  Pelvic Congestion Syndrome: Limited data suggesting GnRH agonists, synthetic progestin, and/or psychotherapy can improve pain. Invasive TX include hysterectomy, embolization of ovarian veins (± internal iliac veins), sclerotherapy, surgical ligation of ovarian veins (no RCT data for any invasive options)
- **Surgical Management:**
  Diagnostic/therapeutic laparoscopy for refractory endometriosis, w/ fulguration of implants. Best shows adhesiolysis ineffective for CPP.
  Hysterectomy ± BSO is last resort for refractory endometriosis. Will not treat non-GYN etiologies of pain

VULVAR PAIN/VULVODYNIA

Definitions and Etiology *(J Reprod Med 2006;51:447; Obstet Gynecol 2016;128:e78)*
- Affects 18–20% of women
- **2015 Consensus Terminology and Classification System** *(Obstet Gynecol 2016;127:745)*
- **Vulvar pain caused by a specific disorder**
  - Infectious (eg recurrent candidiasis, herpes)
  - Inflammatory (eg lichen sclerosus, lichen planus, immunobullous disorders)
  - Neoplastic (eg Paget disease, squamous cell carcinoma)
  - Neurologic (eg postherpetic neuralgia, nerve compression or injury, neuroma)
  - Trauma (eg female genital cutting, obstetric lacerations)
  - Iatrogenic (eg postoperative, chemotherapy, radiation)
  - Hormonal deficiencies (eg genitourinary synd. of menopause, lactational amenorrhea)
- **Vulvodynia – vulvar pain lasting at least 3 mo without clear identifiable cause. May have associated factors. Described using the following factors:**
  - Localized (eg vestibulodynia) or generalized or mixed (localized & generalized)
  - Provoked (eg insertional, contact) or spontaneous or mixed
  - Onset (primary or secondary)
  - Temporal pattern (intermittent, persistent, constant, immediate, delayed)

Clinical Manifestations

- Pain of the external female genital area. Commonly described as: Burning, stinging, irritation, aching, soreness, throbbing.
- The entire vulva may be painful or pain may be centered in a specific area
- Provoked by coitus, vulvar contact w/ tampon, speculum, tight clothing, washing or wiping, sitting, biking, or horseback riding

Diagnostic Workup

- **History:** Assess specifics of pain location, alleviating/inciting factors
- **Pelvic exam:** Gross inspection, single digit exam, speculum exam. Biopsy only needed if there are other indications
- **Cotton swab testing:** Systematic evaluation of location of pain. Testing starts on thighs, followed by labial majora, interlabial sulci, and vestibule at 2-, 4-, 6-, 8-, & 10-o'clock positions. Pain classified as mild, moderate, or severe.
- **Labs:** Wet prep, vaginal pH, yeast culture, STI screening as indicated
- **Diagnosis of exclusion:** Rule out other etiologies (Infectious, dermatologic, neoplastic, neurologic, musculoskeletal, psychological, domestic abuse or relationship discord)

Treatment and Medications

- Most evidence based on expert opinion or small studies
- Extensive pt education & vulvar hygiene (cotton underwear, avoid vulvar irritants/soap on vulva, adequate lubrication for intercourse). Sexual counseling.
- Topical medications: Local anesthetic (lidocaine 5% gel) used immediately before intercourse. Estrogen cream. Tricyclic antidepressants compounded into topical cream.
- Tricyclic antidepressants, anticonvulsants: Avoid polypharmacy, take 3 w to achieve pain control. First line = Amitriptyline (5–25 mg nightly, increase by 10–25 mg qw. Max dose 150 mg daily. Wean medication if discontinuing). Gabapentin well-studied (64% had 80% ↓ in sx. Starting dose 300 mg daily. Increase to maximum of 3600 mg daily split into TID dosing) (*J Reprod Med* 2007;52(1):103).
- Pelvic floor physical therapy ± biofeedback – Particularly effective if vaginismus present
- Surgical intervention as a last resort: Vestibulectomy

FEMALE SEXUAL DYSFUNCTION

Definitions (DSM-5)

- **Female Orgasmic D/O:** Marked delay/absence or ↓intensity of orgasm 75–100% of time
- **Female Sexual Interest/Arousal D/O:** Lack of or ↓ sexual interest//arousal
- **Genitopelvic Pain/Penetration D/O:** Difficulty, fear/anxiety, pain (dyspareunia) or tightening of pelvic floor muscles with/in anticipation of vaginal penetration (vaginismus)
- Each d/o must occur for ≥6 mo and be accompanied by distress or interpersonal difficulty

Epidemiology

- **43% prevalence:** Low sexual desire (22–39%); arousal problems (14–26%); orgasm (21%), sexual pain (7%) (*JAMA* 1999;281:537; *Obstet Gyn* 2008;112:976)

Etiology

- Organic or psychological or a mix of both; more than 1 dysfxn may coexist. Risks: ↓ Age, ↓ educational attainment, ↓ social status, urinary tract sx, sexual trauma
- Medical (depression, anxiety, urinary incontinence, ESRD, anemia, thyroid, DM, substance or EtOH abuse, cancers), meds (SSRIs [most common], beta-blockers, antipsychotics), current relationship, sociocultural factors, estrogen deficiency, abn gyn etiology

Pathophysiology

- ♀ Sexual resp cycle has 4 phases: Desire, plateau, orgasm, resolution (1st described by Masters & Johnson in 1966). Nonlinear model integrates emotional intimacy, sexual stimuli & relationship satisfaction; a sexual encounter may begin w/o desire initially present (*Clin Update Women's Health Care* 2003;11(2):1).

Diagnostic Workup/Studies

- Thorough sexual history includes recording the patient's medical, surgical, social, and psychiatric. Use of prescription and over-the-counter medications
- The Brief Sexual Symptom checklist, a screening questionnaire (*J Sex Med* 2010;337)
- A complete gynecologic evaluation performed, targeting areas that were uncovered in the sexual function history
- Lab eval as clinically indicated: TSH, PRL, etc.

- **Nonpharmacologic therapy (1st line):** Identify rx goals, treat reversible causes; sex therapy w/ requisite exercises (dilators, vibrators) & Eros Therapy (FDA approved), pelvic floor physical therapy, desensitization, relaxation exercises.
- Vaginal lubricants (water or silicone based). Vaginal moisturizers (eg, Replens).
- **Pharmacologic therapy:**
  - Transdermal testosterone: Improves female arousal d/o in short-term, but no data for use >6 mo. Hyperandrogen side effects (hirsutism, acne).
  - Sildenafil: No clear evidence for use of in female arousal d/o (Obstet Gynecol 2011;117:996; Menopause 2006;13:770)
  - Estrogen: Topical vaginal estrogen for vulvovaginal atrophy (see "Menopause" section for dosages). Systemic hormone replacement therapy also available (see "Hormone Therapy" for dosages).

MENOPAUSE

Definitions and Epidemiology (Fertil Steril 2012;97(4):843)

- Final menstrual period (FMP) defined by 12 mo of amenorrhea from a loss of ovarian activity. Perimenopausal transition: Wide fluctuation in hormonal profiles; ↑ irreg cycle length; quantitative FSH of >25 IU/mL on a random sample.
- FMP at <40 y = premature menopause (~1%)
- Growing number of menopausal women. 37.9 million over 55 yo (2010) → 45.9 M (2020).
- Median age of menopause: 51.4 (Am J Epidemiol 2001;153:865). Gaussian distribution 40–58 y.

Etiology

- Reduced quality & quantity of aging follicles → ↓ inhibin & ↓ ovarian estrogen → ↑ FSH → loss of ovarian follicles → depleted ovarian follicle supply→ ovarian senescence
- α- & β-estrogen receptors are located throughout the body; ↓ estrogen → sx

Clinical Manifestations

- **Vasomotor instability (~75%):** Hot flushes & night sweats; most common during late menopausal transition (Stage −1) through early postmenopausal period (Stage +1). Mild (transient heat), mod (heat + sweating + permits continuation of activity), sev (heat + sweating + discontinuation of activity). Mod–sev VMSx = 7 hot flashes/d or 50–60/w. Self-limited w/ resolution in 1st 5 postmenopausal years; 25% symptomatic >5 y.
- **Urogenital atrophy (up to 75%):** Pruritus, recurrent UTI, vaginal neuropathy in the distribution of pudendal nerve, sexual dysfxn, dyspareunia; most common during late postmenopause (Stage +2)
- **Alterations in menstrual patterns:** Chronic anovulation → heavy dysfunctional bleeding during late reproductive stage (Stage −3a) & menopausal transition (Stages −2, −1)
- **Infertility:** Secondary to oocyte depletion
- **Increased cardiovascular dz risk:** ↑ Total cholesterol, ↑ markedly LDL-C.
- **Accelerated bone loss:** Secondary to decreased estrogen. Spine bone density ↓ by 15–30% in 1st 5–7 postmenopausal years; 1–2% per year thereafter. The effect is predominantly on trabecular bone (Hormone Therapy 2010;115(4):844).
- **Decreased collagen support:** ↓ Skin collagen by 30% in 1st 5 y after menopause; ~2% ↓ per year for the 1st 10 y after established menopause.
- Increased endometrial & breast cancer risk d/t unopposed endogenous estrogen

Diagnostic Workup/Studies

- Clinical dx from longitudinal assessment of absence of menses over 12 mo.
- Pelvic exam: May see thin/pale/dry/unrugated vaginal tissue, loss of elasticity, petechial hemorrhages, cervical atrophy, vaginal stenosis/narrowing, urethral caruncle
- Risk assessment for CVD & osteoporosis (lifestyle, FHx, lipid profile). DEXA BMD scan to diagnose osteoporosis, predict fracture risk. See Chap. 1.

Treatment and Medications (Obstet Gynecol 2014;123:202)

- **Perimenopausal transition:** Physical activity, social & mental activities.
- **Vasomotor symptoms (VMSx):** Lifestyle modifications. SSRIs/SNRIs (significant sx ↓ compared to placebo). Paroxetine (7.5 mg/d) is only nonhormone FDA-approved for VMSx. Venlafaxine (37.5 mg/d). Gabapentin (45% ↓ frequency, 54% ↓ severity of VMSx). Hormone replacement therapy (see table).

- **Urogenital atrophy/Sexual Dsfxn/Urinary Dsfxn:** Mild Sx – Vaginal moisturizes regularly, lubricants w/ intercourse, regular sexual activity. Vaginal estrogen (rings, creams, tablets) w/ minimal systemic absorp & increased safety. Systemic HRT (*Obstet Gynecol 2010;115(4):843*).

Treatment for menopausal atrophic vaginal/genitourinary symptoms	
Vaginal estrogen preparations	**Regimen**
Estradiol-17β vaginal ring, 7.5 µg/d	Replace ring q90d
Estradiol vaginal tablet 10–25 µg	Insert 1 tablet daily × 2 w, then twice weekly
Estradiol-17β vaginal cream 2 g/d, Conjugated estrogen cream 0.5–2 g/d	Daily initially, taper to twice weekly
Systemic Hormone Replacement Therapy (see table)	

- Primary & secondary prevention of CHD, stroke, VTE, osteoporosis. Lifestyle changes, Smoking cessation; control of HTN, dyslipidemia, & DM. Calcium suppl (1200–1500 mg daily), Vit D suppl (800 IU daily).

HORMONE THERAPY

Definitions (*Obstet Gynecol 2014;123:202*)
- HT comprises estrogen & progesterone therapy. ET comprises solely estrogen therapy.
- "Timing hypothesis" – timing of initiation of HT in relation to chronologic age/length of menopause affect risk of primary endpoints (*Am J Epidemiol 2007;166:511*); secondary analysis of WHI/observational studies → initiation of HT before 60 y of age or w/i 10 y of menopause may confer maximal cardioprotection for 6 or more years, improved QOL measures over 5–30 y (*Climacteric 2012;15(3):217*).

Indications
- Use HT when benefits of symptom control outweigh risks. Benefit-Risk ratio changes w/ age & sx (eg, VMSx, sleep disturbance, vaginal atrophy, dyspareunia, diminished libido).
- "Timing hypothesis" – Benefits of short-term HT outweigh CV risk when HT initiated close to onset of menopause in appropriate pts (*Hormone Therapy 2010;115(4):847*).
- **Contraindications:** H/o breast/endometrial cancer, CHD, VTE or CVA, active liver dz, or high risk for these complications.
- **Systemic ET contraindicated in any woman with a uterus (must use HT)**

Assessment of the Risk–Benefit Ratio
- **Women's Health Initiative (WHI):** RCT evaluating effects of HT. Women w/ primary CV event had a mean age of 63–64 y & >10 postmenopausal years.
- In a secondary analysis of WHI data: Women aged 50–59 in ET arm had statistically signif reduction in CV endpoints (MI, coronary artery revascularization, & coronary death)

Women's Health Initiative (WHI): Main outcome of HT			
Event	**Relative risk (95% CI)**	**Increased absolute risk per 10 K/persons/y**	**Increased absolute benefit per 10 K persons/y**
CV event (MI)	1.29	7	
Stroke	1.41	8	
Thromboembolism	2.13	18	
Breast cancer	1.26	8	
Colorectal cancer	0.63		6
Hip fracture	0.66		5
Global index	1.15		

Derived from Anderson GL, Limacher M, Assaf AR, et al. Effects of conjugated equine estrogen in postmenopausal women with hysterectomy: The Women's Health Initiative randomized controlled trial. *JAMA*. 2004;291(14):1701–12.

Treatment and Medications
- **HT:** Systemic ET is most effective rx for mod–sev VS; only therapy approved by the FDA for this indication (↓ 75% symptom).
- HT should be guided by use of smallest doses & shortest duration for symptomatic relief.

- **Duration of HT:** Short-term therapy recommended (≤2–3 y). Reassess need annually.
- **Discontinuation of HT:** ~55% of women have recurrence of sx w/ abrupt cessation (*JAMA* 2004;291(14):1701). Taper may not avoid sx recurrence. If recurrent hot flashes try nonhormonal medication. If ineffective, reassess risk:benefit of restarting HT

Hormone therapy regimens			
Treatment	**Dosage/regimen**	**Evidence of benefit**	**FDA approved**
Estrogen-alone or combined with Progestin (Oral MDPA, Progestin IUD in all women with a uterus)			
• Standard dose	Conjugated estrogen 0.625 mg/d	Yes	Yes
	Micronized Estradiol-17ß 1 mg/d	Yes	Yes
	Transdermal estradiol-17b 0.0375–0.05 mg/d	Yes	Yes
• Low dose	Conjugated estrogen 0.3–0.45 mg/d	Yes	Yes
	Micronized estradiol-17b 0.5 mg/d	Yes	Yes
	Transdermal estradiol-17b 0.025 mg/d	Yes	Yes
• Ultralow dose	Micronized estradiol-17b 0.25 mg/d	Mixed	No
	Transdermal estradiol-17b 0.014 mg/d	Mixed	No
Estrogen combined with estrogen agonist/antagonist	Conjugated estrogen 0.45 mg/d and bazedoxifene 20 mg/d	Yes	Yes
Progestin	Depot medroxyprogesterone acetate	Yes	No
Tibolone	2.5 mg/d	Yes	No
Testosterone	Not recommended	No	No
Compounded bioidentical hormones	Not recommended	No	No

From *Obstet Gynecol* 2014;123:202.

PREGNANCY TERMINATION

Epidemiology (*Obstet Gynecol* 2013;121:1394)
- In 2008, 1.2 million abortions occurred in the United States
- 6.2% at 13–15 w GA, 4.0% at ≥16 w, 1.3% at ≥21 w
- Legal upper limit gestational age for abortion varies by state
- US physicians must comply w/ the federal Partial-Birth Abortion Ban Act of 2003: Bans abortions wherein the physician deliberately delivers a living fetus vaginally to the point at which any part of the fetal trunk above the navel is outside the woman's body

Medical Abortion (*Am J Obstet Gynecol* 2003;188(3):664; *Obstet Gynecol* 2014;123:676)
- Utilizes an established medication regimen to induce an abortion up to 63 d of EGA
- 6% of all abortions in US are medication
- Surgical completion of abortion required in case of failure d/t teratogenicity of misoprostol
- **First trimester regimens:** See table below
- **Second Trimester Regimens:** Mifepristone & misoprostol fastest/most effective (mean 6–11 h for completion). Misoprostol alone (mean 9–20 h for completion). Oxytocin-alone regimen only recommended if misoprostol and mifepristone are not available.

Protocols for medical management of pregnancy termination in 1st Trimester			
Common regimens	**EGA**	**Success**	**% of continuing Preg**
Mifepristone 600 mg, misoprostol 400 µg PO 36–48 h later (FDA-approved regimen)	49 d	92%	<1% fail if initiated <49 d; 49% aborted w/i 4 h, 75% w/i 24 h

Common regimens	EGA	Success	% of continuing Preg
Mifepristone 200 mg PO, misoprostol, 800 µg vaginally/buccally/SL 24–48 h later (evidence-based, preferred regimen). More effective, fewer adverse effects, more convenient)	63 d	95–99%	<1% fail if initiated <49 d, 2% if 49–63 d
Methotrexate, 50 mg/m² IM or 50 mg vaginally & misoprostol 800 µg vaginally 3–7 d later	49 d	92–96%	May require up to 4 w for complete abortion to occur, <1% fail if initiated <49 d
Misoprostol, 800 µg vaginally repeated up to 3 dose q3–24h	63 d	88%	<1% if initiated <49 d. 4–10% is 49–72 d

From *Obstet Gynecol* 2014;123:676.

Contraindications to medical abortion	
Avoid medical termination in the following pts	
Contraindications to mifepristone	Confirmed or suspected ectopic Preg, undiagnosed adnexal mass, IUD in situ, current long-term systemic Cort rx, chronic adrenal failure, sev anemia, known coagulopathy or anticoagulant rx, mifepristone intolerance or allergy
Relative contraindications to mifepristone	Severe liver, renal, respiratory dz, uncontrolled HTN, CVD, or severe anemia
Contraindications to misoprostol	Uncontrolled sz d/o or those who have an allergy or intolerance to misoprostol
Other factors	Pt is able to follow up to confirm successful termination, are anxious for completion of abortion, are able to f/u, no language or comprehension barriers to counseling, IUP w/ GA confirmed, hemodynamically stable

From *Obstet Gynecol* 2014;123:676.

Surgical Terminations (*Obstet Gynecol* 2013;121:1394)
- Universal preop antibiotic ppx is effective & inexpensive (↓ 42% decreased risk of postabortal infxn): Doxycycline 100 mg PO 1 h preop & 200 mg PO dose postop.
- Unsensitized Rh negative women should receive Rho(D) Ig w/i 72 h postabortion. 50 µg dose at <13 w GA & 300 µg dose >13 w GA.
- Immediate contraceptive initiation w/ long-acting reversible contraceptives may ↑ contraceptive use, improve continuation, reduce repeat pregnancy, & repeat abortion
- **Potential complications:** Immediate (intraoperatively or in recovery room) or delayed (up to 2 w postop): Retained products of conception, hemorrhage, uterine injury: Cervical tears, uterine perforation, syncope, thromboembolic & cardiorespiratory disorders. Delayed complications also include infxn, persistent intrauterine or ectopic Preg.
- Complication rate lower than induction of labor in 2nd trimester
- **D&C:** Most commonly performed for 7–13 w GA. By convention D&C = <14 w Manual vacuum aspiration – use at <10 w EGA, 60 mmHg suction Electric vacuum aspiration – for all GAs, 60 mmHg suction
- **D&E:** By convention, D&E = >14 w EGA. Mechanically dilate uterine cervix (laminaria, Dilapan, misoprostol, surgical dilators), permitting evacuation of fetal & placental tissue using forceps and vacuum aspirator

ADNEXAL MASSES

Epidemiology (*Obstet Gynecol* 2007;110:201)
- Most adnexal masses are benign
- In the United States, women have 5–10% lifetime risk of undergoing surgery for adnexal mass
- 1.3% of women will be diagnosed with ovarian cancer in their lifetime, most commonly between the ages of 55–64 yo
- Simple cysts ≤10 cm have essentially 0 risk of malignancy even in postmenopausal women

Pathology and Etiology (Obstet Gynecol 2007;110:201)
- **Acute conditions:** Ectopic pregnancy, Ovarian torsion, Tubo-ovarian abscess
- **Functional Cysts:** Premenopausal women – associated with ovulation. Postmenopausal women – induced by high levels of gonadotropins in early menopause. At risk for hemorrhage. Simple, hypoechoic appearance on ultrasound
- **Endometriomas:** Often a/w endometriosis sx. Homogeneous "ground glass" appearance
- **Cystadenomas:** Benign ovarian neoplasm. Serous and mucinous subtypes. Do not spontaneously regress
- **Serous:** Usually >10 cm. Similar US appearance to functional cysts. 10% bilateral
- **Mucinous:** Up to 50 cm. Unilateral. Often multiloculated with variable echogenicity on US
- **Dermoid (Mature teratoma):** 15–25% bilateral. At risk for torsion, rupture. 1–3% risk of malignant transformation. On imaging – calcifications, fat densities, hyperechoic areas
- **Fibromas:** Solid tumor of connective tissue origin. Often misdiagnosed as myoma on imaging. Histology – stellate or spindle-shaped cells in fusiform pattern. No malignant potential
- **Brenner Tumors:** Grossly identical to fibroma. Histology- hyperplastic fibromatous matrix interspersed with nests of epithelioid cells ("coffee bean" pattern)

Clinical Manifestations
- Patients may present with pain (torsion, hemorrhagic cyst), bulk symptoms (large masses), or as an incidental finding
- Symptoms concerning for malignancy: Weight loss, bloating, ↑ abdominal girth, early satiety

Diagnostic Workup/Studies (Obstet Gynecol 2007;110:201)
- Goal of workup is to rule out malignancy
- History, Physical exam
- Family history: Hx of breast, high grade serous ovarian, prostate, pancreatic cancers and melanoma could suggest BRCA mutation (Lifetime risk of ovarian cancer 40%) (BRCA1 mutation), 12% (BRCA2 mutation). Hx of colon & endometrial cancers could suggest Lynch syndrome (Lifetime risk of ovarian cancer up to 24%) (AJOG 2017;4:1)
- **Imaging:** Pelvic US = 1st-line imaging. Imaging features concerning for malignancy: Size >10 cm, papillary or solid components, irregularity, increased blood flow, ascites. Simple cysts up to 10 cm on TV US are likely benign and can be monitored. CT & MRI can be useful for very large masses (Obstet Gynecol 2016;128:e126).
- **Serum Biomarkers:** CA-125, ß-hCG, AFP, LDH useful to help differentiate malignant/benign. Multiple scoring systems available for risk assessment (MIA, ROMA, RMI). OVA1 test FDA approved serum test to assess risk of malignancy.

Abnormal threshold for serum biomarker and multimodal test in women with adnexal masses		
Test	**Premenopausal**	**Postmenopausal**
CA 125	No validated threshold	>35 U/mL
MIA (Multivariate Index Assay)	≥5.0	≥4.4
ROMA (Risk of Ovarian Malignancy)	≥1.31	≥2.77
RMI (Risk of Malignancy Index)	>200	>200

From Obstet Gynecol 2016;128:e126.

Serum biomarkers in ovarian germ cell tumors				
	β-hCG	**AFP**	**LDH**	**CA 125**
Dysgerminoma	+	–	+	–
Endodermal Sinus Tumor	–	+	–	–
Choriocarcinoma	+	–	–	–
Immature Teratoma	–	+	+	+
Embryonal Carcinoma	+	+	–	–

From Obstet Gynecol 2016;128:e126. See also table in Gyn Oncology chapter.

Treatment
- **Expectant management:** Appropriate for benign etiology requiring no f/u (eg functional cyst in premenopausal woman)

- **Continued surveillance:** Appropriate when suspicion for malignancy is low.
  Includes postmenopausal women with simple cysts <10 cm. Most adnexal masses
  fall into this category.
  - No clear guidelines for frequency/duration of surveillance. Per expert opinion,
    repeat imaging every 3–6 mo. Observe stable masses w/o solid components
    for 1 y; stable masses w/ solid components for 2 y.
- **Surgery:** Appropriate if symptomatic, suspected torsion, large suspected
  endometriomas or teratomas. If suspicious for malignancy, refer to Gynecologic
  Oncology for surgical removal
  - Minimally invasive approach preferred in presumed benign adnexal masses
  - Attempt cystectomy rather than oophorectomy in premenopausal women for
    fertility preservation

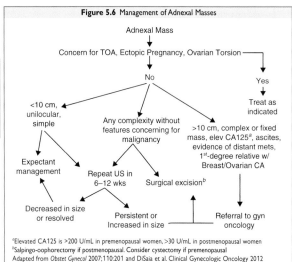

Figure 5.6 Management of Adnexal Masses

[a]Elevated CA125 is >200 U/mL in premenopausal women, >30 U/mL in postmenopausal women
[b]Salpingo-oophorectomy if postmenopausal. Consider cystectomy if premenopausal
Adapted from *Obstet Gynecol* 2007;110:201 and DiSaia et al. Clinical Gynecologic Oncology 2012

Definition
- **Puberty:** Nml physiologic transition from childhood to reproductive & sexual maturity
- **Adrenarche:** Onset of increased adrenal androgen production, leads to pubarche
- **Gonadarche:** Pulsatile GnRH secretion & activation of HPO axis
- **Thelarche:** Onset of, breast dev
- **Pubarche:** Onset of pubic & axillary hair dev
- **Peak Height Velocity (PHV):** Growth spurt characterized by acceleration in growth rate age 9–10, leading to PHV around age 11–12
- **Menarche:** Onset of menstruation (often from effect of E2 on endometrium, no ovulation)

Physiology
- Requires intact HPO axis. Re-emergence of GnRH secretion → ↑ LH ↑ FSH → gonadal maturation & sex-steroid production.
- 20% pubarche precedes thelarche (esp AA). Avg time from thelarche → menarche, 2 y.

Sequence of puberty in girls				
Sequence	Thelarche →	Pubarche →	PHV →	Menarche
Age* AA	9.5	9.5	10.8	12.1
Age H	9.8	10.3	—	12.2
Age C	10.3	10.5	11.5	12.7

*Mean age in years at indicated stage.
AA, African American; H, Hispanic; C, Caucasian; PHV, Peak height velocity.
Data from *J Pediatr* 2006;148:234; *Pediatrics* 2002;110:911; *Stat Med* 1993;12:403.

Tanner stages		
Stage	Breast dev	Pubic hair
1	Prepubertal: Papilla elevation only	Prepubertal: None
2	Breast bud: Elevation of breast & papilla; enlargement of areola	Sparse, long, slightly pigmented hair on labia majora
3	Further enlargement of breast & areola; no separation of contour	Dark, coarse, curled hair, spreading sparsely over mons
4	Areola & papilla form secondary mound above level of breast	Adult-type hair, abundant, limited to mons
5	Projection of papilla only, recession of areola to contour of breast	Adult-type hair, distribution to the medial thigh

Data from *J Pediatr* 2006;148:234; *Pediatrics* 2002;110:911; *Stat Med* 1993;12:403.

Figure 6.1 Tanner staging, female developmental stages

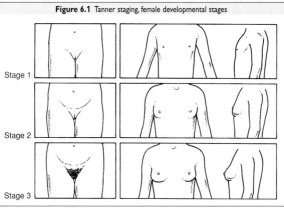

Stage 1

Stage 2

Stage 3

(continued)

Figure 6.1 (Continued)

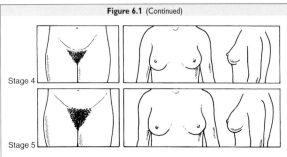

Stage 4

Stage 5

(Modified from Strasburger VC, Brown RT. *Adolescent Medicine: A Practical Guide*. Boston, MA: Little, Brown & Co.; 1991:4.)

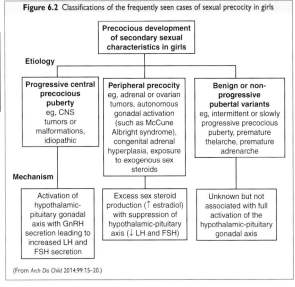

Figure 6.2 Classifications of the frequently seen cases of sexual precocity in girls

Precocious development of secondary sexual characteristics in girls

Etiology

Progressive central precocious puberty
eg, CNS tumors or malformations, idiopathic

Peripheral precocity
eg, adrenal or ovarian tumors, autonomous gonadal activation (such as McCune Albright syndrome), congenital adrenal hyperplasia, exposure to exogenous sex steroids

Benign or non-progressive pubertal variants
eg, intermittent or slowly progressive precocious puberty, premature thelarche, premature adrenarche

Mechanism

Activation of hypothalamic-pituitary gonadal axis with GnRH secretion leading to increased LH and FSH secretion

Excess sex steroid production (↑ estradiol) with suppression of hypothalamic-pituitary axis (↓ LH and FSH)

Unknown but not associated with full activation of the hypothalamic-pituitary gonadal axis

(From *Arch Dis Child* 2014;99:15–20.)

PRECOCIOUS PUBERTY

Definition (*N Engl J Med* 2008;358:2366)
- Dev of breast or pubic hair >2–2.5 SD below mean age. Traditional definition <8 yo. Trend of decreasing age of puberty → now <7 yo in C girls, <6 y in AA girls (*Pediatrics* 1997;99:505; *Pediatrics* 1999;104:936).

Initial Workup
- **Hx:** Onset, family members' ages of puberty, h/o neurologic dz or trauma, exposure to sex steroids, headache, seizures, changes in vision, abdominal pain
- **PE:** Height, weight, growth chart, Tanner staging, fundoscopic exam (papilledema in ↑ intracranial pres), visual field eval (sellar mass lesion), skin exam

- **Bone age eval:** Plain film x-ray of left hand & wrist
- **Lab eval:** Basal LH, LH following GnRH stimulation, FSH, estradiol *(Arch Dis Child 2014;99(1):15–20)*
  LH <0.2 IU/L = premature thelarche or nml
  LH 0.2–0.3 IU/L = true precocious puberty
  LH <5 mIU/L = central (gonadotropin-dependent) precocious puberty

Treatment Goals
- Postpone dev until nml pubertal age, maximize adult height, reduce risk of psychosocial problems w/ early sexual maturation *(Pediatrics 2009;123(4):e752)*

Gonadotropin-*dependent* (Central) Precocious Puberty (GDPP)
- Early maturation of HPO axis with GnRH secretion → LH and FSH secretion → breast & pubic hair dev, w/ usually nml sequence of pubertal events at nml pace, & isosexual (appropriate for gender); pathologic in 10–20% of cases
- **Etiology:** Idiopathic – 90%; dx of exclusion. CNS lesions – tumors, irradiation, hydrocephalus, cysts, trauma, inflamm dz, midline developmental defects. Sev hypothyroidism, specific genetic mutations, sex steroid exposure (repeated exposure to sex steroids from periph sources can induce secondary premature maturation of HPO axis)
- **Dx:** Accelerated linear growth for age (>75% of height at dx), advanced bone age, pubertal levels of FSH, LH, estradiol, ↑ w/ GnRH stimulation test. MRI in all pts to evaluate for CNS lesion. TFTs if clinical concern for hypothyroidism. Evaluate ↓ growth hormone if h/o cranial irradiation. Abdominopelvic US (eval ovarian and uterine vol)
- **Rx:** Treat intracranial lesions or hypothyroidism if present. Idiopathic GDPP, treat if:
  Sexual maturation progresses to next stage w/i 3–6 mo, onset puberty <6 yo, growth velocity <6 cm/y, bone age advanced by 1 y or more, or predicted adult height below target range or decreasing on serial determinations.
  Long-acting GnRH agonist → prepubertal hormone level, prevents pubertal dev, growth acceleration, & bone advancement *(Pediatrics 2009;123(4):e752; N Engl J Med 1981; 305:1546)*. Treat until epiphyses fused or pubertal & chrono ages are appropriately matched. Anticipate return of puberty within 1 y. Monitor q3–6mo

Gonadotropin-*independent* (Peripheral) Precocious Puberty
- Due to excess exposure of sex steroid hormones from gonads, adrenals, or environment. May be contrasexual or isosexual. Pubertal sequence progression may be altered.
- **Etiology:** Functional ovarian follicular cysts – most common cause, w/ transient breast dev & vaginal bleeding 2/2 estrogen withdrawal when cyst regressed, 1+ unilateral or bilateral ovarian cysts >15 mm, bone age nml. Ovarian tumors (rare) – granulosa cell tumor → isosexual, Leydig cell/gonadoblastoma → contrasexual. Adrenal – androgen-secreting tumors, CAH. McCune–Albright syndrome (rare) – triad of periph precocious puberty, café-au-lait spots, fibrous bone dysplasia → recurrent formation of follicular cysts & cyclic vaginal bleeding.
- **Dx:** Low or nml FSH & LH levels, do not ↑ w/ GnRH stimulation. Labs: Testosterone, estradiol, FSH, afternoon cortisol (screen Cushing syn), DHEA, DHEAS, 17-OHP (screen CAH). Abdominopelvic US for ovarian cyst/tumor.
- **Rxs:** Surgical removal (tumor); tamoxifen (SERM) for vaginal bleeding, bisphosphonate for bone dysplasia; aromatase inhibs lack long-term effectiveness; exogenous estrogens as cream, ointment, spray (contrasexual); remove exogenous source; for functional cysts → observation, usually self-limited, surgical removal if persistent or torsion; GnRH agonist ineffective for gonadotropin independent.

Isolated Precocious Puberty
- Isolated premature thelarche or adrenarche with nml bone age suggest Isolated PP. Usually benign nml variants.
- Expectant mgmt w/ re-evaluation at 6 mo. ~20% progress to gonadotropin-dependent precocious puberty. Requires regular exams.
- **Isolated premature thelarche:** Unilateral or bilateral, <8 y, absence of other secondary sexual characteristics, nml linear growth, nml bone age. Estradiol level usually prepubertal – girls typically <3 yo, nonobese. Unk cause.
- **Isolated premature adrenarche:** Isolated pubic &/or axillary hair <8 y. Dx: DHEA-S appropriate for pubic hair stage. Girls typically overweight. 17-OHP & testosterone appropriate for age. Bone age & growth rate ↑ but w/i nml limits. Risk factor for PCOS. Further w/u: ACTH stimulation to r/o CAH when bone age advanced, predicted adult height abnormally low, or serum testosterone & DHEA-S elevated – may be only manifestation of mild CAH.

Rx: Observation, regular exams to detect other signs of precocious sexual dev

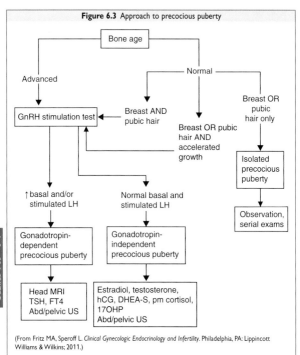

Figure 6.3 Approach to precocious puberty

(From Fritz MA, Speroff L. *Clinical Gynecologic Endocrinology and Infertility*. Philadelphia, PA: Lippincott Williams & Wilkins; 2011.)

DELAYED PUBERTY

Definition (*N Engl J Med* 2012;366:443; *Pediatr Clin North Am* 2011;58:1181)
• Absence of secondary sexual characteristics by age 13 (≥2 SD from mean age), or absence of menses by age 15

Etiology (*J Clin Endocrinol Metab* 2002;87:1613)
• 30% constitutional delay, 26% hypergonadotropic hypogonadism (primary gonadal insufficiency), 20% permanent hypogonadotropic hypogonadism, 19% transient (functional) hypogonadotropic hypogonadism, 5% other causes

Clinical Manifestations
• **Hx:** Anorexia, bulimia, excessive exercise, chronic dzs (eg, celiac dz, Crohns dz), radiation, chemo, meds, nutritional status, psychosocial functioning
• **Sx:** Neurologic sx, inability to smell, headache, weight gain or loss, chronic dz
• **FHx:** Relatives w/ delayed puberty, heights of relatives, age of menarche & fertility status of female relatives, relatives w/ genetic abnormalities (CAH, adenocarcinoma in situ [AIS], gonadal dysgenesis), relatives w/ autoimmune dz

Physical Exam
• Height & weight measurements, growth chart, Tanner staging, examine for stigmata of Turner syn, midline facial defects, scoliosis, thyromegaly
• Arm span greater than height >5 cm sugg delayed epiphyseal closure (2/2 hypogonadism)
• **Neurologic exam:** Optic fundi, cranial nerves, visual fields, sense of smell
• **Pelvic exam:** Clitoral enlargement, hymenal ring patency, degree of vaginal rugation, presence or absence of mucus (indicates degree of estrogen effect), presence of uterus

Workup
- Hx, physical exam, bone age x-ray, labs (LH, FSH, E2)
  Elevated FSH/LH = hypergonadotropic hypogonadism
  Low FSH/LH = hypogonadotropic hypogonadism
- Further w/u if LH, FSH nml:
  PRL – screen for hyperprolactinemia
  TSH, FT4 – screen for thyroid dzs
  MRI – when si/sx CNS lesion present or if indicated by other eval (hyperprolactinemia, Kallmann syn); otherwise may defer until age 15
  CBC, ESR, LFTs – screen chronic dzs (IBD, liver dz, anorexia)
  Pelvic US – determine presence/absence uterus if undetermined by physical exam or ovarian mass
- Usually no apparent alternate cause on initial eval – const del likely dx; no test can reliably differentiate const del from hypogonadotropic hypogonadism; therefore, observe & diagnose isolated hypogonadotropic hypogonadism if endogenous puberty has not begun by age 18; eventual nml progression of puberty confirms const del.

Treatment Goals
- Induce appearance of secondary sexual characteristics or acceleration of growth to mitigate pubertal delay & short stature, & promote nml bone mass
- Predict adult height w/ Bayley–Pinneau tables, although overestimate adult height in const del

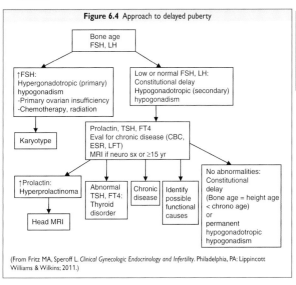

Figure 6.4 Approach to delayed puberty

(From Fritz MA, Speroff L. *Clinical Gynecologic Endocrinology and Infertility.* Philadelphia, PA: Lippincott Williams & Wilkins; 2011.)

Hypergonadotropic (Primary) Hypogonadism
- **Dx:** Elevated LH & FSH due to lack of negative feedback from gonads. Additional w/u: Karyotype, autoimmune dz eval.
- **Etiology:** Primary ovarian insufficiency (idiopathic, resistant ovary syn, autoimmune oophoritis, 17a-hydroxylase deficiency, galactosemia, aromatase deficiency), Gonadal dysgenesis from genetic causes (45, X; 46, XX; 46, XY), ovarian toxins (radiation, chemo, mumps)
  Turner syn: 45X (*Semin Reprod Med* 2011;29:342) – phenotype: Female, short stature, ptosis, low-set ears, micrognathia, short "webbed" neck, broad shield-like chest, hypoplastic areolae, short 4th/5th metacarpals, renal abnormalities (eg, horse-shoe kidney), cardiovascular abnormalities (eg, coarct of the aorta). Risk of aortic dissection & rupture (1.5%). "Streak" gonads consist of fibrous tissue w/o germ

cells. External female genitalia, uterus, fallopian tubes develop normally until
puberty when estrogen-induced maturation fails to occur. 1 in 2,500 live births.
Menstruation & Preg may occur in mosaic karyotype (45, X/46, XX).
Rx: Growth hormone prior to estrogen initiation
Swyer syn: 46, XY complete gonadal dysgenesis. Phenotype: Female, w/ vagina, cervix,
uterus, fallopian tubes, & external genitalia.
Rx: Requires early gonadectomy due to risk of gonadal tumors
Primary ovarian insufficiency: See Chap. 8 (page 8-1).

Permanent Hypogonadotropic (Secondary) Hypogonadism

- **Dx:** Low to nml LH & FSH due to hypothalamic or pituitary disorders
- **Etiology:** GnRH deficiency, CAH, CNS tumors, combined pituitary hormone deficiency,
  chemo, radiation
  Kallmann syn: Anosmia or hyposmia; 1/50,000 females
- **Further w/u:** MRI
- **Rx:** Initial low-dose estrogen titrated to mimic nml puberty to initiate sexual maturation
  After 6–9 mo, cyclic progesterone to induce endometrial shedding
  Transition to combination OCP when breast dev optimized for hormonal replacement
  If fertility desired, pulsatile GnRH or injectable gonadotropin

Transient (Functional) Hypogonadotropic Hypogonadism

- **Dx:** Low LH & FSH due to delayed maturation of HPO axis due to underlying
  condition
- **Etiology:** Systemic illness (IBD, celiac dz, anorexia nervosa or bulimia, hypothyroidism,
  hyperprolactinemia, DM, Cushing dz), CNS disorders (tumors [eg, craniopharyngioma,
  prolactinoma], infxn, trauma), adrenal (Cushing syn, Addison dz), psychosocial
  (excessive exercise, stress, depression), drugs (marijuana)
- **Rx:** Treat underlying cause (treat dz or modify behavior)
- **Const Del:**
  Dx: Low LH & FSH, HA = bone age < chrono age. Adrenarche & gonadarche often
  later than avg; isolated hypogonadotropic hypogonadism has adrenarche at nml age.
  Rx: Expectant observation. If puberty has started (clinically or biochemically) &
  stature not a major concern, reassurance w/ adult height prediction.
  Hormone rx is controversial (goal of preventing developmental psychosocial
  stress). Use low-dose estrogen until puberty progresses, then stop. Progesterone
  not needed as similar long period of unopposed estrogen in early puberty.
  Growth hormone, anabolic steroids, aromatase inhibs not recommended.

AMENORRHEA

Definitions (Ann N Y Acad Sci 2010;1205:23–32; Pediatrics 2006;118:2245; Obstet Gynecol Clin North Am
2003;30:287)

- **Primary amenorrhea:** Absence of menstruation by age 13–14 in absence of
  growth or sexual dev, or age 15–16 in presence of nml growth & sexual dev
- **Secondary amenorrhea:** Absence of menses for ≥3 consecutive menstrual cycles
  in women w/ previously nml menses

Epidemiology

- Primary amenorrhea 1–2% prevalence in US. Amenorrhea not caused by Preg ≤5%
  prevalence during menstrual lives. Most common causes of primary amenorrhea:
  Ovarian failure (48.5%), Müllerian agenesis (16.2%), gonadotropin deficiency (8.3%),
  constitutional delay (6%) (Am J Obstet Gynecol 1981;140:372).

History

- **Hx:** Stress, change in weight, diet, exercise, eating disorder, sugg functional hypothalamic
  etiology
  New meds – evaluate for hyperprolactinemia due to meds (OCPs, danazol, high-dose
  progestin, reglan, antipsychotic drugs)
  New illnesses – sugg chronic illness etiology
  Acne, hirsutism, deepening of voice – sugg hyperandrogenism: PCOS or adrenal
  etiology
  Headache, visual field defects, fatigue, polyuria, polydipsia – sugg CNS lesion
  Hot flashes, vaginal dryness, poor sleep, decreased libido – sugg primary ovarian
  insufficiency
  Galactorrhea – sugg hyperprolactinemia
  H/o postpartum hemorrhage, D&C, endometritis – sugg Asherman or Sheehan syn

Physical exam
- Height, weight (BMI <18.5 at risk for functional hypothalamic amenorrhea; BMI >30 in ~50% pt w/ PCOS).
- Tanner staging if primary amenorrhea. Assess estrogen status: Adequate if breasts present, moist & rugated vaginal mucosa, abundant cervical mucus.
- Assess for presence of uterus, cervix, or signs of obstructed tract
- Assess for signs of excessive testosterone: Hirsutism, acne, acanthosis nigricans
- Evaluate for galactorrhea
- Parotid gland swelling &/or erosion of dental enamel sugg bulimia nervosa
- Evaluate for stigmata of Turner syn

Initial Workup
- History & physical exam. Lab: Urine hCG, TSH, FSH, PRL (↑ by stress, sleep, intercourse, meals, nipple stimulation). If signs of hyperandrogenism: Testosterone, ±17-OHP (CAH), DHEA-S (adrenal etiology). Low E2 + high FSH → POI
- **Progesterone challenge test:** Determine if adequate estrogen present, competent endometrium, patent outflow. Medroxyprogesterone acetate 10 mg PO daily for 7–10 d.
- Withdrawal bleed expected w/i 2–7 d of stopping progesterone:
  - **+ Bleed:** Nml estrogen production & ovarian fxn
  - **− Bleed:** Hypoestrogenic or anatomic outflow tract obst

Etiologies of amenorrhea	
Anatomic defects: Lack of uterus or obstructed outflow 20% of 1° amenorrhea 5% of 2° amenorrhea	Imperforate hymen Transverse vaginal septum Müllerian anomalies AIS Cervical stenosis Asherman syn

Ovarian dysfxn: Ovarian follicles depleted or resistant to stimulation by FSH & LH
50% of 1° amenorrhea
40% of 2° amenorrhea
	Primary ovarian insufficiency (premature ovarian failure)
	Idiopathic
	Resistant ovary
	Chemo, radiation
	Gonadal dysgenesis
	    Turner syn (45,X)
	    X chromo long-arm deletion (46,XXq5)
	    46,XX; 46,XY (Swyer syn)
	Gonadal agenesis
	Autoimmune oophoritis/ovarian failure

Pituitary: Abn FSH/LH production 5% of 1° amenorrhea 19% of 2° amenorrhea	Prolactinoma Other pituitary tumors: Corticotroph adenoma Other tumors: Meningioma, germinoma, glioma Empty sella syn Infarction (Sheehan syn) Radiation Infiltrative lesions: Hemochromatosis, histiocytosis

Hypothalamic: Disruption of pulsatile release of GnRH
20% of 1° amenorrhea
35% of 2° amenorrhea
	GnRH deficiency: Congenital, Kallmann Syndrome
	Functional hypothalamic amenorrhea: Weight loss, excessive exercise, obesity, stress
	    Drugs: Marijuana, tranquilizers
	    Psychogenic: Anxiety, pseudocyesis, anorexia
	Neoplastic: Craniopharyngioma, hamartoma, germinoma, teratoma, metastases
	Brain injury, irradiation
	Infxn: TB, syphilis, meningitis
	Infiltrative dzs: Histiocytosis, hemochromatosis, sarcoidosis, Chronic medical illness

Other endocrinopathies	Hypothyroidism, hyperthyroidism Cushing syn Late-onset adrenal hyperplasia DM Exogenous androgen use
Multifactorial	PCOS
From *Fertil Steril* 2008;90(5 suppl):S219.	

Congenital Anatomic Lesions
- Menses cannot occur w/o an intact uterus, endometrium, cervix, vaginal conduit. Clinical manifestations: Cyclic pelvic &/or lower abdominal pain from accum & subseq dilation of vaginal vault &/or uterus by menstrual bld.
- **Imperf hymen:** Bulging membrane just inside the vagina, often purple-red discoloration
- **Transverse vaginal septum:** Occurs at any level btw hymenal ring & cervix; absence of bulging hymen as septum much thicker. MRI or US to define location and thickness of the septum
- **Vaginal agenesis:** See Chap. 8.
- **Rx:** Surgical correction

Asherman Syndrome (Semin Reprod Med 2011;29:83)
- Acq scarring of the endometrial lining, usually secondary to postpartum hemorrhage or endometrial infxn followed by aggressive D&C. Prevents nml buildup & shedding of endometrial cells → very light or absent menses.
- HSG shows uterine filling defects. No withdrawal bleed following estrogen & progesterone. Hysteroscopic eval demonstrates uterine synechiae.
- **Rx:** Surgical lysis of adhesions by hysteroscopy. Estrogen postoperatively to help promote endometrial regeneration. Some evidence for intrauterine catheter placement.

Primary Ovarian Insufficiency (Premature Ovarian Failure)
See Chap. 8.

Hyperprolactinemia (Curr Opin Obstet Gynecol 2004;16:331; J Reprod Med 1999;44:1075; J Clin Endocrinol Metab 2011;96(2):273)
- **Etiology:** Hypothyroidism, PRL-secreting pituitary adenomas (20% secondary amenorrhea), pituitary or hypothalamic tumors, meds (amphetamines, benzodiazepines, metoclopramide, methyldopa, opiates, phenothiazines, reserpine, tricyclic antidepressants, SSRIs), stress. Occurs due to dopamine receptor antagonism.
- **Clinical manifestations:** ± Galactorrhea, bitemporal field loss
- **Dx:** Elevated serum PRL; r/o hyperthyroidism. Further w/u: MRI to evaluate for pituitary tumor if persistent ↑ PRL or >100 ng/mL
- **Rx:** Dopamine agonist (bromocriptine or cabergoline) or transsphenoidal resxn of CNS lesion

Sheehan Syndrome (Eur J Endocrinol 2014;171(3):311–8)
- Acute infarction & ischemic necrosis of pituitary gland from postpartum hemorrhage & hypovolemic hypotension (requiring multiple pRBC transfusion). More common in low resource settings. Damage to pituitary can be mild or severe, can affect one or more of its hormones
- **Clinical manifestations:** Failed postpartum lactation, fatigue, weight loss, loss of sexual hair. Mean delay in diagnosing syndrome: 20 y.
- **Dx:** Hx, growth hormone, LH, FSH, PRL, ACTH, TSH deficiencies, rare development of diabetes insipidus

Functional Hypothalamic Amenorrhea (N Engl J Med 2010;363:365)
- Abn GnRH pulses → decreased gonadotropin pulsations → low/nml serum LH concentrations → absent LH surge → absence of follicular dev, anovulation, low estradiol
- **Etiology:** Stress, weight change, undernutrition, excessive exercise, anorexia nervosa or bulimia, chronic dz (DM, ESRD, malig, AIDS, malabsorption, IBD), isolated gonadotropin deficiency (Congenital, Kallmann Syndrome), Sheehan syn
- **W/u:** MRI for CNS/hypothalamic/pituitary dz
- **Rx:** Behavior modification if indicated, treat chronic dz, hormonal therapy to prevent bone loss, ovulation induction w/ clomiphene citrate, gonadotropin injection, pulsatile GnRH

Polycystic Ovarian Syndrome (PCOS)
See Chap. 8.

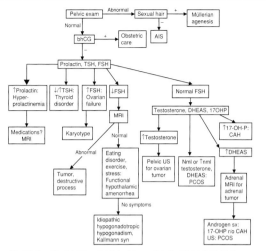

Figure 6.5 Approach to amenorrhea

(From Fritz MA, Speroff L. *Clinical Gynecologic Endocrinology and Infertility.* Philadelphia, PA: Lippincott Williams & Wilkins; 2011.)

ANDROGEN INSENSITIVITY SYNDROME

Definition and Epidemiology (*J Pediatrc Surg* 2005;40:133; *J Clin Endocrinol Metab* 2001;86:4151; Pediatric Disorders of Sex Development. Williams Textbook of Endocrinology, Ac)

- Complete androgen insensitivity syndrome (CAIS, formally called complete testicular feminization)

  Male pseudohermaphrodism from muts in AR & decreased end organ sens. 1.1% incid of CAIS in a premenarchal child w/ inguinal hernias.
- 1 in 20000–99000 individuals with 46,XY

Etiology

- 70% of AR muts are X-linked recessive leading to decreased resp to androgens; 30% de novo sporadic muts. Multi syns.

	Androgen abnormality/insensitivity syndromes				
	Complete	**Incomplete**	**Reifenstein**	**Infertile**	**5α-reductase**
Inheritance pattern	X-linked recessive	X-linked recessive	X-linked recessive	X-linked recessive	Autosomal recessive
Spermatogenesis	–	–	–	↓	↓
Müllerian structures	–	–	–	–	–
Wolffian structures	–	♂	♂	♂	♂
External genitalia	♀	♀ – Clitoromegaly Partial labioscrotal fusion	♂ – Hypospadias	♂	♀
Breasts	♀	♀	Gynecomastia	Gynecomastia	♂

Data from Griffin JE. Androgen resistance—the clinical and molecular spectrum. *N Eng J Med* 1992;326:611–618; Kim HH, Laufer MR. Developmental abnormalities of the female reproductive tract. *Curr Opin Obstet Gynecol* 1994;6:518–525.

Pathophysiology

- Nml male dev only occur if adequate androgen production acting on target tissues (sex differentiation). Muts in AR leads to a defective resp to androgens at all stages of dev. Production of testosterone occurs at ~8–16 w via placental hCG; after 16 w, fetal LH controls circulating androgens.
- Testosterone (produced by Leydig cells in testes) is responsible for Wolffian dev & formation of the epididymis, vas deferens, & seminal vesicles. DHT is responsible for formation of male external genitalia & fusion of labioscrotal folds. Androgens control descent of testes into scrotum → in AIS, testes remain in pelvis.
- Androgens → secondary male sex characteristics at puberty (axillary & pubic hair) & spermatogenesis. MIS is produced normally by Sertoli cells in testes causing regression of Müllerian ducts → no uterus, oviducts, & upper vagina.

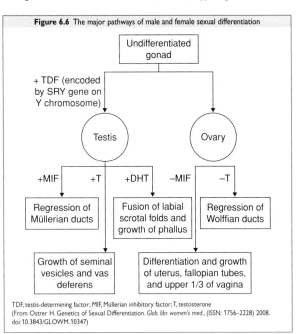

Figure 6.6 The major pathways of male and female sexual differentiation

TDF, testis-determining factor; MIF, Müllerian inhibitory factor; T, testosterone
(From Oster H. Genetics of Sexual Differentiation. *Glob. libr. women's med.*, (ISSN: 1756–2228) 2008. doi:10.3843/GLOWM.10347)

Clinical Manifestations

- Karyotype 46,XY
- Male pseudohermaphroditism: Variety of phenotypes ranging from male infertility to nml female external genitalia. May present w/ ambiguous genitalia or infantile male genitalia. + MIS → short vagina, absent uterus, & cervix.
- Primary amenorrhea/infertility
- **CAIS:** No activity at the AR → nml female phenotype. Nml breast dev w/ pale areola (estrogens produced by testes & circulating androgens fail to antagonize estrogens). Sparse or absent pubic & axillary hair (vellus hair only, if present). Absent uterus. Nml or slightly advanced height, however decreased bone density. 50% w/ inguinal hernias: Gonads (testes) intra-abdominal or in the inguinal rings. Serum testosterone in the range of pubertal male. No issues regarding gender identity or sexual preference given they are not exposed to male androgen levels → brain dev along w/ physical dev is female.
- **PAIS:** Varying degrees of virilization: Due to differing degrees of AR activity (predominantly male or female phenotype). Labial fusion, bifid scrotum, hypospadias, micropenis, &/or clitromegaly. Blind vas deferens. Testes in labioscrotal folds. Nml

- breasts & pubic & axillary hair. Higher rates of bisexuality, homosexuality, & gender identity d/o.
- **Mild AIS:** Phenotypic & genotypic males. Male infertility (oligospermia w/ nml T & LH). Gynecomastia in young men. Minor hypospadias.

Physical Exam
- Female infant or toddler w/ an inguinal hernia → attempt to pass a sterile Q-tip into vagina (consider exam under anesthesia in toddlers). Consider karyotype.
- Adolescent → full physical exam (note breast dev, pubic & axillary hair, & external genitalia including hymenal anatomy), rectal exam to r/o lower vaginal obst.

Diagnostic Workup/Studies
- **CAIS:** ↑ T & ↑ LH. Diff:
  MRKH syn or Müllerian agenesis; distinguish by karyotype; XX genetic females; nml testosterone; presence of pubic & axillary hair (absent in CAIS)
  Swyer syn = XY complete gonadal dysgenesis. No breast dev & short stature; XY genetic males.
- **PAIS:** Nml T & ↑ LH (*Clin Endocrinol Metab* 2006;20:577), MRI (gold std) or pelvic US to document internal anatomy, localize testes, r/o testicular tumors, genetic testing and karyotype, genetic counseling for parents.
  Differential diagnoses (DDx)
  Partial gonadal dysgenesis
  17β-Hydroxysteroid dehydrogenase deficiency
  5α-Reductase deficiency
  Mixed gonadal dysgenesis w/ mosaic Turner syn (45,XO/46,XY)
  Defect in LH receptor

Treatment
- Prophylactic gonadectomy in CAIS b/c of ↑ rate of malig degeneration & formation of dysgerminomas/gonadoblastomas after pubertal dev, then estrogen replacement
- Incid of 0.5% malig in CAIS, 5.5% in overall AIS pop; as high as 50% in PAIS if gonads in nonscrotal position (intra-abdominal location inc risk for malig). If dx prior to puberty, serial US monitoring for pelvic masses (*Acta Endocrinol* 1990;123:416; *Int J Gynecol Pathol* 1991;10:126; *J Clin Endocrinol Metab* 2005;90:5295)
  Rate of malig in pts w/ AIS prior to puberty is 0.8% (CAIS) & 5.5% (overall)
  (*Endocrine Rev* 2006;27:468; *J Pathol* 2006;208:518)
- Hormone replacement
  CAIS → Estrogen replacement during late adolescence/early adulthood to aid final Tanner 5 breast dev, help build bone, Vit D, regular weight-bearing exercise; DEXA or bisphosphonates prn
  PAIS → large doses of androgens to promote phallic growth (if phenotypically male)
- ± Vaginal dilators for increased vaginal length; d/c once regular vaginal intercourse
- ± Genital reconstructive surg when pt voices desire to proceed
- Multidisciplinary support including a mental health provider, social worker, geneticist

CONGENITAL ADRENAL HYPERPLASIA (CAH)

Definition and Epidemiology (*Ferri's Clinical Advisor* 2017;313:e2–313.e4)
- Autosomal recessive disorders of cortisol &/or aldosterone biosynthesis, result in **cortisol deficiency, ± aldosterone deficiency, & androgen excess.** There are two forms:
  - **Classic CAH** (sev form, 1/15–16000 live births)
    a. salt wasting (67%)
    b. nonsalt losing (simple virilizing; 33%)
  - **NCAH** (mild or late onset); asymptomatic or postnatal

Pathology and Pathophysiology
- Caused by a mut in cortisol producing enzymes
- ↑ Corticotrophin → adrenal hyperplasia
- ↑ Cortisol precursors which are diverted to the biosynthesis of sex hormones → androgen excess → ambiguous genitalia in newborn girls, rapid postnatal growth in both sexes
- Aldosterone deficiency → salt wasting → FTT, hyponatremic hypovolemia, shock
- HyperK
  Classic CAH – abn cortisol, sex hormone, ± aldosterone production
  NCAH – nml cortisol & aldosterone, but mild to mod ↑ sex hormones

- **Muts:**
    - **CYP21** (CYP21A2; 95% of cases; codes for adrenal 21-hydroxylase) → *CYP21* mut → **21-hydroxylase deficiency** → inadeq cortisol synthesis → inadeq negative feedback to hypothalamus & pituitary → increased ACTH secretion → adrenal gland hyperplasia. Adrenal steroids are converted to adrenal androgens.
    - **CYP11B1** mut → **11β-hydroxylase deficiency** → ↑ 11-deoxycortisol & 11-deoxycorticosterone → salt retention → hypervolemia, HTN
    - **HSD3B2** mut → 3β-hydroxysteroid dehydrogenase deficiency → sev adrenal insufficiency, ↑ ACTH → ↑ pregnenolone, 17-hydroxypregnenolone, & DHEA → mild virilization, ± salt wasting

Clinical Manifestations
- Salt-losing adrenal crisis in neonat period for 3/4ths newborns w/ classic CAH.
- **46,XX female pseudohermaphroditism:** Nml uterus, fallopian tubes & ovaries but varying levels of ambiguous genitalia depending on degree & type of enzyme deficiency
- **Ambiguous genitalia:** Classic CAH – most common cause in 46,XX, newborn ambiguous genitalia (clitoral hypertrophy, labioscrotal fusion – partial or complete, common urogenital sinus). Boys have no overt sx except hyperpigmentation & penile enlargement. NCAH – presents in adolescence; rapid growth, premature pubic or axillary hair, hirsutism.
- **Hyperandrogenism:** Hirsutism, acne, oligomenorrhea/amenorrhea, polycystic ovaries, precocious puberty
- **Infertility:** 80% women w/ simple virilizing & 60% women w/ salt-wasting CAH are fertile. A/w infertility in males *(Endocrinol Metab Clin North Am 2001;30:207)*
- Metabolic syn/insulin resistance/obesity
- **Short stature:** Untreated, long-term sex hormone exposure leads to advanced skeletal age & premature epiphyseal fusion. Mean adult height = 10 cm below nml pop.
- Issues of gender & sexuality *(Endocrinol Metab Clin North Am 2001;30:155)*
- Iatrogenic Cushing syn

Workup
- **Serum electrolytes, aldosterone, & plasma renin:** HyperK, ↓ aldosterone, hyperreninemia (use age-specific reference for renin)
- **Random 17-OHP:** >242 nmol/L (nml 3 nmol/L) at 3 d in full-term infants. False positives in premature infants. Use weight & gestational age–based reference ranges.
- **Adrenocorticotrophin (ACTH)-stimulation test:** 250 μg cosyntropin followed by measurement of 17-OHP 60 min later. 17-OHP level >10 ng/mL (30.3 nmol/L)
- **Early morning (before 08:00 h) 17-OHP:** >2.5 nmol/L in children & >6 nmol/L in women during follicular phase r/o NCAH
- Genetic analysis, neonat screening, or gene-specific prenatal dx
- Abdominal US to eval adrenal glands or uterus in cases of ambiguous genitalia

Treatment
- **Glucocorticoids** (short acting in children to avoid growth suppression). Stress dosing during febrile illness, Surg, trauma, etc. (Double or triple daily dose.)
    - *Hydrocortisone:* 12–18 mg/m² divided in 2 or 3 doses. Longer-acting glucocorticoids can be used in adults.
    - *Prednisone:* 5–7.5 mg QD in 2 doses or *dexamethasone* 0.25–0.50 mg QHS. Good in Preg (does not cross the placenta). Goal early morning 17-OHP 12–36 nmol/L.
- Mineralocorticoids to normalize electrolytes and plasma renin
    - **Fludrocortisone** 100–200 μg QD
- NaCl suppl (salt-losing CAH) 1st 6–12 mo of life
- Infertility → ovulation induction
- Hirsutism → antiandrogens (w/ OCPs as antiandrogens are teratogens)
- **Prenatal rx:** Mat dexamethasone suppresses fetal HPA axis & ↓ genital ambiguity
    Start prior to 8 w of gest when masculinization of external genitalia begins CVS or amniocentesis for gender, if male or unaffected female → d/c steroids
    85% of prenatally treated female infants are born w/ nml or slightly virilized genitalia
- **Neonat rx:** Hydrocortisone dose ≤25 mg/m² QD. Monit weight, length, adrenal steroid conc, plasma renin, & electrolytes
- **Surgical mgmt of ambiguous genitalia** (controversial): Age 2–6 mo in virilized girls; technically easier than at later ages (std of care) vs. later ages when psychosexual identity is established
- **Psychological counseling**

Innervation of Bladder and Urethra (Compr Physiol 2015;5:327–96)

Control of micturition					
Target	Effect	Nerve	Type	Transmitter	Receptor
Bladder (detrusor)	Contraction/voiding	Pelvic plexus efferents (S2–4)	Parasymp	Ach	M3 muscarinic
	Relaxation/filling	Hypogastric (T11–L2)	Symp	NE	β3-Adrenergic
Urethral sphincter	Contraction/filling	Hypogastric	Symp	NE	α1-Adrenergic
External urethral sphincter	Contraction/voluntary retention	Pudendal (S2–4)	Somatic	ACh	Nicotinic cholinergic

- **CNS involvement (pontine micturition center)** – Afferent signal through spinothalamic tracts & dorsal columns → intensity of signal reaches threshold of consciousness triggering void when socially acceptable → efferent signal through reticulospinal & corticospinal tracts

Anatomy
- EAS – Striated muscle innervated by **hemorrhoidal branch** of pudendal nerve, voluntary squeeze
- IAS – Continuation of smooth circular muscle of rectum under autonomic control, constant contraction contributes **70–80%** of resting anal tone
- Levator ani complex – Defines prox border of anal canal – PR muscle – striated musc sling originating from pubic bone supporting the rectum, innervated via direct branches from **S3, S4, & pudendal nerve**, constant tone at rest creates the **anorectal angle (~90°)**

Mechanism of Normal Defecation
- Rectum acts as reservoir → receptors in PR sense distention → IAS reflexively relaxes to sample contents & then contracts RAIR → voluntary relaxation of pelvic floor (PR) & EAS straightens anorectal angle by >15° & allows passage of contents

POP 7-1

Definitions
- Loss of support of the anter, apical, or postcompartments of the vagina that result in protrusion of pelvic organs into or out of the vaginal canal (bladder, rectum, small bowel, sigmoid, colon, or uterus/cervix)
- **Anterior:** Cystocele: Prolapse of bladder into the vagina
- **Apical:** Uterine prolapse: Prolapse of uterus & cervix into the vagina or vaginal vault prolapse: Prolapse of the vaginal vault or cuff after hysterectomy
- **Posterior:** Rectocele: Prolapse of rectum into the vagina

Epidemiology (Obstet Gynecol 2010;116:1096)
- Risk of POP requiring Surg by the age of 85 is ~19%
- POP is the 3rd most common indication for hysterectomy following leiomyomata & endometriosis

Pathophysiology (Cochrane Database Syst Rev 2010;4:3)
- Risk factors – Preg, childbirth, obesity, congen or Acq connective tissue abnormalities, denervation or weakness of the pelvic floor, aging, hysterectomy, menopause & factors a/w chronically raised intra-abdominal pres, & race (Black & Asian w/ lowest risk, Hispanic w/ highest risk)

- 3 levels of support of the vagina *(Am J Obstet Gynecol 1992;166:1717)*
  - **Level I:** Apical & uterine support comprised of cardinal & uterosacral ligament attachment to the cervix & upper vagina → defects in this support complex may lead to apical prolapse
  - **Level II:** Lateral support of the vagina including paravaginal attachments (pubocervical fascia & arcus tendineus fasciae pelvis) contiguous w/ the cardinal/uterosacral complex at the ischial spine → defects in this support may lead to lateral, paravaginal, & anter wall prolapse
  - **Level III:** Support of distal 3rd of the vagina comprised of perineal body, superficial & deep perineal muscles, & fibromuscular connective tissue → defects in this support may lead to anter & post vaginal wall prolapse, gaping introitus, & perineal descent

Clinical Manifestations

- **Assoc sx** (Note: Many women may be asymptomatic and stage of prolapse does not correlate well with symptoms):
  Bulge, pelvic heaviness, backache, urinary incontinence, frequency or urgency, difficulty in initiating & maintaining urinary flow, incomplete emptying, sexual dysfxn, incontinence of stool or flatus, constip, or need for splinting
- **Physical exam:**
  Perform a full physical exam to determine pathology outside of the pelvis
  Vaginal exam:
  Routine external & bimanual exam while in lithotomy position
  Elicit bulbocavernosus reflex & anal wink reflex to determine if sacral pathways are nml
  Ask the pt to Valsalva while gently spreading the labia to determine overall prolapse
  Inspect each compartment of the vagina separately w/ the pt performing max Valsalva. Use 1 blade of the speculum to assist in visualizing the anter or post-compartment individually. During assessment determine the location & degree of prolapse relative to the hymenal ring.
  Perform a rectovaginal exam to assess post wall defects, enterocele, & determine anal sphincter strength
  A PVR by catheterized specimen will help determine adequate emptying. Will also provide opportunity for urinalysis.

Pelvic Organ Prolapse Quantification (POP-Q)

- Provides an objective site-specific system for determining location & staging of POP w/ the hymen as the fixed point of reference
- Negative numbers indicate support above the hymen where a positive value indicates prolapse beyond the hymen

---

Figure 7.1 A (Left): POP-Q. There are site points labeled Aa, Ba, C, D, Bp, and Ap that correspond to points above or below the hymenal remnants and are stated in centimeters above (negative) or below (positive) that point. The genital hiatus (gh), perineal body (pb), and total vaginal length (tvl) are also listed as lengths in centimeters. They are used to quantify pelvic organ support anatomy. **B (Right):** Grid for recording quantitative description of pelvic organ support.

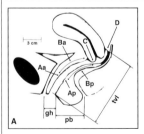

anterior wall **Aa**	anterior wall **Ba**	cervix or cuff **C**
genital hiatus **gh**	perineal body **pb**	total vaginal length **tvl**
posterior wall **Ap**	posterior wall **Bp**	posterior fornix **D**

(From *Am J Obstet Gynecol* 1996;175:10.)

Stages of Prolapse
- **Stage 0:** No prolapse is demonstrated
- **Stage I:** Most dependent portion of prolapse is >1 cm above the hymen
- **Stage II:** Most dependent portion of prolapse is ≤1 cm prox or distal to the hymen
- **Stage III:** Most dependent portion of prolapse is >1 cm below the hymen but extends no further than 2 cm, ≤TVL − 2 cm
- **Stage IV:** >TVL − 2 cm

Diagnostic Workup/Studies
- Physical exam is generally sufficient to determine type & stage of prolapse
- Urodynamic studies may be useful to determine occult urinary incontinence

Treatment: Nonsurgical Management
- Assurance & observation
- Pelvic floor muscle exercises (Kegel exercises)
  Minimal risk & low cost, but no high-quality evid supporting prevention or rx of prolapse
- Pessary
  Indications: Poor operative candidate, desire to avoid Surg, used as diagnostic tool to determine if urinary incontinence resolves w/ restoration of anatomy
  Continuation rate 50–80% after 1 y of use (*Int Urogynecol J* 2011;22:637)
  Risk: Vaginal erosion in 9% of users (*Int Urogynecol J Pelvic Floir Dysfunct* 2006;17:155)

Treatment: Surgical Management
- **Apical support** (uterine or vault prolapse):
  Sacrocolpopexy: Mesh (typically polypropylene) suspension of the vagina or uterus to the anter longitudinal ligament of sacrum via abdominal, laparoscopic, or robotic-assisted approach
    Risks: Mesh erosion 2–11% (*Obstet Gynecol* 2004;104:805), GI complications including SBO, other abdominal surgical complications, de novo stress incontinence, thus need to consider concomitant anti-incontinence procedure (*NEJM* 2006;354:1557)
  Sacrocolpoperineopexy: Same technique as above, w/ addition of post arm of mesh extending to the perineal body
  Uterosacral ligament suspension: Suspension of the vaginal cuff after hysterectomy to the bilateral uterosacral ligaments at the level of the ischial spines
    Risks: Ureteral obst ranges from 3–11% (*Am J Obstet Gynecol* 2000;183:1402; *JAMA* 2016;311:1023–34), reoperation for symptomatic prolapse in 3–9% (*Am J Obst Gynecol* 2010;202:124; *JAMA* 2016;311:1023–34) mostly anterior compartment failures
  Sacrospinous ligament fixation: Suspension of the vaginal apex to the sacrospinous ligament either unilaterally or bilaterally, typically using an extraperitoneal approach
    Risks: Anterior prolapse rate 6–28%, pudendal & inferior gluteal vessels & nerves lie behind the sacrospinous ligament & may be injured during procedure causing hemorrhage or postop gluteal pain
  Iliococcygeal suspension: Attaches the vaginal apex to the fascia of the iliococcygeus muscles bilaterally
    Risks: No randomized trials that support the use of this procedure & may shorten vagina
- **Anter compartment defect:**
  Anter colporrhaphy: Midline plication of endopelvic fibromuscularis of the anter vagina w/ removal of excess vaginal mucosa, ± graft reinforcement
    Benefits: Easy to perform
    Risks: Only 50% anatomic cure
  Paravaginal repair: Same as above w/ addition of lateral dissection to the arcus tendineus or obturator fascia w/ reinforcement sutures placed in these structures. Can be performed by laparoscopic, vaginal, or abdominal approaches.
- **Postcompartment defect:**
  Postcolporrhaphy: Midline plication of the rectovaginal fibromuscularis in the postvagina w/ removal of excess vaginal mucosa
    Benefits: Cure rate is 76–96%
    Risks: Excessive removal of vaginal mucosa can result in vaginal narrowing & dyspareunia, 25% rate of postsurgical dyspareunia alone
  Site-specific repair: Identification of isolated defects in the rectovaginal fibromuscularis & subseq repair
- **Obliterative procedures in nonsexually active individuals:**
  Complete colpocleisis – Removal of vaginal epithelium w/ suturing of the anter & postvaginal walls together, thus obliterating the vaginal lumen & effectively closing the vagina

> Le Fort colpocleisis – Partial excision of the anter & postvagina w/ closure of the vaginal lumen distal to the cervix (uterus in situ), lateral tracts left patent to allow for egress of cervical & vaginal mucus or discharge

- **Mesh augmentation & mesh kit procedures:**
  - **Biologic:** Autologous (self), allograft (donor), or xenograft (porcine/bovine)
  - **Synthetic:** Types I–IV based on pore size, type I monofilament most used due to large pore size & decreased rates of infxn
  - **Mesh kits:** Various types of kits: There is an FDA warning about the increased risk of complications including mesh erosion, GI involvement, pain, & need for reoperation. ACOG recommends vaginal mesh be reserved for high-risk pts including those w/ recurrent prolapse &/or medical comorbidities precluding a lengthier Surg

  (Obstet Gynecol 2011;118:1459–64)

URINARY INCONTINENCE

Definition
- **Involuntary leakage of urine:**
  - **Stress urinary incontinence (SUI):** Complaints of involuntary leakage of urine w/ cough, sneezing, or exertional maneuvers that ↑ abdominal pres
  - **Urge urinary incontinence (UUI):** Complaints of involuntary leakage of urine w/ sensation of urgency, often referred to as OAB
  - **Mixed urinary incontinence (MUI):** Combination of both SUI & UUI
  - **Continuous urinary incontinence:** Complaint of continuous leakage
  - **Overflow incontinence:** Complaint of involuntary loss of urine preceded by an inability to empty the bladder (a/w overdistention & urinary retention due to obst or neurologic causes)

Epidemiology
- Prevalence of 25–55% in Western countries
- May be as high as 77% in nursing home pts & 40% in postmenopausal women
- Many women will not address this issue w/ their physicians due to embarrassment. May lead to signif impairment in QOL

Etiology
- Age, childbearing, obesity, medical diagnoses (diabetes, stroke, spinal cord injury)
- Hysterectomy & menopause w/ inconsistent results

Pathophysiology (N Engl J Med 1985;313:800; Obstet Gynecol 2005;105:1533)
- Impairment in the physiologic voiding mech
- Functional incontinence – incontinence occurring b/c of factors unrelated to the physiologic voiding mech
  - Remember mnemonic **DIAPPERS** (**D**elirium, **I**nfxn, **A**trophic urethritis & vaginitis, **P**harmacologic [diuretics, sedatives, anticholinergics, CCB, α blockers], **P**sychologic [depression], **E**ndocrine [calcium, gluc], **R**estricted mobility, **S**tool impaction)
- Genitourinary etiologies include filling & storage disorders (SUI, UUI, MUI), fistulae (vesicovaginal, ureterovaginal, or urethrovaginal), congen (ectopic ureter, epispadias)

Clinical Manifestations
- **Hx:** Provides the most insight to cause, type, & rx. Include the following: Voiding frequency, nocturnal voiding frequency, number of episodes of incontinence & vol a/w episodes, number of pads used, bowel incontinence, bulge sx, diet (including caffeine & EtOH intake), medical & surgical hx, obstetrical & gynecologic hx, neurologic conditions (diabetes, multi sclerosis, disk dz, & stroke), pulm conditions, smoking, & meds
- Consider having the pt keep a voiding diary over 24 h to 3 d, includes timing and amount of fluid intake, voids, voided volume, leakage episodes and activity during leakage
- **Physical exam:** Complete full physical exam including gynecologic, rectal, & genital/lower neurologic exam. Include POP-Q (see POP section)
- **Urethral mobility:** May be assessed w/ the *Q-tip test* & helps aid in the dx of stress incontinence (Obstet Gynecol 1971;38:313–15)
  - A Q-tip is placed in the urethra to the level of the vesical neck & assessment of the change of axis is performed while asking the pt to Valsalva.
  - An angle of >30° is indicative of urethral hypermobility
- Cough stress test
- PVR to determine if urinary retention an issue <150 mL adequate bladder emptying
  (N Engl J Med 2012;366:1987–97)

- **Lab test:** Clean midstream or catheterized urine sample for **urinalysis & culture prn.** Bld testing including BUN, Cr, gluc, & calcium

Subsequent Workup

- **Urodynamic testing:** A test that evaluates stress incontinence, detrusor instability, 1st sensation, desire to void, bladder compliance, & bladder capacity. Recommended in the following circumstances: (1) Dx unclear, (2) Surg being considered, (3) marked POP present which may have underlying de novo incontinence, or (4) a neurologic condition exists.
    More accurate diagnosis of incontinence type and may change treatment plan in up to 27% of pts (*Int Urogynecol J Pelvic Floor Dysfunct* 2008;19:1235)
    Measurements:
    Uroflowmetry: Measures urine volume voided over time, assesses ability to empty bladder, assesses abnormal voiding
    Filling cystometry: Measures detrusor fxn including sensation, compliance, capacity, & evid of uninhibited detrusor contractions Pres catheters are placed in the bladder & vagina or rectum while the bladder is retrofilled. Detrusor activity is determined by Pves (pres in bladder) – Pabd (pres in abd, measured by vaginal/rectal catheter). Individual measurements are recorded throughout the tracing including *LPP, 1st desire & maximal bladder capacity* → ISD – Valsalva LPP <60 cmH$_2$O
    Pressure-flow study: Measures both bladder pressure and urinary flow to determine cause of abnormal voiding. Most commonly abnormal in setting of anterior prolapse
    Urethral pressure profile: Evaluate for ISD, dual sensor catheter is used to determine *MUCP & functional urethral length* → **ISD** – MUCP is 20 cmH$_2$O or less
- **Cystourethroscopy:** May be req for eval of microscopic hematuria, irritative voiding sx w/o evid of infxn & persistent hematuria in women >50 yo, or suspicion of suburethral mass

Treatment

- **Behavioral approaches:** 50% reduction in incontinence episodes (*Obstet Gynecol* 2002;100:72–8)
    Lifestyle modification: Weight loss, caffeine, EtOH, or fluid intake reduction, decreased weight bearing, smoking cessation, & constip relief, "bladder diet"
    Bladder training: May aid in UUI & MUI
    Kegel exercises: Strengthen the voluntary periurethral & perivaginal muscles, may be augmented w/ biofeedback training or electrostimulation via a pelvic floor physical therapist
- **Pelvic floor muscle training (PMFT)**
    Conservative therapy for both prevention and treatment of UI and POP
    Goal is to strengthen pelvic muscles that support the bladder neck and urethra rest
    PMFT associated with 50% resolution of SUI (*Neurol Urogyn* 2015;34:300–8)
    PMFT decreased episodes of UUI by 60–80% and may be more effective as anticholinergics (*JAMA* 1998;280:1995–2000)
- **Medical management:**
    Estrogen may ↑ urethral bld flow, α-adrenergic receptor sens, & build collagen but is not proven to help in incontinence & some trials suggest incontinence may be worsened
    Antichol medication is often used for UUI or MUI
- **Nonsurgical rx:**
    Incontinence pessary: Help w/ SUI during exercise-need fitting
    Urethral plugs: Help w/ SUI during exercise-need fitting
- **Surgical rx:**
    See sections under stress & detrusor instability

OVERACTIVE BLADDER AND URGE INCONTINENCE

Treatment

- **Medical management** generally involves antichol or antimuscarinic meds
    Antichol may be best for MUI
    Side effects of anticholinergics include dry mouth, constip, blurred vision (contraindicated in pts w/ narrow-angle glaucoma)

Medications for mixed or urge incontinence		
Name	Drug type	Dosage
Oxybutynin IR (Ditropan)	Antimuscarinic	2.5–5 mg PO TID
Oxybutynin ER (Ditropan XL)	Antimuscarinic	5–10 mg PO daily
Oxybutynin patch (Gelnique)	Antimuscarinic	1 patch 5 mg twice weekly
Tolterodine (Detrol/ Detrol LA)	M_3 – selective antimuscarinic	1–2 mg PO BID (short acting) 2–4 mg PO daily (long acting)
Trospium chloride (Sanctura)	Antimuscarinic quaternary amine	20 mg PO BID
Trospium ER (Sanctura XR)	Antimuscarinic quaternary amine	60 mg PO daily
Darifenacin ER (Enablex)	M_3 – selective antimuscarinic	7.5–15 mg PO daily
Solifenacin (Vesicare)	M_3 – selective antimuscarinic	5–10 mg PO daily
Fesoterodine ER (Toviaz)	M_3 – selective antimuscarinic	4–8 mg PO daily
Imipramine (Tofranil)	Antichol, α-adrenergic	10–25 mg PO daily – QID
Mirabegron (Myrbetriq)	β_3-adrenergic	25–50 mg once daily

- **Surgical management:** Used for refractory urge incontinence
- **Botulinum toxin type A (Botox) injection:**
  Inhibits periph cholinergic nerves by inhibiting ACh release from presynaptic terminal.
  Intra-detrusor injections typically by cystoscopy → reduce detrusor stimulation/ contractions and prevent bladder contractions
  May cause postinjection urinary retention requiring self-catheterization
  May have up to a 73% continence rate *(Eur Urol 2004;45:510)*
- **Sacral nerve modulation (SNM):**
  2 approaches: (1) Staged surgical procedure. First a permanent sacral lead is placed in sacral foramen #3 under fluoroscopy. If ≥50% improvement in symptoms, pt returns for implantation of pulse generator (which usually lasts 2–7 y).
  (2) Percutaneous nerve eval. Done in office with no anesthesia to determine response. If perc nerve stim → ≥50% improvement in symptoms, then pt to OR for permanent lead and pulse generator placement in one procedure.
  Botox and SNM both reduced urge incontinence in RCT (Botox slightly better and more improved quality of life). UTI more common after Botox (35% vs. 11% for SNM). SNM device revision needed in 3% *(JAMA 2016;316: 1366–74)*.

STRESS INCONTINENCE

Treatment
- **Medical management** not generally useful
  Pessary or urethral plugs can be attempted
  Duloxetine and imipramine have been used with minimal improvement
- **Surgical management:**
  Retropubic colposuspension (Burch & MMK):
  Previously considered the gold std for SUI
  Involves suspension of the pubocervical fibromuscularis to pubic symphysis periosteum (MMK) or Cooper's ligament (Burch)
  Midurethral slings: Standard of care for surgical treatment of SUI according to AUGS and SUFU. Cure rates from 62–98% with TOT and 71–97% with TVT (tension-free vaginal tape; retropubic sling) *(Cochrane Database Syst Rev 2015)*
  Risks: Mesh exposure rates of 1.7%
  Retropubic sling (TVT)
  Has largely replaced colposuspension & thought to be as effective
  Polypropylene mesh (most common material) is placed under the midurethra w/ minimal tension through the retropubic space
  Risks: Bladder, ureteral, urethral, bowel, or bld vessel injury thus mandating cystoscopy postplacement

Transobturator sling (TOT)
Directed bilaterally through the obturator foramen & underneath the midurethra
Designed to reduce complications of retropubic trocar placement, lower rates
of bladder perforation, voiding dysfunction, vascular injury, operating time.
Slightly higher rates of postoperative pain and de novo dyspareunia *(Am J Obstet Gynecol* 2010:202:481)
Risks: Bladder, ureteral, & bld vessel injuries are less than the retropubic sling
approach; however, pts may experience more groin pain

Minislings (single-incision slings):
Newer slings which include 1 transvaginal incision & either placed into an H
position (obturator internus muscle) or a U position (urogenital diaphragm)
Risks: Higher risk of reoperation *(Eur Urol* 2011;60:468–80)

- **Facial bladder neck slings:**
Utilizing fascia from the rectus muscle or elsewhere to perform a retropubic bladder
neck sling → preserved for complicated cases

OVERFLOW INCONTINENCE

Definition and Etiology
- Involuntary loss of urine due to inability to adequately empty the bladder
Detrusor underactivity: Smooth muscle damage, fibrosis, low estrogen peripheral
neuropathy (diabetes, B12 deficiency, alcoholism)
Bladder outlet obstruction: External compression of urethra from fibroids,
advanced POP, fecal impaction, prior anti-incontinence procedures
Medications: Anticholinergics, antimuscarinics
Neurologic disorders: Spinal cord disorders that interfere with normal bladder
reflexes including multiple sclerosis, diabetic neuropathy, CNS trauma, stroke,
Parkinson, normal pressure hydrocephalus

Clinical Manifestations
- Inability to void or fully empty bladder voluntarily
- Loss of small amounts of urine w/o sensation of emptying
- Medication hx important to exclude causes of urinary retention

Physical Exam and Workup/Studies
- UA/Urine culture to r/o infection
- Nonpainful bladder that is palpable after voiding
- Signif PVR (typically >300 mL)
- Urodynamics

Treatment
- Therapy directed at treating the underlying cause
- CIC or indwelling catheter to ↓ overdistention
- Sacral nerve stimulation – see OAB section, above
- α-Blockers are not FDA approved for use in women, but have been useful in BPH in males

BYPASS INCONTINENCE AND UROGENITAL FISTULAE

Definition and Etiology
- Leakage of urine from extraurethral sources ("extraurethral incontinence")
Urogenital fistulae – VVF, ureterovaginal fistula: Most common cause in developed
countries is gynecologic surg (0.1% of all hysterectomies, 1.1% following radical
hysterectomy). Intraoperative risk factors include uterus weight >250 g, longer
operative times, concurrent ureteral injury.
Obstetrical trauma (pressure necrosis) is most common cause in developing countries
(2% of obstructed labor) *(Lancet* 2006;368:1201)
Other causes include radiation, trauma, malig, complications of parturition
Ectopic ureter
Urethral diverticulum

Clinical Manifestations
- Continuous leakage of urine common in urogenital fistula
- Pts w/ urethral diverticula may complain of pre- or postvoid "dribbling"
- May present with recurrent UTIs, vaginal candidiasis, perineal irritation

Diagnostic Workup/Studies (*Female Pelvic Med Reconstr Surg 2012;18:71*)
- Most diagnosed with physical exam
- Urinalysis, urine culture to r/o infection
- Dye test – Sterile colored fluid (eg, indigo carmine, methylene blue) instilled into bladder. A clean tampon is placed into the vagina and then checked for die.
- Voiding cystourethrogram – 1st-line imaging
- Cystourethroscopy – Helpful to determine location in bladder
- Intravenous pyelogram may be performed if there is a suspicion for ureteral fistula
- CT/MRI may be used to further characterize size & location

Treatment
- Surgical rx to correct the anatomic abnormality, best outcomes with recognition and repair of the injury at primary surgery
    - If injury not identified, recommended to wait 6–12 w for granulation tissue to dissipate
- May consider conservative management of small VVF w/ prolonged bladder drainage
- Genitourinary fistulas may be repaired vaginally, laparoscopically, or abdominally depending on size, location, & surgeon skill set
    Vaginal repair preferred for uncomp VVF
        Latzko procedure – partial colpocleisis w/o excision of fistulous tract
        Layered closure – surrounding tissues mobilized, fistulous tract excised, multilayers closed w/ absorbable interrupted sutures
        Martius flap – transposition of labial fat pad, useful for large VVF w/o adequate vaginal tissue
    Abdominal or laparoscopic repair may be needed for prox, complex VVF & uretero-vaginal fistulae

INTERSTITIAL CYSTITIS

Definition
- Also known as IC/BPS (interstitial cystitis/bladder pain syndrome)
- Syndrome characterized by chronic pelvic pain, urinary urgency & frequency, dyspareunia, nocturia, and bladder discomfort associated with filling and relieved by voiding

Epidemiology
- Prevalence 2.6–6.5% of women in US (*J Urol 2011;186:540*)
- Up to ~40% women w/ chronic pelvic pain

Pathophysiology
- Poorly understood, potential theories include mast cell activation, upregulation of sensory nerves, altered bladder wall permeability
- May be triggered by caffeine, alcohol, citrus fruits, tomatoes, and spicy foods

Diagnostic Workup/Studies (*J Urol 2014;193:1545*)
- Rule out UTI & other causes of chronic pelvic pain
- American Urological Association definition "an unpleasant sensation perceived to be replated to the urinary bladder, associated with lower urinary tract symptoms of more than 6 w duration, in the absence of other identifiable causes"
- Bladder diary may show frequent small voids
- Cystourethroscopy w/ hydrodistention ± bx showing increased mast cells
- Bladder filled to near capacity, emptied, & then inspected for petechial hemorrhages, Hunner ulcers (diagnostic), glomerulations (not diagnostic)
- Potassium sens test – instillation of nml saline into bladder followed by KCl solution, positive if pain present w/ KCl instillation (low spec)

Treatment (*J Urol 2014;193:1545–53*)
- 1st-line treatment include: Education, avoidance of bladder irritants including spicy foods, coffee, tea, carbonated beverages, tomatoes. Self-care practices and behavioral modifications and stress management.
- 2nd-line treatment include: Manual physical therapy, multimodal pain management with medication, and behavioral therapy. Amitriptyline, Cimetidine, Hydroxyzine, and pentosan polysulfate as oral medications. Intravesical treatment including DMSO, heparin, and lidocaine
- 3rd-line treatment include: Low pressure hydrodistention can improve sx in 50–70% of pts, but may be short lived (*Int Urogynecol J Pelvic Floor Dysfunct 2008;19:1379–84*)

- 4th-line treatment include: Interdetrusor botulinum toxin A and sacral neuro-modulation
- 5th-line treatment include cyclosporine A
- 6th-line treatment include major surgery with urinary diversion, cystoplasty with and without cystectomy

ANAL INCONTINENCE

Definition and Epidemiology
- Involuntary passage of flatus or stool, pts prefer term accidental bowel leakage (ABL)
- Fecal incontinence – inability to prevent passage of stool until socially acceptable
- Prevalence 2–17% general pop, up to 50% of nursing home residents *(NEJM 2007;356:1648)*
- **Risk factors:** Female sex, pelvic radiation, obstetric trauma, neurologic d/o, prev anorectal Surg, chronic diarrhea (IBD, IBS, celiac sprue), fecal impaction, urinary incontinence, nursing home placement, smoking, obesity, diabetes

Etiology
- Anal sphincter weakness: May be due to traumatic (child birth, surgery) or atraumatic causes (spinal cord injury, diabetes, systemic sclerosis)
    - Obstetric anal sphincter injury (OASIS) is the most established risk factor
    - Pts with a history of OASIS may be offered a cesarean delivery *(Am J Obstet Gynecol 2003;189:1251–6)*
- Impaired rectal sensation: Patients sense reduced sphincter resting pressure. Associated with diabetes, multiple sclerosis, dementia, meningomyelocele, spinal cord injuries
- Decreased rectal compliance: Leads to increased frequency and may contribute to incontinence. Due to radiation proctitis, ulcerative proctitis
- Overflow: Fecal retention and fecal impaction inhibit the internal anal sphincter tone allowing leakage of liquid stool around impaction. Secondary to impaired mental function, immobility, recto hyposensitivity, inadequate fluids, and fiber
- Pseudoincontinence – Fecal soiling only (rectovaginal fistula, external hemorrhoids, incomplete rectal emptying)

Clinical Manifestations
- Direct questioning or written questionnaires are important
- Detailed hx including onset, frequency, severity, consistency of stool, presence of bld, pus, or mucus, pad use, effect on QOL, bloating, fecal urgency, straining, insensible loss of stool, fecal soiling
- Thorough medication hx important (laxatives, meds causing constip [anticholinergics, iron, narcotics, etc.] can lead to overflow incontinence)

Physical Exam
- Inspection of perineum & anus – external hemorrhoids, dermatitis, nml perineal skin creases, rectal prolapse, scars from prev lacerations or episiotomies, patulous anus (indicative of denervation), fissures
- Dovetail sign – loss of anter perineal creases (disruption of EAS)
- Inspection w/ squeeze to evaluate symmetry of folds & mvmt of perineum
- Inspection w/ bearing down to evaluate excessive perineal descent (>3 cm)
- Perineal sensation – dull & pinprick sensation should be tested in S2–4 dermatomes
- Anocutaneous reflex – cotton swab touched over bulbocavernosus muscles should elicit contraction of EAS bilaterally
- Digital rectal exam – evaluates resting tone, contraction of EAS & PR, areas of tenderness, fecal impaction, masses

Diagnostic Workup/Studies
- Daily stool diary, validated questionnaires
- Rule out systemic & metabolic causes (infectious, autoimmune, malig, endocrine)
- Stool studies in pts with diarrhea
- **Flexible sigmoidoscopy:** Indicated for pt <40 to assess for masses or mucosal inflammation
- **Colonoscopy:** Indicated for *any* pt >40 yo or w/ concerning sx (weight loss, melena/ hematochezia, chronic diarrhea), family h/o colon cancer, HNPCC or Lynch syn, evaluate for IBD, celiac sprue
- **Endoanal US:** Useful when there is clinical suspicion for anal sphincter injury, evaluates structure *only* (best *1st-line test for poor anal squeeze*)

- **Anal manometry:** Useful study in pts w/ nml anal tone who reports *abn* sensation to defecate, evaluates rectal sensation, compliance, & RAIR, evaluates fxn *only*
- **Other studies:** Electromyography (mapping EAS defects), pudendal nerve conduction studies, defecography (evaluates perineal descent, anorectal angle, rectocele, etc.), dynamic pelvic MRI, colonic transit studies

Treatment *(NEJM 2007;356:1648)*
- Management directed at primary cause
- Modification of stool consistency & deliv
    - Increased fiber intake increases solid stool bulk & may facilitate emptying (may worsen diarrhea in some pts) *(Gastroenterology 1980;79:1272)*
- Pelvic floor exercises: Kegel
- Biofeedback: Performed using visual, auditory or verbal feedback with an EMG probe in the anorectum to display pressure changes. Wide range of success from 38–100% *(Curr Obstet Gynecol Rep 2014;3:155–64)*
    - Improves rectal sensation & sphincter contraction, sensorimotor coordination and enhanced perceived rectal distension *(Dis Colon Rectum 2007;50:417–27)*
- **Surgical management:**
    Sacral neuromodulation (SNM) – see OAB section, an effective minimally invasive procedure. >85% therapeutic success and >30% continence at 5 y *(Dis Colon Rectum 2013;56:234–45)*

    Overlapping anal sphincteroplasty – 70–80% short-term improv; however, only 20–58% at 5 y *(Am J Gastroenterol 2004;99:1585–604)*

    Risks: Wound infection rates of 6–35%
    Note: Long-term studies have not shown a difference in outcomes btw end-to-end vs. overlapping sphincteroplasty for perineal laceration repair after vaginal delivery, although at 1 y end-to-end assoc w ↓ incontinence (Obstet Gynecol 2012;120:803)
    End colostomy is an effective treatment for difficult cases and may result in improved QOL

    Rectal prolapse repair – transrectal, transabdominal, or laparoscopic rectopexy

    Other options – Percutaneous tibial nerve stimulation, injectables with bulking agents, and artificial anal sphincter

INFERTILITY EVALUATION

Definitions and Epidemiology (Fertil Steril 2008;90:S60)
- **Infertility:** No preg after 1 y of regular unprotected intercourse in <35 yo. Consider earlier workup after 6 mo in >35 yo. Affects 7–8% of US women (Fertil Steril 2006;86:516).
- **Fecundity:** Probability that a single menstrual cycle results in live birth

Causes of infertility	
Diagnosis	**% affected**
Ovulation disorders	17
Tubal dz	23
Endometriosis	7
Male factor	24
Unexplained	26
Other	3
From JAMA 2003;290(13):1767–70.	

History (Fertil Steril 2004;82:S169)
- Ob Hx: Gravidity, parity, preg outcomes/assoc complications
- Gyn Hx: Age @ menarche, cycle length & characteristics, dysmenorrhea, moliminal sx
- Prev methods of contraception, abn pap smears & any subseq rx, use of OPK, STIs & PID
- Infertility Hx: Duration of infertility, frequency & timing of intercourse, results of any prev eval & rx, H/o thyroid dz, pelvic or abdominal pain, galactorrhea, hirsutism, dyspareunia
- Medical and surgical Hx: Focus on abdominal, pelvic, and gyn surgery
- Medications and allergies: Include supplements and over the counter rx
- Social Hx: Occupation, exercise, stressors, tobacco, EtOH, drug use, other toxic exposures
- Family Hx: Birth defects, mental retardation, infertility, early menopause
- Partner's reproductive Hx: Previous children conceived, testicular trauma, chronic medical conditions, meds, toxic exposures, drug use, employment hx

Physical Examination
- Weight, height, BMI, vitals
- General exam: Tanner stage and signs of androgen excess
- Targeted exam: Thyroid, breast, abdominal, and gyn (digital and speculum)

Diagnostic Evaluation
- **Ovulatory fxn:** Oligomenorrhea (>35 d btw menses) or amenorrhea (>3 mo btw menses). Luteal phase (cycle day 21 or 7 d after ovulation) serum prog 3–6 ng/mL confirms ovulation. Urinary LH (commercial ovulation predictor kits) generally reliable & correlate w/ serum LH. Serum FSH & estradiol (cycle day 3), TSH, and prolactin as initial eval. If ovarian reserve issue suspected, anti-Müllerian hormone (AMH), antral follicle count, and clomiphene citrate challenge test (CCCT) as additional eval.
- **Anatomy assessment:**
  - *Hysterosalpingogram (HSG)* evaluates tubal patency & uterine cavity, endometrial polyps, submucosal fibroids. Inject radiopaque contrast via cervical canal → visualize endocervical canal, endometrial cavity, lumen, & tubal patency (via dye spill into pelvis). Rx doxycycline 100 mg PO BID for 5 d if h/o PID or dilated tubes (Obstet Gynecol 2009;113(5):1180).
  - *Sonohysterography* (saline infusion sonogram) more accurate than HSG, as accurate as hysteroscopy for cavity assessment.
  - *Transvaginal ultrasound (TVUS)* shows uterine cavity contours & small intrauterine lesions. 3D TVUS useful for uterine anomalies.
  - *Hysteroscopy* for definitive dx + rx of submucosal fibroids, adhesions, polyps, and septums.
  - *Laparoscopy* definitive for tubal & pelvic pathology (endometriosis).
  - *Chromopertubation* (the injection of dye through cervical canula w/ direct intra-abdominal observation of tubal spill for eval of tubal occlusion) & rx of fimbrial agglutination or adhesion
- **Partner assessment (Male factor infertility):** See below

PREMATURE OVARIAN INSUFFICIENCY (POI)

Definition and Epidemiology (Obstet Gynecol 2009;113:1355; Lancet 2010;376:911)
- Dev of hypergonadotropic hypogonadism in a woman <40 yo. 0.3% of repro age ♀; 5–10% ♀ w/ secondary amenorrhea.

Etiology
- Accelerated follicular atresia due to genetic syn (Turner XO → oocyte apoptosis; fragile X premutation → oocyte toxic prot). Autoimmune ovarian failure secondary to systemic autoimmune dz (check for type 1 DM, thyroiditis, hypoadrenalism). Ovarian toxins (chemo w/ alkylating agents, XRT, smoking, infxn such as mumps or CMV).
- Abn follicular stimulation due to defects in steroidogenic enzymes or defects in ovarian gonadotropin receptors (eg, FSH receptor mutation)
- Result is ↓ ovarian estrogen production → ↓ negative feedback on pituitary → ↑↑ FSH, LH

Clinical Manifestations
- Primary or secondary infertility? Irreg menses vs. primary or secondary amenorrhea?
- Fragile X – mental retardation, ataxia, premature ovarian failure
- Turner syn – short stature, shield chest, web neck, low hairline, low set ears, aortic coarct, streak ovaries
- ↓ Estrogen w/ primary infertility → impaired secondary sexual dev, dyspareunia (secondary to vaginal dryness), decreased bone density
- ↓ Estrogen w/ secondary infertility → hot flashes, night sweats, emotional lability, dyspareunia, decreased bone density

Initial Workup
- ↓ Estrogen → ↑ FSH, ↑ LH. POI if:
  FSH >10 mIU/mL (except during the midcycle preovulatory LH surge)
  FSH > LH w/ E2 <50 pg/mL (×2 if ↑ FSH) = absent/nonfunctioning follicles
- Clomiphene citrate challenge test – check FSH on cycle day 3 & 10 after 100-mg clomiphene PO daily on cycle day 5–9; ↑ FSH after clomid sugg low ovarian reserve
- AMH – Secretion by small preantral & early antral follicle granulosa cells reflects size of primordial follicle pool, declines w/ age, undetectable at menopause. Early marker of ovarian reserve and is not cycle dependent. AMH >1 but <3.5 ng/mL → adequate ovarian reserve with likely good response to ovarian stimulation
- AFC by TVUS – high variability, useful if equivocal labs
- Genetics: Karyotype for all patients with POI and testing for Fragile X Premutation (FMR1 mutated in 14% of familial POI)

Follow-up Studies
- Antiadrenal and anti-21 hydroxylase antibodies for asymptomatic autoimmune adrenal insufficiency (3% of spont POI)
- Anti-islet cell Ab (given association w/ type 1 DM)
- TSH, Free T4, antithyroid peroxidase and antithyroglobulin antibodies
- Bone mineral density to detect osteopenia

Treatment and Medications
- HRT to ↓ sx of estrogen deficiency & prevent bone loss
- Daily calcium (1200–1500 mg) + Vit D (600–800 IU) for bone health
- Exogenous androgen – unclear role in mgmt; no high-quality evid
- IVF using donor oocytes – controversial in women w/ Turner syn given pregnancy risk

POLYCYSTIC OVARY SYNDROME (PCOS)

Definition (Nat Rev Endocrinol 2011;74:219)
- A d/o of ovarian fxn characterized by anovulation, elevated androgen levels, & polycystic ovaries. A/w obesity & insulin resistance (metabolic syn). Different diagnostic criteria used:
  1990 NIH – NICHD: Hyperandrogenism or hyperandrogenemia, oligoanovulation, & exclusion of other endocrine disorders (need all 3)
  2003 Rotterdam Criteria: 2 of following 3: Clinical or biochemical hyperandrogenism, oligo- anovulation, polycystic ovaries. Other endocrine disorders must be excluded.
  2006 Androgen Excess – PCOS Society: Clinical or biochemical hyperandrogenism w/ oligo-/anovulation and polycystic ovaries (need all 3)

Epidemiology and Pathophysiology
- 6–10% of women, depending on diagnostic criteria. Uncertain etiology, but hyperandrogenism may cause ovulatory dysfxn & abn gonadotropin secretion.
- Androgen excess → follicular arrest & ↑ LH. Hyperinsulinemia may also → follicular arrest & phenotypic features.
- Presentation may include excess body or facial hair, frequent shaving/plucking, irreg menstruation, infertility, alopecia, acne, obesity, metabolic syn

Physical Exam
- Assess weight & BMI, hair pattern/growth, thyroid, galactorrhea (prolactin-secreting tumor), acanthosis nigricans
- Deep voice, male pattern facial/body hair, clitoromegaly may suggest androgen-secreting tumor or congenital adrenal hyperplasia

Diagnostic Workup
- Document oligo- or anovulation by Hx, midluteal serum progesterone, or urinary LH testing
- Labs: Consider testing for serum androgens esp if no clinical hyperandrogenism – or – if frank virilization. TSH, FSH/Estradiol & prolactin if pt anovulatory. 75 g, 2-h GLT for women w/ hyperandrogenism w/ anovulation + acanthosis nigricans + obesity (BMI >30 kg/m^2, or >25 in Asian pop) + FHx of T2DM or GDM (Fertil Steril 2012;97(1):28)
- TVUS ovaries: ≥12 follicles in each ovary measuring 2–9 mm in diameter, &/or ovarian volume >10 mL indicates polycystic ovaries
- Endometrial bx if long Hx of oligomenorrhea due to ↑ endometrial cancer

Treatment (Fertil Steril 2008;89:505)
- Exercise & weight loss may restore ovulatory cycles, improv symp, and improv fertility – 1st-line rx
- In women not attempting preg, low-dose combination OCP (w/ prog of low androgenicity) may ↓ hyperandrogenism & risk of endometrial cancer, and restore ovulatory cycles
- Clomiphene citrate (7% risk of twins) and Letrozole (if BMI >30) as 1st-line agents for ovulation induction (NEJM 2014;371(2):119)
- Addition of Metformin may help women with glucose intolerance improve fertility rates; Addition of spironolactone may help women with hyperandrogenism unresponsive to OCPs
- Ovulation induction w/ exogenous gonadotropins is 2nd-line therapy. IVF is 3rd-line therapy.

TUBAL FACTOR INFERTILITY

Definition and Epidemiology (Curr Opin Infect Dis 2004;17(1):49;2005)
- Infertility caused by obliteration of the fallopian tube, usually by prior pelvic infxn. 20–30% of infertility may be tubal factor. Very common.

Etiology
- Obliteration of the fallopian tube or damage to fimbriae by infectious or inflamm process. Most cases caused by prev hx of PID.
- Less common causes are inflammation related to endometriosis, inflamm bowel dz, & surgical adhesions
- Iatrogenic causes include hx of tubal ligation for contraception or salpingectomy

Clinical Manifestations
- Usually asymptomatic but may have dysmenorrhea & dyspareunia if endometriosis
- Hx of PID or prior pelvic Surg
- Increases risk of ectopic pregnancy

Diagnostic Workup/Studies
- HSG – diagnostic, but also may ↑ fertility if minimal adhesive dx
- Consider laparoscopy w/ chromopertubation if endometriosis suspected
- Chlamydia and Gonorrhea testing to assess for current infection or test of cure

Treatment and Medications (Fertil Steril 2012;97:539)
- Prox tubal obst → tubal cannulation, assoc w/ best outcomes
- Hydrosalpinges → salpingectomy or prox tubal occlusion improves IVF Preg rates.
- Tubal ligation → tubal reanastomosis if >4 cm of residual tube, dependent of method of tubal ligation (Clips > rings > Pomeroy method > electrocautery)

RECURRENT PREGNANCY LOSS (RPL)

Definition (N Engl J Med 2010;363:1740)
- 3 or more consecutive preg losses before 20 w gest; some recommend w/u after 2 consecutive losses, esp if age >35 yo or pt requests

Epidemiology and Etiology
- 15–20% of pregnant women miscarry, <1% of all pregnant women will have RPL
- 10–50% of very early (<10 w) miscarriages due to aneuploidy
- Autoimmune dz, uterine or cervical abnormalities, endocrine factors, infection, & thrombophilias

Evaluation
- Determine actual gestational age at time of miscarriage rather than time of onset of sx
- Ask about hx of thrombosis or prev fetal death, dysmenorrhea, or menorrhagia (may suggest uterine abn); chronic medical conditions such as thyroid dz, diabetes, or autoimmune dz such as lupus; smoking, toxins, obesity, EtOH use, excessive caffeine use

Diagnostic Workup (Int J Gynaecol Obstet 2002;78:179)
- Parental karyotype for balanced translocation, Robertsonian translocation, and mosaicism
- Antiphospholipid Ab syn w/u w/: Lupus anticoagulant, β_2 glycoprotein Ab (IgM/IgG), & anticardiolipin Ab (IgM/IgG). Need 2 positive tests 6–8 w apart to make dx.
- Consider thrombophilia w/u *only* if pt has a Hx of thromboembolism. Test for Factor V Leiden, prothrombin G20210A mut, prot C/ S, antithrombin III deficiency.
- Evaluate uterine cavity using Pelvic US, HSG, hysteroscopy, or sonohysterography
- No dx is made in 50% of cases of recurrent Preg loss (Fertil Steril 2012)

Treatment (N Engl J Med 2010;363:1740)
- If antiphospholipid antibodies, anticoagulation & low-dose ASA can ↓ miscarriage rates
- If genetic abnormality may consider preimplantation genetic screening
- If uterine septum → hysteroscopic resxn. Repair of bicornuate or unicornuate uterus not necessary as obstetric outcome often good & repair has higher risk.
- No rx for women w/ thrombophilias thus far has been found beneficial

MÜLLERIAN ANOMALIES

Definitions and Epidemiology (Hum Reprod Update 2011;17:761)
- An anomaly of the uterus, tubes, or upper vagina due to failure of dev, fusion, or resorption of Müllerian structures
  5–6% of women (arcuate uterus 3.9%, septate uterus 2.3%, bicornuate 0.4%, unicornuate 0.3%, didelphys 0.3%). ↑ To 8% w/ infertility. ↑ To 13% w/ recurrent miscarriage. ↑ To 25% w/ mixed infertility & recurrent miscarriage.

Etiology (Fritz MA, Speroff L. *Clinical Gynecologic Endocrinology & Infertility*. Philadelphia, PA: Lippincott Williams & Wilkins; 2011)
- **Sporadic:** Multifactorial & polygenic. 46 XX (92%); sex chromo mosaicism (8%)
- **Risk factors:** Hypoxia during Preg, MTX, DES, thalidomide, radiation, viral infxn
- Vertical fusion failure (canalization) → urogenital sinus & Müllerian tubercle separate
- Lateral fusion failure (duplication) → failure to merge bilateral Müllerian ducts
- Dev of the uterus, fallopian tubes, & upper vagina:
  2 Müllerian (paramesonephric) ducts form from celomic epithelium beside Wolffian (mesonephric) ducts. In *absence* of SRY gene on Y chromo & subseq AMH, Müllerian ducts proliferate & grow caudally & medially extending from vaginal plate of urogenital sinus to beside developing ovary. In *absence* of testosterone, Wolffian ducts involute. Canalization of the ducts occurs w/a cranial lumen opening into peritoneal cavity. The paired ducts fuse/resorb in the midline forming the body of the uterus & the unfused lateral arms from the fallopian tubes.
- Dev of urogenital sinus forms *lower* vagina, bladder, urethra
  Urogenital sinus develops from the ventral portion of the cloaca (terminal hindgut; confluence of the urethra, rectum, & vagina). The caudal aspect of the paramesonephric ducts fuses w/ the urogenital sinus to form the vagina & cervix.

Figure 8.1 Types of congenital uterine anomalies

Classification of Müllerian Anomalies

Hypoplasia/agenesis

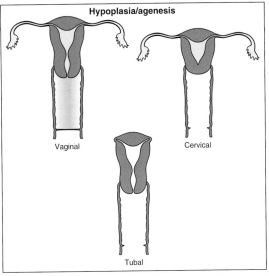

Vaginal

Cervical

Tubal

Unicornuate

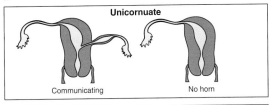

Communicating

No horn

Didelphys

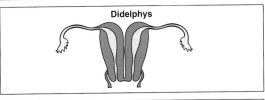

Bicornuate

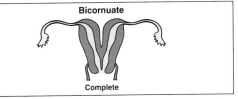

Complete

(continued)

Figure 8.1 (Continued)

Classification of Müllerian Anomalies

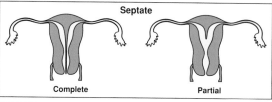

Septate

Complete

Partial

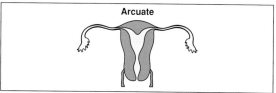

Arcuate

(From Fritz MA, Speroff L. *Clinical Gynecologic Endocrinology & Infertility*. Philadelphia, PA: Lippincott Williams & Wilkins; 2011.)

Clinical Manifestations *(Curr Opin Obstet Gynecol 2010;22:381; Fertil Steril 2008;89:219)*
- Most often asymptomatic w/ nml secondary sex characteristics
- Sx *can* include primary amenorrhea or changes in menstrual cycle (uterine or vaginal malformations); dysmenorrhea or cyclic acute ± chronic pelvic pain
  Abn vaginal bleeding; foul-smelling vaginal discharge (worse at the time of menses); difficulty inserting a tampon; pelvic mass (from hematometra/hematocolpos); dyspareunia; infertility; recurrent preg loss (esp septate uterus)
- Preg complications (higher rates of SAB, preterm birth, fetal malpresentation, labor dystocia, PPROM, placental abruption of previa, IUGR, & increased c-section risk) *(Am J Obstet Gynecol 2011;205:558)*

Risk of pregnancy outcome by uterine anomaly			
	Preg loss (%)	Premature delivery (%)	Fetal survival (%)
Bicornuate uterus	40		62
Septate uterus	>60		6–28
Uterine didelphys	35	19	60
Unicornuate uterus	44	25	43

Data from Ribeiro SC. Müllerian duct anomalies: Review of current management. *Sao Paulo Med J.* 2009;127:92.

Specific anomalies *(Obstet Gynecol 2013;121:1134)*
- **Vaginal agenesis/MRKH**
  Müllerian agenesis of upper vagina, ± uterus/tubes → blind pouch vagina. Affects 1 in 5000 ♀. Nml ovarian & sex dev. ↑ GU tract, skeletal, & ant abd wall anomalies. Usually dx'd during eval for primary amenorrhea, painful intercourse, or pelvic pain
- **Vaginal atresia**
  15% are segmental. Nml uterus, cervix, upper vagina. Primary amenorrhea. Hematocolpos → cyclic pelvic pain. Ddx: Imperf hymen, transverse septum. Segmental has ≥1 cm btw the upper & lower vaginal tract.
- **Transverse vaginal septum**
  Defect in resorption, affects 1/3000–1/80000 women. Presents like vaginal agenesis.
- **Longitudinal vaginal septum**
  Defect in resorption → Preg loss, preterm deliv, dyspareunia, dysmenorrhea. Inc risk of urinary anomalies and endometriosis

- **Uterine didelphys**
  - Defect in lateral fusion w/ double uterus & cervix ± double vaginas → postmenarchal dysmenorrhea, abd pain, palpable abdominal mass. Linked w/ ipsilateral renal agenesis (OHVIRA/Herlyn–Werner–Wunderlich syn); 75% have septate vagina
- **Unicornuate uterus**
  - Only 1 Müllerian duct formed, w/ absent/incomplete contralateral side. 5% of all uterine anomalies; 1 in 4020 ♀. 74% have rudimentary horn, generally not communicating w/ hemiuterus. 40% w/ renal anomalies. 15% w/ endometriosis. Rarely extrapelvic or absent ovaries. Recommend removal of rudimentary horns prior to Preg. Obstetric complications: Ectopic preg (2.7%), late 1st & early 2nd tri SAB (35%), preterm deliv (20%), 3rd trifetal demise (3.8%), placenta accreta, postpartum atony.
- **Cervical atresia**
  - 4 categories: (1) Agenesis, (2) fragmentation, (3) fibrous cord, (4) obst; 50% also w/ vaginal agenesis. 33% w/ uterine anomalies. ↑ Endometriosis, hematosalpinx, & pelvic adhesive dz.

Diagnostic Workup/Studies *(Fertil Steril 2008;89:219)*
- **Goal:** Identify dilated/obstructed uterus &/or mass, pelvic anatomy, distance of an obstructed vagina from the perineum, thickness of a vaginal septum or atretic segment, & presence/absence of urinary tract anomalies
- Physical exam including pelvic ± rectal exam (adol/young adults). Exam under anesthesia ± vaginoscopy (pediatric pop).
- MRI or 3D Transvaginal US most sensitive imaging test for uterine anomalies. Vaginoscopy for vaginal/cervical anomalies, Laparoscopy and HSG useful for uterine anomalies
- Evaluate for GU anomalies (20–30% of pts)

Treatment and Medications *(Fertil Steril 2008;89:1)*
- **Uterine/vaginal obst** → immediately relieve obst surgically
  - If unable to proceed to OR immediately, place Foley catheter to avoid urinary retention. Consider percutaneous drainage, laparoscopic drainage, continuous OCPs to suppress endometrial growth until surgical repair.
- **Vaginal anomaly** → surgical or mechanical repair. If not emergent, medical/surgical intervention when emotionally mature/reproductive age. Vaginal dilators are used postop to prevent stenosis. Overall pts have a satisfactory sex life similar to the nml pop. Discuss Preg options, IVF, surrogacy. Pts need multidisciplinary support including mental health providers & social work.
  - Surgical mgmt vs. Progressive perineal dilation: Dilators are *1st-line therapy* as surgical neovagina ↑ stenosis & multi reoperations. More successful if greater depth of vaginal dimple, increased frequency of dilation, & sexual intercourse.
  - Surgical procedures:
    - Vecchietti procedure (abdominal or laparoscopic technique w/ gradual traction on the vaginal dimple) → creation of a neovagina in 6 mo for 90% of pts. Must use vaginal mold continuously for the 1st 3 mo postop.
    - McIndoe neovagina (dissection btw the urethra & rectum) → place split-thickness skin graft
    - Davydov neovagina (abdominal or laparoscopic-assisted technique w/ dissection of rectovesical space, mobilization of the peritoneum, creation of vaginal fornices, & attachment of the peritoneum to the introitus)
    - Williams' vulvovaginoplasty (uses a vulvar flap to make a vaginal tube). Dilation is needed for a long period. Abn angle of neovagina.
    - Rotational flaps (use pudendal thigh, gracilis myocutaneous, labia minora, & other fasciocutaneous reconstruction). Also can create vagina from bowel.
- **Septum** → hysteroscopic resxn of uterine or longitudinal vaginal septum. Low or midtransverse vaginal septum approached vaginally; high septum & segmental vaginal atresia combine vaginal & abdominal approach.
- **Bicornuate uterus** → Strassman metroplasty unifies both cavities. Inc risk of uterine rupture in labor.
- **Rudimentary horn, obstructed hemivaginas, etc.** → laparoscopic resxn
- **Cervical atresia** → hysterotomy & uterovaginal anastomosis vs. hysterectomy
- **Didelphys, bicornuate** → rarely require repair
- **Uterine septum** → outcomes improved w/ resxn if 1st trimester loss or desires IVF

MALE FACTOR INFERTILITY

Definition and Epidemiology (Fertil Steril 2006;86:S202)
- Inability of a male to achieve a Preg w/a fertile female after 1 y of intercourse
- 20% due to purely male factors. Additional 30–40% combined male & female factors.
- **Risk factors:** Toxic exposure to chemicals, radiation, or heat; Hx of varicocele, mumps, hernia repair, pituitary tumor, anabolic steroid use, testicular injury, impotence

Etiology
- **Endocrine disorders**
  Hypogonadotropic (secondary) hypogonadism (1–2%)
  Congenital: Klinefelter syn (XXY), Kallmann syn (abn neuronal migration resulting in anosmia & hypothalamic hypogonadism)
  Acquired: Tumors – macroadenoma, craniopharyngioma; Infiltrative dz – sarcoidosis, TB, hemochromatosis; Lymphocytic hypophysitis or infundibulitis; Vascular – infarction, aneurysm; hypothalamic/pituitary dz or drugs that affect them; Drugs & EtOH, Androgen excess
  Hypergonadotropic (primary) hypogonadism (30–40%)
  Congenital: Klinefelter syn (XXY, 1 in 500–700), cryptorchidism, androgen receptor or synthesis disorder (5-α-reductase), myotonic dystrophy
  Acquired: Cancer, infxn (viral orchitis, mumps), drugs (alkylating chemo agents, antiandrogen agents), torsion, radiation, smoking, hyperthermia, antisperm antibodies; Varicocele – dilation of the pampiniform plexus of spermatic veins in scrotum (left more common than right).
- **Genetic disorders of spermatogenesis (10–20%):** Y chrom microdeletions/substitutions, autosomal and X chromosome defects, epigenetic changes
- **Post-testicular defects (10–20%):** Cryptorchidism, dz of epididymis or vas deferens (infxn, vasectomy, CF), cryptorchidism, testicular cancer, retrograde ejaculation, and erectile dysfunction
- **Idiopathic (40–50%)**

Clinical Manifestations and Workup
- **Assess Hx:** Prior pregnancies fathered, coital frequency & timing, childhood illness (mumps orchitis), developmental/pubertal Hx, systemic medical illnesses, prior surgeries (hernia repair), toxic exposures, meds, Hx of STIs, genital trauma, sexual dysfxn
- **Physical exam:** Assess secondary sexual characteristics: Body habitus, hair distribution, gynecomastia. Examine penis including location of urethral meatus. Palpate testes & estimate testicular volume w/ Prader orchidometer. Assess presence/consistency of vas deferens & epididymidis, presence of varicocele. Digital rectal exam to assess masses.
- **Semen analysis:** Collect after 2–7 d of abstinence; 2 samples 1 mo apart; see reference values table below, & also eval leukocyte count, microscopic debris/agglutination, immature germ cells

Semen analysis reference values	
On at least 2 occasions:	
Ejaculate volume	>1.5 mL
Sperm conc	>15 million/mL
Total sperm count	>39 million/ejaculate
Motility	>40%
Progressive motility	>32%
Nml morphology	>5% nml
Vitality (live, membrane intact) (Methods Mol Biol 2013;927:13–19)	>60%

Data from Human Repro 2010;16:231–245 and World Health Organization reference values for human semen characteristics and Methods. Mol Biol. 2013;927:13–9.

- **After initial w/u:** Urology consult if indicated. Additional semen studies (sperm autoantibodies, biochemistry, culture, sperm–cervical mucus interaction, sperm fxn tests [sperm analysis, acrosome rxn, zona-free hamster oocyte penetration test, human zona pellucida binding test, sperm chromatin & DNA assays]). Endocrine eval: Testosterone, LH, FSH, prolactin. Postejaculatory urinalysis in pt w/ low volume semen to rule out retrograde ejaculation. Transrectal & scrotal US to identify obst & nonpalpable varicocele. Genetic testing – CFTR gene (a/w congen absence of vas deferens), karyotype to detect chromosomal abnormalities (a/w impaired testicular fxn), PCR to detect Y chromo microdeletions (a/w isolated spermatogenic impairment).

Treatment and Medications
- Treat underlying etiology if known. Improve coital practice – intercourse q2d during most fertile interval (3 d prior to & including day of ovulation).
- Sperm aspiration for obstructive azoospermia – TESE or MESA followed by IVF w/ ICSI (see below)
- Use ARTs as described below, ICSI useful for male factor infertility, consider sperm donor

OVULATION INDUCTION AND ASSISTED REPRODUCTION

Definition
- Use of medication to stimulate nml ovulation in pts w/ oligo/anovulation (18–25% of couples presenting for infertility of ovulatory disorder)

Clomiphene Citrate (Clomid) (Fertil Steril 2004;82:90)
- **Indications:** Initial rx of oligo- or anovulation, also for unexplained fertility & age-related decline in fertility. Contraindication: Preg.
- **Mech of action:** Estrogen agonist/antag – antag properties predominate, competitively binds estrogen receptors in hypothalamus → ↑ GnRH by hypothalamus → ↑ FSH, LH by pituitary → follicular growth & ovulation
- Administer 50–150 mg PO daily for 5 d, starting cycle day 2–5 of menstrual cycle. Combined w/ timed intercourse or intrauterine insemination. Monitor for ovulation using BBT, urine LH, elevated progesterone in midluteal phase, or US demonstrating preovulatory follicle prior to ovulation & subseq follicular collapse.
- Success rate for ovulation 60–80% – absence of ovulation or no Preg w/ known ovulation over 6 mo indicates failure of rx; many pts go to IVF if clomiphene citrate unsuccessful; Must counsel patients on 7–9% chance of twins. Low risk of OHSS

Letrozole (NEJM 2015;371:119)
- Aromatase inhibitor used in oncology for estrogen receptive cancers but growing data about off-label use for ovulation induction
- Administer 2.5–7.5 mg/d on cycle days 3–7 and monitor for ovulation like Clomid
- In PCOS women w BMI >30, higher live birth rate (20 vs. 10%) and lower twin rate (3.4 vs. 7.4%)

Gonadotropin Injection (Fertil Steril 2008;90:S13)
- Many protocols based on nml physiology of menstrual cycle
- **Mech of action:** FSH stimulates granulosa cell proliferation & follicle dev. LH stimulates theca cell production of androgen (converted to estrogen by granulosa cells). hCG stimulates follicular maturation of oocyte from prophase I through metaphase II & ovulation; may be used as alternative to LH for stimulation of ovulation.
- **Typical administration:** Gonadotropins (hMG or FSH) administered SQ or IM shortly after menstruation (–day 3 of cycle) → hCG, LH, or GnRH agonist once follicle growth reaches target size (18–20 mm). Timed intercourse, intrauterine insemination or oocyte retrieval typically 34–36 h following hCG administration. Progesterone or hCG for corpus luteum support following conception.
- **Monitoring:** Transvaginal US to assess follicular dev (diameter >18 mm) & endometrial thickness prior to stimulation of ovulation w/ hCG. Estradiol level correlates w/ follicular maturation (E2 >200 pg/mL per follicle). Progesterone level prior to hCG administration to determine premature LH surge.
- Complications of gonadotropins include multi gest (↑ w/ lower mat age & higher number of embryos transferred) & OHSS

Intrauterine Insemination (IUI) (Cochrane Database Syst Rev 2012;4:CD003357)
- **Advantages:** Most cost-effective intervention prior to proceeding w/ IVF. Disadvantages: Requires patency of at least 1 fallopian tube.
- **Indications:** Sexual dysfxn (coitus can be avoided), cervical factor infertility, male factor infertility, unexplained fertility, endometriosis. Contraindications: Preg, bilateral fallopian tube occlusion, active pelvic infxn.

- **Procedure:** Wash ejaculated semen specimen to remove prostaglandins. Concentrate sperm in culture media. Inject sperm suspension directly into upper uterine cavity using a small catheter threaded through the cervix – timed to occur just prior to ovulation (check urine LH).
- Cumulative Preg rate of 5–20%, usually attempt 3–6 cycles before proceeding w/ IVF

In Vitro Fertilization (IVF) *(Cochrane Database Syst Rev 2012;18:CD003357)*
- **Advantages:** Highest chance of success. Disadvantages: Expensive, higher risks of multi gest & OHSS given use of gonadotropins.
- **Indications:** Tubal factor infertility, failure of less invasive therapies, male factor infertility, diminished ovarian reserve, ovarian failure (egg donor use), uterine factor infertility (surrogacy). Contraindications: Mat dz in which Preg contraindicated (eg, malig), active pelvic infxn.
- **Procedure:** Controlled ovarian hyperstimulation as above → follicle aspiration – usually transvaginally under US guidance. Oocytes mixed w/ prepared sperm in vitro, fertilization occurs w/i next 18 h. Embryo(s) transferred into uterine cavity on cycle day 3–5. Preg test (serum hCG) 10–12 d following transfer.
- Live birth rate of 45% – decreases w/ advancing mat age

Intracytoplasmic Sperm Injection (ICSI) *(Fertil Steril 2008;90:S187)*
- **Advantages:** Assists fertilization process by direct injection of sperm into oocyte. Disadvantages: Technically demanding, high cost.
- **Indications:** Male factor infertility, select rare types of female infertility (morphologic anomalies of oocytes or zona pellucida inhibiting nml fertilization process). Contraindications: Same as for IVF.
- **Procedure:** Controlled ovarian hyperstimulation & follicular aspiration as outlined above
- Direct injection of single spermatozoon into cytoplasm of human oocyte
- Live birth rate of 30%, long-term fetal outcomes unknown

Assisted Hatching (AH) *(Human Repro 2000;15;1061)*
- Hatching is natural process in which embryo expands and "breaks through" zona pellucida to implant in endometrium
- AH is a lab procedure whereby zona is mechanically opened
- Believed to improve % of embryos that implant in subset of poor embry quality patients/older women

FERTILITY PRESERVATION

Epidemiology *(Semin Reprod Med 2011;29(2):147)*
- The probability of a cancer dx in a premenopausal female is 11%
- Survival for many types of childhood malignancies is >80%
- Rx for many of these cancers can lead to infertility, so consideration of future reproductive desires important *before* Surg, chemo, or XRT

Pathophysiology
- Primary oocytes are arrested in prophase of the 1st meiotic division at birth with continuous apoptosis depleting the pool of primary follicles
- Alkylating chemo agents affect resting follicles & carry a high risk of ovarian failure
- Antimetabolites affect only metabolically active oocytes & granulosa cells, leading to a lower risk of ovarian failure
- Radiation also affects developing oocytes; dose of 24 Gy → ovarian failure
- Intensive multiagent chemo & total body irradiation needed for bone marrow stemcell xplant results in >90% risk of permanent ovarian failure

Approaches
- **Nonsurgical:** Sperm cryopreservation or embryo cryopreservation are established methods for fertility preservation *(Fertil Steril 2005;83:1622)*. Experimental techniques: If embryo cryopreservation is not possible due to lack of partner or desire to avoid creation of surplus embryos, some centers are capable of oocyte cryopreservation after a COH cycle. Some centers perform cryopreservation & in vitro maturation of oocytes from nonstimulated ovaries if a COH cycle is not possible.
- **Surgical:** Ovarian transposition surg can move an ovary out of pelvis or abd if a pt is to undergo radiation. Ovarian tissue cryopreservation is a still experimental procedure where ovarian tissue is harvested, frozen, then thawed & retransplanted or individual follicles are isolated & grown in vitro. Cortical strips can be either transplanted back into pelvis or to abd or forearm. Fxn has been reported up to 7 y from transplantation *(Fertil Steril 2010;93(3):762)*.

- Fertility preserving surgeries for gynecologic malignancies:
    - **Cervical cancer** → Trachelectomy in pts w/ tumor <2 cm & w/o lymph node metastasis; cerclage must be placed at time of surg. Inc risk of 2nd tri loss & preterm deliv.
    - **Endometrial cancer** → Progesterone therapy if well-differentiated tumor w/o lymph node involvement. Initial resp rate >60% in selected pts. Definitive therapy w/ hysterectomy should be performed as recurrence risk >50%.
    - **Ovarian cancer** → Unilateral salpingo-oophorectomy & lymph node dissection in malig germ cell tumor or early stage epithelial ovarian cancer

PREIMPLANTATION GENETIC TESTING

Definition (Fertil Steril 2008;90:S136)
- New technology for pts undergoing ART w/ goal of assessment for gene mut & aneuploidy prior to implantation to establish unaffected Preg
- **Preimplantation genetic diagnosis (PGD):** Genetic testing of embryo when 1 or both of genetic parents are known to carry a specific gene mut or balanced chromosomal rearrangement
- **Preimplantation genetic screening (PGS):** Screening of embryo for aneuploidy in chromosomally nml couples

Indications
- Avoid preg termination w/ fetus at risk for heritable debilitating dz, or medically indicated sex selection
- Reduce recurrent preg loss in pts w/ known balanced chromosomal translocations

Procedure
- Small opening created in zona pellucida, cell or polar body extracted using small suction pipette, genetic analysis performed by PCR to assess gene defects, FISH for chromosomal anomalies
- 1st & 2nd polar bodies may be removed from oocytes after retrieval if genetic mother carrying detectable mut
- Trophoblastic cells may be aspirated from embryo 3 d following fertilization

Counseling
- Embryo bx & culture may lower viability of Preg (NEJM 2007;357:9). Unanticipated birth of affected offspring – unprotected sex resulting in Preg, xfer of wrong embryo, misdiagnosis. Disposition of embryos found to have genetic anomalies & not used for xfer. False-positive results may result in discard of potentially nml embryos. Confirmatory prenatal testing after PGD still recommended if desired, due to risk of early embryo mosaicism with result different from fetus – offer routine aneuploidy testing in pregnancy, CVS or amniocentesis.

OVARIAN HYPERSTIMULATION SYNDROME (OHSS)

Definition and Epidemiology (Fertil Steril 2008;90:S188)
- Life-threatening complication of ovulation induction characterized by ovarian enlargement due to multi ovarian cysts & acute fluid shift out of intravascular space. Occurs in 0.2–6% ovulation induction cycles.
- **Risk factors:** Prior Hx of OHSS, age <35 y, low body weight, PCOS, higher doses of exogenous gonadotropins, high absolute or rapidly rising serum E2 levels. Preg increases likelihood, duration, & severity of OHSS.

Pathophysiology
- Main trigger: hCG – physiologic or exogenous
- Ovarian enlargement due to stimulation by gonadotropins → ↑ ovarian hormones & vasoactive substances (cytokines, angiotensin, VEGF) → ↑ capillary permeability & acute 3rd space sequestration
- Massive extracellular exudative fluid accum & sev intravascular volume depletion & hemoconcentration → multiorgan system failure

Clinical Manifestations
- **Signs/sx:** Bloating, abdominal discomfort & distention, emesis, diarrhea, rapid weight gain, tense ascites, hemodynamic instability, respiratory difficulty (tachypnea), oliguria, HoTN, other signs of intravascular hypovolemia

- **Lab findings:** Hemoconcentration (↑ Hct, leukocytosis, thrombocytosis), electrolyte imbalance (HoNa, hyperK, metabolic acidosis), ↑ Cr, ↑ liver enzymes
- **Life-threatening complications:** Acute renal failure, ARDS, heart failure, hemorrhage from ovarian rupture, thromboembolism

Treatment
- **Self-limited:** Rx mostly for symptomatic relief & stabilization
- **Outpt mgmt for mild cases:** Analgesia for pain, oral hydration, monitoring for progression. Serial labs, serial US, daily weights. No intercourse, no strenuous activity to reduce risk of cyst rupture or ovarian torsion.
- **Hospitalization & ICU care – supportive:** Fluid mgmt – strict I&O, IV fluids (D5 NS MIVF 25% albumin prn) to maintain urine output & BP. Thoracentesis, culdocentesis, & paracentesis under US guidance as needed. Ppx against thromboembolism – venous support stockings, pneumatic compression devices, prophylactic anticoagulation. ICU admission for mgmt of thromboembolic complications, pulm compromise, or renal failure. Cardiac: Invasive monitoring of CVP, PCWP. Pulm: Oxygen suppl, assisted ventilation, thoracentesis. Renal: Low-dose dopamine for renal compromise → renal vessel dilation → ↑ renal bld flow. May require short-term dialysis.

Prevention (Fertil Steril 2010:94:389)
- Carefully monit after gonadotropins, esp for rapidly rising E2 levels, E2 >2500 pg/mL, or US evid of emergence of large number of intermediate-sized follicles (10–14 mm). Use minimum dose & duration of gonadotropin therapy necessary to achieve therapeutic goal. Delay administration of hCG until estradiol levels plateau or ↓. Use GnRH agonist (eg, leuprolide) instead of hCG (can only be used in antagonist cycles). Use cabergoline (dopamine agonist) to reduce ovarian resp to FSH.

Common Obstetric Terms
- **Gravidity:** Number of times a woman has been pregnant (including current Preg)
- **Parity:** Preg outcomes, using TPAL system. *Term* deliveries/*Preterm* deliveries/*Abortions*/*Living* children. Deliv refers to a single event, not the number of births (ie, multiples count as 1 deliv event). Eg G3P0112 = currently in 3rd preg, after 1 abortion & 1 preterm deliv of twins (both alive)
  - **T** = Term: ≥37 w0d
  - **P** = Preterm: 20 w0d–36 w6d
  - **A** = Abortus: Spont or induced losses <20 w0d
  - **L** = Living: Living children at the time of the encounter
- **EDD:** Accurate dating is crucial, EDD is 280 d (±13 d; or 40 w) from LMP. Initial EDD assigned by LMP. Dating can be confirmed by US if menses are irreg, LMP uncertain, if conception occurred while on contraception or if there is a size-dates discrep. US most accurate prior to 12 w & should be compared to LMP. Later sono dating less accurate (±2 w in 2nd trimester, ±3 w in 3rd trimester).

Guidelines for redating based on ultrasonography		
Gestational age range[a]	**Method of measurement**	**Discrepancy between ultrasound dating and LMP dating that supports redating**
≤13 6/7 w	CRL	
• ≤8 6/7 w		More than 5 d
• 9 0/7 w to 13 6/7 w		More than 7 d
14 0/7 w to 15 6/7 w	BPD, HC, AC, FL	More than 7 d
16 0/7 w to 21 6/7 w	BPD, HC, AC, FL	More than 10 d
22 0/7 w to 27 6/7 w	BPD, HC, AC, FL	More than 14 d
28 0/7 w and beyond[b]	BPD, HC, AC, FL	More than 21 d

AC, abdominal circumference; BPD, biparietal diameter; CRL, crown–rump length; FL, femur length; HC, head circumference; LMP, last menstrual period.

[a]Based on LMP.

[b]Because of the risk of redating a small fetus that may be growth restricted, management decisions based on third-trimester ultrasonography alone are especially problematic and need to be guided by careful consideration of the entire clinical picture and close surveillance.

- **Viability:** 24 w0d +
- **Periviable:** 22 w0d–23 w6d
- **Previable:** <22 w (institution/location variation)
- **Early term:** 37 w0d–38 w6d
- **Full term:** 39 w0d–40 w6d
- **Late term:** 41 w0d–41 w6d
- **Post term:** ≥42 w0d, ↑ stillbirth risk (*JAMA* 2013;309:2445)
- **Primigravida:** 1st Preg
- **Nulliparous** (nullip): No prior birth events (regardless of outcome)
- **Primiparous:** Gave birth once (ie, >20 w, or once for "T + P" in TPAL system)
- **Multiparous:** Gave birth more than once (parity does not include ABs)
- **Grand multipara:** Woman who has delivered 5 or more times
- **NT:** Nuchal translucency thickness on 1st trimester sono, ↑ in Down syn
- **Triple screen:** uE3 + hCG + AFP to evaluate for Trisomy 21, Trisomy 18, NTDs
- **Quad screen:** Triple screen + inhibin A
- **Cell Free Fetal DNA:** After 10 wga, test for trisomy 13, 18, 21 and Y chromosome. Detection rate of Down syndrome 99% (in those who receive result), screen positive rate 0.5%
- **IUGR** = Mild estimated fetal weight (EFW) <10%ile for gestational age, severe IUGR <5th%, AC <5%tile can be used as surrogate for IUGR
- **GTT** (screening): 50 g oral gluc → 1 h serum gluc → 135–140 cutoff
- **GTT:** 100 g oral gluc after fasting → 1, 2, 3 h postgluc (<180, 155, 140, 95)
- **Fundal height (FH):** FH-measurement from pubic bone to top of fundus correlates w/ GA after 20 w (20 w = umbilicus, add 1 cm/w after that). FH misses 30% IUGR.

Summary of prenatal care by gestational age (Perinatal Care 8th Edition)	
GA	**General mgmt & special screening by approximate weeks GA**
1st trimester (Weeks 0–14)	Complete H&P w/ careful review of Ob-Gyn Hx, Med/Surg Hx, FHx, meds, nutrition, social hx, Trauma Hx Determine viability and confirm EDD, via US Social services (if high risk), social & IPV screening Prenatal 1st visit labs (CBC, T&S, HBsAg, RPR, Rubella, HIV, ±Hgb electrophoresis, ±HCV, ±CF, HbA1c if suspect DM [or do early GLT], GC/CT, Pap, UA/C&S, PPD [or QuantiFERON]) Offer aneuploidy screening: See Genetic Screening Visits every 4 w to check fetal heart tones
2nd trimester (Weeks 14–28)	15–22 w6d: AFP, Quad screen, or 2nd part of integrated/sequential screen. 18–22 w: Sono for fetal anatomy, placentation, AFI, adnexae, CL 25–28 w: 3rd trimester labs → ±GTT, CBC, recheck RPR, T&S, HIV if ↑ risk). Rhogam for Rh negative. Visits every 4 w for FH, fetal heart tones. Plan contraception & breastfeeding.
3rd trimester (Weeks 28–42)	28–36 w: Visits q2–3w >36 w: Weekly visits 35–37 w: Perineal swab for GBS; clinic sono for presenting part; deliv planning & counseling; GC/CT rpt if high risk. If CHTN, GHTN, DM, GDMA2, other high-risk factors: ±Fetal testing 1–2×/w (BPP or NST starting 32–36 w, depending on problem). 25–33 w: Visits q4w to check for FH & fetal heart tones; 33–37 w: q2w; 37 w – deliv: Visits qw; induce after 41 w, or continue to 42 w0d w/ antenatal testing

Considerations in Routine Prenatal Care

- **OB review of systems:** Every encounter ask about VB, LOF, CTX, & FM
  1st FM (quickening): 16–18 w if multiparous, 18–20 w if nulliparous
- **Physical:** BP, weight (current & interval change), FHR, & FH at each visit. Complete PE & pelvic exam at 1st prenatal visit.
  FHR: Detected by Doppler at 10–12 w & by fetoscope at 18–20 w (w/ nml BMI)
- **Cervical exam:** Assess dilation, effacement, station near term
- **Psychosocial screening:** Tobacco use, EtOH/substance use, DV, nutrition, psychosocial situations, job-related risks, depression, & high-risk behaviors
  Tobacco: Encourage tobacco cessation each visit; ~50% of ♀ quit smoking during or before their Preg. ~50% resume smoking w/i 1 y postpartum. A/w IUGR, low birth weight, placental abruption, placenta previa, PPROM, ectopic Preg & perinatal mortality. Children of smokers – ↑ asthma, colic, obesity, & SIDS. Counsel using 5 A's strategy (Ask, Advise, Assess, Assist, Arrange). Nicotine replacement not well assessed, but likely safer than smoking. Insufficient evidence regarding safety of bupropion & varenicline preg/lactation.
  EtOH: No safe threshold. A/w mental retardation, neurologic deficits, fetal EtOH syn (esp w/ chronic EtOH use; growth restriction, facial anomalies, & CNS deficits).
  Marijuana: Encourage cessation, concerns for impaired fetal neurodevelopment. Lactation insufficient evidence (discouraged)
  DV: Red flags include unwanted Preg, late presentation for PNC, substance abuse, poor weight gain, & multisomatic complaints.
  Depression: ACOG recommends screening at least 1× in pregnancy with standardized/validated tool. Screening insufficient without appropriate f/u, tx, Tools include EPDS, PHQ-9. See Chap. 1.
  Substance abuse: Validating screening tools for opioid use and opioid use disorder in pregnancy (4Ps, NIDA Quick Screen, Craft). See Chap. 1.
- **GDM screening:** 2-step approach w/ GLT then GTT. See Chap. 17. 24–28 w. Opt out for extremely low risk considered (age <25, BMI <25, <23 in Asian Americans) no FHx of DM, no personal h/o gluc intolerance, no h/o adverse obstetrical outcomes a/w DM or LGA infant, no co-morbidity & not of an ethnic group w/ ↑ risk DM.
- Screening strategy for detecting early GDM → consider testing in all women who are overweight or obese + 1 or more RF (physical inactivity, 1st-degree relative with DM, high-risk race/ethnicity, prior infant 4000+ g, prior GDM, HTN, HDL <35, triglyceride >250, PCOS, A1C >/= 5.7%, h/o cardiovascular dz (Obstet Gynecol 2017;130:e17)

- **Vaccines:** See Chap. 1. Influenza vaccine recommended for all pregnant women (any trimester). TDaP recommended between 27–36 w during EACH pregnancy (↑ transplacental IgG immunity for neonate) or postpartum if >10 y since last dose (MMWR 2011;60:1424). Postpartum vax for rubella or varicella if nonimmune. Limited data on HPV vaccine in pregnancy. Indications for pneumovax not changed in pregnancy. HepB safe in pregnancy.
- **GBS screening:** 35–37 w or if deliv anticipated (every Preg) (Obstet Gynecol 2011;117:1019). See Chap. 10. Swab lower vagina, introitus, & rectum. Cx valid for 5 w. For pts w/ sev PCN allergy (anaphylaxis/angioedema/urticarial) → request clindamycin & erythromycin sens testing. Must be sensitive to BOTH clinda and erytho to use either of these antibiotics.

Physiologic Changes of Pregnancy (Best Pract Res Clin Obstet Gynaecol 2008;(5):801)
- **Cardiovascular:** ↓ SVR → ↑ HR. BP ↓ early (−10% by 7–8 w) → nadir at 24 w → gradual ↑ to term. CO ↑ in 1st trimester → peaks in 2nd trimester at 30–50% above nonpregnant values. By term, uterus receives 17% (450–650 mL/min) of CO. See Chap. 12.
- **Respiratory:** O_2 consump ↑ 30–50 mL/min (2/3 due to mat requirement, 1/3 for fetal). Tidal vol ↑ to 500–700 mL (prepregnancy of 200 mL). Respiratory rate unchanged. Minute ventilation ↑ from 7.5–10.5 L/min. Functional residual capacity ↓ by 500 mL. Vital capacity unchanged. See Chap. 13.
- **Renal:** Renal bld flow ↑ 35–60%. Kidneys ~1 cm larger w/ ↑ in bld vol; renal pelves, calyces, & ureters ↑ in size in resp to progesterone. GFR ↑ 40–50%, peaks at 180 mL/min by the end of 1st trimester. See Chap. 14.
- **Gastrointestinal:** Progesterone → ↓ esoph sphincter tone → GERD. Delayed gastric emptying & ↑ intestinal transition time. Increased constip. See Chap. 15.
- **Hematologic:** Plasma vol ↑s rapidly. 10% ↑ by 7 w → plateau at 32 w ~50% above nonpregnant → dilutional anemia of Preg. Red cell mass ↑ 18–25% secondary to ↑ erythropoietin. Nml Preg Hgb 11–12 g/dL. WBC ↑ in 1st trimester → plateau at 30 w. Nml Preg WBC 5000–12000/mm³. See Chap. 16.
- **Endocrine:** ↑ Hepatic production of thyroid-binding globulin → ↑ total T4. Free T4 essentially unchanged (except for transient ↑ from hCG's thyrotropin-like activity in 1st trimester). TSH falls in 1st trimester, then normalizes. No real change in mat thyroid status. Pancr islet cells undergo hyperplasia → ↑ insulin secretion. Placental factors ↓ mat insulin sens. Pituitary ↑ volume 135%, but no optic nerve compression. Prolactin levels peak at term. See Chap. 17.

NUTRITION IN PREGNANCY

Weight Management
- **Caloric intake:** Encourage balanced diet
    1st trimester: No additional caloric intake from baseline
    2nd trimester: ↑ 340 kcal/d from baseline
    3rd trimester: ↑ 452 kcal/d from baseline
    Breastfeeding: Increase by 300–500 kcal/d

Institute of Medicine recommended weight gain during pregnancy by BMI		
Category	BMI (kg/m²)	Weight gain
Underweight	<18.5	12.7–18 kg (28–40 lb)
Nml weight	18.5–24.9	11.3–15.8 kg (25–35 lb)
Overweight	25–29.9	6.8–11.3 kg (15–25 lb)
Obese	≥30	0.45–9.1 kg (11–20 lb)

From Obstet Gynecol 2013;121:210–12.

- **Obesity in Preg:** Inc risk of SAB (OR 1.2), recurrent miscarriage (OR 3.5), pre-eclampsia, cardiac dysfunction, GDM, stillbirth, cesarean delivery, wound dehiscence, endometritis, failed trial of labor, VTE. Consider HbA1C or early GLT (Obstet Gynecol 2015;126:112).
- **Exercise in Preg:** ACOG recommends at least 20–30 min/d (on most or all days). Avoid activities w/ high risk for abdominal trauma (eg, horseback riding, skiing/snowboarding), or Scuba diving. Absolute contraindications to aerobic exercise: Hemodynamically significant heart dz, restrictive lung dz, cervical insufficiency/cerclage, multiple gestation at r/o PTL, persistent 2nd or 3rd trimester bleeding, previa >26 wga, PTL, ROM, pre-eclampsia, PIH, severe anemia (Obstet Gynecol 2015;126:e135)

Food Warnings
- **Methylmercury:** High levels can cause CNS damage & mild dysfxn in fetus. Avoid: Shark, swordfish, king mackerel, or tilefish. Limit albacore tuna to 6 oz/w. Encourage 12 oz (~2 servings) of low mercury fish weekly.
- **Caffeine:** Mod consump safe (<200 mg/d) not major contributing factor in miscarriage or preterm birth. One 8 oz coffee = ~95 mg caffeine (*Am J Obstet Gynecol* 2008;198:279). No clear evid for caffeine ↑ risk of IUGR (*JAMA* 1993;269:593).
- **Vit A:** Limit to 750 µg/d (*Lancet* 2010;375:1640). Deficiency common in developing countries. Supplements improve night blindness & anemia w/o teratogenicity. >3000 µg/d (10000 IU) → ↑ fetal malformations. See "Teratogens."
- **Food-borne illness:** Encourage good hand hygiene & thorough cooking
  Listeriosis: Hot dog, lunch meats, cold cuts, unpasteurized soft cheeses, refrigerated meat spreads & pate, unwashed raw produce
  Brucellosis: Unpasteurized milk & cheese made from raw milk.
  Toxoplasmosis: Undercooked meats & contaminated vegetables > cat feces.
- **Pica:** Consuming nonfood substances (*J Am Diet Assoc* 1991;91:34). More common in Preg. Avoid pica & screen for iron-deficiency anemia (unclear mech).

Nutrients in Pregnancy

Macro- and micronutrients in pregnancy			
	Nonpregnant	**Pregnant**	**Comments**
Prot	0.8 g/kg/d	1.1 g/kg/d	Vegetarian women may be advised to supplement specific amino acids not found in vegetable prot sources
Carbs	130 g/d	175 g/d	
Iron	15 mg/d	30 mg/d	If anemic, need btw 30–120 mg daily
Calcium	1000 mg/d	1000 mg/d	Body mobilizes calcium stores in Preg so ↑ intake generally not needed
Folic acid	0.4 mg/d preconception	0.4–4 mg/d	See Folic acid below

- **Folic acid:** ↓ Risk NTDs. NT forms during week 4 of gest → start folate prior to Preg. Low-risk women, use 0.4 mg/d (common dose in prenatal vitamins). Women w/ h/o NTD in prior Preg → 4 mg/d (72% ↓ in recurrence risk). If on antiepileptic drugs, pregestational diabetes or multiple gestation pregnancy also ↑ folate dose.
- **Vit D:** Deficiency common in Preg (newborn levels dependent on mat levels), esp vegetarians, limited sun exposure & dark-skinned ethnicity. Deficiency = maternal serum 25-OH-D <20. No routine screening for Vit D in Preg. Suppl w/ 1000–2000 IU/d (*Obstet Gynecol* 2011;118:197).

CLINICAL PELVIMETRY

Pelvic Anatomy
- **Pelvis:** Sacrum, coccyx, & *innomin* bones. Innomin = *ilium, ischium,* & *pubis* → join sacrum at *sacroiliac jnts* & each other at *symphysis pubis*
- **Linea terminalis** (aka innomin line): Divides false & true pelves
  False pelvis: Above linea terminalis, bounded by lumbar vertebra, iliac fossa, & anter abdominal wall
  True pelvis: Clinically important for parturition; it includes:
  Post: Anter surface of the sacrum
  Lateral: Inner surface of ischial bones
  Anter: Pubic bones & ascending rami of ischial bones

Planes and Diameters of the Pelvis
- **Obstetric Conjugate** (OC; aka AP diameter): Obstetrically relevant diameter. Shortest distance btw the promontory of the sacrum & the symphysis pubis. Measured indirectly by subtracting 1.5–2 cm from the *diagonal conjugate* (>10 cm).
- **Diagonal conjugate:** Distance btw lower margin of symphysis to sacral promontory. Measured clinically w/ examining hand to calculate OC (≥11.5 cm).
- **Transverse diameter:** Distance btw linea terminalis on either side. At right angle to obstetrical conjugate. Largest diameter of pelvis.
- **Interspinous diameter:** In midpelvis. Smallest pelvic diameter, but usually >10 cm.
- Inlet considered contracted if diameters smaller than normal

Figure 9.1 Pelvic shapes

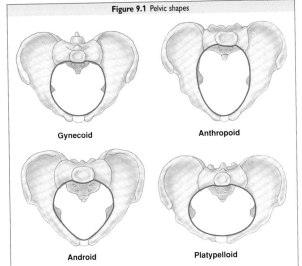

Gynecoid

Anthropoid

Android

Platypelloid

From Klossner NJ, Hatfield NT. *Introductory Maternity & Pediatric Nursing*. 4th ed. Philadelphia, PA: Wolters Kluwer Health; 2017.

Normal AP and transverse diameters of pelvis by shape				
	Gynecoid	**Anthropoid**	**Android**	**Platypelloid**
AP diameter	12 cm	>12 cm	12 cm	12 cm
Transverse diameter	11 cm	<12 cm	11 cm	10 cm
Description	"Ideal"	Upright oval	Heart shaped	Sideways oval

Pelvic Shapes
- **Caldwell & Moloy classification:** Describes 4 ideal types, recognizing there are variations in pelvic shape. Characterized primarily by the transverse & interspinous diameter.
  Gynecoid: Deemed "ideal" w/ wide pelvic inlet & outlet & straight sidewalls
  Anthropoid: Narrow transverse diameter but wide AP diameter
  Platypelloid: Wide inlet & outlet w/ narrow AP diameter & sacral inclination
  Android: Straight sidewalls w/ narrow subpubic arch & narrow incline of sacrum

Pelvimetry in OB Practice
- **Clinical:** Clinical exam of pelvis to predict CPD. Poor predictor of CPD
- **Radiologic pelvimetry:** X-ray or MRI to predict CPD. No impact on mat or neonat morbidity or mortality (*Cochrane Database Syst Rev* 2000:CD000161).
- No evid to recommend C/S for concerns for CPD based on clinical/radiographic pelvimetry.

COMMON PRENATAL COMPLAINTS

Nausea and Vomiting (*Obstet Gynecol* 2018;131:935)
- **NVP:** 50–70% of pregnancies. ↑ hCG & estrogen → NVP. Typically presents <9 w ± abdominal pain. If abd pain & fever → broader diff. 50% resolves by 14 w; 90% by 22 w (*Am J Obstet Gyn* 2000;182:931). PNV 3 mo bf conception may reduce incidence.
  Therapy: Small, frequent meals w/ bland low-fat foods (BRAT diet). Use of ginger can be effective. Encourage hydration.
  1st-line meds: Vit B6 (10–15 mg TID–QID) or Vit B6 & doxylamine 10 mg
  2nd-line meds: Promethazine, metoclopramide, or ondansetron

- **Hyperemesis Gravidarum (HEG):** NVP significant enough to cause dehyd, metabolic alkalosis, ketonuria, weight loss (>5%), hypokalemia. <1% of pregnancies. Risks: Multi gest, FHx, or personal Hx in prior Preg.
- **W/u:** Labs may show elevated transaminases (<300), Amylase, & lipase; hypochloremic metabolic alkalosis; suppressed TSH & ↑ thyroxine; ketones on UA
- **Therapy:** IV hydration (w/ dextrose ± thiamine), enteral nutrition (eg, tube feeding), hospitalization for monitoring & suppl as above

Carpal Tunnel Syndrome (CTS) (Muscle Nerve 2006;34:559)
- **Incid** btw 2 & 35%; most often in 3rd trimester. Risks: H/o CTS in prior Preg, age >30, nulliparous, edema. Caused by compression of median nerve related to edema in Preg. Sx include numbness, pain, paresthesias of thumb, index, & middle fingers, often worse at night. Exacerbated by flexion or extension of wrist, improved by mvmt of hands.
- **Exam:** ± Median nerve sensory deficit. Phalen test: Pain reproduced w/ prolonged (>60 s) flexion of wrists. Tinel test: Pain reproducible w/ percussion at wrist over median nerve.
- **Rx:** Low salt diet, physical therapy, wrist bracing, Tylenol → consider Cort injections for refrac cases. Surgical intervention generally not indicated, sx improve w/i 1 y of deliv (4–50% persist after 1 y).

Round Ligament Pain
- **Anatomy:** Origin at uterine fundus → inguinal canal, terminates in labia majora
- **Presentation:** Lower abdominal pain (more common in right lower quadrant). Exacerbated by mvmt, often reported as "shooting pain into vagina." Case reports of association w/ endometriosis, lipomas, & varicosities. Dx depends on ruling out other etiologies (eg, torsion, appendicitis, preterm labor).
- **Rx:** Typically self-limited. Advise acetaminophen, rest, hydrotherapy, & reassurance. Belly-band can be helpful.

Lower Extremity Edema
- **Physiologic changes** in Preg predispose to edema dev. SVR ↓, venous return impeded by gravid uterus. Water retention mediated by ↓ plasma osmolality due to osmolar reset of vasopressin & thirst thresholds (Br J Obstet Gynaecol 1985;92:1131).
- **Rx:** Elevation of feet & support stockings. Counsel women to report nonsymmetric edema or nondependent edema as these can be signs of pathology such as DVT or preeclampsia.

Low Back Pain (Obstet Gynecol 2004;104:65)
- Up to 70% report LBP during Preg. Risks: LBP outside of Preg, in a prev Preg, or w/ menstruation.
- **Presentation:** Attributed to changes in posture & joint laxity. Pain exacerbated by mvmt, relieved by rest. ± Assoc neurologic sx.
- **Exam:** Eval motor/sensory fxn & reflexes to detect radiculopathy. Paraspinal or joint tenderness to palpation & ↓ range of motion. Imaging not indicated in the absence of progressive neuro signs or trauma.
- **Rx:** Avoid excessive weight gain, lifting heavy objects, prolonged standing, bending from waist. Recommend shoes w/ arch support & sleeping on side w/ pillow btw knees. Use of good body mechanics when lifting & getting out of vehicles is critical. Exercise, acupuncture, support belts may be helpful adjuncts

Lower-Extremity Varicosities
- **Pathophysiology:** Femoral venous pres ↑ in Preg up to 24 mmHg secondary to uterine compression on IVC. Pressures closer to 8 mmHg (pregravid state) in lateral recumbent position (Surg Gynecol Obstet 1950;90:481).
- **Presentation:** Sx vary from cosmetic complaints to a range of discomfort. Throbbing pain that may worsen w/ advancing Preg, weight gain, & standing.
- **Rx:** Periodic elevation of feet & support stockings. Surgical correction during Preg generally avoided unless sev sx.

Vulvar Varicosities
- **Pathophysiology:** 4% lifetime prevalence, most often occurring during Preg b/c of ↑ venous pressures & ↑ pelvic bld flow. "Vulvar veins lack valves"
- **Presentation:** Often asymptomatic & noted only on exam. Pelvic discomfort & swelling worsened with standing or intercourse.
- **Mgmt:** Reassurance – most vulvar varicosities regress postpartum. Vulvar support belt for sev sx or local excision for thrombosis. Vaginal deliv not contraindicated despite theoretical risk of hemorrhage w/ laceration.

Hemorrhoids

- **Pathophysiology:** Arise w/i plexus of inferior & superior hemorrhoidal veins. ↑ Venous pressures in Preg → engorgement both internally & externally → venous stasis → thrombosis & pain/swelling.
- **Presentation:** Painless bleeding w/ defecation or anal pruritus. Sev pain or complaints of a palpable lump can occur w/ thrombosis. External hemorrhoids visualized as dilated veins; thrombosis felt on palpation during rectal exam.
- **Rx:** Supportive w/ local anesthesia, hydration, & stool softeners. Topical anesthetics or steroid creams (external and/or suppositories) along w/ sitz baths can provide local relief. Thrombosis can be treated w/ excision under local anesthesia.

Leg Cramps

- **Pathophysiology:** Exact cause unclear, distinguish from RLS (strong urge to move legs, pain, achy)
- **Presentation:** Often nocturnal, muscle spasm of the calf
- **Mgmt:** No evidence to suggest use of Magnesium, Vit C, Ca, Vit B, more data needed (RLS often caused by iron deficiency, worsens in pregnancy). Nonpharmacologic methods (massage, yoga, heat, dorsiflexion), with limited trials

Constipation

Common medications for treatment of constipation				
Type	**Name**	**Mech**	**Maximal dose**	**Side effects**
Bulk laxative	Psyllium (Metamucil)	Increases colonic residue, stimulates peristalsis	Titrate up to 20 g	Bloating, flatus
Osmotic laxative	Magnesium hydroxide (MOM)	Draws water into intestines	15–30 mL up to BID	Hypermagnesemia
	Magnesium citrate		150–300 mL prn	
	Sodium phosphate (Fleet)		10–25 mL w/ 12 oz water prn	Hyperphos
Poorly absorbed sugars	Lactulose	Poorly absorbed, draw water into intestines	15–30 mL 1–2 times a day	Bloating, flatus
	Sorbitol			
	Polyethylene glycol (Miralax, GoLytely – electrolytes)		17–36 g 1–2 times a day	Less bloating & discomfort
Stimulant laxative	Senna	Stimulates intestinal motility or secretion	187 mg daily	Melanosis coli
	Bisacodyl (Dulcolax)		5–10 mg QHS	Cramping
	Docusate sodium (Colace)	Ionic detergents allow incorporation of water into stool	100 mg BID	Diarrhea
Enema/ suppository	Tap-water enema	Distends rectum to initiate evacuation, lubrication	500 mL daily	Electrolyte abnormalities can occur if retained
	Soapsuds enema		1500 mL daily	
	Mineral oil enema		100 mL daily	
	Bisacodyl suppository	Topical stimulation of colonic muscle	10 mg daily	Cramping
Prokinetic	Tegaserod (Zelnorm)	5-HT$_4$ agonist	6 mg BID	Diarrhea

Adated from *NEJM* 2003;349:1360–8.

Common medications for treatment of diarrhea			
Name	**Mech**	**Dosage**	**Side effects**
Loperamide (Imodium)	Inhibits peristalsis, increases sphincter tone	2 mg PO TID Max 8 mg/d	Constip, nausea
Diphenoxylate–atropine (Lomotil)	Inhibits circular smooth muscle	5 mg PO QID	CNS effects, nausea
Hyoscyamine sulfate	Antichol	0.325 mg BID	Constip, dry mouth

From Lentz GM. Anal incontinence: Diagnosis and management. In: Lentz GM, ed. *Comprehensive Gynecology.* 6th ed. Philadelphia, PA: Mosby; 2012:503–18.

FETAL ULTRASOUND: ANATOMY AND ECHOCARDIOGRAPHY

- **First Trimester US** confirms IUP, evaluate for ectopic, eval vaginal bleeding/pelvic pain, establish/confirm due date, dx/eval multiple gestation, confirm viability, adjunct to CVS/embryo transfer/IUD removal, eval pelvic/adnexal mass/uterine abnormalities, screen for fetal aneuploidy, eval for hydatidiform mole *(Obstet Gynecol 2016;128(6):1459).*
- **Second Trimester US** includes fetal presentation and number, amniotic fluid volume (AFV), cardiac activity, placental position, fetal biometry, and anatomic survey
- **Amniotic fluid volume:** Described subjectively or by semiquantitative methods
  Amniotic fluid index: Division of uterus into 4 quadrants and measure deepest vertical pocket of fluid in each, then add four measurements together. Width of pocket at least 1 cm. Normal 5–25 cm.
  SDP (Single deepest pocket): Vertical depth (cm) of deepest pocket of fluid not containing cord or fetal extremities (Nml 2–8 cm).
- **Placental location:** Describing location (anter/post) & relation to internal os. Endovaginal US should be performed if internal cervical os not clearly visualized. Placental abnormalities (eg, previa) should be followed up w/ 3rd trimester US.
- **Umbilical cord:** Identify number of arteries and insertion site
- **CL:** Not currently a rec for low-risk pop. Recommendations for CL screening are evolving. Screening CL at anatomy US after 16 w GA is reasonable. Endovaginal US w/ empty bladder more accurate.
- **GA:** Most accurate in 1st trimester (CRL). 2nd trimester determination (fetal biometry) includes:
  BPD: Measured at level of thalamus & cavum septum pellucidum
  HC: More reliable than BPD if head shape flattened or rounded
  AC: Measured at junction of umbilical vein, portal sinus, & stomach. Can compare to BPD to determine symmetric macrosomia or IUGR.
  FL: Long axis of femur not including the distal & prox epiphysis
- **EFW:** Combination of BPD, HC, AC, & FL to determine EFW
  EFW compared to known values to establish %ile & establish macrosomia/IUGR

Fetal Anatomy Assessment *(Obstet Gynecol 2016;128(6):1459)*
- Routinely performed at 18–20 w GA. Thorough assessment of fetal structures.
  Head, face, neck (lateral cerebral ventricles, choroid plexus, midline falx, cavum septum pellucidi, cerebellum, cisterna magna, upper lip). **Chest** (heart – 4 chamber view and outflow tracts), **Abdomen** (stomach, kidneys, urinary ladder, umbilical cord insertion site, and vessel number), **Spine** (cervical, thoracic, lumbar and sacral spine), **Extremities** (legs, arms), **Fetal sex**
- **Aneuploidy screening:** US alone not adequate for trisomy 21 (T21) or other aneuploidy. Presence or absence of fetal anomalies a/w T21, such as cardiac anomalies & duodenal atresia, confers ↑ or ↓ risk, respectively. ↑ NT on 1st trimester US identifies ↑ risk of aneuploidy. **Soft markers:** Echogenic bowel, EIF, short femur or humerus, or dilated renal pelvis. Absence of "soft markers" for Down syn on US ↓ a priori risk of T21 or mat serum screening risk by 50%.

Fetal Echocardiography *(Circulation 2014;129:2183)*
- **Congenital heart disease:** Leading cause of mortality & morbidity. Prenatal dx offers planning for infant & intervention at birth.
- **Indications:** Used as adjunct to routine US screening, btw 18–22 w
- **Mat indications:** Diabetes, autoimmune antibodies (eg, Anti-SSA/SSB), familial inherited cardiac d/o, 1st- or 2nd-degree relative w/ CHD or syndromes w/ CHD,

IVF, metabolic dz (eg, phenylketonuria), cardiac teratogen exposure, rubella exposure 1st trimester
- **Fetal indications:** Abn cardiac screening exam, abn HR or rhythm, fetal chromosomal anomaly, extracardiac anomaly, hydrops, ↑ NT, monochorionic twins, unexplained sev polyhydramnios

CONGENITAL ANOMALIES

Definitions and Terminology
- **Terminology:** Description related to etiology
  Malformation: Due to an intrinsic process in embryonic dev (prior to 8 w)
  Deformation: Due to intrauterine process unrelated to fetus (tumor, multi gest)
  Disruption: Due to interference w/ nml dev (eg, amniotic band syn)
  Dysplasia: Due to abn growth of cells into tissues
- **Patterns of anomalies:** Multi anomalies can be described by overarching descriptors
  Syndrome: Assoc anomalies due to single pathologic etiology (eg, Turner syn)
  Sequence: Group of anomalies related to a common upstream pathologic cause (eg, Potter's sequence: Renal agenesis → oligohydramnios → bone fractures).
  Developmental field defect: Due to disruption of dev in a particular region of the embryo that leads to disruption in related areas (eg, bladder exstrophy)
  Association: Group of anomalies unrelated pathologically occurring more commonly than one would expect by chance (eg, VACTERL association)

Teratogens
- **Definition:** An agent or factor that causes an anomaly in the developing fetus. Ex:
  Mat illness: Due to toxic metabolites or antibodies from mother crossing placenta
  Pregestational diabetes: 6–7% risk (2× nml pop) of congenital anomalies including NTD, congenital heart disease (CHD), & caudal agenesis (rare but 15–20% a/w DM)
  Systemic lupus erythematosus: A/w fetal congen complete heart block
  Infxn: TORCH infxns, varicella, or parvovirus B19
  Meds: Thalidomide & its association w/ limb reduction is classic example
  Environmental: Lead, ionizing radiation, fever, hyperthermia, & mercury consump

Embryologic development by organ system		
System	**Embryology**	**Timing**
Neural tube	Neural plate → neural folds → fuse to form neural tube	Weeks 3–4
Cardiovascular	Primitive heart tube → looping & division → formation of primitive structures (BC, outflow tracts, sinus venosus, PA, & PV) → septum primum/secundum separate RA & LA → endocardial cushions divide atria & ventric → BC becomes RV & PV becomes LV separated by musc ventricular septum → outflow tract septates & divides & remodeling forms semilunar valves	Weeks 4–8: Week 4 primitive heart tube is formed & begins looping → weeks 4–5 atria divided by septum primum → week 6 ventricles divided → weeks 7 & 8 outflow tract divided
Pulm	Bronchial tree & assoc pulm arteries undergo branching & division	Weeks 3–16: Surfactant production starts at 20 w
Gastrointestinal	Physiologic herniation of abdominal contents into extraembryonic coelom to allow space for growth of abdominal organs	Weeks 9–11: Physiologic herniation resolved by 12 w
Genitourinary	Pronephros → mesonephros → ureteric bud → invades metanephric blastema to make metanephros → kidney → migrates caudally. Metanephros fuses w/ cloaca to make bladder	Develops weeks 4–6. Producing urine by week 11 Bladder fusion begins at week 5

Neural Tube Defects (Int J Gynaecol Obstet 2003;83:123)

- **Epidemiology:** 1.4–2 per 1000 pregnancies; 2nd most common anomaly worldwide.
- **Etiology:** Genetic, environmental, or a/w syndromes (eg, Meckel syndrome)
    - **Genetic:** ↑ Risk for pts who have a child w/ prior NTD; 5% of NTD have familial assoc.
    - **Environmental:** Diet (low folic acid consump), teratogen exposure (anticonvulsants, Vit A), mat diabetes w/ poor 1st trimester gluc control, high mat core temperature in the 1st trimester.
- **Pathophysiology:** Failure of closure of neural tube
    - **Cranial defects:** Eg: Anencephaly, encephalocele, exencephaly, iniencephaly. All cranial defects except small encephaloceles (failure of skull formation w/ extrusion of brain into membranous sac) are lethal. **Spinal defects:** Often a/w ventriculomegaly (often require shunt placement)
    - **Spina bifida:** Failure of fusion of caudal portion of neural tube
    - **Meningocele:** Failure of fusion, meninges exposed
    - **Meningomyelocele:** Failure of fusion, meninges, & neural tissue exposed
- **Clinical manifestations:** Higher lesions generally indicate worse prog
    - **Bladder/bowel:** Dysfxn common, even w/ lower spinal lesions. Bladder dysfxn → UTIs, stones, & significant morbidity. Sexual dysfxn common.
    - **Neuro:** Sensory & motor handicap correlated w/ level of lesion; ventriculomegaly a/w ↓ intelligence quotient
- **Dx:** ↑ Amniotic fluid & mat serum AFP (MSAFP)
    - **Screening:** 89–100% of pregnancies w/ NTD have ↑ MSAFP
    - Other causes of ↑ MSFAP: (1) Incorrect GA, (2) multi gestations, (3) abdominal wall defects, (4) abnorm placentation (eg, accreta), (5) IUFD, (6) Finnish nephrosis, (7) sev skin anomalies such as lethal ichthyosis.
    - ↑ MSAFP risk factor for placental abruption
    - US able to identify many causes – done after MSAFP collection, usually 18–22 w
    - **US:** 97% sens & 100% spec for NTD in experienced centers
    - **Dx:** 2% of pts w/ positive MSAFP have fetus w/ NTD. Confirmatory test can be an amniocentesis for AFP and if elevated, AF acetylcholinesterase
- **Prevention:** Avoid of teratogens & suppl w/ folic acid prior to and during preg (see *Nutrition*)
- **Rx:** Deliv at hospital w/ NICU support; consideration of fetal surg vs. postpartum repair
    - Breech presentation common in fetus w/ NTD necessitating Cesarean deliv; vaginal deliv should be considered if fetus in cephalic presentation.

Other Neurologic Anomalies

- **Ventriculomegaly:** ↑ Vol of cerebral ventricles on US (≥1 cm on anatomy US)
    - **Isolated:** Often found to be a/w NTD or other malformations after birth
    - **Associations:** Can be related to infxn (toxoplasmosis, CMV, lymphocytic choriomeningitis virus), genetic syndromes, or aneuploidy
    - **W/u:** Amniocentesis should be offered for aneuploidy/infxn w/u. F/u 3rd trimester scan should look for progression or other identifiable causes
- **Hydrocephalus:** Pathologic ventriculomegaly from ↑ pres
- **Choroid plexus cysts (CPC):** Cystic sonolucent lesions w/i choroid plexus
    - 1–2% of normal pregnancies. Isolated CPC not a/w aneuploidy & typically resolve by 3rd trimester. CPC with other anomalies ↑ risk aneuploidy, esp trisomy 18

Cardiovascular Anomalies

- **Nonimmune hydrops fetalis (NIHF):** Cardiac anomalies cause up to 40% of NIHF.
    - **Manifestations:** Pts can present w/ fundal height > dates & ↓ FM. US: Ascites pleural effusions, pericardial effusions, skin edema (late finding), polyhydramnios, and/or placentomegaly.
    - **Associations:** Structural heart dx, tachyarrhythmias, or bradyarrhythmias
- **Hypoplastic left heart syndrome (HLHS):**
    - **Anatomy:** Underdeveloped LV w/ hypoplasia, stenosis, or atresia of aortic valve, MV, &/or aorta. Survival dependent on PDA & ASD to allow for flow from RV to aorta.
    - **Dx:** US: small or nonfunctioning LV, small aortic root, small aortic arch, ↑ or absent Doppler velocities through the aortic valve, abn MV, and/or restricted or reversed flow through the foramen ovale (usually right to left flow in utero)
    - **Associations:** Trisomy 18, Trisomy 13, Turner syn, or sporadic
    - **Mgmt:** Identification can allow for birth planning (administration of prostaglandins to ensure persistent PDA) & poss fetal intervention. Dilation of AS can reverse HLHS physiology. In utero atrial septostomy can allow for ASD creation.

- **AVSDs:** Atrial & ventricular septal defects w/ singular, multileaflet atrioventricular valve. Diagnosed on US, confirmed w/ echo. AVSDs a/w aneuploidy.
- **Conotruncal anomalies:** Tetralogy of Fallot, persistent truncus arteriosus. Should prompt testing for DiGeorge syn (microdeletion of chromo 22q11, detectable by FISH).
- **Tachyarrhythmias:** Treated by giving rate-controlling agents to mother or directly to fetus.

Thoracic Anomalies
- Congenital pulmonary airway malformation (CPAM)
  - Sporadic lesion due to abnormalities in branching of pulm tree → cystic or solid lung lesions. Classified based on size cystic or solid components. Different types confer varying risks of regression, progression, or malig transformation.
    - **Type 1:** Large (>2 cm) multiloculated cysts
    - **Type 2:** Smaller uniform cysts
    - **Type 3:** Not grossly cystic → "adenomatoid" type
- **Congenital diaphragmatic hernia (CDH):** Defect in diaphragm → herniation
  - Dx: Solid (on right due to liver) or cystic (on left due to bowel) mass on US
  - Occurs as isolated finding, as part of a sequence, or w/ aneuploidy (10–20%).
  - Prognosis: Left-sided lesions more common. Right-sided lesions confer worse prog (liver herniation). ↑ Fetal lung vol improves prog. Can lead to NIHF & dextroposition.
  - Further w/u includes fetal echo, fetal karyotype or microarray, & poss MRI.

Gastrointestinal Anomalies
- **Omphalocele:** Defect in abdominal wall holding herniated abdominal wall contents.
  - **Dx:** Diagnosed on US after week 12 GA (before week 12 herniation of contents physiologic). Hernia covered by amnion & peritoneum; herniation at site of cord insertion. Classified by whether or not defect contains liver (liver-containing defect never nml regardless of GA). Causes elevated MSAFP.
  - **Associations:** 50% association w/ cardiac lesion (fetal echo recommended); Beckwith–Wiedemann syn, OEIS syn, & amniotic band syn. Association w/ aneuploidy in nonliver containing lesions (chromo analysis recommended).
- **Gastroschisis:** Evisceration of abdominal contents through abdominal wall defect
  - **Dx:** Seen as full thickness abdominal wall defect, generally to right of cord insertion (nml cord insertion is seen on US). Bowel may become thickened & matted w/ increasing GA. No overlying peritoneum.
  - **Associations:** No ↑ risk of chromosomal aneuploidy but a/w other GI problems. ↑ Risk of recurrence w/i families.
- **Echogenic bowel:** ↑ Echogenicity (brightness) of bowel noted on US.
  - **Etiology:** A/w intestinal bleeding events, aneuploidy, CF, growth restriction, infxn microarray & idiopathic (most common).
  - **Aneuploidy:** 3–25% association w/ aneuploidy, primarily trisomy 21. Offer amniocentesis for chromosomes/microarray, CF & CMV testing.

Genitourinary Anomalies
- **Renal agenesis:** Ureteric bud fails to develop & induce differentiation of kidney
  - **Etiology:** Can be unilateral or bilateral. Bilateral usually due to embryonic issue; unilateral difficult to distinguish agenesis from dysplasia & hypoplasia.
  - **Dx:** Bilateral renal agenesis diagnosed w/ nonvisualization of kidneys, bladder, & oligohydramnios. Unilateral diagnosed by absent or abn kidney location (amniotic fluid nml). Full fetal bladder is good indicator of renal fxn.
  - **Prog:** Bilateral renal agenesis incompatible w/ life due to pulm hypoplasia. High rate of IUFD due to cord accidents from oligohydramnios.
  - **Associations:** 50% association w/ other anomalies; high rate of single umbilical artery
- **VACTERL:** Vertebral anomalies, Anal atresia, Cardiac defects, TE fistula, Renal defects, Limb defects
- **Müllerian anomalies:** Defects in female reproductive tract including separate or absent reproductive systems. See Chap. 8.
- **OEIS complex (Cloacal exstrophy):** Omphalocele, Exstrophy of the bladder, Imperf anus, Spinal defects
  - **Etiology:** Due to abnormalities of cloaca – blind pouch from which rectum & urogenital sinus develop. Typically sporadic & not a/w aneuploidy.
- **Bladder exstrophy:** Diagnosed w/ absent bladder filling, low-set umbilicus, lower abdominal mass increasing in size throughout Preg. Independent of OEIS complex, can be other assoc abdominal wall, musculoskeletal & genital deficits.

Musculoskeletal Anomalies
- **Skeletal dysplasias:** Qualitatively or quantitatively abn bones on prenatal US
  - **Dx:** FL or HL <5%ile based on GA
  - **Etiology:** Constitutionally short fetus (isolated abn FL), IUGR (a/w small AC), or skeletal dysplasia. Can be marker of aneuploidy.
  - **W/u:** Interval growth in 3–4 w can show normalization of FL or nml interval growth. Comparison to other parameters (AC, BPD, HC) can reveal IUGR. If continued short FL compare to qualitative description of other bones.
    - → **SMA (spinal muscular atrophy)** → SMN1 gene. Degeneration of anterior horn in spinal cord and motor nuclei, results in progressive muscle weakness/atrophy. All women should be offered screening (ACOG).
    - → **Achondroplasia** → Most common bone dysplasia. AD condition. Disproportionate short stature, long bone shortening, macrocephaly. Normal cognition.
    - → **Osteogenesis Imperfecta** → Inherited connective tissue disorder. Severely affected patients suffer from multiple fractures with minimal/no trauma. In its most severe form, infants die in perinatal period.
- **Talipes equinovarus (clubfoot):** Excessive plantar flexion w/ foot facing medially.
  - **Etiology:** Primarily idiopathic or isolated (familial recurrence); can be due to aneuploidy (trisomy 18), deformation (extrinsic).

GENETIC SCREENING

Maternal Serum Aneuploidy Screening (Obstet Gynecol 2016;127(5):e123; 2017;129:e41)
- Aneuploidy screening should be offered to all pts. Counseling includes what is being screened for, potential results, advantages/disadvantages (including cost) & how the results might impact their decisions about the preg.
- Reported as "risk" of aneuploidy (w/ regard to trisomy 21 & trisomies 13/18) compared to age-matched reference, not as positive or negative (except for cell-free fetal DNA, see below). Overall: 5% positive screen rate for maternal serum screening (predetermined)
- **Screening parameters:** Combination of values used in various screening approaches
  - **Nuchal translucency:** Defined anatomic area behind fetal neck measured sonographically as width (mm) btw ~11–14 w. ↑ in aneuploidy & other conditions. Lower false positive rate if combined w/ serum markers. Useful in multiples when serum markers not accurate (Inc also a/w congenital heart defects). If NT ≥3.5 mm w/ normal fetal karyotype → targeted US and fetal echo.
  - **Nasal bone:** Absent nasal bone a/w significantly increased risk of Down syndrome
  - **Serum markers:** Preg hormones used in combination to calculate risk (AFP, β-hCG, PAPP-A, inhibin A, UE3)
- **1st trimester screening:** NT, PAPP-A & β-hCG in mat serum at 11–14 w. Comparable detection rates to 2nd trimester screen but higher screen positive rate in women >35 yo. Advantages: Time for CVS as diagnostic test & earlier termination options. Disadvantages: More costly approach. In case of sequential strategy, pts must wait for results until 2nd trimester.
- **2nd trimester screening:** AFP, hCG, unconjugated estriol (UE3), and inhibin A in screen at 15–22 6/7 w. Detection 69% for triple screen, 81% for quadruple screen. Advantages: Does not rely on NT (operator dependent test). Serum markers may suggest other problems (eg, ↑ AFP for NTD).
  - Disadvantages: Only screening → amniocentesis for dx. Given later GA, if anomaly found, options may be more limited.

Second trimester maternal serum analytes			
	AFP	**UE₃**	**hCG**	**Inhibin A**
T21	↓	↓	↑	↑
T18	↓	↓	↓	↓
NTD	↑	N/A	N/A	N/A

- Triple Screen → hCG, unconjugated estriol, MSAFP (detection rate for Down syndrome is about 70%, 5% of pregnancies have positive screening result)
- QUAD screen → Add inhibin A to triple screen, improves detection rate for Down syndrome to about 80%

- **Combined approaches:**
  - **Integrated screening:** Integrates 1st & 2nd trimesters → results given in 2nd trimester. 94–96% detection rate w/ full integrated screen.
  - **Sequential screening:** 1st & 2nd trimester screens performed w/ results reported after 1st & then altered after 2nd trimester. Benefits: Allows CVS for those at highest risk 95% detection rate by 2nd trimester.

Cell-free Fetal DNA (Obstet Gynecol 2015;126:e31)
- **Definition:** Free fetal DNA in mat circulation likely from syncytiotrophoblast cells, extracted from mat serum & proportion of target fetal genetic material measured by sequencing. Comprises 3–13% of total cell free maternal DNA after 10 w. Imbalance of genetic material sugg extra or missing chromo.
- Single bld test w/ >99% sens & spec for T21 & T18. Lower sensitivities for T13 and sex chromosome abnml, but >99% spec. Rapidly evolving technology. Does NOT detect balanced DNA defects (eg, triploidy).
- **Applications:** Aneuploidy, sex determination (presence of Y chromo), Rh typing. Performed after 10 w.

All pts can be offered cfDNA screening, including low risk OB population (Obstet Gynecol Surv 2016;71(8):477).

Screening for Hemoglobinopathies
- See Chap. 16
  - **Alpha-thalassemia:** HbEP unable to detect alpha-thalassemia, if of Southeast Asian ancestry w/ microcytic anemia, nml iron studies, & nml HbEP offer DNA testing for abn alpha-globin gene. If positive, partner requires screening.
  - **Dx:** If both parents are carriers & have described genetic mutations → offer CVS or amniocentesis for fetal genetic testing

Other Inherited Diseases (Obstet Gynecol 2017;129:e41)
- **CF:** Autosomal recessive condition due to >1700 of mutations in CFTR gene. Routine testing for common mutations offered to all pts (regardless of ethnicity) after appropriate education regarding the implications of testing & results. Detection of test related to prevalence in pop. Pts w/ personal Hx or FHx of CF or related conditions should undergo genetic counseling to determine if expanded mut screens are warranted. If pt positive, partner should be screened & consider amniocentesis/CVS.
- **Fragile X:** Most common *inherited* form of MR. Due to ↑ triplet repeats on FMR1 gene. Offer carrier testing in FHx of fragile X-related disorders, unexplained MR, autism or premature ovarian failure. Variable penetrance based on number of triplet repeats and may impact future generations with increased severity (anticipation). Only test for FMR1 triplet rpt is diagnostic test using CVS or amniocentesis for known carriers.
- **Tay-Sachs:** Ashkenazi Jewish, French Canadian, or Cajun descent
- **Familial dysautonomia or Canavan dz:** Ashkenazi Jewish descent
- Offer other screening tests (musc dystrophy, Huntington's) based on FHx. Lengthy carrier panels are available.

AMNIOCENTESIS AND CHORIONIC VILLUS SAMPLING (CVS)

Invasive Prenatal Diagnostic Testing
- Definitive diagnoses for specific conditions. Discuss the difference btw screening & diagnostic tests, risks & benefits, alternate screening tests & interpretation of results.

Amniocentesis (Obstet Gynecol 2007;110:1459)
- **Definition:** Removal of AF using transabdominal approach, typically w/ US guidance. Both diagnostic & therapeutic indications. Genetic amniocentesis preferred at 15–20 w.
- **Diagnostic amniocentesis:** Usually for prenatal genetic testing, but several applications:
  - **Genetics:** Allows for culture of fetal cells & dx of aneuploidy via karyotype FISH or CGH
  - **Infxn:** AF can be used for cell count, gluc, & culture for suspected chorio or can be used to perform diagnostic tests for infxn, such as PCR for CMV
  - **Hemoglobin:** Fetal hemoglobin can be obtained for eval of fetal anemia, fetal bld type, or eval of hemoglobinopathies
  - **Other indications:** Can be used to test fetal lung maturity or for NTDs.

- **Therapeutic amniocentesis:** Amnioreduction (removal of AF) can be therapeutic for pts w/ twin-to-twin xfusion syn & preterm CTX from polyhydramnios
- **Risks:** Higher w/ if performed from 11–13 w, not recommended. 1 in 300–500 Preg loss, lower at experienced centers. Direct fetal injury. 1–2% vaginal spotting or leakage of fluid; <1:1000 for chorio. AF cells can fail to culture leading to nondiagnosis after amniocentesis. Small risk of transmission of HCV or HBV but data limited. Small risk of transmission of HIV if pt on antiretroviral therapy/ undetectable viral load. Rh-negative women should get anti-D Rhlg prior to procedure to prevent sensitization.

Chorionic Villus Sampling (CVS)
- **Definition:** Removal of chorionic villi via transabdominal (TA) or transcervical (TC) catheter w/ needle under US guidance. Typically used for dx using karyotype analysis, FISH, or genetic testing for specific alleles. Performed 9–16 w gest.
- **Risks:** Complication rate of TA-CVS lower than rates of TC-CVS. Fetal loss (0.7–1.3%) higher than amniocentesis but background rate of fetal loss at earlier GA is higher. Rates of loss at similar GAs are the same btw amniocentesis & CVS. U Limb reduction or oromandibular defects after 9 w, risk = 6 in 10000 (similar to risk in general pop). Rh-negative women should get anti-D Rhlg prior to procedure to prevent sensitization.
- **Counseling:** Offer to pts interested in 1st trimester diagnostic testing. Advantage of CVS is early GA at dx = more options.
- **Chromosomal Microarray** (*Obstet Gynecol* 2016;128:e262) can be sent on fetal cells. Often reflex if the karyotype is normal → look for smaller DNA errors as well as the large changes. Different from karyotype. Adding microarray to karyotype identifies ~5% additional DNA errors.

ANTENATAL FETAL TESTING

Goal of Testing

- **Goal:** Prevention of fetal demise via detection of abnormal fetal physiology and/or alteration in fetal behavioral states that reliably correlate with abnormal fetal oxygenation and acid/base status

Indications for antenatal testing	
Maternal conditions	**Pregnancy-related conditions**
• Pre-existing hypertension	• Gestational hypertension
• Pregestational diabetes mellitus (Type 1 or Type 2 DM)	• Preeclampsia
• Thyroid disease (poorly controlled)	• Gestational diabetes mellitus (on medications)
• Hemoglobinopathies	• Fetal growth restriction
• Chronic renal disease	• Oligohydramnios
• Systemic lupus erythematosus	• Post term pregnancy
• Cyanotic heart disease	• Isoimmunization
• Antiphospholipid antibody syndrome	• Multiple gestation
	• Prior fetal demise

Data from *J Obstet Gynaecol Can* 2007; 29:S3-56, *Obstet Gynecol* 2014;124:182–92.

Testing Modalities (Obstet Gynecol 2014;124:182–92)

- **Fetal movement count** ("kick counts") (Cochrane Database Syst Rev 2007:CD004909)
- Variable protocols, usually 10 movements over 2 h is reassuring, 3–7×/w; insufficient evidence to recommend this method of surveillance
- **Nonstress test**
  Fetal Heart Rate (FHR) monitoring with external transducer for at least 20 min (occasionally up to 40 min or longer)
  Maternal position: Lateral recumbent position or semi-Fowler
  Reactive: At least 2 15 bpm × 15 s accelerations, if >32 w (or 10 × 10, if <32 w)
  Nonreactive: Insufficient FHR accelerations over 20-min period
  Performance for prediction of stillbirth within 1 w: Sens 99.7%, Spec 45%
  Brief (<30 s), nonrepetitive (<3 in 20 min) variable decelerations do not affect negative predictive value. Decelerations lasting >1 min are associated with fetal compromise and need for OB intervention
- **Biophysical profile** (NST + Real-time ultrasonography performed over 30 min)
  5 Components (2 points each if present; 0 if absent):
  1. Breathing: Continuous fetal breathing (1 episode lasting >30 s)
  2. Movement: 3 or more fetal limb or discrete body movements
  3. Tone: 1 or more episodes of extension/flexion of a limb or opening/closing of a hand
  4. Amniotic fluid: Adequate amniotic fluid → single deepest vertical pocket >2 cm
  5. NST: Reactive NST
  8–10/10 = normal, 6/10 = equivocal (repeat in 6–24 h), ≤4/10 = abnormal (consider deliv). Prediction of stillbirth within 1 w: Sens 99.92%, Spec 50%.
  Modified biophysical profile: (NST + Amniotic fluid volume assessment). NST is an immediate assessment of fetal acid–base status, AFI is an assessment of uteroplacental function.
- **Contraction stress test** (oxytocin or nipple stimulation to produce 3 contractions in 10 min of >40 s, w/ continuous FHR monitoring)
  Negative = No late or significant variable decelerations
  Positive = Late decelerations after 50% or more of contractions (even with insufficient contractions)
  Equivocal = intermittent decels or contractions q2min
  Unsatisfactory = Uninterpretable fetal heart tracing or <3 contractions in 10 min
  Prediction of stillbirth within 1 w: Sens 99.96%, PPV 70%
- **Umbilical artery Doppler velocimetry** (US measurement, *only* indicated in fetuses w/ growth restriction)
  Low resistance system should allow forward flow throughout entire cardiac cycle
  Normally grown fetuses should have high-velocity diastolic blood flow. Growth-restricted fetuses demonstrate decreased umbilical artery diastolic flow, due to obliteration of small arteries in the placenta. The normal progression in fetal compromise: Elevated S/D → AEDF → REDF
  Absent or reverse end-diastolic flow is associated with increased perinatal mortality (5× greater w/ reversed flow) (Lancet 1994;344:1664)

- **Middle cerebral artery Doppler velocimetry**
  US measurement of peak systolic velocity (increased in fetal anemia), indicated if risk factors for fetal anemia.
  Velocity >1.5 MoM has Sens for mod/sev anemia 100%, false positive rate 12% (N Engl J Med 2000;342:9). Optimal screening interval likely 1–2 w starting at 18–20 w.

FETAL LUNG MATURITY TESTING BY AMNIOCENTESIS

General Considerations
- Not routinely performed, but can be considered for planned delivery between 32–39 w. If delivery indicated before 39 w for maternal or fetal indications there is no indication to test. No indication to test for poor dating (Obstet Gynecol 2013;121:911–15).
- Before 32 w → low likelihood of maturity
- Test performance worsens at earlier GAs
- All tests more accurately predict absence of respiratory distress (w/ mature result) than predict respiratory distress (w/ immature result) (Obstet Gynecol 2001;97:305)

Specific Assays
- **Lamellar body count** (direct assessment) or optical density at 650 nm (indirect assessment) of surfactant production
  >50000/μL or optical density (OD) >0.15 sugg maturity. May vary by institution. Falsely elevated in presence of blood.
- **L/S ratio** (L/S about equal until ~35 w, then lecithin increases)
  Threshold value for "mature" varies by institution. Generally mature at >2 (2–3.5)
- **PG measurement** (appears ~35 w & rapidly increases)
  Quantitative or qualitative measurement. Not affected by mec or blood.
- **Foam stability index:** Measures functional surfactant. >47 signifies maturity.
- **Surfactant/albumin ratio,** TDx-FLM II (phased out by manufacturer in 2011)

NEWBORN RESPIRATORY DISTRESS

Epidemiology (Am Fam Physician 2007;76:987; Breathe 2016;12(1):30–42)
- 7% of infants. Most common causes: Transient tachypnea of the newborn, respiratory distress syndrome, mec aspiration syndrome
- Less common causes: Delayed transition, infection, persistent pHTN, pneumonia, nonpulmonary causes (anemia, CHD)

Signs and Symptoms
- Tachypnea (>60 breaths/min), nasal flaring, poor feeding, grunting, sub- or intracostal retractions, inspiratory stridor, apnea, cyanosis

Transient Tachypnea of the Newborn
- Incidence of 5.7 per 1000 term births (Br J Obstet Gynaecol 1995;102(2):101)
- Delayed resorption and clearance of alveolar fluid from lung → decreased pulm compliance → tachypnea, hypoxemia
- Onset within 2 h of birth; usually resolves in <72 h
- Clinical diagnosis, CXR: Diffuse parenchymal infiltrates
- Management: supportive with supplemental O_2, usually self-limited

Respiratory Distress Syndrome (Hyaline Membrane Disease) (Peds 2010;126(3):443)
- Most common before 28 w gestation
  1/3 of infants 28–34 w gestation
  <5% of infants after 34 w gestation
- Surfactant deficiency causing atelectasis → V/Q mismatching → hypoxemia
- Increased likelihood for newborns of diabetic mothers (Semin Fetal Neonatal Med 2009;14(2):111)
- CXR: Reticular ground glass, & air bronchograms
- Management: Surfactant admin, CPAP

Meconium Aspiration Syndrome
- Mec-stained amniotic fluid = 2–10% of those get mec aspiration syndrome; meconium = irritative, obstructive, medium for bacterial culture in the lungs
- Usually term or post-term infants; significant respiratory distress immediately after delivery
- CXR: Patchy atelectasis or consolidation

General Management

- Diagnostic CXR; CBC, blood gas, blood culture
- Supplemental oxygen therapy, w/ positive pressure support or assisted ventilation if necessary
- Supportive care w/ fluid/electrolyte management & neutral thermal environment
  Oral feeding often withheld w/ respiratory rate >80 breaths/min
- Empiric ampicillin & gentamicin if risk factors for sepsis or refractory/persistent symptoms
- Surfactant administration may be required

GROUP B STREPTOCOCCAL DISEASE

Definition and Epidemiology (MMWR 59(RR10):1; Obstet Gynecol 2011;117:1019–27)

- Intrapartum vertical transmission of GBS is the leading cause of infectious morbidity/mortality in neonates; incid is ~0.25/1000 births
- Caused by GBS infection of fetal mucosal surfaces by GBS in amniotic fluid or birth canal
- 10–30% of pregnant women are colonized w/ GBS in GI tract or vagina
- Risk factors for invasive GBS disease include:
  <37 w at delivery, ruptured amniotic membranes for >18 h, intra-amniotic infection, GBS bacteriuria, and history of prior infant with GBS disease

Clinical Manifestations

- Early GBS disease: 24 h–6 d pp; late GBS disease >1 w–3 mo pp
- Sepsis, PNA, & meningitis in the 1st w of life
- Fatal in 2–3% full-term infants & 20–30% of preterm newborns <33 w gestational age

Screening and Diagnosis

- Pregnant women should routinely be screened by rectovaginal swab at 35–37 w.
  Culture results are valid for up to 5 w, then should be repeated at >5 w.
- If PCN allergic – need Clindamycin and Erythromycin disc sensitivity on culture
- NAAT for GBS is currently only indicated in women w/ (1) culture data unknown, (2) at term, & (3) w/o prolonged rupture of membranes or fever
- Women with GBS bacteriuria in current pregnancy, or prior affected infant with GBS → treat regardless, no need to screen

Treatment

- Indications for intrapartum antibiotic prophylaxis:
  Positive rectovaginal culture
  GBS bacteriuria (exempt from routine screening)
  History of prior invasive GBS disease (exempt from routine screening)
  GBS Unknown AND any of the following:
  Preterm (<37 w), prolonged rupture of membranes (≥18 h), maternal fever (>100.4°F), positive intrapartum NAAT
- Intrapartum ppx NOT indicated at the time of cesarean deliv at any GA for women delivered *prior to labor w/ intact membranes*

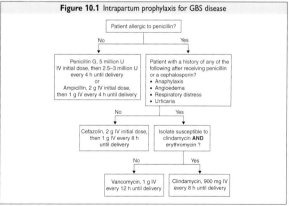

Figure 10.1 Intrapartum prophylaxis for GBS disease

Definitions
- **Labor:** Regular uterine contractions & cervical change
- **1st stage of labor:** Onset of labor → full cervical dilation (10 cm)
  - **Latent phase:** Early labor until acceleration of rate of cervical change (<6 cm)
  - **Active phase:** Period of accelerated cervical change until full dilation (6–10 cm)
  - **Historically, minimum rate of cervical change:** Nulliparous ~1.2 cm/h, multiparas, ~1.5 cm/h (*N Y Acad Med* 1972;48:842)
  - **Contemporary rates of change:** Nulliparous 0.5–0.7 cm/h, multiparas 0.5–1.3 cm/h (*Obstet Gynecol* 2010;116:1281–7)
  - **Labor curve:** Friedman (1955) described ideal labor progress at term; Zhang (2010) showed women enter active phase at 6 cm, w/ variable labor course & no deceleration phase
  - **Definition of arrest of labor in 1st stage** (*Obstet Gynecol* 2014;123:693–711):
    Spontaneous labor: ≥6 cm dilation with membrane rupture and one of the following: 4 h or more of adequate contractions (eg >200 Montevideo units) OR 6 h or more of inadequate contractions and no cervical change
- **2nd stage of labor:** Full cervical dilation → deliv of the infant
  - **Prior to diagnosis of arrest of labor in 2nd stage** (*Obstet Gynecol* 2014;123:693–711): Allow <u>at least</u> 2 h of pushing in multiparous women (3 h in nulliparous). Longer durations may be appropriate on individualized basis (eg, epidural, malposition) with documented progress.
- **3rd stage of labor:** Delivery of the infant → delivery of the placenta (approximately 30 min)
- **4th stage of labor:** 1–2 h immediately following deliv of the placenta
- **Cervical assessment:** Cervical dilation is measured in cm. Cervical effacement is documented as percentage of full-length (4 cm) cervix lost (0% is full length & 100% is paper thin). Fetal station is descent of the *bony* fetal presenting part in centimeters above or below the mat ischial spine (−5–+5 cm scale).
- **Fetal lie:** Relationship between long axis (spine) of fetus to that of the mother (longitudinal or transverse)
- **Fetal presentation:** Fetal presenting part – cephalic (head), breech (footling, complete, frank), face, or shoulder
- **Fetal position:** Orientation of the presenting part relative to the mat pelvis
  Cephalic presentation w/ occiput documented on maternal left/right, rotated post/anter/transverse (eg, ROA). The sacrum may be used for fetuses in breech presentation, the acromion for transverse lie, the mentum for face presentations

---

Figure 10.2 Presentation: Cephalic and types of breech

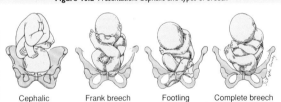

Cephalic   Frank breech   Footling (incomplete) breech   Complete breech

(Modified from Cruikshank DP . Breech, other malpresentations, and umbilical cord complications. In: Scott JR, Gibbs RS , Karlan BY, et al, eds. *Danforth's Obstetrics and Gynecology*. 10th ed. Philadelphia, PA: Wolters Kluwer; 2008.)

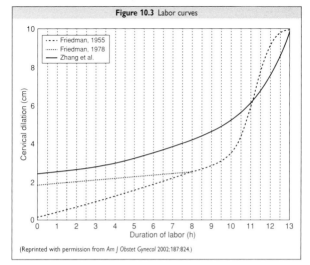

Figure 10.3 Labor curves

Cervical dilation (cm) vs Duration of labor (h)
- --- Friedman, 1955
- ···· Friedman, 1978
- — Zhang et al.

(Reprinted with permission from *Am J Obstet Gynecol* 2002;187:824.)

Median (and 95%ile) h in labor (4–10 cm)		
	Nulliparas	**Multiparas**
Spontaneous labor	3.8 (11.8)	2.4 (8.8)
Induced labor	5.5 (16.8)	4.4 (16.2)
Active phase (6–10 cm) was similar amongst all groups, w/ median ~1 h		

Data from Harper LM, Caughey AB, Odibo AO, et al. Normal progress of induced labor. *Obstet Gynecol.* 2012;119(6):1113–8.

Cardinal Movements of Labor – Described in Relationship of Fetal Vertex
- **Engagement:** Passage of widest diameter (BPD) below pelvic brim
- **Descent:** Passage of presenting part downward into pelvis
- **Flexion:** Allows optimal descent by presenting smallest cranial diameter
- **Internal rotation:** Movement of the fetal head from transverse to anteroposterior
- **Extension:** Movement of the fetal head under the pubic symphysis & out the introitus
- **External rotation ("restitution"):** Movement of the head to align w/ torso
- **Expulsion:** Delivery of the fetal body

Management of Labor
- Physical exam on presentation: Mat VS; cervical dilation, effacement, fetal station, fetal presentation, rupture of membranes (±mec), presence of vaginal bleeding, & estimated fetal weight (by Leopold maneuver)
  Fetal heart assessment (intermittent in low-risk, or continuous in high-risk pts) & uterine tocometry to assess fetal status & contractions
- Laboratory evaluation: CBC, Type & Screen, RPR
- IV access, clear liquid diet (*Obstet Gynecol* 2017;129:e20–8)
- Walking & upright positioning in early labor may ↓ the 1st stage by 1 h (*Cochrane Database Syst Rev* 2013;10:CD003934)
- Assess desire for pain control, w/ or w/o regional anesthesia
- GBS status (prophylaxis if indicated)

Management of Delivery
- Pushing may begin w/ full cervical dilation or be delayed until presenting part descends ("laboring down"); pushing generally accompanies contractions. Delayed pushing ↑ length of the 2nd stage by ~1 h, but no difference in episiotomy or laceration incidence, APGARS <7 or NICU admissions (*Cochrane Database Syst Rev* 2015;10:CD009124). Pushing should not be delayed if there is an indication to expedite delivery (eg, infection, preeclampsia, nonreassuring fetal status).

- No indication for routine episiotomy. If necessary, mediolateral recommended over midline due to ↑incidence of OASIS with midline *(Obstet Gynecol 2016;128:e1–15)*
- Warm compresses to the perineum may ↓ incid of 3rd/4th-degree lacerations *(Cochrane Database Syst Rev 2011;12:CD006672)*
- In women w/o epidural anesthesia, pushing while upright was a/w ↑ risk of EBL >500 cc & ↓ abn FHTs w/o signif impact on length of 2nd stage *(Cochrane Database Syst Rev 2012;5:CD002006)*
- Delivery of the fetal head:
  - Care should be taken to control speed of delivery & to protect the anterior vaginal wall, urethra, & clitoris
  - The perineum should be eased over the fetal head
  - The head should be allowed to restitute
  - Gentle downward traction of the head to deliver the anterior shoulder (difficulty w/ this maneuver should prompt consideration of shoulder dystocia)
  - The body should be delivered w/ gentle upward traction, supporting the perineum
- The cord should be clamped & cut → delayed cord clamping is recommended for all vigorous preterm and term infants for 30–60s, ↓ risk of fetal/neonatal anemia, but ↑ need for phototherapy *(Obstet Gynecol 2017;129:e5–10; Cochrane Database Syst Rev 2008:CD004074; BMJ 2011;343:d7157)*. Delaying cord clamping in premature infants <37 w may also ↓ risk of NEC, IVH & neonatal transfusion *(Cochrane Database Syst Rev 2012;4:CD003248)*
- Active management of 3rd stage w/ suprapubic pressure & controlled cord traction may ↓ maternal hemorrhage *(Cochrane Database Syst Rev 2011;11:CD007412)*
- Consider delivery onto maternal abdomen ("skin to skin") to promote immediate breastfeeding & bonding *(Cochrane Database Syst Rev 2012;5:CD003519)*
- Give oxytocin in the 3rd stage to ↓ postpartum hemorrhage *(Cochrane Database Syst Rev 2001;(4):CD001808)*
- Inspect the placenta to identify anomalies & to ensure no evidence of retained products
- Fetal cord blood gas analysis & postpartum hemorrhage (see sections below)

INDUCTION OF LABOR (IOL)

Definition and Epidemiology
- Stimulation of uterine contractions with intent to cause vaginal delivery prior to onset of spontaneous labor
- 23.2% of births in 2009 were after IOL *(National Vital Statistics Report 2011)*
- Cervical ripening (CR): Softening, thinning, & dilating of the cervix to facilitate successful induction of labor and decrease time to delivery

Indications
- Maternal–fetal risk of continuing pregnancy
- Prior to 41 w0d, IOL should be performed based on maternal–fetal indications. IOL at ≥41 w0d should be performed to reduce risk of cesarean delivery and perinatal morbidity/mortality *(Obstet Gynecol 2014;124:390–6)*
- **Contraindications:** Any contraindication to vaginal delivery (eg, vasa previa or complete placenta previa, malpresentation, umbilical cord prolapse, prior classical cesarean, active genital herpes infection, prior myomectomy entering endometrial cavity)

Simplified Bishop Score for determining successful IOL				
Points scored	0	1	2	3
Dilation (cm)	0	1–2	3–4	≥5
Station	−3	−2	−1 or 0	+1 or +2
Effacement (%)	0–30	40–50	60–70	≥80

Total score: Successful IOL (Sens/Spec)
>4: 59.2/67.9   >5: 40.6/82.6   >6: 18.8/94.2
Note: Cervical consistency (firm, soft) & position (anter, post) are included in the "full" Bishop Score, but do not add predictive power beyond the simplified score above
Unfavorable cervix = BS ≤6, BS **≥8 = favorable with probability of SVD equal to that of spontaneous labor** *(Obstet Gynecol 2009;114:386–97)*

Data from Laughon SK, Zhang J, Troendle J, et al. Using a simplified Bishop score to predict vaginal delivery. Obstet Gynecol. 2011;117(4):805–11.

- Overall, multiparas are less likely than nulliparous to fail induction or require cesarean deliv at a given Bishop Score

Methods of Cervical Ripening (CR) & Induction of Labor (IOL) (Obstet Gynecol 2009;114:386–97)

- **Oxytocin** – Most commonly used induction agent
  Various dosing regimens; titrate to contractions q2–3min
  Low-dose regimen (start 0.5–2 mU/min w/ 1–2 mU/min ↑ q15–40min)
  High-dose regimen (start 6 mU/min w/ 3–6 mU/min ↑ q15–40min)
  Note: High-dose regimen decreases time to deliv, but increases rate of tachysystole w/ FHR changes (Cochrane Database Syst Rev 2012;3:CD001233)
- **Misoprostol (PGE$_1$)** – CR or IOL
  Oral misoprostol as effective as vaginal misoprostol for CR/IOL (fewer 5-min Apgars <7)
  Dosage 25 μg PO q2h or 50 μg PO q4h (Cochrane Database Syst Rev 2014;(6):CD001338)
  Vaginal misoprostol may be used for CR/IOL at dose of 25–50 mcg PV q4h
  Contraindication: Prior uterine surgery (cesarean section and myomectomy) due to elevated risk of uterine rupture
- **Dinoprostone (PGE$_2$)** – CR or IOL
  Vaginal insert contains 10 mg of dinoprostone → releases mean dose of 0.3 mg/h
  Dosed q24h
  Upon removal of insert, quickly eliminated from maternal circulation
- **Amniotomy alone** (Cochrane Database Syst Rev 2000;(4):CD002862)
  Insufficient evidence regarding efficacy
  ↑ Need for oxytocin augmentation vs. vaginal prostaglandin
- **Balloon catheter** (Cochrane Database Syst Rev 2012;3:CD001233) – CR or IOL
  2 types: Single vs. double balloon (cervical and vaginal balloon), no difference in efficacy between the 2 types
  Placement of balloon catheter w/ 30–60 cc of saline through internal os into extra-amniotic space
  When used with PG or oxytocin ↓ cesarean delivery rate and ↓time to delivery
- **Membrane stripping** (Cochrane Database Syst Rev 2005;(1):CD000451)
  Manual detachment of inferior pole of fetal membranes during vaginal exam
  Causes significant increases in phospholipase A$_2$ and prostaglandin F$_{2alpha}$
  Increases likelihood of spontaneous labor within 48 h and reduces continuation of pregnancy past 41 w
- **Sexual intercourse:** Insuff evid. Likely ineffective (Obstet Gynecol 2007;110(4):820–6; Cochrane Database Syst Rev 2001;(2):CD003093).
- **Breast stimulation:** Decreased postpartum hemorrhage compared to no intervention. No difference in rates of cesarean when compared to no intervention or oxytocin. Not effective in women w/ unfavorable cervix (Cochrane Database Syst Rev 2005;(3):CD003392).

Complications of Induction

- Tachysystole (>5 contractions in 10 min). Rx: Stop/↓ uterine stimulation, consider tocolysis
- Uterine tetany (contraction lasting >2 min). Rx: Stop/↓ uterine stimulation, consider tocolysis
- Cord prolapse (w/ amniotomy). Rx: Cesarean deliv.
- HypoNa (w/ extended infusion of oxytocin). Rx: Stop oxytocin infusion, consider free water restriction, recheck, & resume
- Cesarean delivery ↑ compared to spontaneous labor, but elective IOL at 41+ w, compared w/ expectant mgmt may ↓ c-section (Cochrane Database Syst Rev 2012;6:CD004945)

INTRAPARTUM FETAL MONITORING

Background

- Justification for intrapartum FHR monitoring based on expert opinion & medicolegal precedent
- Continuous FHR monitoring a/w (1) reduction in neonatal seizures, w/o significant differences in cerebral palsy, infant mortality or other std measures of neonatal well-being; & (2) ↑ in cesarean deliv & instrumental vaginal births when compared to intermittent auscultation or no monitoring (Cochrane Database Syst Rev 2006;3:CD006066)

Methods of Monitoring
- FHR:
    - External via Doppler US
    - Internal via fetal scalp electrode (FSE)
- Contractions:
    - External pressure transducer (qualitative)
    - Intrauterine pressure catheter (IUPC; quantitative).
    - Measurement in MVU: Add up peak minus baseline uterine pres for each contraction over 10 min; >200 MVU considered adequate for labor (Obstet Gynecol 1986;68:305)

Definitions (Obstet Gynecol 2008;112:661)
- **Baseline:** Avg FHR, exclusive of accelerations, decelerations, & marked variability, minimum of 2 min during a 10-min interval, rounded to nearest 5 bpm
    - Tachycardia: Baseline >160 bpm
    - Bradycardia: Baseline <110 bpm
- **Variability:** Beat-to-beat fluctuations in the baseline FHR, exclusive of accelerations & decelerations. Measured from peak to trough of rapid fluctuations.
    - Absent: Amplitude undetectable
    - Minimal: Amplitude between 1–5 bpm
    - Moderate: Amplitude between 6–25 bpm
    - Marked: Amplitude >25 bpm
- **Accelerations:** Increased FHR ≥15 bpm for ≥15 s (before 32 w, use ≥10 bpm & ≥10 s). Time from baseline to peak HR is <30 s. Prolonged acceleration lasts 2–10 min.
- **Decelerations:** ↓ In FHR
    - Early deceleration: Symmetric. Nadir w/ peak of contraction. Baseline to nadir takes >30 s.
    - Late deceleration: Symmetric. Nadir after peak of contraction. Baseline to nadir >30 s.
    - Variable deceleration: ↓ ≥15 bpm from baseline lasting at least 15 s. Baseline to nadir <30 s.
    - Prolonged deceleration: ↓ ≥15 bpm from baseline lasting 2–10 min
- **Sinusoidal Pattern:** Smooth, sine wave-like undulating pattern in FHR baseline. Cycle frequency 3–5 min. Lasts ≥20 min.

Fetal heart tracings in labor		
Category	Definition	Interpretation
I	Baseline FHR btw 110–160 • w/ mod variability • w/o late or variable decelerations • w/ or w/o accelerations • w/ or w/o early decelerations	Nml & requires no additional action. Accelerations (particularly >2 in 30 min) are highly predictive of favorable fetal acid–base status (Am J Obstet Gynecol 1982;142:297; Am J Obstet Gynecol 1979;134:36).
II	Any tracing not Category I or Category III	Indeterminate significance & requires close follow-up. Trial of supportive measures reasonable (see Category III).
III	**Includes either:** Absent baseline FHR variability with any of following: • Late decelerations during >50% of contractions over 20 min • Variable decelerations w/ >50% of contractions over 20 min • Bradycardia OR • Sinusoidal pattern	Abn & requires immediate eval. Initial intrauterine resusc: • Change mat position • Administer mat oxygen • D/c labor stimulation • Consider tocolytics • Correct mat HoTN or compromised placental perfusion If supportive measures fail to correct the Category III pattern, deliv may be indicated.

Sample Fetal Heart Tracings

Figure 10.4 Fetal heart rate variability

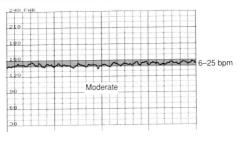

6–25 bpm

Moderate

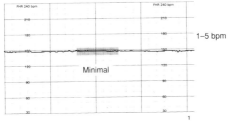

1–5 bpm

Minimal

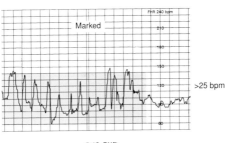

Marked

>25 bpm

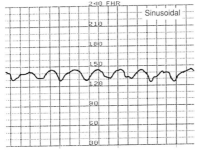

Sinusoidal

(From Menihan CA, Kopel E. *Electronic Fetal Monitoring: Concepts and Applications.* 3rd ed. Philadelphia, PA: Wolters Kluwer; 2018.)

Figure 10.5 Fetal heart rate accelerations and decelerations

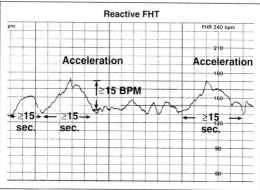

Reactive FHT

Acceleration   Acceleration

≥15 BPM

≥15 sec.   ≥15 sec.   ≥15 sec.

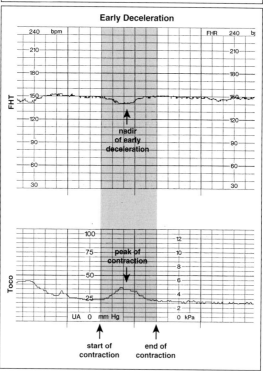

Early Deceleration

FHT

nadir of early deceleration

peak of contraction

Toco

UA 0 mm Hg

start of contraction   end of contraction

(continued)

Figure 10.5 (Continued)

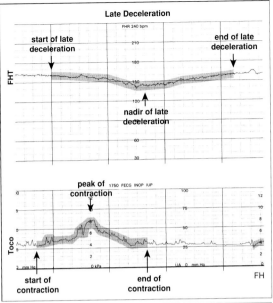

Late Deceleration

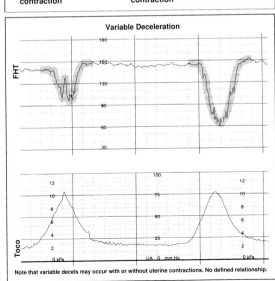

Variable Deceleration

Note that variable decels may occur with or without uterine contractions. No defined relationship.

INTRAPART MONIT 10-11

OPERATIVE VAGINAL DELIVERY

Definition and Epidemiology (Obstet Gynecol 2015;126:e12–24)
- Delivery using forceps or vacuum. In 2013, 3.3% of vaginal births were operative (National Vital Statistics Report, 2015)

Indications
- Prolonged 2nd stage of labor
- Suspicion of immediate or potential fetal compromise
- Shortening of 2nd stage of labor for maternal benefit (eg, maternal exhaustion, cardiac dz)

Prerequisites
- Cervix fully dilated and retracted
- Ruptured membranes
- Engaged fetal head
- Known fetal position
- Estimated fetal weight
- Adequate pelvis and anesthesia
- Empty maternal bladder
- Informed consent obtained (discussion of risks and benefits of procedure)
- Ability to perform cesarean delivery in the event of failed operative delivery

Contraindications
- <34 w GA for vacuum (elevated risk of IVH)
- Fetal bone demineralization disorder (eg, osteogenesis imperfecta)
- Fetal bleeding disorder (eg, hemophilia, von Willebrand dz) OR maternal anticoagulation w/ agent that crosses the placenta (eg, warfarin)
- Unknown fetal head position or fetal head unengaged
- Macrosomia is NOT a contraindication; caution for shoulder dystocia is advised

---

Figure 10.6 Placement of vacuum cup on fetal head

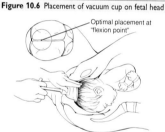

Optimal placement at "flexion point"

(Reprinted with permission from Scott JR, Gibbs RS, Karlan BY, et al. *Danforth's Obstetrics and Gynecology.* 10th ed. Philadelphia, PA: Wolters Kluwer; 2008.)
Placement of vacuum is 2 cm anterior to posterior fontanelle, centered over the sagittal suture

---

Figure 10.7 Correct placement of the forceps blades on the OA fetal head

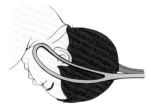

(Reprinted with permission from Scott JR, Gibbs RS, Karlan BY, et al. *Danforth's Obstetrics and Gynecology.* 9th ed. Philadelphia, PA: Lippincott Williams & Wilkins; 2003.)
Placement of forceps: Sagittal suture is midline of the shanks; posterior fontanelle is 1–2 cm from the shanks

Complications of Operative Delivery
- Neonatal
  - Vacuum: Scalp laceration, cephalohematoma (11–16%), subgaleal hematoma (2.6–4.5%), intracranial hemorrhage (0.2%), retinal hemorrhage (up to 75% → disappear w/i weeks) (BMJ 2004;329:24; Ophthalmology 2001;108:36)
  - Forceps: Superficial laceration, cephalohematoma (6%), facial nerve palsy, ocular trauma, skull fracture, intracranial hemorrhage (Obstet Gynecol 2015;126:e12–24)
- Maternal (BMJ 2004;329:24)
  - Vacuum: Perineal laceration: 3rd degree (9.6%), 4th degree (6.2%)
  - Forceps: Perineal laceration: 3rd degree (12.5%), 4th degree (9.8%)
- Routine episiotomy is not recommended due to potential of poor healing and prolonged discomfort. Risk of persistent pelvic floor dysfunction is difficult to quantify. Maternal laceration is more likely w/ operative delivery, but should be weighed against risks of cesarean. Complications are highest w/ multi instruments (ie, vacuum plus forceps), thus use of more than 1 instrument in contraindicated. If 1 fails → typically proceed w/ cesarean delivery.

VAGINAL BIRTH AFTER CESAREAN

Definitions (Obstet Gynecol 2010;116:450)
- TOLAC: Trial of labor after prior cesarean
- VBAC: Vaginal birth after cesarean
- ERCD: Elective repeat cesarean delivery

Selection of Candidates
- Appropriate candidate: History of 1–2 cesarean deliveries via low transverse OR low vertical hysterotomy. Unknown scar location is NOT contraindication to TOLAC unless high suspicion for classical hysterotomy.
- Inappropriate candidate: Previous classical or T-incision, prior uterine rupture, extensive transfundal uterine surgery (eg, myomectomy), and patients with any contraindication to vaginal delivery
- Overall success rate of TOLAC is 60–80%
- ↑ Rate of successful TOLAC: Prior vaginal birth, spontaneous labor
- ↓ Rate of successful TOLAC: Recurring indication for prior c/s (labor dystocia), increased mat age, nonwhite ethnicity, GA >40 w, maternal obesity, preeclampsia, short interval pregnancy, fetal macrosomia
  - <60% probability of VBAC, could be ↑ morbidity w TOLAC compared w ERCD; counsel patient and manage expectations for success
- Online NICHD VBAC success rate calculator – https://mfmu.bsc.gwu.edu/PublicBSC/MFMU/VGBirthCalc/vagbirth.html

Maternal risks associated with TOLAC			
	ERCD (%)	TOLAC w/ 1 prior c-section (%)	TOLAC w/ 2+ prior c-sections (%)
Endometritis	1.5–2.1	2.9	3.1
Operative injury	0.42–0.6	0.4	0.4
Bld xfusion	1–1.4	0.7–1.7	3.2
Hysterectomy	0–0.4	0.2–0.5	0.6
Uterine rupture	0.4–0.5	0.7–0.9	0.9–1.8
Mat death	0.02–0.04	0.02	—

Neonatal risks associated with TOLAC		
	ERCD (%)	TOLAC (%)
Stillbirth 37–38 w	0.08	0.38
Stillbirth >39 w	0.01	0.16
Hypoxic ischemic encephalopathy	0–0.13	0.08
Respiratory morbidity	1–5	0.1–1.8
Hyperbilirubinemia	5.8	2.2
Transient tachypnea of newborn	6.2	3.5

Neonatal death (<1 mo) no signif change; perinatal death (<1 w) 0.01% w/ ERCD; 0.13% w/ TOLAC

- Misoprostol should NOT be used for TOLAC induction given elevated risk of uterine rupture: 24.5/1000 *(NEJM 2001;345:3)*
- Continuous fetal monitoring should be employed
- Maintain high suspicion for signs/sx of uterine rupture, including: New onset uterine pain, loss of fetal station, new fetal heart race tracing abnormalities (most common), vaginal bleeding, & mat hemodynamic instability
- Staff (OB & anesthesia) must be immediately available for emergent c-section

FETAL CORD BLOOD GAS ANALYSIS

Purpose *(Obstet Gynecol 2006;108:1319)*
- Provides an assessment of neonatal metabolic status
- May be useful to determine whether an asphyxia event (acidemia + metabolic acidosis + hypoxia) accompanied neonatal depression
- If nml, rules out asphyxia at time of deliv as a cause of neonatal complications
- Collect 1–2 mL of bld from both umbilical vein & artery in heparinized syringes. Can collect from clamped cord for up to 60 min w/ valid result. If samples are not immediately sent to laboratory, store on ice for up to 60 min.

Pathophysiology
- Interruption of umbilical cord blood flow leads to retention of fetal CO_2 (ie, respiratory acidosis) → prolonged respiratory acidosis → mixed respiratory/metabolic acidosis → metabolic acidosis

Indications/Sentinel Events
- Cesarean delivery for suspected fetal compromise, abnormal FHR tracing, maternal thyroid dz, maternal infection, multifetal gest, uterine rupture, shoulder dystocia, severe placental abruption, umbilical cord prolapse, amniotic fluid embolus, maternal cardiovascular collapse, fetal exsanguination (eg, vasa previa, fetomaternal hemorrhage)

Normal values	
Term	**Preterm**
pH: 7.15–7.38	pH: 7.14–7.40
pCO_2: 49.2–50.3	pCO_2: 49.2–51.6
HCO_3^-: 22–23.1	HCO_3^-: 22.4–23.9
BE: −2.7−−3.6	BE: −2.5−−3.3

From *Clin Obstet Gynecol* 1993;36(1):13–23.

- Approach to interpretation of fetal blood gas:
  - If pH is lower than nml limits, ACIDEMIA exists
  - If pCO_2 is higher than nml limits, RESPIRATORY ACIDOSIS exists
  - If BE is more negative than nml limits, METABOLIC ACIDOSIS exists
- Fetal umbilical artery acidemia:
  - If pH <7.0, or base deficit ≥12 mmol/L, or both → ↑ probability that neonatal encephalopathy, if present had an intrapartum hypoxic component. Respiratory acidosis alone unlikely cause of neonatal complications
  - If pH >7.20 → ↓ probability that intrapartum hypoxia is responsible for neonatal encephalopathy
  - APGAR score of <5 at 5 and 10 min
- **Criteria to define acute intrapartum hypoxic event sufficient to cause cerebral palsy:**
  - Arterial cord pH <7 w/ base excess −12 or worse
  - Early onset of mod or sev encephalopathy
  - CP of spastic, quadriplegic, or dyskinetic type
  - Exclusion of other identifiable etiologies
- Key resource for evaluating neonatal encephalopathy is *Neonatal Encephalopathy and Neurologic Outcome*, 2nd Edition (2014) *(Obstet Gynecol 2014;123:896)*

ROUTINE POSTPARTUM CARE

In Hospital Care

- **Monitoring:** Frequent VS (q15min × 2 h; q shift [8–12 h] thereafter); assess uterine size & tone, perineal integrity, abdominal incisions; note quantity of vaginal bleeding; high vigilance for intra-abdominal or pelvic hemorrhage & urinary retention
- **Pain:** NSAIDs & cold compresses to the perineum, w/ opioids reserved for breakthrough or postsurgical pain *(Cochrane Database Syst Rev 2011;(5):CD004908)*
- **Constipation:** Stool softeners & laxatives as needed & w/ opioids; longer stool softener rx for 3rd/4th-degree laceration repairs
- **Urinary retention:** Mobilize early to facilitate voiding; use intermittent or indwelling catheter if unsuccessful
- **Malodorous lochia/discharge:** Inspect perineum for wound breakdown or retained sponge. Assess for fever, fundal tenderness, and consider postpartum endometritis.
- **HA:** Most likely are tension, but consider preeclampsia & postdural puncture HA *(Am J Obstet Gynecol 2007;196:318)*. See Chap. 18.
- **Fever:** DDx: UTI, wound infxn, mastitis/breast abscess; breast engorgement; endometritis; septic pelvic thrombophlebitis; clostridium-difficile; drug or anesthesia reaction, pneumonia, DVT/PE
- Fever workup: CBC, CXR, UA, UCx, Breast & Pelvic examination, Fundal Check (assess for tenderness), wound examination (if applicable), assess for DVT (unilateral erythema, edema, tenderness [Homan's sign])
- Discharge w/i 24–48 h after Uncomp vaginal deliv & 48–96 h after routine cesarean deliv

Clinic Follow-up Care

- Postpartum visit recommended for all women at 4–6 w postpartum & 7–14 d complicated vaginal delivery (eg, 3rd/4th degree lacerations)
- **GHTN/preE:** BP check in office within 7 d of discharge *(Obstet Gynecol 2013;122(5):1122–31)*
- **Hx should assess:** Mat–infant bonding, including feeding; breast complaints; mat mood/coping & social supports; urinary & fecal continence; resumption of intercourse & contraceptive plan
- **Exam should include:** VS (including weight & BP); breasts, abd, & pelvis

Postpartum Contraception

- Mean resumption of ovulation in nonlactating women occurs 45–94 d (25 d at earliest) postpartum *(Obstet Gynecol 2011;117(3):657)*
- **Exclusive** breastfeeding is 92–98% effective as contraception in the 1st 6 mo postpartum if amenorrhea and baby is feeding q4h during day and q6h at night *(Contraception 1989;39:477)*
- Sterilization (by tubal ligation) may be performed immediately (within ~24 h) postpartum or as an interval procedure (6 w after delivery) *(Obstet Gynecol 2013;121:392–404)*
- Barrier methods may be used on resumption of intercourse
- Progestin-only methods safe to initiate postpartum in any woman w/o a contraindication, & do not influence breast milk production *(Contraception 2010;82:17)*
- IUD (copper or levonorgestrel) may be placed either immediately postpartum (w/i 10 min of deliv of placenta) or 6–8 w postpartum *(Obstet Gynecol 2016;128:e32–7)*
- Estrogen-containing contraceptives may be initiated 21 d postpartum in women w/o additional risk factors for VTE, & otherwise may be considered at 6 w postpartum. CDC & ACOG recommend 4-6-w delay before starting estrogen-containing contraceptives in breastfeeding women depending on VTE risk profile *(MMWR 2011;60:878; Obstet Gynecol 2006;107:1453)*. Estrogen may suppress breast milk production.
- Key Resource: CDC Medical Eligibility Criteria for Contraceptive Use *(MMWR Recomm Rep 2016;65(No. RR-3):1–104. doi: http://dx.doi.org/10.15585/mmwr.rr6503a1)*

BREASTFEEDING

Physiology and Initiation

- Copious milk secretion begins w/ progesterone withdrawal 2–7 d postpartum. Longer in nulliparous & after cesarean deliv *(Pediatrics 2003;112:607)*. Maintenance of lactation depends on adequate frequency of breastfeeding &/or pumping *(Obstet Gynecol 2007;109:479)*. During the 1st 2 w, feeding initiated on infant demand (8–12× daily).
- Initiation of successful breastfeeding (unless medical issues take precedence; *Pediatrics 2012;129:e827*):
    Maintain direct skin-to-skin contact btw mother & infant until 1st feeding is completed

Avoid commercial formulas & sugar water
Avoid use of pacifier
Room-in newborns w/ mother
Discharge w/ contact information for breastfeeding support

Benefits (Obstet Gynecol 2013;122:423–8; Obstet Gynecol 2016;127:e86–92)
- Full-term infant: ↓ Incid of otitis media; atopic dermatitis, & asthma; GI & lower respiratory tract infections; diabetes (weak association); obesity; childhood leukemia; SIDS
- Preterm infant: ↓ Incid of nec enterocolitis, sev retinopathy of prematurity Improved neurodevelopmental outcomes (Pediatrics 2012;129:e827)
- Mat: ↓ Incid of breast & ovarian cancer; & dev of type 2 diabetes

Relative Contraindications (Obstet Gynecol 2007;109:479; Pediatrics 2012;129:e827)
- Contraindicated:
  Mat use of illicit drugs or uncontrolled EtOH use
  Mat infxn w/ brucella, HIV, HTLV-I, or HTLV-II
  Mat active, untreated varicella, TB, or herpes simplex w/ breast lesions
  Infant galactosemia
- Breastfeeding does NOT ↑ the risk of vertical transmission of hepatitis C (Clin Infect Dis 1999;29:1327)
- Infants born to hepatitis B positive mothers should receive HepBIg & be vaccinated at birth; breastfeeding is safe thereafter (Obstet Gynecol 2002;99:1049)

Lactational Mastitis
- **Dx:** Fever >38.0°C + swollen, red, indurated breast in breastfeeding mother
- Labs not necessary, milk culture only in sev or refrac case
  US only if abscess suspected
- Typical pathogens are group A streptococci & MSSA
- **1st-line antibiotic:** Dicloxacillin (500 mg QID) × 10–14 d
  PCN-allergic or MRSA: Clindamycin (300 mg QID) or TMP/SMX (1–2 BID)
- Continue breastfeeding to completely empty breasts, NSAIDs, & warm compresses
- **DDx:** Breast abscess, obstructed milk duct, galactocele, inflamm breast cancer

Breastfeeding and Maternal Medications
- **LactMed:** Comprehensive database on pharmaceuticals & lactation
  http://toxnet.nlm.nih.gov/cgi-bin/sis/htmlgen?LACT

AFFILIATED OBSTETRICAL PROVIDERS

Midwives			
	Education/training	**Accreditation**	**Other**
CNM	APRN: Registered nurse, plus Master's/Doctoral degree	American College of Nurse-Midwives	Licensed in 50 states
CM	Master's degree in midwifery	American College of Nurse-Midwives	Licensed in NY, NJ, RI; authorized in DE, MO
CPM	No formal requirements (can be DEM or CNM/CM) Written exams & eval of skills Must have some out-of-hospital practice	North American Registry of Midwives	Regulated variously in 26 states
DEM	No formal education require- ments unless req by state law Informal/formal workshops or apprenticeships	None	Legal status varies Practice outside hospital setting

From American College of Nurse-Midwives; www.midwife.org

Doulas
- **Definition:** Women who provide continuous, nonmedical intrapartum/postpartum support to laboring women
- Scope of practice includes emotional support, attention to physical comfort, nonmedical advice, & advocacy
- Credentialing/certification varies by organization

Definition (*Hypertension in Pregnancy*, ACOG Task Force, 2013) (see Chap. 12)
- **Chronic HTN:** SBP ≥140 or DBP ≥90 prior to preg, prior to 20 w gest, or persisting longer than 12 w postpartum
- **Gestational HTN:** SBP ≥140 or DBP ≥90 after 20 w w/o proteinuria
- **Preeclampsia:** New onset HTN (SBP ≥140 or DBP ≥90 ×2 ≥4 h apart) w proteinuria >20 w. Proteinuria defined as ≥300 mg/24 h (or 1+ urine dip or urine protein:creatinine ratio of ≥0.3). If severe features are present, proteinuria is **not needed for the diagnosis**.
    Severe features: SBP ≥160 or DBP ≥110; thrombocytopenia <100000; elevated liver fxn tests ≥2× upper limit of normal; severe RUQ pain; renal insufficiency (Cr >1.1 or doubling of baseline value); pulmonary edema; new-onset cerebral/visual symptoms
    Eclampsia: Preeclampsia with seizures
- **Chronic HTN w/ superimposed preeclampsia:** CHTN w/ sudden increase in HTN w/ new onset or worsening proteinuria or CHTN with new onset of severe features
- All BP should be taken on 2 occasions 4 h apart (after pt has been seated quietly for several minutes, cuff level w/ heart). Also see HELLP (Chap. 15) & Eclampsia (Chap. 18).
See detailed discussion and Management of Hypertension in Chap. 12.

Epidemiology and Etiology
- Preeclampsia found in ~7% of pregnancies. True cause unk.
- **Risk factors:** Nulliparity, prior preg w/ preeclampsia, CHTN, renal disease, thrombophilia, multifetal pregnancy, IVF, FHx preeclampsia, Diabetes, obesity, SLE
- **Poss causes:** Endothelial damage, altered metabolism, inflammation, oxidative stress

Clinical Manifestations
- **Preeclampsia:** HTN, HA, visual changes (scotomata, photophobia), edema, abdominal pain (specifically epigastric or RUQ). But often times asymptomatic.

Physical Exam
- **Perform full neurologic exam:** Evaluate for HA, visual changes, clonus
- Palpate abd to assess abdominal tenderness (specifically RUQ as this could be a sign for subcapsular liver hematoma)
- Visualize/palpate extremities to evaluate for periph edema

Diagnostic Workup/Studies
- CBC, CMP (evaluate liver & renal fxn), assessment of proteinuria (by urine spot prot to Cr ratio, urinalysis, or 24-h urine collection)
- CT/MRI can show cerebral edema in the post hemispheres, a form of PRES (Postreversible encephalopathy syn)

Treatment and Medications
- **Acute HTN** (*Obstet Gynecol* 2015;125:521)
    Labetalol: 20 mg IV, rpt at 10-min intervals, double dose w/ max dose of 80 mg at 1 given time; total max dose of 300 mg (eg, 20 mg → 40 mg → 80 mg → 80 mg → 80 mg)
    Hydralazine: 5–10 mg IV over 1–2 min, rpt at 20-min intervals. Max dose of 30 mg.
    Nifedipine: 10 mg PO, rpt at 20-min intervals. If next BP severe, can give 20 mg PO.
    Nitroprusside: 0.20–4 µg/kg/min IV drip, titrate to effect. Only in critical illness.
    Nicardipine: 2.5 mg/h IV titrating, do not exceed 15 mg/h
    DO NOT USE: ACEI or ARB
    Goal: ↓ Risk of mat stroke but maintain pres for placental perfusion
- **Oral treatments**
    Labetalol: 100–800 mg PO BID–TID (max dose 2400 mg/24 h)
    Methyldopa: 250 mg PO BID (max dose 3 g/24 h)
    Nifedipine XR: 30–90 mg PO daily (max dose 120 mg/24 h)
- **Preeclampsia with severe features, or chronic HTN w/ superimposed preeclampsia with severe features**
    Magnesium sulfate for seizure prevention ($MgSO_4$): Given during stabilization prior to expectant management, during delivery, and 24 h postpartum. Bolus 4–6 g IV w/ maintenance of 1–2 g/h for sz prevention, titrate and consider no bolus if pt has renal failure
    Monitor closely for pulm edema as $MgSO_4$ is a smooth muscle relaxer
- **Timing for delivery:**
    Chronic HTN: No earlier than 38 w if well-controlled
    Gestational HTN: 37 w
    Preeclampsia:
        Without severe features: 37 w, or ≥34 w if IUGR <5%ile or oligohydramnios

With severe features: At 34 w if severe HTN is only feature. Otherwise deliver after 48 h of BMZ if other severe features present.
CHTN with superimposed preeclampsia: At 37 w if no severe features. Otherwise same as preeclampsia with severe features.

HYDROPS FETALIS

Definition and Epidemiology (Am J Obstet Gynecol 2015;212(2):127)
- Accum of fluid in 2 or more of the following extravascular compartments: Heart (pericardial effusion), lungs (pleural effusion), abd (ascites), and subcutaneous tissue (edema with skin >5 mm). Polyhydramnios and placental thickening can also be seen but are no longer diagnostic criteria.
- **Immune Hydrops:** Fetal anemia causes immune hydrops if secondary to Rh isoimmunization or other RBC isoimmunization
  - RhD– Mom w/ RhD+ fetus has 16% chance of having isoimmunization
  - ↓ 2% w/ postpartum anti-D immune globulin administration
  - ↓ To 0.1% w/ additional administration in the 3rd trimester (Transfus Med Rev 1988;2:129)
  - 6/1000 live births undergo Rh isoimmunization
  - 2nd Preg more affected than 1st (1st usually mildly affected, if affected at all, as 1st Ig produced is IgM which DOES NOT cross placenta)
  - Anti-Kell antibody leads to decreased production of RBCs in addition to RBC destruction
- **Nonimmune Hydrops:** Hydrops from all other causes (accounts for 90% of fetal cases of hydrops in US). 1/1500–1/3800 births affected

Etiology
- **Immune:** Fetal anemia/hypoxia leads to heart failure
  Maternal RBC Ag neg + fetus RBC Ag⁺ → antibodies cross placenta → antibodies bind to fetal bld → hemolysis of fetal bld → release of bilirubin & fetal anemia → fetal cardiac failure & damaged myocardium → fluid accum → hydrops fetalis
- **Nonimmune:** CV (heart defect, arrhythmia), chromosomal (aneuploidy, rearrangements, deletions, duplications), hematologic (anemia from thalassemia), infectious (TORCH), thoracic (mass effect from CDH, CPAM, other tumor), Twin–twin transfusion, urinary tract abnormalities (nephrotic hypoproteinemia), GI (infarction of bowel), lymphatic dysplasia, tumors (chorioangioma), skeletal dysplasia, syndromic, inborn errors of metabolism.

Clinical Manifestation
- US findings can include pericardial effusion, pleural effusion, ascites, skin edema, polyhydramnios, placentomegaly
- **Fetal HR tracings:** Sinusoidal pattern indicative of fetal anemia
- **Mirror syndrome:** Mother gets edema and hypertension that mimics the hydropic fetus

Physical Exam
- Mother may appear edematous if experiencing mirror syn
- Infant can range from hyperbilirubinemic to pale, limp, edematous

Diagnostic Workup/Studies
- **Immune:** All women have Rh(D) typing & Ab screening at 1st prenatal visit → if antibodies present, indirect Coombs test provides Ab titer
  Titer <1:32 (some institutions start at <1:16), fetus at low risk
  - Repeat titer every 4 w
  - If remains <32 (or <16) deliver at term vs. if ≥32 (or >16) proceed w/ w/u below
  Titer ≥1:32, fetus at potential risk for anemia → test father's Ag and genotype
  - Homozygous: Fetus at risk. MCA Doppler q1–2w starting at 18 w
  - Heterozygous: Perform amniocentesis for fetal Ag typing
    - Fetus Ag⁺: MCA Doppler q1–2w at 18 w
    - Fetus Ag neg: Fetus not at risk, return to routine care
- **Nonimmune:**
  Detailed history: FHx, medications, infection
  Perform detailed US & fetal ECHO
  Obtain MCA Doppler to assess fetal anemia
  Offer amniocentesis (chromosomal microarray; PCR for CMV, parvo, toxo, lysosomal enzyme testing)
  Obtain mat blood for type and screen, CBC, DNA testing for alpha-thalassemia if MCV <80 fL, serologic tests for CMV, parvovirus B19, toxoplasmosis, syphilis

Treatment

- **Immune:** If fetus at risk with + Ag and MCA PSV >1.5 MoMs, check fetal HCT with PUBS and transfuse if HCT <30
- **Nonimmune:** Prognosis depends upon etiology. Uncertain etiology has 40–50% risk of IUFD. Termination should be discussed in many cases.
  - Parvovirus: PUBS and IUT
  - Fetal Arrhythmia: Maternal anti-arrhythmic agents
  - Fetal cardiac compression from cystic chest mass: Fetal shunt
  - Fetal cardiac compression from solid chest mass: Possible fetal surgery
  - Chorioangioma: Possible laser therapy of tumor vessels
  - Twin–twin transfusion syndrome: Placental laser therapy

INTRAUTERINE GROWTH RESTRICTION

Definition and Epidemiology (Obstet Gynecol 2013;121:1122)
- Defined as sonographic EFW <10th percentile
  Risk of poor outcome (eg, stillbirth) generally increases with degree of growth restriction

Etiology
- **Maternal factors:**
  Behavioral: Smoking, substance use, decreased nutritional intake
  Medical: Diabetes, renal insufficiency, autoimmune disease, cyanotic cardiac disease, hypertensive disorders, obesity
  Teratogen exposure
  Extremes of maternal age
- **Fetal factors:**
  Chromosomal or genetic cause, fetal infection, constitutional, multiple gestations
- **Placental factors:**
  Poor implantation, placenta previa, umbilical cord abnormalities

Clinical Implications
- In utero: Fetal demise, preterm delivery, maternal HTN
- Neonat morbidity: Neonatal demise, hypoglycemia, hyperbilirubinemia, hypothermia, IVH, necrotizing enterocolitis, seizures, sepsis, RDS
- Perinatal morbidity & mortality is increased, particularly below 3%ile EFW

Physical Exam
- Lagging fundal height compared to gestational age. Nml fundal height measurements from 20–36 w are defined as 1 cm/w of gest ±2 cm. FH <3 cm of expected should prompt ultrasound.

Diagnostic Workup/Studies
- Goal: Identify true placental insufficiency causing IUGR vs. constitutional or other
- US:
  - Fetal biometry: Head circumference, biparietal diameter, abdominal circumference, & femur length
  - EFW <10% = IUGR
  - Fluid assessment with MVP or AFI: Oligohydramnios (AFI <5 cm or MVP <2 cm) correlates w/ an increased risk of fetal death
  - Umbilical artery Doppler: Measurement of velocity of flow through umbilical artery during systole & diastole
  - Peak systolic velocity is elevated in IUGR → indicates ↑ placental resistance. W/ progression of IUGR, diastolic flow ↓ as placental resistance ↑ → AEDF or REDF
- Maternal Labs: CMV, Toxoplasmosis serology if fetal findings on ultrasound
- Amniocentesis for genetic testing if birth defects or early IUGR

Management
- Growth ultrasounds repeated every 3–4 w
- Weekly antenatal testing:
  - Twice weekly NST, or once weekly BPP with NST, or weekly NST with weekly AFI
    - Umbilical artery Doppler weekly
- **Delivery**
  - Abnormal Doppler:
    - REDF: Deliver after 32 w
    - AEDF: Deliver after 34 w
    - >95th percentile: 34–37 w

- Normal Doppler: ≥39 w
  - For delivery <37 w, BMZ ×2 doses prior to delivery. Delivery <32 w should have MgSO₄ for fetal neuroprotection

Earlier delivery (≤34 w) considered for the most severe cases (eg, REDF), after steroids for FLM and with MgSO₄ for fetal neuroprotection (for ≤32 w GA)

MULTIPLE GESTATION

Definition and Epidemiology (*Obstet Gynecol* 2016;128(4):926)
- Pregnancy in which more than one fetus implants in the uterus
- Multiple gestations account for 3% of all births
- Significant rise in twins and triplets since 2002, likely secondary to ART

Etiology
- Zygosity – number of eggs initially fertilized
  Monozygotic = one egg fertilized by one sperm; splitting of initial zygote
  Dizygotic = two eggs fertilized by two sperm; two separate fertilization events
- Chorioamnionicity (esp important for monozygotic twins)
  Chorionicity: Number of placentas (di = 2, mono = 1)
  Amnionicity: Number of amniotic sacs around embryos (mono = both embryos in 1 sac)
  Determined by timing of embryonic splitting for monozygotic twins:
  0–4 d after fertilization → dichorionic diamniotic twins
  4–8 d after fertilization → monochorionic diamniotic twins
  8–12 d after fertilization → monochorionic monoamniotic twins
  >12 d post fertilization → conjoined twins

Physical Exam
- Uterine size > dates

Diagnostic Workup/Studies
- Best test is US in early Preg → easily determines chorioamnionicity
  1st trimester twin peak sign = dichorionic gest

Figure 11.1 A: Monochorionic diamniotic twins have fused amniotic membranes with no intervening placental tissue (<1 mm thick). **B:** Dichorionic diamniotic twins show twin peak sign with membrane separation and intervening chorion.

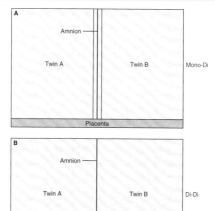

Complications
- **Discordance:** One twin larger than the other; clinically signif when greater than 20%. Calculate discordance % as: [(larger EFW − smaller EFW)/larger EFW] × 100.
- **Multiples of all types:**
    Maternal complications: Hyperemesis, GDM, HTN, anemia, hemorrhage, cesarean, postpartum depression, preeclampsia
    Fetal complications: Preterm delivery, IUGR, birth defects, genetic defects, IUFD
- **Monochorionic diamniotic twins:** Twin to twin transfusion syndrome (TTTS)
    Due to bld vessel anastomoses w/i single placenta w/ pressure diff
    Occurs in ~15% of monochorionic diamniotic twin gestations
    Donor twin: Oligohydramnios, smaller twin
    Recipient twin: Polyhydramnios, larger twin
    Stages of TTTS (J Perinatol 1999;19:550)
        1. Polyhydramnios/oligohydramnios
        2. Poly/oli, donor bladder absent
        3. Poly/oli, abn Doppler
        4. Poly/oli, hydrops of recipient
        5. IUFD of one or both fetuses
- **Monochorionic monoamniotic twins:** Cord entanglement & subseq cord accident

Management
- **Dichorionic twins**
    Early US for chorionicity, detailed ultrasound at 18–22 w, growth every 4–6 w, delivery at 38 w
- **Monochorionic diamniotic twins:**
    Early US for chorionicity, US for TTTS f/u every 2 w at 16 w, growth every 4 w, delivery at 34–37 w
- **Monochorionic monoamniotic twins:**
    Early US for chorionicity, US for TTTS f/u every 2 w, growth every 4 w, admission at 24–28 w, delivery at 32–34 w
- **TTTS:**
    Laser photocoagulation of vessel anastomosis (stage II or worse)
    Serial amnioreduction
    Selective reduction with bipolar cautery
- **Delivery considerations:**
    Vaginal delivery contraindicated with breech of presenting fetus
    Vaginal delivery of twins with possible breech extraction of twin B is acceptable if twin B is >1500 g and <20% larger than twin A
    Cesarean section recommended for all higher-order multiples and should be considered for mo/mo twins

CERVICAL INSUFFICIENCY & SHORT CERVIX

Definition and Epidemiology (Obstet Gynecol 2014;123:372)
- Inability of cervix to maintain a Preg until term in the absence of contractions in the 2nd trimester
- Weakened cervical tissue leading to loss of Preg, often 2nd trimester

Etiology
- **Congen:** Collagen dz, Müllerian anomalies, h/o DES exposure in utero
- **Acq:** Surgical cervical trauma (LEEP, conization, mechanical dilation), obstetric lacerations
- Abnormality in cervical remodeling (4 steps: Softening, ripening, dilation, repair)

Clinical Manifestation
- Asymptomatic/painless cervical dilation/effacement
- Often h/o painless dilation & deliv in the 2nd trimester w/ prior pregnancies

Physical Exam
- Speculum exam can show a dilated cervix
- Digital exam reveals soft, effaced, & possibly dilated cervix

Diagnostic Workup/Studies
- When performing fetal anatomy US at 16–24 w, CL should be evaluated. TVUS is the gold standard if a short cervix suspected.

Treatment and Medications
- **For short cervix:** Vaginal progesterone 200 mg micronized or 90 mg gel daily
- **For short cervix or cervical insufficiency:** Cervical cerclage *(Obstet Gynecol 2014;123:372)*
    Surgical stitch placed circumferentially around the cervix
    McDonald: "Purse-string" placed at cervicovaginal junction
    Shirodkar: Requires dissection of the vesicovaginal & rectovaginal fascia to the level of the internal os
- **When to treat:**
    Singleton Preg w/:
        No prior spont preterm births and short cervix → offer vaginal progesterone suppl if CL ≤20 mm at ≤24 w
        Prior spont preterm birth (start progesterone injections weekly from 16–36 w, check CL every 1–2 w from 16–23 w6d) → cerclage if CL ≤25 mm at ≤24 w
        Dilated cervix <24 w → consider exam indicated cerclage on individual basis
        History of successful cerclage in prior pregnancy or second trimester loss from painless cervical dilation → consider history indicated cerclage in first trimester
    Multiples show no improv w/ progesterone & worse outcomes w/ cerclage

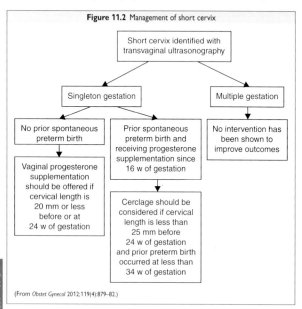

Figure 11.2 Management of short cervix

Short cervix identified with transvaginal ultrasonography

Singleton gestation

Multiple gestation

No prior spontaneous preterm birth

Prior spontaneous preterm birth and receiving progesterone supplementation since 16 w of gestation

No intervention has been shown to improve outcomes

Vaginal progesterone supplementation should be offered if cervical length is 20 mm or less before or at 24 w of gestation

Cerclage should be considered if cervical length is less than 25 mm before 24 w of gestation and prior preterm birth occurred at less than 34 w of gestation

(From *Obstet Gynecol* 2012;119(4):879–82.)

PRETERM PREMATURE RUPTURE OF MEMBRANES

Definition and Epidemiology *(Obstet Gynecol 2016;128(4):e165)*
- **PROM:** Rupture of membranes before the onset of active labor ("premature" to labor)
- **PPROM:** Premature rupture of membranes <37 w (preterm GA *and* prior to labor)
- Occurs prior to 1/3 of preterm births

Etiology
- No consensus on the cause of PPROM – thought to be on spectrum of preterm labor
- Risk factors include intra-amniotic infxn, uterine overdistention, smoking, connective tissue disorders, 2nd & 3rd trimester bleeding, nutritional deficiency, prior preterm deliv, symptomatic contractions, short cervix, smoking, drug use, amniocentesis (leakage after amniocentesis more likely to stop & not lead to deliv)

Clinical Manifestation
- Leakage of amniotic fluid prior to labor
- If accompanied by mat fever or tachy, uterine fundal tenderness, fetal tachy, purulent or malodorous fluid there should be concern for intra-amniotic infxn

Physical Exam
- Sterile speculum exam *(Obstet Gynecol 1992;80:630; Am J Obstet Gynecol 2000;183:1003)*
- Avoid digital exam, esp if preterm. Single digital exam decreases latency to deliv.

Diagnostic Workup/Studies
- **Clinical dx:**
    Leakage of fluid per vagina that is consistent w/ amniotic fluid (see below)
    Signs of infxn should prompt deliv, regardless of prematurity, to ↓ risk of mat & neonat sepsis
    Sterile speculum exam: Pooling of fluid in the vaginal vault sugg ROM
    US: Oligohydramnios is often present, though not diagnostic
    NST: Fetal tachy is often present w/ intra-amniotic infxn
    Oligohydramnios → variable decelerations
- **Lab tests:**
    Ferning: Place fluid from vaginal vault on a dry slide; salts in the amniotic fluid produce a delicate ferning pattern under microscope.
    pH: Amniotic fluid has a basic pH → turns pH paper blue (nitrazine test)
    Also nitrazine positive: Bld, bact vaginosis, semen.
- Diagnostic procedures
    Indigo Carmine amniotic infusion "tampon test"
        Indigo Carmine injected into the amniotic sac via amniocentesis
        Tampon inserted vaginally to detect blue color indicating leakage of amniotic fluid
    If amniocentesis performed to assess chorioamnionitis, get cell count, gram stain, gluc, & cx (aerobic/anaerobic/myco- and ureaplasma)

Management
- **Previable (<24 w):** May be managed outpt until viability. Latency antibiotics can be considered.
    Major complications: Limb contractures, pulm hypoplasia, maternal infection. Termination via D&E or induction should be discussed
- **Early preterm (24–34 w):**
    Antenatal corticosteroids (recommended for pregnant women between 24–34 w)
    Admit to inpt observation in nearly all cases
    Avoid tocolytics (even through steroid window)
    Collect GBS culture
    Magnesium for neuroprotection if delivery prior to 32 w0d is imminent
    Latency antibiotics:
        ↑ Duration of Preg ("latency period") on avg 1 w
        ↓ Neonat morbidity (respiratory distress, NEC)
        Does not ↑ incid of chorio
    Induction at 34 w gest or w/ signs of preterm labor, chorio, abruption, fetal distress

---

Latency antibiotics regimen*

Ampicillin 2 g IV q6h × 48 h → Amoxicillin 250 mg PO q8h × 5 d
AND
Erythromycin 250 mg IV q6h × 48 h→ Erythromycin 333 mg PO q8h (or 250 mg q6h) × 5 d

*Other regimens can be employed (eg, azithromycin instead of erytho). For severe PCN allergy, use erythro alone. Augmentin should NOT be used in place of amp (inc risk of NEC).
Data from Mercer BM, Miodovnik M, Thurnau GR, et al. Antibiotic therapy for reduction of infant morbidity after preterm premature rupture of the membranes. A randomized controlled trial. National Institute of Child Health and Human Development Maternal-Fetal Medicine Units Network. JAMA. 1997;278(12):989–95.

- **≥34–<37 w:**
    Unless contraindications exist to vaginal deliv, induction may be attempted
    Consider steroids between 34 w0d–36 w6d to ↓ respiratory morbidity in newborns
    After 34 w, no difference in neonat sepsis btw induction & conservative mgmt, but trend toward ↓ neonat morbidity w/ induction
    More likely to see variable decelerations during labor → ↑ CD for fetal intolerance
    GBS status should be assessed during latency & appropriate therapy in labor
- **≥37 w:**
    Move toward delivery
    GBS status should be assessed during latency & appropriate therapy in labor

PRETERM LABOR

Definition and Epidemiology (Obstet Gynecol 2016;128(4):e155)
- Preterm Labor (ctx + cervical dilation) occurring after 20 w and before 37 w gest
- Preterm deliv occurs in roughly 12% of pregnancies

Etiology
- Poorly understood, but risk factors include multi gest/uterine overdistention, bact infxn, placental abruption, cervical insufficiency, prior preterm labor, ruptured membranes

Clinical Manifestation
- Physical exam findings of labor including persistent uterine contractions leading to changes in cervical effacement & dilation
- Rupture of membranes is common

Physical Exam
- Painful uterine contractions leading to cervical change, and eval for PPROM, abruption, etc

Diagnostic Workup/Studies (Obstet Gynecol 2012;120:964)
- **Pelvic exam:**
  Sterile speculum and digital exam to evaluate cervical dilation
  Collect fFN swab (from 22 w–34 w)
  GBS swab if deliv is not imminent & has not been collected previously
  Sterile vaginal exam to directly assess cervix (must be after fFN collected!)
- **Labs:**
  fFN: Basement membrane peptide present in amniotic membranes. Can be tested via cervical swab – not reliable w/ vaginal bleeding, recent (<24 h) intercourse or vaginal exam. If negative, 95% do *not* deliver in 14 d (Br J Obstet Gynecol 1996;103:648)
  Amnio: Consider amniocentesis to rule out chorioamnionitis with maternal fever, maternal elev WBC, uterine tenderness, maternal tachycardia, fetal tachycardia
- **US:**
  Transvaginal US measurement of cervical length <25 mm is associated with preterm delivery

Treatment and Medications (Obstet Gynecol 2012;119:1308)

Tocolytic medications				
Category	**Example**	**Contraindication**	**Mat effects**	**Fetal effects**
Beta-mimetics	Terbutaline	Tachycardia-sensitive mat cardiac disease, poorly controlled DM	Tachycardia, hypotension, tremor, palpitations, pulmonary edema, hypokalemia Hyperglycemia	Tachycardia
Magnesium sulfate	Magnesium sulfate	Myasthenia gravis	Flushing, muscle weakness, pulm edema, respiratory depression, cardiac arrest	Hypotonia, respiratory depression
CCBs	Nifedipine	Hypotension, pre-load-dependent cardiac lesions (Aortic Insuf)	Dizziness, flushing, hypotension	None
NSAID	Indomethacin	PLT dysfunction, hepatic dysfunction, GI ulceration, renal dysfunction, asthma with hypersensitivity to aspirin	nausea, GERD, gastritis	Closure of ductus arteriosus, oligohydramnios

- **Prior to 37 w gest but greater than 32 w gest:**
  Administer corticosteroids for fetal lung maturation if delivery likely within 7 d (steroid course if <34 w, only give between 34 w0d–36 w6d if they have not received steroids before)
  Tocolytics such as nifedipine PO only to allow for Cort administration (48 h) or mat xfer – no pharmacotherapy proven to stop preterm labor
  GBS prophylaxis if culture unknown

- **Prior to 32 w gest:**
  - Give steroid course if delivery likely within 7 d (Can use rescue course of BMZ once during pregnancy up to 34 w if it has been more than 7 d since the prior course)
  - Magnesium sulfate administration for fetal neuroprotection (N Engl J Med 2008;359:895)
  - Can use indocin until 32 w. CCB and beta-mimetics should be used with caution while using magnesium.
  - GBS prophylaxis if culture unknown
- **Prevention of recurrent preterm birth:**
  - 17-OH progesterone caproate (250 mg IM weekly) starting at 16 w until 36 w (30% reduction in recurrent preterm deliv) (N Engl J Med 2003;348:2379)
  - Serial cervical length measurements starting at 16–24 w/ poss cerclage placement if cervical length <25 mm. See short cervix, above (Am J Obstet Gynecol 2009;201:375).

POSTPARTUM HEMORRHAGE (PPH)

Definition and Epidemiology (Obstet Gynecol 2017;130:e168)
- Cumulative blood loss ≥1000 mL or blood loss with S and Sx's of hypovolemia within 24 h after the birth process
- Common, w/ incid 2–3% of all births in the US (Am J Obstet Gynecol 2010;202:353). Clinically, excessive bld loss causing symptomatic anemia (palps, SOB, lightheadedness) &/or signs of hypovolemia (tachy, HoTN, hypoxemia)
- Major cause of mat mortality (1.7/100,000 live births in US)
- **Primary (early) PPH:** W/i 24 h of deliv
- **Secondary (late) PPH:** From 24 h–12 w after deliv

Etiology
- **Risk factors:** Prolonged labor, high parity, chorio, general anesthesia, multiples, poly, macrosomia, uterine fibroids, operative vaginal delivery, episiotomy, succenturiate placenta, fetal death, abruption, anticoagulation
- **Causes primary (early) PPH:**
  - Uterine atony, lacerations, retained placenta, abnormally adherent placenta, DIC, uterine inversion
- **Causes secondary (late) PPH:**
  - Subinvolution of placenta, retained POCs, infection, inherited coagulation defects (vWD)
- Bleeding may not be apparent if intra- or retroperitoneal bleed, or if genital tract hematoma

Prevention
- Active management of the third stage: Oxytocin, uterine massage, umbilical cord traction
- Oxytocin can be administered before or after placental delivery

Physical Exam
- Bimanual exam to assess for atony or retained placental tissue
- Thorough inspection of the genital tract for laceration or hematoma
- Tachycardia & HoTN seen when bld loss approaches 1500–2000 cc

Diagnostic Workup/Studies
- Identify origin of bleeding:
  - Visualize cervix & vagina to evaluate for lacerations
  - Bimanual uterine massage to assess for uterine atony
  - Bedside US to view poss retained products
  - Manual evacuation of uterine cavity for poss extraction of retained products
  - Place Foley catheter (distended bladder may contribute to poor uterine tone)
- **Labs:** Bld type & cross, CBC, PT/INR, PTT, fibrinogen. 5 mL of bld in red top tube at bedside → clot in 8–10 min if fibrinogen >150 mg/dL.

Treatment
- **Uterine Atony:**
  - Bimanual examination with removal of clot and uterine massage
  - Foley to decompress bladder
  - Oxytocin (Pitocin) – Onset of action: ~1 min (IV), 3–5 min (IM).
  - Add other uterotonics – Misoprostol, methylergonovine, prostaglandin (see table)
  - Uterine tamponade balloon with uterine artery embolization if other measures fail
  - Operative intervention with D and C for possible retained POCs, uterine artery ligation, B-lynch suture, and hysterectomy as last resort.

Uterotonic treatment for atony					
Agent	Dose	Route	Dosing frequency	Side effects	Contra-indications
Oxytocin (Pitocin)	10–40 U in 1 L crystal-loid or 10 U IM	IV, IM/IU	Continuous	N/V, emesis, hypona-tremia	Hypersensitivity to oxytocin
Misoprostol (Cytotec)	600–1000 ug	oral, Sublin-gual, buccal, rectal	Single dose	N/V, diar-rhea, fever, chills	None
Methyler-gonovine (Methergine)	0.2 mg	IM,	Every 2–4 h	HTN, N/V	HTN, pre-eclampsia
Prostaglandin $F_{2\alpha}$ (Hemabate)	0.25 mg	IM IU	Every 15–90 min (8 dose max)	N/V, diar-rhea, flushing, fever, HA, chills	Asthma; active car-diac, pul-monary or hepatic dz

- **Trauma:**
  Rapid identification of vaginal clitoral, high vaginal, and cervical lacerations
  Hematomas (labial, vaginal broad ligament, and retroperitoneal): Most can be managed conservatively. Incision and drainage for rapid expansion. Consider embolization.
- **Retained Placenta:**
  US used for diagnosis: See echogenic mass in canal
  Manual removal is first step
  Banjo curette to remove adherent tissue (US guidance recommended)
- **Acute Coagulopathy:**
  Consider abruption and AFE in DDx
  Initiate massive transfusion protocol
- **Uterine Inversion:**
  Bimanual exam shows firm mass below the cervix with inability to palpate fundus abdominally
  Avoid detachment of placenta
  Manually replace uterus, may need uterine relaxation
  Surgical approach: When manual replacement fails, perform laparotomy and grasp uterus with babcocks. Possible need for incision of posterior cervix.

Medical Therapies for PPH
- See uterotonic section previously
- Crystalloid replacement in 3:1 ratio (fluid:EBL)
- Tranexamic acid: Antifibrinolytic agent. Given 1 g IV during hemorrhage when other agents fail.
- Massive transfusion: More than 10 units of PRBCs in 24 hours, or more than 4 U PRBCs within 1 h of delivery, or replacement of the complete blood volume.
  - Transfusion ratio of PRBC:FFP:PLT = 1:1:1
  - Cryo used for low fibrinogen levels
  - Complications: Hyperkalemia from PRBCs, citrate toxicity with low calcium, febrile nonhemolytic reactions, acute hemolytic transfusion reaction, acute transfusion reactions related to lung injury
- Recombinant factor VII: Will improve hemostasis, but increased risk of thrombosis. Reserved for extenuating circumstances.

Procedural Therapies for PPH
- Uterine massage for atony (external, bimanual)
- Manual extraction of placenta
- D&C/Suction curettage of the uterus for retained placenta
- Uterine tamponade: Balloon catheter placement (Foley or Bakri balloon, or lap packing) for tamponade, esp lower uterine segment atony
- Uterine compression sutures (eg, B-Lynch) or mattress sutures
- Uterine artery embolization (interv radiol): Have to be hemodynamically stable
- Exploratory laparotomy
  Compression sutures: B-Lynch, Hayman, Pereira (physically ↑ uterine tone)
  Vessel ligation: Uterine arteries (O'Leary sutures), hypogastric arteries (↓ perfusion)
- Hysterectomy (definitive therapy)

Figure 11.3 Management of uterine atony with bimanual massage

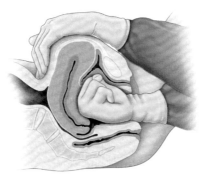

(Reprinted with permission from Casanova R, *Beckmann & Ling's Obstetrics & Gynecology*. 8th ed. Baltimore, MD: Wolters Kluwer, 2018.)

Figure 11.4 Initial surgical management of uterine atony

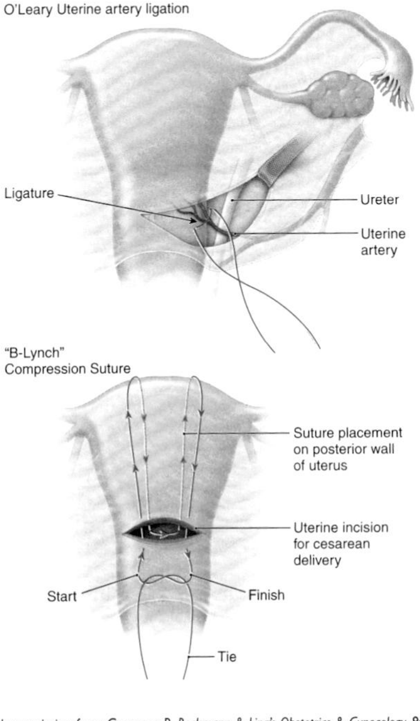

O'Leary Uterine artery ligation

Ligature

Ureter

Uterine artery

"B-Lynch" Compression Suture

Suture placement on posterior wall of uterus

Uterine incision for cesarean delivery

Start   Finish

Tie

(Reprinted with permission from Casanova R, *Beckmann & Ling's Obstetrics & Gynecology*. 8th ed. Baltimore, MD: Wolters Kluwer, 2018.)

Example postpartum hemorrhage protocol

Assessments	Meds/Procedures	Blood bank
Routine measures		
Assess for risk for PPH Quantify EBL routinely	Oxytocin IM or IV Fundal massage	Type & screen or crossmatch
Bld loss: >500 mL vaginal or >1000 mL cesarean or VS changes (by >15% or HR >110, BP <85/45, O$_2$ sat <95%)		
Notify nursing & anesthesia Continuous VS & calculation of EBL Bimanual & visual exam of genital tract, placenta, & (if intra-op) uterus, strict I/Os	Notify anesthesia team. Ensure adequate IV access. ↑ Oxytocin rate. Fluid resusc Continue bimanual uterine massage Methergine 0.2 mg IM if not hypertensive. May rpt if good resp, otherwise use another uterotonic. Empty bladder, place Foley	Crossmatch 2 units of pRBCs if not already done. Request FFP when requesting 3rd unit pRBC.
Continued bleeding w/ total bld loss under 1500 mL		
Mobilize 2nd obstetrician, rapid resp team (per hospital) Continue q5–10min VS, EBL Reexamine uterus, genital tract for bleeding source Send labs, including coagulation panel Consider uterine inversion, amniotic fluid embolism	Hemabate 0.25 mg IM &/or Misoprostol 800–1000 μg PR 2nd IV access vaginal birth Move to OR • Repair lacerations Consider D&C for retained placenta Place intrauterine balloon for tamponade Consult interventional radiology for selective embolization Cesarean birth Inspect broad ligament, post uterus, retained placenta B-Lynch suture Place intrauterine balloon for tamponade	Notify bld bank of OB hemorrhage 2 units RBCs to bedside, transfuse for clinical signs & *anticipated loss* (not lab values) Use bld warmer for xfusion Consider thawing 2 units FFP, use if transfusing >2 units RBCs at 1:1 Determine availability of additional RBCs & other bld products
Bld loss over 1500 mL, or >2 units pRBCs given or VS unstable or suspicion of DIC		
Prepare for postpartum hysterectomy. Call 2nd anesthesia provider, OR staff Rpt labs including coags/ABG Consider central line Social worker/family support – Keep family updated	Activate massive hemorrhage protocol B-Lynch suture Uterine artery ligation Hysterectomy Fluid warmer Upper body warming device Sequential compression devices	Transfuse aggressively Near 1:1 pRBC:FFP 1 platelet pack per 6 units pRBCs & as needed If coagulopathy unresponsive after 10 units pRBCs & coagulation factor replacement, consider rFactor VIIa

From The California Maternal Quality Care Collaborative, Obstetric Hemorrhage Care Summary 2010.

PLACENTAL ABRUPTION

Definition and Epidemiology *(Semin Perinatol 2009;33:189–95)*
- Partial or complete separation of a normally implanted placenta from the uterine wall before delivery and after 20 w
- **Incid:** 0.49–1.8%.
- **Risk factors:** Prior abruption, HTN, cocaine, tobacco, multiple gestation, PPROM, chorio, abd trauma

Pathophysiology
- Decidual hemorrhage → decidual cells release tissue factor → thrombin (uterotonic) is formed, upregulates apoptosis, induces expression of inflamm cytokines → tissue necrosis *(Am J Obstet Gynecol 2004;191:1996)*

Clinical Manifestation and Physical Exam
- **Acute:** Vaginal bleeding, abdominal/back pain, contractions (high frequency, low amplitude), abdominal/uterine tenderness, bright red bld in vaginal vault
- **Chronic:** Intermittent vaginal bleeding, often in small amounts, dark/old bld in vagina
- **Couvelaire uterus:** Purple tinged uterus due to bld in myometrium seen at cesarean
- **Placenta:** Gross retroplacental clots & histologic decidual necrosis or placental infarction
- **Fetus:** Fetal distress can be seen on NST

Diagnostic Workup/Studies
- Clinical dx by Hx, exam & suspicion. US is not a good predictor of diagnosis, but can be used.
- Continuous electronic fetal monitoring & uterine tocometry: Frequent uterine contractions (tetany) & nonreassuring fetal heart tracing
- **US:** 25–50% sens
  Retroplacental clot: Elevated region of placenta → if seen, likelihood of abruption HIGH (Acute blood loss is hyperechoic while chronic is hypoechoic)
  Thickened placenta that moves w/ mat mvmt
- **Labs:** CBC, T&C, coags, Kleihauer–Betke (Rh-mother)
  ↑ Early mat serum AFP: 10× risk of abruption if AFP not a/w a fetal anomaly (*Prenat Diagn* 2007;27:240)
  ↓ Fibrinogen (<200 mg/dL) = indicates possible coagulopathy

Treatment and Medications
- Large-bore IV placement & fluid/bld resusc as necessary
- **Term:** Deliv. If nonreassuring fetal heart tones → emergent CS
- **Preterm:** Generally delay deliv if fetal well-being is reassuring
  Many chronic abruptions will not require deliv
  Antenatal steroids if deliv anticipated prior to 37 w gest
  Tocolysis not used in women w/ acute abruption
  Antenatal testing & serial growth ultrasounds w/ expectant mgmt
  Be prepared w/ uterotonics in the postpartum period

PLACENTA PREVIA

Definition and Epidemiology
- Placenta overlying or proximate to internal cervical os (definitions have varied)
  Complete: Placenta completely covers os (>20–30%)
  Low-lying placenta: Placenta edge in the lower uterine segment, <2 cm from internal os. The terms "partial previa" (partly covering the internal cervical os) and "marginal previa" (placental edge within 2 cm of internal os, but not covering) are no longer used. Measurement (cm from int os) preferred for management decisions.
- **Incid:** 0.4% of pregnancies over 20 w (*J Matern Fetal Neonatal Med* 2003;13:175)
- ↑ W/ increasing parity, cigarette smoking, h/o placenta previa, prior uterine Surg, & prior CD
  1–4% in the preg following a CD; up to 10% if ≥4 CDs

Etiology
- **Trophoblastic implantation:** Scarred endometrium may ↑ this process
- Increased need for placental oxygen or nutrient deliv (smokers, multi gest, higher altitude residence)
- ↑ Risk of previa at earlier gestational age as the unidirectional growth of trophoblastic tissue toward fundus (trophotropism) is limited. Lower uterine segment ↑ w/ gestational age → Over 90% of placenta previa identified in the 2nd trimester resolve at term

Clinical Manifestation and Physical Exam
- **Painless vaginal bleeding** in the 2nd & 3rd trimesters
- DO NOT perform digital cervical exam on a pt suspected to have a previa, perform US to confirm
- A sterile speculum exam is used to visually assess cervical dilation

Diagnostic Workup/Studies
- Identification of placenta during routine US, usually performed from 18–22 w
- Transvaginal US is the gold standard for diagnosis
- Prior CSs + previa = look carefully for evid of placenta accreta (below)

- Pelvic rest (no intercourse or digital exams for duration of preg)
- **Outpt mgmt:** Small bleeds resolved for >7 d, live close to the hospital, & are highly compliant
- **Inpt mgmt:** Actively bleeding placenta previa, ≥2–3 episodes of vaginal bleeding
    If pt can be stabilized & deliv is not needed immediately for fetal distress:
        Large-bore IV × 2 for access
        Baseline labs (H/H, platelet count, type & screen, coags)
        Antenatal steroids should be administered <37 w gest
- CD at 36 w0d–37 w6d gest *(Obstet Gynecol 2013;121:908)*

VASA PREVIA

Definition and Epidemiology *(Am J Obs Gynecol 2018;218:B2)*
- Umbilical vessels in membranes cross over internal os or within 2 cm of internal os
- Prevalence: 1:2500 deliveries *(OBG Survey 2004:245)*
- Type 1: From a velamentous cord insertion (vessels not surrounded by Wharton's jelly)
- Type 2: From vessels btw lobes of a bilobed or succenturiate lobed placenta

Clinical Manifestation
- Vaginal bleeding w/ rupture of membranes → fetal vessel laceration
- Sinusoidal fetal HR (indicating fetal anemia) or bradycardia

Diagnostic Workup/Studies
- Placental cord insertion needs to be identified at second trimester US
- Transvaginal US is gold standard. Color Doppler demonstrates FHR of blood vessel <2 cm from internal os.

Treatment and Medications *(Am J Obstet Gynecol 2015;213(5):615)*
- Pelvic rest (no intercourse or digital exams)
- Antenatal corticosteroid between 28–32 w
- Antepartum hospitalization at 30–34 w for closer surveillance
- Scheduled CD at 34–37 w

PLACENTA ACCRETA

Definition and Epidemiology
- Abn placental implantation: Placental villi attach to the myometrium or grow through it instead of being contained by decidual cells
- Incid of accreta 1/533 pregnancies; incidence increasing parallel to increasing CS rate
- Risk of accreta ↑ w/ myometrial tissue damage (prior myomectomy, ablation, uterine artery embolization, multiple D&C procedures), placenta previa, & increasing number of CDs. Other risks: Older maternal age, smoking, advanced parity.

CS and risk for placenta accreta *(Obstet Gynecol 2006;107:1226)*		
Cesarean section #	Risk w/ no placenta previa	Risk w/ placenta previa
1	0.03%	3.3%
2	0.2%	11%
3	0.1%	40%
4	0.8%	61%
5	0.8%	67%

Pathology
- **Accreta:** Chorionic villi attached to myometrium
- **Increta:** Chorionic villi invade the myometrium just up to the serosa
- **Percreta:** Chorionic villi protrude through the uterine serosa and can invade other organs

Clinical Manifestation
- Often diagnosed prior to delivery on imaging (US or MRI)
- Placenta does not detach after deliv → PPH

Diagnostic Workup/Studies
- Women w/ placenta previa or low lying anter placenta & prior uterine surg → sono for accreta. US sensitivity 77–87%, specificity 96–98%, PPV 65–93%, NPV 98% *(Obstet Gynecol 2012;120:207)*

- Ultrasonographic findings suggestive of placenta accreta:
  Loss of hypoechoic boundary btw placenta & bladder or thin myometrium <1 mm
  Placental lacunae or vascular spaces w/ turbulent flow
  Irreg bladder wall w/ extensive vascularity
  Loss of retroplacental clear space
- Consider color Doppler sono, 3D sono, & MRI. Cystoscopy if bladder invasion suspected

Subsequent Workup
- If accreta identified, pt should be seen by a team of physicians (Anesthesia, General Surg or gynecologic oncology, Interventional Radiology, Uro) to prepare for cesarean hysterectomy
- Monitor closely for vaginal bleeding & abdominal pain throughout preg

Treatment and Medications
- CD at 34 w0d–35 w6d, be prepared for hyst (Obstet Gynecol 2013;121:908)
- Steroids for fetal lung maturity should be individualized
- PPH w/ extreme blood loss likely. Maintain IV access & T&C for bld products. Consider internal iliac artery balloon catheters, postsurgical embolization.

UTERINE INVERSION

Definition and Epidemiology
- **Complete:** Internal lining of fundus extrudes through cervical os
- **Incomplete:** Portion of fundus extrudes to the cervix but not through the os
- 1 in 2500 deliveries (J Reprod Med 1989;34:173)

Etiology
- Not completely understood but risk factors include: Excessive umbilical cord traction during 3rd stage of labor, uterine atony, uterine malformations, abnormal placentation (eg, placenta accreta)

Physical Exam
- Visualization of endometrial lining through the cervical os (meaty, red tissue)
- Palpation of bulge in vagina on bimanual exam
- Inability to palpate fundus of uterus
- Persistent vaginal bleeding

Treatment and Medications
- Manually reinvert the uterus w/ constant/gentle pres of vaginal hand, in a cephalad direction, on the fundally inv portion of the uterus. Reinversion becomes more difficult w/ delay. Bleeding ↑↑↑
- General anesthesia & tocolytic agents may be needed to assist w/ replacing the uterus
  Magnesium sulfate 4–6 g IV
  Terbutaline 0.25 mg IV or SQ
  Nitroglycerine 50 µg IV
  Halogenated anesthesia (isoflurane, sevoflurane)
- Obstetrical emergency if reinversion is not successful → laparotomy → elevate fundus by round ligaments & restore cephalad with a hand below in the vagina. May need to incise posterior cervix.

AMNIOTIC FLUID EMBOLISM

Definition and Epidemiology
- Presence of amniotic fluid in mat circulation, occurring usually during labor or immediately postpartum
- Rare, incidence of 1–12/100,000 births. Unpredictable & unpreventable

Pathophysiology
- Poorly understood. Amniotic fluid enters mat circulation → precipitation of dic & shock in mother (cardiogenic vs. distributive)
- Risk factors: Operative delivery, placenta previa, placenta accreta, abruption, multiple gestations, polyhydramnios

Clinical Features
- Great variability in clinical manifestation, but classically acute onset of hypotension, hypoxia, & coagulopathy

- Nonspecific sx include chills, N/V, agitation, tonic–clonic seizures
- Can lead to cardiac arrest and need for resuscitative measures

Diagnostic Workup/Studies
- **Clinical dx:** HoTN, hypoxemia, cardiorespiratory failure
- **Lab eval:** CBC, T&C, PT/INR, PTT, Fibrinogen, CMP. AFE is a clinical diagnosis.
- **Ddx:** Placental abruption, uterine rupture, peripartum cardiomyopathy, sepsis, PE, anaphylaxis, MI, anesthetic complication, eclamptic seizure

Treatment and Medications
- If deliv has not yet occurred, emergent (often bedside) deliv of the fetus is warranted. Delivery of a fetus >23 w improves maternal outcomes.
- Supportive rx: Correct hypoxemia (intubate if necessary), CPR if cardiopulmonary arrest, hemodynamic support with BCLS and ACLS protocols, reverse coagulopathy with massive transfusion protocol. Transfer to ICU

MALPRESENTATION

Definition and Epidemiology
- Fetal presentation refers to the presenting part of the fetus (lowest or nearest cervix). Poss presentations include:
  Cephalic presentation divided into vertex, brow, face
  Breech presentation divided into frank, complete, footling
- Breech presentation occurs in 3–4% of term pregnancies
- See Chap. 10, Figure 10.2.

Breech presentations		
Frank breech	**Footling breech**	**Complete breech**
Fetal hips flexed, fetal knees extended; "butt 1st"	Fetal foot or knee is below the breech; "foot 1st"	Fetal hips flexed, fetal knees flexed

Etiology and Diagnosis
- Uterine anomalies (bicornuate, septum), fibroids, placentation defects (previa), multiparity, poly/oligohydramnios, contracted mat pelvis, fetal or neuro defect, short umbilical cord
- Presenting part is felt w/ vaginal exam, identified on Leopold maneuvers. Verify w/ US.

Treatment
- Breech & mentum post face presentations → usually CD. *Planned* vaginal breech deliv a/w ↑ perinatal mortality, neonat morbidity & mortality than planned CD (5% vs. 1.6%) (*Lancet 2000;356:1375*).
- **External cephalic version** may be attempted (at >37 w) to convert a breech presentation to a cephalic. Use parenteral tocolysis (terbutaline) improves success. Inadequate data for ECV in pts with prior CS scar. Contraindicated in pregnancies where CD is indicated (eg, placenta previa) (*Obstet Gynecol 2016;127:e54*).

FETAL MECONIUM

Definition and Epidemiology
- Fetal mec stool usually passed in the 1st days of life. If prior to deliv → meconium-stained amniotic fluid, which if breathed by fetus can → respiratory distress from mec aspiration syn
- Meconium-stained amniotic fluid in ~9% of live births w/ 0.1% mec aspiration syn
- Most common in pregnancies reaching 41–42 w gest (post-term)
- More likely during labor c/b fetal hypoxia → possibly indicating fetal stress resp

Pathology
- Aspiration of mec by the fetus → dz in neonat lungs → causing hypoxemia and acidosis
- Injury from mechanical obst of the airway, inflamm damage caused by irritation in the lungs, or by inactivation of surfactant w/i alveoli

Clinical Manifestations
- Dark brown to green amniotic fluid when membranes rupture or after (describe as thin, mod, thick)
- Note color & presence or absence of particulate matter

- Mec aspiration can occur during deliv – mec aspiration syn is dx w/ neonat respiratory distress in setting of mec stained delivery and absence of other causes of distress

Treatment and Medications
- Amnioinfusion does not prevent mec aspiration syn
- Peds should be at deliv when mec is noted on rupture of membranes
- To prevent aspiration, nonvigorous neonates should *not* be initially stimulated at the perineum. Allow peds to evaluate & perform tracheal suction w/ laryngoscope.

INTRAAMNIOTIC INFECTION

Definition and Epidemiology (Obstet Gynecol 2017;130:e95)
Intraamniotic infection; also referred to chorioamnionitis
- Infxn and/or inflammation of any combination of amniotic fluid, placenta, fetus, fetal membranes, or decidua
- Complicates 2–5% of all births in US
- Risk factors – ↑ Duration of membrane rupture, GBS positivity, prolonged labor, multi vaginal exams, internal monitoring

Etiology
- May be transmitted via ascending infxn from lower genital tract, transplacentally from mat bld stream, or iatrogenically (eg, via amniocentesis)
- **Typical organisms:** This is a polymicrobial infection. *Ureaplasma, Mycoplasma hominis* (more common in ascending infections), GBS, *Escherichia coli, Listeria monocytogenes* (more common w/ transplacental spread from mat infxn)
- **Sequelae:** Neonatal pneumonia, meningitis, sepsis, and death. Maternal endomyometritis, hemorrhage, peritonitis, sepsis, and death (rare).

Physical Exam
- Documented maternal fever: Oral temp ≥39.0°C. If temp b/w 38.0°C–39.0°C, repeat 30 min later. If repeat ≥38.0°C, then fever is confirmed.
- Rule out other causes of maternal fever (eg, epidural, dehydration, PGE2 use, extrauterine causes of infection)
- Fetal tachycardia >160 bpm × 10 min or longer
- Purulent fluid from cervical os

Diagnostic Workup/Studies
- Objective diagnosis is a positive amniotic fluid culture or gram stain. However, most diagnoses are clinical.
- Suspected intraamniotic infection if maternal fever + 1 of the following: Maternal leukocytosis, purulent cervical drainage, or fetal tachycardia
- Confirmed intraamniotic infection: Amniocentesis proven + gram stain, low glucose or + amniotic fluid culture, placental pathology with infection. This is clinically often not made or made only after delivery.

Treatment and Medications
- Acetaminophen for fever control → ↓ incid of neonat encephalopathy
- Antibiotics recommended
- Not an indication for cesarean delivery
- **IV Abx (continue from diagnosis to delivery, then determine postpartum treatment need)**

Antibiotics for intrauterine infection/chorioamnionitis	
Primary Regimen	• Ampicillin 2 g IV q6h + Gentamicin 1.5 mg/kg IV q8h until deliv • With mild PCN allergy, substitute cefazolin 2 g IV every h for ampicillin • With severe PCN allergy, substitute clindamycin 900 mg IV every 8 h for ampicillin
Alternative Regimens	• Ampicillin–Sulbactam 3 g IV every 6 h • Piperacillin–tazobactam 3.375 g IV every 6 h • Cefotetan 2 g IV every 12 h • Cefoxitin 2 g IV every 8 h • Ertapenem 1 g IV every 24 h
Postdelivery	• **Vaginal:** May not need additional antibiotics • **Cesarean:** One additional dose of antimicrobial therapy after delivery is recommended. Add clindamycin 900 mg IV or metronidazole 500 mg IV for one additional dose

ENDOMYOMETRITIS

Definition and Epidemiology
- Infxn of the endometrial, parametrial, or myometrial tissue usually >24 h after deliv (low-grade mat fever common during this period). Clinical suspicion guides dx.
- Incid varies w/ mode of deliv:
  Vaginal deliv: 0.2–0.9%; higher if chorio was present
  CD: 5–30%; decreased w/ perioperative prophylactic Abx

Etiology
- Similar to chorioamnionitis (ascending infxn from lower genital tract). Also introduced infxn from surgical trauma. Usually polymicrobial.
- Infxn from genital tract can invade the surgical wound

Physical Exam
- Maternal fever, uterine tenderness, purulent lochia, malaise, chills

Diagnostic Workup/Studies
- ↑WBC (although commonly elevated in labor & postpartum)
- Largely clinical dx & depends on context/suspicion. Imaging generally unnecessary unless suspecting pelvic abscess or larger/progressing infxn.
- Cx for chlamydia & gonorrhea could be considered if not already obtained
- Routine endometrial culturing is not helpful secondary to genital tract contamination

Treatment and Medications
- Gentamicin 5 mg/kg IV q24h + Clindamycin 900 mg IV q8h. IV Abx until asymptomatic/afebrile for 24–48 h; no data exist to support continued oral antibiotic rx. Clinical response guides antibiotic coverage/spectrum (eg, broaden if no response in ~24 h or clinically worsening) and duration of treatment.
- Acetaminophen/Ibuprofen for mat fever. Breastfeeding okay.

Epidemiology

- CVD = Leading cause of death in women in US (*Circulation 2017;13:e1349*)
- ↑ Incid of CVD in Preg due to ↑ age at 1st Preg & ↑ prevalence of risk factors (DM, HTN, obesity) (*J Am Coll Cardiol 2010;56:1149*)
- Hypertensive disorders occur in 6–8% of pregnancies (*Am J Obstet Gynecol 2000;183:S1*). Other CVD complicates 0.2–4% of pregnancies (in western countries) (*Am J Obstet Gynecol 1998;179:1643*)
- Hypertensive is at risk of premature birth, small for gestational age, and associated morbidity and mortality (*Circulation 2002;105:2179*)

Maternal Cardiac Risk Estimation

- **Prepregnancy counseling:** Risk of Preg depends on specific heart dz & current clinical status. Risk assessment should be performed prior to Preg, including medication review.
- **Mat risk assessment:** WHO risk classification integrates all known mat CV risk factors; Other risk models: ZAHARA I and CARPREG (*Heart 2014;100:1373*)
- Fetal risks of maternal CVD: Higher rate SAB, IUGR, IUFD, PTB, and perinatal mortality; If Fam History of Congenital Heart Dz → get fetal echo

WHO maternal cardiac risk classification		
WHO class	**Definition & mgmt**	**Example**
1	Low risk, limited cardiology follow-up in Preg	Mild Pulm Sten, PDA, MV pro-lapse, isolated ectopic atrial or ventricular beats, repaired ASD/VSD
2	Low or mod risk, cardiology follow-up every trimester	Most arrhythmias, repaired tetralogy of Fallot, unrepaired ASD/VSD, repaired coarc, Marfan or bicuspid aortic valve (BAV), no root dilation
3	High risk, frequent cardiology follow-up	Mild LV dysfunction, hypertro-phic cardiomyopathy, mechan-ical valve, cyanotic heart dz, complex congenital heart dz, Marfan or BAV root dilated 40–45 mm
4	Very high risk, Preg "contraindi-cated." Recommend termination of Preg, otherwise frequent cardiology follow-up.	Pulm arterial HTN, sev ventri-cular dysfxn (NYHA III–IV or EF <30%), sev MS or AS, Marfan dilated aortic root >45 mm, BAV root diameter >50 mm

From *Heart* 2006;92(10):1520–5.

Cardiac disease in pregnancy score (CARPREG)
1 point earned for each of the following:
NYHA functional class >II or cyanosis
Left heart obst w/ MV area <2 cm^2, AVA <1.5 cm^2, or L ventricular outflow tract gradient >30 mmHg
LVEF <40%
H/o prior cardiac event or arrhythmia
Risk of cardiac complication (eg, pulm edema, tachy/bradyarrhythmia req rx, MI, stroke, cardiac death): 0 points = 5%; 1 point = 27%; >1 point = 75%

From *Circulation* 2001;104(5):515–21.

CARDIOVASCULAR CHANGES IN PREGNANCY

Blood Volume (*Eur Heart J* 2011;32:3147)
- Plasma vol ↑ 40% from 6–32 w gest to 4700–5200 mL
- RBC mass ↑ by 20–30% (from ↑ production of RBCs)
- Plasma vol ↑ more than RBC vol, causing physiologic hemodilution → anemia
- ↑ Erythrocyte 2,3-diphosphoglycerate conc, ↓ affinity of mat Hgb for O_2 → facilitates dissociation of oxygen from Hgb → preferential xfer of O_2 to fetus

Hemodynamic Profile
- CO ↑ 30–50% during Preg (50% of that during 1st 8 w)
  Turning from supine to left lateral recumbent position → release of vena caval compression by gravid uterus can ↑ CO by 25–30%
- Uterine bld flow ↑ 10-fold to 500–800 mL/min (17% of total CO at term)
- Renal bld flow ↑ by 50%. No change in perfusion to brain or liver
- ↑ HR at 5 w → max ↑ 15–20 beats/min by 32 w to term
- ↓ BP from 7 w to nadir 5–10 mmHg systolic & 10–15 mmHg diastolic by 24–32 w, then ↑ toward nonpregnant values at term

Heart Sounds
- Benign systolic flow murmur develops in more than 95% of pregnant women: ↑ CO → turbulent flow over pulmonic or aortic valve
- Audible 1st btw 12–20 w w/ regression usually by 1 w postpartum

Intrapartum Hemodynamic Changes
- **1st stage labor:** 12–31% ↑ CO. 2nd stage: 49% ↑ CO. ≈2-fold ↑ from nonpregnant.
- Contractions cause 300–500 mL xfer of bld from uterus to general circulation
  SBP & DBP ↑ by 35 & 25 mmHg, respectively

Maternal hemodynamic profiles in the 3rd trimester			
	Nonpregnant	**Pregnant**	**Change**
Cardiac output (L/min)	4.3 ± 0.9	6.2 ± 1	+43%
Heart rate (beats/min)	71 ± 10	83 ± 10	+17%
Systemic vascular resistance (dyne-sec cm^{-5})	1530 ± 520	1210 ± 266	−21%
Pulse volume recording (dyne-sec cm^{-5})	119 ± 47	78 ± 22	−34%
Central venous pressure (mmHg)	3.7 ± 2.6	3.6 ± 2.5	—
Colloid osmotic pressure (COP) (mmHg)	20.8 ± 1	18 ± 1.5	−14%
Pulmonary capillary wedge Pressure (PCWP) (mmHg)	6.3 ± 2.1	7.5 ± 1.8	—
COP–PCWP (mmHg)[a]	14.5 ± 2.5	10.5 ± 2.7	−28%

[a]Important factor in dev of pulm edema throughout Preg.
From *Obstet Gynecol* 1989;161:1439.

Postpartum Hemodynamic Changes
- **60–80% ↑ CO w/i 10–15 min of vaginal deliv:** Release of venocaval obst, autotransfusion of uteroplacental bld, rapid mobilization of extravascular fluid → *watch for pulm edema.* CO returns to prelabor value by 1-h postpartum
- Important to monit women w/ CVD closely until at least 24 h after deliv
- CV measurements (SV, SVR, CO) take up to 24 w to return to prepregnancy values

ECG Changes in Pregnancy
- Majority of pregnant pts have a nml ECG (*Eur Heart J* 2011;32:3147)
- Change in heart position 2/2 rise of diaphragm (rotated to left) → 15–20° L axis deviation; mimics LV hypertrophy
- **Common ECG changes:** Transient ST segment & T wave changes; Q wave & inv T wave in lead III; attenuated Q wave in lead AVF; inv T wave in leads V_1, V_2, & occ V_3
- Premature beats & sustained tachyarrhythmia ↑ in Preg. Ventricular & atrial ectopy in up to 50–60% of pregnant women. Symptomatic exacerbation of paroxysmal SVT in Preg in 20–44% of cases (Rx: Vagal maneuvers → adenosine).
- VT rare in Preg but Rx similar to nonpregnant (cardioversion → beta blocker or verapamil)
- 15% of pregnant women w/ CHD develop arrhythmia. Most palps are benign, but warrant a Holter monit.

CHRONIC HYPERTENSION (CHTN)

Definitions

Hypertension definitions			
Category	Systolic (mmHg)		Diastolic (mmHg)
Nonpregnant (JNC 8 Classification)			
Nml	<120	AND	<80
Pre-HTN	120–139	OR	80–89
Stage 1 HTN	140–159	OR	90–99
Stage 2 HTN	≥160	OR	≥100
Pregnant (GHTN vs. CHTN depends on timing)			
HTN	≥140, <160		≥90, <110
HTN (severe feature range)	≥160		≥110

Data from James PA, Ortiz E, et al. 2014. Evidence-based guideline for the management of high blood pressure in adults: (JNC8). *JAMA*. 2014 Feb 5;311(5):507.

- **CHTN:** Blood pressure ≥140/≥90 based upon the average of 2 or more properly measured readings at each of 2 or more office visits after an initial screening
- **CHTN in Preg:** Use of antihypertensive medication prior to Preg, OR onset of HTN before Preg, OR HTN prior to 20 w0d gest OR HTN that persists beyond 12 w postpartum

Epidemiology and Etiology

- **Nonpregnant:** 10–15% Caucasian adults (>age 18), 25% AA adults, increase with age
- **Pregnant:** Occurs in up to 5% of pregnant women. Hypertensive disorders overall represent the most common medical complications of Preg (incid 6–8%)
- **Essential (95%)**
- **Secondary:**
  Renal (4%): Renal artery stenosis, parenchymal, PCKD
  Endocrine (0.5%): Pheo, primary aldosteronism (Conn), Cushing
  Anatomic (0.2%): Coarct of the aorta
  Other: Collagen vascular dz, sleep apnea

Gestational complications of CHTN		
	HTN (%)	Sev HTN (≥160/110) (%)
Superimposed PEC	10–25	50
Placental abruption	0.7–1.5	5–10
Preterm deliv	12–34	62–70
SGA infant	8–16	31–40

From Sibai SM. Chronic Hypertension in Pregnancy. *Obstet Gynecol* 2002;100:369.

Workup

- **H&P:** Including fundoscopic, cardiac, abdominal, vascular, & neurologic exams
- **Studies:** Electrolytes, BUN/Cr, gluc, Hgb/Hct, UA, lipids, ECG, ± Echo
- **W/u for secondary causes:** Severe or resistant HTN, onset before puberty, age <30 if nonobese non-Black pt without FH or risk factors, hypokalemia, elevated Cr
- **Additional w/u for Preg:** Baseline PEC labs (Hgb, Plt, Cr, AST/ALT, 24-h urine prot)

Complications

- **Nonpregnant:** Mostly long term, including TIA/CVA, CAD, CHF, CKI
  ↑ Of 20 mmHg SBP or 10 mmHg DBP doubles CV complications (*Lancet* 2002;360:1903)
- **Pregnant:** Additional mat risks: Pulm edema, hypertensive encephalopathy (PRES), retinopathy, cerebral hemorrhage, acute renal failure
  Additional fetal risks: Perinatal mortality ↑ 3–4×

Treatment

- **Rx goals nonpregnant** (*JAMA* 2014;311(5):507)
  Age ≥60 initiate pharmacologic treatment to lower BP at SBP ≥150 or DBP ≥90 to treat to goal <150/90; can allow SBP <140 if well tolerated
  Age <60, initiate pharmacologic treatment at SBP ≥140 or DBP ≥90 to lower BP <140/90
- **CKD or DM:** Rx goal SBP <140 and DBP <90 regardless of age
- **Rx goals pregnant:** <160/105 (*N Engl J Med* 2015;372(5):407)

For SBPs ≥140–<160, and DBP ≥90–<105, weigh maternal benefits of BP to control heart disease, CKD, etc. in those with pre-existing organ damage with fetal risks of uteroplacental insufficiency

Medication for treatment of CHTN		
Drug	**Mechanism of action**	**Notes**

ACE inhibitor[a,b]
    Captopril
    Enalapril
    Lisinopril
	Inhibits angiotensin converting enzyme, preventing conversion of Angiotensin I to Angiotensin II	Alternative 1st-line for non-Black adults without CKD
		1st-line for adults WITH CKD
		Used in atherosclerosis, DM, CKI, CHF, post-MI
		Generally **avoided in pregnancy**, however, some safety data emerging *(Am J Obstet Gynec 2017;129:174)*
		Side effect: Dry cough, angioedema 2/2 inhibition of breakdown of bradykinin

Angiotensin receptor blocker[a,b]
    Eprosartan
    Candesartan
    Losartan
    Valsartan
    Irbesartan
	Blocks angiotensin II action at receptors, therefore preventing secretion of ADH and reducing secretion of aldosterone, as well as preventing vasoconstriction	Alternative 1st-line for non-Black adults without CKD
		1st-line for adults with CKD
		Avoid in pregnancy

β-Blockers
    Atenolol
    Metoprolol
    Labetalol
	Selective β1 blockers act on cardiac muscle, slowing heart rate
	Labetalol is β1 and β2 blocker. β2 controls smooth muscle relaxation, so blocking can cause bronchospasm
		Used w/ angina, post-MI, CHF
		Labetalol: Drug of choice in Preg. No known teratogenicity, avoid in asthmatics, pts w/ CHF.
		Avoid atenolol in Preg: ↑ risk for IUGR
		Avoid atenolol & metoprolol postpartum: Concentrate in breast milk

Calcium channel blockers[a,c]
    Amlodipine
    Diltiazem Extended release
    Nitrendipine
    Nifedipine
	Nondihydropyridine (Diltiazem) – smooth muscle dilator and negative inotrope
	Dihydropyridine (Nitrendipine, Nifedipine) – selective to smooth muscle dilation (minimal inotropic effect)
	Amlodipine is both
		Alternative 1st line for adults without CKD
		Used w/ DM & vascular dz in Preg
		No known teratogenicity

Thiazide diuretic[a,c]
    Bendroflumethiazide
    Chlorthalidone
    Hydrochlorothiazide
    Indapamide
	Reduces sodium absorption in distal convoluted tubule; unrelated, increases calcium reabsorption, and decreases magnesium reabsorption	1st line for adults WITHOUT CKD
		Reduces plasma vol expansion in Preg
		D/c if evid of reduced uteroplacental perfusion

Hydralazine	Increases cGMP to directly vasodilate	Side effect of tachycardia, palpitations, flushing
Methyldopa	Central α2 agonist	Drug with the most safety data in pregnancy, however, poor at controlling blood pressure

[a]In a general non-Black population initial Rx should include thiazide, CCB, ACE or ARB.
[b]In population with CKD Rx should include ACEI or ARB to improve kidney outcome (regardless of race or DM).
[c]In a general Black population (including DM) initial Rx should include thiazide or CCB.
(JAMA 2014;311(5):507; Obstet Gynecol 2013;122:1122).

- Goals of treatment: Preventing acute complications of hypertension, maintain a healthy pregnancy as long as possible, minimize risks to the fetus
- Lifestyle modifications preconception: Weight loss, diet (low saturated & total fat, low sodium), exercise, ↓ EtOH
- A successful prepregnancy BP regimen generally can be continued in Preg except ACEI/ARB
- Need serial growth scans for CHTN in pregnancy (every ~4 w). Serial fetal testing (NST, AFI) generally twice weekly from 28–34 w (depending on severity)
- Delivery timing (Obstet Gynecol 2011;118:323–33):
  - No Meds, BP controlled, no IUGR → 38–39 w
  - Well controlled on Meds → 37–39 w
  - Difficult to control BP, multiple agents, severe range BP → 36–37 w

HYPERTENSIVE CRISIS

Definition
- **Hypertensive emergency:** Elevated BP w/ target organ damage
- **Hypertensive urgency:** SBP ≥180 or DBP ≥110 w/ minimal or no target organ damage

Treatment of Nonpregnant Patients – Goal <160/100
- **Hypertensive emergency:** ↓ MAP by 25% in minutes to 2 h using IV agents
- **Hypertensive urgency:** ↓ MAP 25% in hours using oral agents

IV & oral agents for treatment of hypertensive crisis of nonpregnant patients			
IV agents		**Oral agents**[a]	
Agent	**Dose**	**Agent**	**Dose**
Nitroglycerin	17–1000 µg/min	Labetalol	Initial 100 mg BID; max 800 mg TID
Labetalol[b]	10–80 mg q10min or 2–4 mg/min	Clonidine	0.2 mg load → 0.1 mg qh Max dose 0.7 mg
Hydralazine[b]	10–20 mg q4–6h	Hydralazine	Initial 10 mg QID; max 300 mg daily
		Captopril	6.25 or 12.5 mg (if not volume overloaded); max 100 TID

[a]Sublingual nitroglycerine is not used for acute HTN due to reported serious CV morbidity.
[b]Recommended for use in acute sev HTN in Preg though dosing intervals different.

Treatment of hypertensive crisis of pregnant patients (Obstet Gynecol 2017;129:e90)		
Always institute fetal monitoring, when pt is pregnant with viable fetus		
Labetalol	**Hydralazine**	**Nifedipine**[a]
• BP >160/110 persist for 15 min, give **20 mg IV labetalol** over 2 min • Recheck BP in **10 min** • If BP >160/110, give **40 mg IV labetalol** over 2 min • Recheck BP in **10 min** • BP >160/110, give **80 mg IV labetalol** over 2 min • Recheck BP in **10 min** • BP >160/110, move to hydralazine algorithm, starting with **10 mg IV** • Can use constant infusion 1–2 mg/min IV	• BP >160/110 persist for 15 min, give **5–10 mg IV hydralazine** over 2 min • Recheck BP in **20 min** • If BP >160/110, give **10 mg IV hydralazine** over 2 min • Recheck BP in **20 min** • If BP >160/110, give **20 mg IV hydralazine** over 2 min • Recheck BP in **20 min** • BP >160/110, move to labetalol algorithm, starting with **40 mg IV** • Can use constant infusion 0.5–10 mg/h	• BP >160/110 persist for 15 min, give **10 mg Oral nifedipine** • Recheck BP in **20 min** • If BP >160/110, give **20 mg Oral nifedipine** • Recheck BP in **20 min** • If BP >160/110, give **20 mg Oral nifedipine** • Recheck BP in **20 min** • BP >160/110, move to labetalol algorithm, starting with **40 mg IV** • Can us 30 mg XL, or 10–20 mg q2–6h

If moving from 1 algorithm to the next, obtain MFM consult, or internal medicine, anesthesia, or critical care input	
Once BP threshold reached, repeat BP every 10 min for 1 h, every 15 min, for 1 h, every 30 min for 1 h, and every h for 4 h	

[a]Immediate release oral (not sublingual) nifedipine used as 2nd-line agent for treatment of severe hypertension while awaiting IV placement due to risk of overcorrecting hypertension and maternal rebound tachycardia.

PREGNANCY-RELATED HYPERTENSION

Definitions (And see Chap. 11; *Obstet Gynecol* 2013;122:1122)

Gestational hypertensive disorders			
Dz	**BP**	**Proteinuria***	**Notes**
Gestational HTN	SBP ≥140 or DBP ≥90 Sev: SBP ≥160 or DBP ≥110 On 2 occasions at least 4 h apart & no more than 7 d apart	<300 mg prot in 24-h urine OR Protein/Creatinine <0.3	1st diagnosed beyond 20 w gest
Preeclampsia without severe features	SBP ≥140 or DBP ≥90 On 2 occasions at least 4 h apart & no more than 7 d apart	≥300 mg prot in 24-h urine OR Protein/Creatinine ≥0.3	1st diagnosed beyond 20 w gest gHTN plus proteinuria Absence of any severe features (see below)
Preeclampsia with severe features	SBP ≥160 or DBP ≥110 On 2 occasions at least 4 h apart while the pt is on bed rest. BP should be measured seated upright. OR Need to institute antihypertensive medications prior to 4 h	≥300 mg prot in 24-h urine OR Protein/Creatinine ≥0.3 *Can also diagnose PEC w/ SF without proteinuria, in presence of severe range BP and any severe feature at right	Elevated BP plus a severe feature: Sev-range BP (as left) Thrombocytopenia (<100,000/uL) Serum Cr >1.1 mg/dL or twice baseline in absence of pre-existing kidney disease Elevated LFTs (2× upper limit normal) Persistent RUQ pain Pulmonary edema New onset cerebral/visual symptoms (headache, scotomata)
Superimposed PEC	CHTN + PEC	New onset proteinuria (≥300 mg 24-h urine, or Protein/Creatinine ≥0.3) or sudden increase in proteinuria from baseline	Severe features same as above

Epidemiology (*Obstet Gynecol* 2003;102:181)
- **Risk factors for Preg-related HTN:** Nulliparity, multifetal gest, obesity, AMA, family or personal hx PEC, CHTN, renal dz, DM, vascular & CTD, abn uterine artery Doppler, antiphospholipid Ab syn, thrombophilia, SLE, IVF, AA race
- **gHTN:** 6–17% in nulliparous & 2–4% multiparous women
- **PEC:** 4–8% of all pregnancies; up to 18% in women w/ a h/o PEC
- **Eclampsia:** 1 in 2000–3448 pregnancies

Other disorders associated with HTN in pregnancy	
Diagnosis	**Definition**
Eclampsia	Seizures not attributed to another cause in a woman w/ PEC
HELLP	**H**emolysis, **E**levated **L**iver enzymes, **L**ow **P**latelets (sev PEC variant)
AFLP	**A**cute **F**atty **L**iver of **P**regnancy. Very elevated LFTs (>500), low gluc, Not always hypertensive

Etiology/Pathophysiology (AJOG 2015;213:S9.e1)

- Potential causes: Abn trophoblast invasion of uterine bld vessels, immunologic intolerance btw fetoplacental & mat tissues, maladaptation to the CV/inflamm changes of Preg, dietary deficiencies, genetic abnormalities
- Failure of remodeling of spiral arteries during placental invasion
- Endothelial activation of inflammatory response and upset of angiogenic balance and maintenance of endothelial structure and function of syncytiotrophoblasts
- Proangiogenic – VEGF and PIGF
- Antiangiogenic – sFlt1 (pronounced "S-Flit-One") inhibits VEGF and PIGF
- Excessive antiangiogenic activity in nonpregnant experimental animals creates a PEC-like syndrome

Prevention

- High risk: H/o PEC, multifetal gestation, CHTN, DM, renal Dz, autoimmune Dz
- Moderate risk: Nulliparity, obesity, 1st-degree family history PEC, Black, low socioeconomic status, age ≥35, previous pregnancy >10 y, low birth weight or SGA
- If high-risk, or has several moderate-risk factors, recommend ASA starting after 12 wga, and before 16 wga, continuing until delivery (Ann Int Med 2014;161:819)
- There may be a dose–response relationship, with greater risk reduction with up to 150 mg ASA daily (RR PEC 80 mg = 0.52 vs. RR PEC 150 mg = 0.07) (AJOG 2017;216:110)

Clinical Manifestations of PEC

- **Cerebral:** HA, dizziness, tinnitus
- **Visual:** Diplopia, scotomata, blurred-vision, amaurosis
- **GI:** Nausea, vomiting, epigastric/RUQ pain, hematemesis
- **Renal:** Oliguria, anuria, hematuria

Initial Workup

- Collect baseline bld work at 1st prenatal visit (if high risk) or at time of dz presentation Hgb, Plt, Cr, AST/ALT, 24-h urine prot (if patient will not complete 24-h collection, get Protein/Creatinine ratio). Rpt if ↑ clinical concern.
- Fetal eval: NST/AFI, growth US in 3rd trimester (umbilical artery Doppler if IUGR)

Management/Treatment

Management & treatment of PEC			
	Mat surveillance	**Fetal surveillance**	**Deliv**
gHTN	No hospitalization Monit for sev gHTN or PEC	Daily kick counts Serial NST/AFI or BPP (1–2×/w) Serial fetal growth US (q4w)	37 0/7–38 6/7 w gest Sev gHTN managed as sPEC
PEC without severe features	Candidate for outpatient management if able to follow-up twice weekly Monit for severe features Evaluate for organ dysfxn Weekly labs	Daily kick counts Serial NST/AFI or BPP (1–2×/w) Serial fetal growth US (q3–4w)	37 0/7 w gest
PEC with severe features OR Superimposed PEC w/ sev features	Evaluate organ dysfxn Serial labs (q6h → daily if stable) MgSO₄ sz ppx Antihypertensive meds for BPs	Daily fetal assessment Serial NST/AFI or BPP (2×/w) Serial fetal growth US (q3w) Betamethasone for fetal benefit <34 w gest[d] (possibly up to 37 wga based on ALPS trial)	34 0/7 w gest or if develops contra-indication to expectant management[b]

	Mat surveillance	Fetal surveillance	Deliv
Eclampsia	Stabilize mother Rx: IM: "Give 2 high fives" – 5 mg MgSO₄ IM to each buttock IV: MgSO₄ loading dose 4–6 g → 2 g/h	Fetal brady frequently occurs during eclamptic sz → managed by mat resusc Continuous monitoring	Deliv "in timely fashion" Method dependent on gestational age, presentation, cervical dilation, & mat stability Cesarean NOT always indicated
HELLP/AFLP	Stabilize mother MgSO₄ for sz ppx Supportive therapy postpartum	Continuous monitoring	Delivery 48 h after initiation of beta-methasone if maternal stability allows[a]

[a] NOT ELIGIBLE to delay delivery for 48 h until steroids complete: Severe hypertension refractory to treatment, eclampsia, suspected placental abruption, nonreassuring fetal testing, pre/nonviable fetus, pulmonary edema, evidence of DIC, significant renal dysfunction.

[b] NOT ELIGIBLE for expectant mgmt. after beta complete include the above plus unable to control blood pressures on maximum doses of 2 medications, severe persistent symptoms (headache, epigastric pain, visual disturbances), HELLP syndrome (or thrombocytopenia <100,000, transaminitis), significant renal dysfunction, severe oligohydramnios, reversed end-diastolic flow (umbilical artery Doppler), labor or premature rupture of membranes.

From Am J Obstet Gynecol 2011;205(3):191–8; Obstet Gynecol 2013;122:1122.

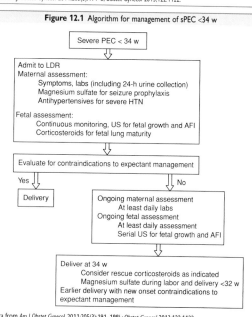

Figure 12.1 Algorithm for management of sPEC <34 w

Severe PEC < 34 w

Admit to LDR
Maternal assessment:
  Symptoms, labs (including 24-h urine collection)
  Magnesium sulfate for seizure prophylaxis
  Antihypertensives for severe HTN

Fetal assessment:
  Continuous monitoring, US for fetal growth and AFI
  Corticosteroids for fetal lung maturity

Evaluate for contraindications to expectant management

Yes → Delivery

No → Ongoing maternal assessment
  At least daily labs
Ongoing fetal assessment
  At least daily assessment
  Serial US for fetal growth and AFI

Deliver at 34 w
  Consider rescue corticosteroids as indicated
  Magnesium sulfate during labor and delivery <32 w
Earlier delivery with new onset contraindications to expectant management

Data from Am J Obstet Gynecol. 2011;205(3):191–198.; Obstet Gynecol 2013;122:1122.
NOT ELIGIBLE to delay delivery for 48 h until steroids complete: Severe hypertension refractory to treatment, eclampsia, suspected placental abruption, nonreassuring fetal testing, pre/nonviable fetus, pulmonary edema, evidence of DIC, significant renal dysfunction. NOT ELIGIBLE for expectant mgmt. after beta complete include the above plus unable to control blood pressures on maximum doses of two medications, severe persistent symptoms (headache, epigastric pain, visual disturbances), HELLP syndrome (or thrombocytopenia <100,000, transaminitis), significant renal dysfunction, severe oligohydramnios, reversed end-diastolic flow (umbilical artery Doppler), labor or premature rupture of membranes.

Intrapartum Management
- PEC with SF/Eclampsia is *not* an indication for immediate cesarean deliv; IOL by obstetric indications
- Maternal precautions: Frequent BP monitoring, seizure precautions
- Fetal precautions: Continuous fetal monitoring
- $MgSO_4$ to prevent sz (Lancet 2002;359:1877)

  $MgSO_4$ superior to other antiepileptics (diazepam, phenytoin, or lytic cocktail) in PEC. Lower rate of recurrent seizures (RR = 0.41 [95% CI, 0.32–0.51]). Lower rate of mat death (RR = 0.62 [95% CI, 0.39–0.99]). Use intrapartum & 12–24 h postpartum. NNT for sPEC: 71; NNT for nonsevere PEC: 400.

  Magnesium tox: Monit closely throughout rx. Lower dose (eg, 1 g/h) or consider checking levels if renal impairment. Therapeutic level: 4–6 mEq/L. Loss of patellar reflexes: 8–10 mEq/L. Respiratory depression: 12 mEq/L. Mental status changes: >12 mEq/L. Cardiac arrest: >24 mEq/L.

  Rx of magnesium tox: D/c magnesium, obtain ECG, obtain serum level, give calcium gluconate: 1 g IV over 5 min, supportive therapy & close monitoring

Dosing magnesium sulfate		
IM	Loading dose	5 g IM each buttock
	Maint dose	5 mg IM q4h
IV	Loading dose	4 g IV over 10–20 min; 6 g for fetal neuro protection <32 wga
	Maint dose	1–2 g/h IV

Postpartum Management
- Continue to monit BPs closely. BP decreases w/i 48 h, but may ↑ 3–6 d postpartum. Monitor 72 h postpartum in hospital, then check at home daily, and 1 w postpartum BP check in clinic.
- If magnesium initiated intrapartum, continue until 12–24 h postpartum or until adequate diuresis has been documented (fluid balance net negative)
- Follow labs daily until clinically stable & trending toward nml (consider repeat 24-h urine postpartum in setting of extreme proteinuria)
- **Postpartum HTN** (Am J Obstet Gynecol 2012;206(6):470): Persistence of gHTN, PEC, CHTN vs. de novo dev. Treat w/ magnesium sulfate × 24 h or until clinical improv w/ PEC. Prevalence: 0.3–27.5%.

  Ddx for postpartum HTN includes PEC spectrum, pre-existing or undiagnosed HTN, hyperthyroidism, primary hyperaldo, pheo, renal artery stenosis, cerebral vasoconstriction syn, cerebral venous thrombosis/stroke, thrombotic thrombocytopenic purpura/hemolytic uremic syn
- **Long-term counseling:** Preeclampsia increases risk of cardiovascular disease later in life (risk is higher when delivered preterm, or if fetus IUGR); encourage healthy weight, aerobic exercise, healthy diet, and avoid tobacco

Management of Maternal Complications/Sequelae
- **Convulsions:** See Eclampsia in Chap. 18
- **Pulm edema:** Diurese w/ furosemide (10–40 mg IV) → monit urine output, intubation if necessary
- **Acute renal or liver failure, liver hemorrhage, DIC, stroke:** Supportive therapy → consider transfer to ICU

Complications/Sequelae

Progression to preeclampsia with mild gHTN	
Weeks' gest	% who developed PEC
34–35	37.3
32–33	49.3
30–31	50
<30	52.1

From Am J Obstet Gynecol 2001;184(5):979–83.

Pregnancy outcomes in women with PEC		
Outcome	Nonsevere[a] (%)	Sev[b] (%)
Preterm deliv	14–25.8	33–66.7
SGA infant	4.8–10.2	11.4–18.5
Placental abruption	0–3.2	1.4–6.7

Outcome	Nonsevere[a] (%)	Sev[b] (%)
Perinatal death	0–1	1.4–8.9
Mat mortality	Rare	0.2
Mat morbidity[c]	Rare	5

[a]Rates similar to normotensive & gHTN pregnancies.
[b]Rates similar to sev gHTN.
[c]Convulsions, pulm edema, acute renal or liver failure, liver hemorrhage, DIC, stroke.
From *Obstet Gynecol* 2003;102(1):181–92.

CORONARY ARTERY DISEASE/ACUTE CORONARY SYNDROME

Definition and Epidemiology (*Circulation* 2012;125:188; *Clin Cardiol* 2012;35(3):141)
- CAD → MI, angina pectoris (AP), or both
- **ACS:** Acute coronary syndrome-Atherosclerosis → plaque rupture → thrombosis → acute myocardial ischemia. Other causes of ischemia: Coronary artery spasm, embolism, aortic dissection, vasculitis, myocarditis.
- **STEMI:** ST segment elevations in ≥1 mm in 2 anatomically contiguous leads; OR ≥2 mm in V2 and V3 OR new left bundle branch block and presentation consistent with ACS
- **NSTEMI/Unstable Angina:** ST segment depressions or deep t wave inversions without Q waves OR possibly no ECG changes
- **Risk factors:** Age, smoking, HTN, hyperlipidemia, DM, FHx
- **Prevalence:** CAD: ♂ 8.3%, ♀ 6.1%. MI ♂ 4.3%, ♀ 2.2%. AP: ♂ 3.8%, ♀ 4%; 1 of 6 deaths in US in 2008 due to CAD; ↑ mortality in women <55 yo

Presentation and Physical Exam
- Angina + dyspnea, diaphoresis, N/V, palps, lightheadedness
- Women often present w/ nonclassic sx (eg, GI distress)
- Signs of ischemia or heart failure: S3, S4, new murmur, ↑ JVP, crackles

Diagnostic Studies
- **ECG:** See definitions for STEMI vs. NSTEMI above, repeat ECG 10–15 min if not dx
- **Cardiac enzymes:** Troponin = most sensitive & specific. Detectable 4–6 h after injury, peaks 24 h after injury, ↑ up to 10 d. CK-MB = less sensitive/specific.
- **Labs:** Electrolytes, CBC, consider coagulation studies

Acute Treatment
- **Any ACS:** Assess and stabilize ABCs, treat sustained arrhythmias (ACLS), O_2 >90%
  Aspirin: 325 mg chew/swallow or PR (withhold if dissection on differential)
  Nitrates: 0.4 mg nitroglycerin tablet q5min ×3 doses OR aerosol spray SL; only give nitrates if persistent chest pain, HTN, or signs of heart failure WITHOUT signs of hemodynamic compromise or history of PDE inhibitor
  Beta-Blocker: Metoprolol 25 mg PO once vs. 5 mg IV q5min ×3 doses IF no signs of heart failure or hemodynamic compromise, reactive airway disease, cocaine use
  Morphine: 2–4 mg IV q5–15min for persistent discomfort or anxiety
  Atorvastatin: 80 mg as early as possible if not already on statin
- **STEMI:** Primary PCI by 120 min; antifibrinolytics if no PCI within 120 min, symptoms <12 h, and no contraindications; add antiplatelet therapy (clopidogrel vs. ticagrelor) to ASA and anticoagulant therapy (UFH vs. LMWH)
- **NSTEMI/Unstable angina:** Can be managed by invasive or noninvasive approach. Add antiplatelet therapy to ASA for all patients; anticoagulant therapy with UFH or LMWH.
- Specific choice of antiplatelet agent and anticoagulant depends on primary intervention and patient comorbidity

Pregnancy Considerations (*Eur Heart J* 2011;32:3147)
- Risk of MI 3–4× higher compared to nonpregnant women. ACS: 3–6/100000 deliveries → mortality 5–10%. All stages of gest, but more common in 3rd trimester. Most commonly involves anterior wall. Consider alternate etiologies such as spontaneous coronary artery dissection (SCAD) or coronary vasospasm (*Heart* 2016;15:102)
- Preg can be considered if CAD & no residual ischemia or LV dysfxn
- **Rx:** PCI for STEMI. AVOID ACEI & ARB. Clopidogrel or GPIIb/IIIa limited data.
- **Intrapartum mgmt:** SVD generally preferred. AVOID methergine for postpartum hemorrhage: May induce coronary artery vasospasm.
- **Cardiac arrest** rare (1:30,000 Preg) but important modifications exist:
  After 20 w perform CPR with manual pushing of uterus leftward
  Perform cesarean delivery at 4 min of arrest to alleviate aortocaval compression, improve venous return, and improve maternal outcomes (*Circulation* 2017;135:e1195)

PULMONARY HYPERTENSION

Definition and Epidemiology
- Mean PA pres >25 mmHg at rest or >30 mmHg w/ exertion
- **Idiopathic pHTN:** 1–2 per million. Mean age of onset: 36 (men older than women). Female:male 1.7–3.5:1.

Classification of pulmonary hypertension	
Group	**Etiology**
1	Pulmonary arterial hypertension (PAH)
	1.1 Idiopathic
	1.2 Heritable
	1.3 Drug- and toxin-induced
	1.4 Associated with CTD, CHD, portal HTN, infection
	1′ Pulmonary veno-occlusive disease/capillary hemangiomatosis
	1″ Persistent pulmonary hypertension of the newborn
2	Pulmonary hypertension due to left heart disease
	2.1 LV systolic dysfunction
	2.2 LV diastolic dysfunction
	2.3 Valvular disease
	2.4 Congenital outflow tract obstruction and cardiomyopathies
3	Pulmonary hypertension due to lung disease and/or hypoxia
	3.1 COPD
	3.2 Interstitial lung disease
	3.3 Other pulmonary disease
	3.4 Sleep disordered breathing
	3.5 Alveolar hypoventilation disorders
	3.6 Chronic exposure to high altitude
	3.7 Developmental abnormalities
4	Chronic thromboembolic pulmonary hypertension (CTEPH)
5	Pulmonary hypertension with unclear multifactorial mechanisms
	5.1 Hematologic (anemia, splenectomy, myeloproliferative disorders)
	5.2 Systemic (sarcoidosis, vasculitis)
	5.3 Metabolic (glycogen storage disease, Gaucher disease)
	5.4 Others (tumor, chronic renal failure, mediastinitis)

From *J Am Coll Cardiol* 2013;62:S34.

Diagnosis
- Dyspnea, syncope, or chest pain on exertion, sx of right-sided heart failure
- Prominent P2, right-sided S4, RV heave, PA flow murmur, PR, TR
- **Signs of RV failure:** JVD, periph edema, ascites, hepatomegaly
- **Definitive dx w/ cardiac cath:** ↑ RA, RV, & PA pres, ↑ PVR, ↓ CO, nml PCWP
- **W/u:** Echocardiogram to determine if left heart dz explains degree of pHTN. Hx and exam guide workup which may include PFTs, V/Q scan, overnight oximetry, polysomnography

Treatment
- Oxygen, diuretics, dig, anticoagulation
- **Vasodilators:** CCB, prostacyclin, prostacyclin analogues, endothelin-1 receptor antag
- Lung xplant if refrac
- **Preconception counseling:** Women w/ pHTN discouraged from Preg; if Preg occurs, termination should be offered (*Obstet Gynecol* 2017;129:511; *Eur J Heart Fail* 2016;18:1119)
- **Antepartum:** Antepartum mgmt often requires hospitalization and multidisciplinary care with availability of ECMO advised if possible; on L&D RV filling is important; modest elevations in CVP → increasing RV dysfxn & rapid deterioration

Prognosis
- **Nonpregnant:** 2.5-y median survival if untreated; if respond to nifedipine: 95% 5-y survival; nifedipine nonresponder (requiring prostacyclin): 54% 5-y survival; lung xplant: 45–55% 5-y survival
- **Pregnant pop:** 17–33% mortality w/ sev pHTN & Eisenmenger syn; mod pHTN (PAP <40 mmHg) up to 30% develop cardiac failure or die w/i 3 mo postpartum (*Obstet Gynecol* 2017;129:511; *Eur J Heart Fail* 2016;18:1119); death occurs in last trimester & in 1st months after deliv from hypertensive crisis, pulm thrombosis, refrac right heart failure. 75% mortality occurs postpartum.

VALVULAR HEART DISEASE

Etiology

Pregnancy concerns with valvular heart disease		
Valvular abnormality	**Pathophysiology**	**Preg considerations**
MS rheumatic heart dz, congen, myxoma, thrombus, valvulitis, or infiltration	Valve stenosis impedes bld flow from LA to LV in diastole	↑ CO cannot be achieved → pulm congestion Relative tachy shortens diastole & ↓ LV filling
MR Leaflet abnormalities, ruptured chordae tendineae, papillary muscle dysfxn, left ventricular dilation, annulus dilation, progression of MV prolapse, rheumatic heart disease	↑ Regurg → LA enlargement → greater volume into LV → dilation & impaired contractility	↓ SVR promotes forward flow ↑ SVR in PEC may impair forward flow ↑ CO exacerbates LV vol overload Catecholamine release during L&D impairs forward flow
AS CHD (congen stenosis), rheumatic heart dz	Pres overload → concentric LVH	Sensitive to loss of preload a/w hypotension
AI/AR Valve dz, root dz	LV compensates for loss of forward flow w/ ↑ in LVEDV	SVR reduction → improv in cardiac performance
Aortic diseases Bicuspid aortic valve (BAV), Marfan's, Ehlers–Danlos syndrome (EDS), Loeys–Dietz syndrome	Often underlying genetic disorder (not for BAV) affecting connective tissue with specific clinical phenotype and cardiac manifestation	Underlying disease can lead to AR dilation → increased risk of aortic dissection in Preg; Risk of Preg related to risk of aortic dissection which depends on underlying disease, degree of AR dilation, personal or family history

Clinical Manifestations and Diagnostic Studies
- **Clinical:** Dyspnea, pulm edema, Afib
- **Diagnosis:** ECG, CXR, echocardiogram, cardiac cath

Physical exam	
Valvular abnormality	**Physical exam findings**
MS	Low-pitched, diastolic rumble at apex. Loud S1. Opening snap (high-pitched early diastolic sound)
MR	High-pitched, holosystolic murmur at apex, radiating to axilla Obscured S1
AS	Harsh, systolic, cres–decres murmur at RUSB radiating to carotids & down left sternal border Delayed carotid upstroke Can hear ejection click at LLSB in cases of AS due to BAV
AI/AR	High-pitched, diastolic decrescendo murmur at LUSB PMI diffuse & laterally displaced

Classification of Key Disease (*J Am Coll Cardiol* 2014;63:e57)

Classification of mitral stenosis			
Stage	**Definition**	**Valve area (cm²)**	**Consequences and symptoms**
A	At risk for MS	4–6	None
B	Progressive MS	>1.5	Mild–Mod LA enlargement, nl pulmonary artery pressure (PAP)
C	Asymptomatic severe MS	1–1.5	Severe LA enlargement, ↑ PAP
D	Symptomatic severe MS	<1	Stage C + ↓ exercise tolerance, or exertional dyspnea

Classification of aortic stenosis			
Stage	Definition	Valve anatomy*	Consequences and symptoms
A	**At risk for AS** BAV or aortic valve sclerosis	Vmax <2	None
B	**Progressive AS** Mild–mod leaflet calcification, or reduction in systolic motion, or rheumatic valve changes with fusion	**Mild:** Vmax 2–2.9; ΔP <20 **Moderate:** Vmax 3–3.9, ΔP 20–39	Early LV diastolic dysfxn may be present, no symptoms
C	**Asymptomatic severe** Severe leaflet calcification or congenital stenosis	Vmax ≥4 or ΔP ≥40 or AVA ≤1	**Stage C1:** LV diastolic dysfunction but nl LVEF **Stage C2:** LVEF <50%
D	**Symptomatic severe** Severe leaflet calcification with severely reduced motion		Exertional dyspnea or decreased exercise tolerance, exertional angina, exertional pre/syncope
D1	High-gradient AS	Vmax ≥4 or ΔP ≥40 or AVA typically ≤1 (but may be larger with mixed AS/AI)	LV diastolic dysfunction, LV hypertrophy ± Pulm HTN
D2	High-gradient AS with reduced EF	AVA ≤1 with resting Vmax <4 or ΔP <40 Dobutamine stress echo Vmax ≥4 at any flow rate	LVEF <50% HF, angina, Pre/syncope
D3	Symptomatic severe low-gradient AS	AVA ≤1 with resting Vmax <4 or ΔP <40 Stroke volume index <35 mL/m²	Increased LV wall thickness, small LV chamber, restrictive diastolic filling, LVEF ≥50% HF, angina, Pre/syncope

*Vmax = maximum aortic velocity (m/s); ΔP = pressure gradient (mmHg); AVA = aortic valve area (cm²).

Pregnancy Considerations/Prognosis (Eur Heart J 2011;32:3147)
- **MS:** Decompensation depends on severity, heart failure ↑ w/ mod or sev MS. 15% dev A Fib. Mortality: 0–3%. W/ mod or sev MS, counsel against Preg w/out repair. Offer termination in early Preg. Avoid signif tachy to allow time for LV filling in diastole.
- **AS:** Morbidity related to severity, heart failure in 10% & arrhythmias in 3–25% of women w/ sev AS, mortality low. Get preconception exercise testing. Peak gradient <40 mmHg → typically Uncomp prenatal courses. Severe symptomatic AS warrants valve replacement, possibly in surgery after early delivery via c/s. Avoid acute drop in PVR.
- **Mitral regurg or aortic regurg:** Regurgitant lesions well tol in Preg due to increased plasma volume and decreased afterload. Prepregnancy eval for sx, echo w/ ascending aorta diameter, LV dimension & fxn; exercise testing for mod to sev; preconception Surg for sev regurg, sx, or LV dysfxn due to ↑ heart failure risk
- **Aortic Disease:** Pregnancy prognosis depends on specific disease pathology

Treatment/management		
Valvular abnormality	Medical rx (generally same in pregnant & nonpregnant)	Surgical rx
MS	Na restriction, diuretics, β-blockers, anticoagulation (if Afib)	Replacement vs. percutaneous valvotomy. Only intervene during preg if NYHA Class III/IV, or Pulm Art Press >50 mmHg
MR	Only if nonoperative; ↓ afterload: ACEI, hydralazine/nitrates; ↓ preload: Diuretics, nitrates; ↑ inotropy: Dig; consider anticoagulation	Repair → replacement typically delayed until after pregnancy

Valvular abnormality	Medical rx (generally same in pregnant & nonpregnant)	Surgical rx
AS	If symptomatic, diuretics. If dev A Fib, Beta blockers, or Ca Channel blockers for rate control	Valve replacement if severe symptomatic AS; valvuloplasty in young adults w/o calcification; During preg perc valvuloplasty in noncalcified valves w/ min regurg; if life threatening, deliver early and open repair
AI/AR	Only if not operative; ↓ afterload w/ LV dysfxn or dilation	Valve replacement typically delayed until after pregnancy
Aortic disease	Minimal medical intervention	Marfan's: Valve replacement recommended at 40–45 mm; BAV/Others: Valve replacement at 50 mm; Replacement before Preg related to risk of dissection, rate of dilation over time

Labor and Delivery Considerations (*Circulation* 2017;135:e1195)
- Pain → tachy that can exacerb valvular pathology (particularly MS and AS)
- Contractions → ↑ venous return therefore pulm congestion
- Consider telemetry in patients w/ history of arrhythmias or symptomatic women with ↓ EF
- Abrupt elevation of PAPs in the immediate postpartum period from autotransfusion
- Cesarean delivery reserved for obstetric indications with exception of aortic disease; may recommend cesarean delivery or assisted 2nd stage if critical aortic root dilation (>40 mm in Marfan's, >50 mm in others) or severe symptomatic aortic stenosis

Endocarditis Prophylaxis (*Circulation* 2017;135:e1195)
- **Cardiac conditions a/w infxn that warrant abx ppx:** Prosthetic cardiac valve, or other prosthetic material; prev infective endocarditis; unrepaired cyanotic CHD; repaired CHD w/ residual defect at adj to the site of a prosthetic patch or device; cardiac transplant with valve regurg due to structurally abnl valve

Types of Prosthetic Valves (*Circulation* 2015;132:132)
- **Mechanical:** Durable but require anticoagulation; ↑ miscarriage & thromboembolic events including stroke, valve thrombosis (warfarin lowers risk of thrombosis compared to heparins, but increases risk of miscarriage and IUFD). ↑ Risk of death
- **Bioprosthetic:** Less durable, but do not require anticoagulation; Preg does not appear to alter lifespan of valve, but risk that may need replacement during pregnancy (*J Am Heart Assoc* 2014:3)

Medical management of prosthetic valves		
	Mechanical valve	**Bioprosthetic valve**
Nonpregnant	Warfarin + ASA	Warfarin + ASA × 3 mo → ASA (w/o risk factors*)
Pregnant	Heparin/LMWH during Preg; can consider warfarin after organogenesis given improved outcomes w/ mechanical valves (continue during 1st trimester for high-risk patients); heparin at 36 w → d/c 4–6 h prior to deliv; LMWH or warfarin postpartum	No anticoagulation after initial postsurgical ppx

Endocarditis ppx & anticoagulation generally indicated for all prosthetic valves.
*Risk factors = AFib, ↓ EF, prior embolic event, hypercoagulable state.
Data from ACC/AHA guidelines for the management of patients with valvular heart disease. A report of the American College of Cardiology/American Heart Association. Task Force on Practice Guidelines (*J Thorac Cardiovas Surg.* 2014;148:e1–132. *J Am Coll Cardiol.* 2017;70:252.)

PERIPARTUM CARDIOMYOPATHY

Definition and Epidemiology (Eur J Heart Fail 2010;12:767)
- **Definition:** Heart failure w/i the last month of Preg to 5 mo postpartum
- Incid 1 in 2500–4000 live-births (in US); incid strongly related to geographic region
- **Diagnosis:** Criteria based on risk for idiopathic DCM: Absence of prior heart dz; no alternative cause; echocardiographic evid of LV dysfxn (EF <45% or fractional shortening <30%, LVED dimension >2.7 m^2)
- **Differential Diagnosis:** Unmasked DCM, unmasked valvular heart disease, cHTN assoc heart disease, Preg assoc MI, HIV/AIDS cardiomyopathy, PE

Pathophysiology
- Exact cause under investigation; similar genetic predisposition as to dilated CM (N Engl J Med 2016;374:233). Theories include prolactin, oxidative stress, inflammation, autoimmune
- Risk Factors: HTN, DM, smoking, AMA, multiparity, multifetal gestations, malnutrition. Cardiac myocyte damage leads to systolic dysfunction

Clinical Manifestations and Diagnostic Studies
- **Findings:** Dyspnea, cough, orthopnea, tachy, hemoptysis, elevated JVP, S3 present, elevated BNP
- **CXR:** Cardiomegaly, pulm edema, pleural effusions
- **ECG:** Look for Afib, bundle branch block
- **Echocardiogram:** ± LV dilation, EF <45%, regional or global LV HK, poss RV HK, poss mural thrombi; repeat before discharge, at 6-w PP, 6 mo, and annually
- **Cardiac MRI:** More accurate measurement of chamber volumes and ventricular function

Treatment
- Antepartum: β-Blockers improve cardiac fxn & survival in stable, euvolemic pts, diuretics for volume overload, consider risks/ benefits of ACEI/ARBs
- Intrapartum: Consider telemetry, vag delivery preferred for well compensated, encourage epidural, consider assisted 2nd stage; if require pressors or mechanical support, prefer CS; careful with IVF
- Postpartum: Treat as HF (Eur J Heart Fail 2008;10:933), early diuresis; possible role for bromocriptine (inhibits prolactin secretion); use with anticoagulation; discuss risks and benefits of breast feeding (prolactin secretion) (Eu J Heart Fail 2010;12:767)
- OK to use implantable defibrillators in Preg (Circulation 1997;96:2808)

Management of peripartum cardiomyopathy	
Goal	**Drug**
↓ Preload	Diuretic
↓ Afterload	Hydralazine or nitroglycerine (antepartum), ACEI (postpartum)
Relieve pulm congestion	Diuretic
↑ Contractility	Inotropes
Rate control w/ AF	Beta blocker, Ca Channel blocker, Dig
Anticoagulation	Heparin/LMWH (antepartum), warfarin (postpartum)

Prognosis
- **Peripartum:** Mortality 6–10%; cardiac explantation 4–7% (Circulation 2005;111(16):2050; N Engl J Med 2000;342(15):1077); w/i 6 mo, $\frac{1}{2}$ of pts demonstrate resolution of LV dilation → good prog, the other $\frac{1}{2}$ → 85% 5-y mortality
- **Subseq Preg:** Recurrence up to 50% (Circulation 1995;92(Suppl 1):1; N Engl J Med 2001;344(21):1567; Ann Intern Med 2006;145(1):30)

  >8% mortality if LV dysfxn has not resolved → discourage Preg if EF <25% at time of dx or persistent LV dyxfxn with EF <50%; <2% mortality if LV dysfxn has resolved

Definitions

- Total lung capacity (TLC) = sum of Forced Vital Capacity (FVC) + Residual Volume (RV); total volume of air in the lungs at full inhalation
- FVC = sum of Inspiratory Reserve Volume (IRV), Tidal Volume (VT), and Expiratory Reserve Volume (ERV); total volume of air exhaled after max insp with max exp effort
- Functional residual capacity (FRC) = sum of ERV + RV; volume after tidal exhalation
- Forced expiratory volume in 1 s (FEV_1) = volume of air exhaled in 1st s of maximal expiratory effort. FEV_1/FVC: % of total expiration in 1st s.

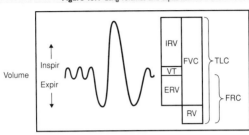

Figure 13.1 Lung volumes and capacities

(From Hyatt RE, Scanlon PD, Nakamura M. *Interpretation of Pulmonary Function Tests: A Practical Guide.* 4th ed. Philadelphia, PA: Wolters Kluwer; 2014)

Spirometry (Am Fam Physician 2004;69(5):1107)

- Indicated for dx of pulm dz, follow-up of known dz, preoperative eval of pts w/ known pulm dz or prior to thoracic procedures
- Pt inhales maximally, then exhales w/ maximal effort as long as poss (at least 6 s). Contraindicated if Valsalva would be poorly tolerated. Time & vol vs. flow graphed. Rpt 3× for reliability/pt effort.
- FVC, FEV_1, FEV_1/FVC compare to % predicted values based on height/weight, age, sex, race
- **Interpretation of spirometry:** Ensure reliability & good pt effort (ie, valid study). If FVC, FEV_1 nml & FEV_1/FVC >70% → nml spirometry. If FVC nml or ↓, FEV_1 ↓ & absolute FEV_1/FVC <70% → obstructive physiology. If parameters correct after bronchodilator → reversible airway dz. If FVC ↓, FEV_1 ↓ or nml & absolute FEV_1/ FVC >70% → restrictive physiology. Refer to pulm lab for lung volumes & DL_{CO}.
- **Obstructive diff dx:** Asthma, chronic obstructive pulm dz (chronic bronchitis, emphysema)
- **Restrictive diff dx:** Intrinsic lung dz (acute pneumonitis, interstitial lung dz)
  Extrinsic dz (mechanical abnormality of chest wall/pleura preventing expansion)
  Neuromuscular d/o of respiratory muscles
  Abdominal mass (incl pregnancy), ascites

Peak Flow Measurements

- Peak flow meter measures current PEFR; compare to personal best. Assesses relative obst & sx control. Does NOT establish dx – for surveillance only. Use in conjunction w/ asthma action plan.
- See http://reference.medscape.com/calculator/peak-expiratory-flow for expected peak flow calculator

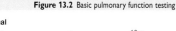

Figure 13.2 Basic pulmonary function testing

Normal

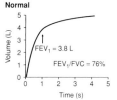
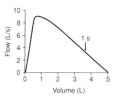

$FEV_1 = 3.8$ L

$FEV_1/FVC = 76\%$

1 s

Obstructive

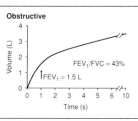
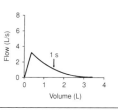

$FEV_1/FVC = 43\%$

$FEV_1 = 1.5$ L

1 s

Restrictive

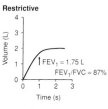
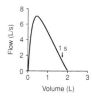

$FEV_1 = 1.75$ L

$FEV_1/FVC = 87\%$

1 s

(From Hyatt RE, Scanlon PD, Nakamura M. *Interpretation of Pulmonary Function Tests: A Practical Guide.* 4th ed. Philadelphia, PA: Wolters Kluwer; 2014.)

RESPIRATORY CHANGES IN PREGNANCY

General (*Clin Chest Med* 2011;32:1)
- **Upper airway:** Mucosal hyperemia, edema, glandular hypersecretion. May contribute to disordered breathing in sleep from obst. ↑ Mallampati score, ↑ neck circumference. "Rhinitis of Preg" present during last 6 w of Preg, disappears postpartum in absence of allergy or other pulm pathology.
- **Chest wall:** Compliance decreased. Widened subcostal angle, increased anteroposterior dimension mediated hormonally by relaxin. Changes peak at 37 w. Diaphragmatic excursion increased. Max inspiration/expiration pressures same as prior to Preg.

Lung Function
- Minute ventilation ↑ 20–50% by term (most ↑ during 1st trimester). ↑ Progesterone & ↑ CO_2 production (V_{CO2}) ↑ central stimuli for hyperventilation. Physiologic dyspnea of Preg may be awareness of ↑ stimulus to breathe. VT ↑ with **unchanged** RR.
- Oxygen consump (V_{O2}) is increased; respiratory exchange rate (V_{CO2}/V_{O2}) unchanged vs. minimally increased
- FRC ↓ by diaphragm elevation, ↓ chest wall recoil, ↓ abd pull. (Note: Obesity → ↓ FRC & ↑ RV [air trapping]. In Preg, ↓ FRC w/ ↓ RV.) Airway resistance unchanged.
- (IC; IRV + VT) increases 5–10%. TLC is unchanged or ↓ minimally at term.
- FEV_1, FEV_1/FVC, flow/vol curve not significantly changed. Abn spirometry sugg pathology.
- DL_{CO} no change. Increased cardiac outpt offset by decreased Hgb.

Intrapartum/Postpartum Changes
- Hyperventilation ↑ w/ pain/anxiety. Analgesia mitigates this. Minute ventilation varies widely.
- Hypocarbia can cause placental vasoconstriction → hypoperfusion
- Postpartum, all above changes resolve, except for widened subcostal angle.

ARTERIAL BLOOD GAS (ABG) ANALYSIS

Procedure
- Sterile prep area overlying radial, femoral, brachial, dorsalis pedis, or axillary artery
- Consider local anesthesia over puncture site. Assess for collateral circulation.
- Obtain 2–3 mL bld in heparinized syringe. Remove air bubbles, place on ice for transport.
- Consider indwelling arterial catheter for serial ABGs.

Considerations in Pregnancy (Clin Chest Med 2011;32(1))
- ↓ pCO_2 from hyperventilation. ↓ Serum bicarb compens for chronic respiratory alkalosis. ↑ pH (7.42–7.46).
- Chronic alkalosis stimulates ↑ 2,3-DPG w/ shift of Hgb dissociation curve; aids in placental O_2 exchange. ↑ pO_2 facilitates placental O_2 exchange. PO_2 significantly lower supine vs. sitting. High metabolic rate can cause rapid desaturation if apneic.

Definitions
- **Acidemia:** Arterial pH lower than nml (<7.35)
- **Alkalemia:** Arterial pH higher than nml (>7.45)
- **Metabolic acidosis:** Process that decreases serum HCO_3 → ↓ pH (bicarb deficit)
- **Respiratory acidosis:** Process that increases serum pCO_2 → ↓ pH (hypoventilation)
- **Metabolic alkalosis:** Process that increases serum HCO_3 → ↑ pH (bicarb excess)
- **Respiratory alkalosis:** Process that decreases serum pCO_2 → ↑ pH (hyperventilation)

Normal Values
- Nonpregnant: pH, 7.35–7.45; pCO_2, 32–45 mmHg; pO_2, 72–104 mmHg; HCO_3, 22–30 mEq/L

Mean Maternal ABG values in pregnancy					
N = 20	**12 w**	**24 w**	**32 w**	**38 w**	**Postpartum**
pH	7.46	7.44	7.44	7.43	7.41
pCO_2	29.4 (0.4)	29.5 (0.7)	30.3 (0.5)	30.4 (0.6)	35.3 (0.7)
pO_2	106.4 (1.1)	103.1 (1.6)	102.4 (1.2)	101.8 (1)	94.7 (1.5)

From Br J Anaesth 1976;48(10):1001–4.

Diagnosis (Longo DL, Fauci AS, Kasper DL, et al. Harrison's Principles of Internal Medicine, 18th ed. McGraw-Hill Education; 2011)
- Obtain ABG & electrolytes simultaneously. Use HCO_3 from electrolytes.
- Determine whether simple or mixed d/o by assessing whether expected compensatory resp is present. "Compens" cannot change alkalemia to acidemia or vice versa. If apparent insuff or overexuberant compens, mixed d/o likely exists.
- If acidosis present, calculate AG: (Na − [Cl + HCO_3]) w/ adjustment for albumin (nml AG ≈ 2.5 × albumin)

Predicted changes for acid–base disorders	
Disorder	**Compensation**
Metabolic acidosis	$PaCO_2 = (1.5 \times HCO_3) + 8 \pm 2$
Metabolic alkalosis	$PaCO_2$ will ↑ 6 mmHg per 10 mmol/L ↑ in [HCO_3]
Respiratory acidosis	
Acute	[HCO_3] will ↑ 0.2 mmol/L per mmHg ↑ in $PaCO_2$
Chronic (>3–5 d)	[HCO_3] will ↑ 0.4 mmol/L per mmHg ↑ in $PaCO_2$
Respiratory alkalosis	
Acute	[HCO_3] will ↓ 0.1 mmol/L per mmHg ↓ in $PaCO_2$
Chronic (>3–5 d)	[HCO_3] will ↓ 0.4 mmol/L per mmHg ↓ in $PaCO_2$

- Consider $\Delta AG/\Delta HCO_3$ ratio to determine if simple high AG metabolic acidosis (ratio btw 1 & 2). If ratio >2, likely additional metabolic alkalosis. If <1, likely additional nongap metabolic acidosis.
- Ddx guides clinical assessment & final dx:
    For high AG metabolic acidosis: Renal failure, lactic acidosis, toxins, ketoacidosis. W/o high AG: Renal tubular acidosis, GI loss.
    For metabolic alkalosis: Exogenous alkali, extracellular fluid contraction w/ hypoK, extracellular fluid expansion w/ hypoK/Mineralocort excess
    For respiratory acidosis: Hypoventilation (obst, CNS depression, neuromuscular d/o, impaired gas exchange)
    For respiratory alkalosis: Hyperventilation (secondary to hypoxia, Preg, pain, sepsis, drugs)

PNEUMONIA

Definitions (Am J Respir Crit Care Med 2005;171:388; Clin Infect Dis 2016;63(5):e61–111)
- **CAP:** PNA Acq as outpt
- **HAP:** PNA developing >48 h after admission, not incubating at time of admission
- **VAP:** PNA developing >48–72 h after intubation
- **Risk factors for MDR infxn:**
    High prevalence of MDR pathogens in community or inpt unit; chronic heart, lung, liver, renal dz; functional or surgical asplenia; malig; immunocompromise or immunosuppression; recent use of Abx (PO or IV) w/i last 90 d, alcoholism, child in daycare

Diagnosis
- **Signs & sx:** Cough, dyspnea, pleuritic chest pain, sputum production (fewer reported by elderly); tachypnea, fever, decreased oxygen sat, abn lung exam; ↑ WBC. Imaging: New lung infiltrate on XR or CT
- **Microbiology:** Consider induced sputum, influenza assays, urine strep or legionella assays; bld cx if febrile (& prior to Abx); bronchoscopy/washings. Limited sens for cx; consider diff (include pt factors for uncommon causes) & often treat empirically.

Common etiologies of pneumonia	
Bacteria	Mycoplasma, *Strep pneumoniae*, *Chlamydia pneumoniae*, *Haemophilus influenzae*, *Moraxella catarrhalis*, *Legionella*, *Klebsiella*, *Staphylococcus aureus*, *Pseudomonas*, *Escherichia coli*, *Enterobacter*, *Serratia*, *Acinetobacter*, mycobacteria
Viruses	Influenza, parainfluenza, RSV, CMV, HSV, SARS, adenovirus, human metapneumovirus
Fungi	PJP, *Aspergillus*, *Cryptococcus*, *Candida*, mucormycosis
Other	Chemical pneumonitis (acid/bile/other irritant), parasites (strongyloides, toxoplasmosis)

Treatment: Empiric Antibiotic Selection (Clin Infect Dis 2007;44:S27–72; Clin Infect Dis 2016;63(5):e61–111)
- Multip decision tools to assess severity of dz on presentation; PSI may be most rigorous (N Engl J Med 1997;336(4):243). Calculator available at http://pda.ahrq.gov/clinic/psi/psicalc.asp.
- For CAP
    W/o risk factors for MDR: Macrolide (erythro-/clarithro-/Azithro) **OR** doxycycline
    W/ risk factors for MDR or inpt CAP: Respiratory quinolone (moxi-/gemi-/Levo) **OR** β-lactam plus macrolide (amox-clav + azithro)
- For HAP/VAP
    W/o risk factors for MDR: Antipseudomonal/anti-MSSA (Pip-tazo, cefepime, levofloxacin)
    W/ risk factors for resistant GNRs: Add aminoglycoside (amikacin, gent, tobra) to above
    W/ risk factor for MRSA: Add anti-MRSA (vanc, linezolid) to above
    If *Legionella* is suspected, add macrolide or use quinolone instead of aminoglycoside
- For aspiration w/ concern for bact infxn
    Clindamycin (preferred), ampicillin/sulbactam or imipenem; may use metronidazole if added on to an MDR regimen above. Consider d/c Abx if no infiltrate 48–72 h after aspiration event.

- In outpts, 5 d **w/** or w/o MDR risk factors; may dose Azithro × 3 d b/c of long half-life
- In inpts, reassess clinical status after 2–3 d of rx

    If improved & neg cx, consider d/c Abx or continue for 7–8 d w/o pseudomonal/ MRSA coverage. If cx +, tailor Abx & consider rx for 7–8 d (15 d if *Pseudomonas*, 21 d if *S. aureus*).

    If no improv, consider broadening/adjusting Abx, search for alt infxn, dx, or pathogens

- Suspected PNA in Preg is rarely treated, outpt given increased morbidity & mortality. Low threshold for inpt rx.

Prevention

- Avoid intubation & reintubation. Ensure ventilator circuit is well maintained.
- If risk for aspiration, keep head of bed >30 deg
- Enteral feeding preferred to parenteral feeding to ↓ risk of bact translocation from gut
- Minimize time w/ NGT in place to ↓ risk of nosocomial sinusitis
- Formal eval & diet changes for pts w/ difficulty speaking/swallowing
- Postoperatively, consider incentive spirometry, optimize pain control, avoid routine NGT
- Pneumococcal vax if >65 yo or w/ high-risk medical illness. Splenectomy vax if indicated. Flu vax for all pts.

Pneumonia in Pregnancy *(Crit Care Med 2005;33(10) Suppl)*

- Pregnancy increases risk of maternal complications of CAP (10% resp failure, pulmonary edema), and fetal risks (PTL, PTB)
- Most common pathogens: *Strep. pna, H. influenzae*, varicella
- Risk factors: Asthma, anemia, antenatal steroids
- Do not withhold CXR or CT, if clinically indicated, but shield abdomen. Est fetal absorption 0.0005–0.01 mGy for CXR, 0.01–0.66 for CT chest (Est. fetal threshold 50–100 mGy <2 w, 200 mGy @ 2–8 w, 60 mGy 8–15 w, 250 mGy 16–25 w) *(Obstet Gynecol 2017;130:e210)*
- Treatment: Same as nonpregnant, goal Pao_2 >60–70 mmHg
- Varicella pna more severe in pregnancy: 40% maternal mortality without tx. Diffuse nodular densities, reticular infiltrates. Tx: IV acyclovir. Fetal congenital varicella syndrome 1.2–2%. Neonatal varicella in 17–30% if primary maternal infection 5 d before or 2 d after delivery, 31% neonatal mortality rate.

PULMONARY EDEMA

Definition/Diagnosis

- Inappropriate accum of fluid in pulm interstitium & alveoli
- **Sx:** Dyspnea, orthopnea. Signs: Tachypnea, desaturation, rales, rhonchi, wheezes, respiratory failure, S3 gallop. Imaging: Peribronchial thickening, prominent vascular markings, Kerley B lines, alveolar infiltrates.

Etiology

- Fluid accum/retention OR redistribution into tissues from vasoconstriction/dilation
- **Cardiogenic:** Left ventricular dysfxn → elevated hydrostatic pres in pulm veins, extravasation of fluid into lung tissue
- **Noncardiogenic:** Iatrogenic volume overload (postoperative or during prolonged obstetrical admission); direct lung injury (chest trauma, aspiration, PNA, oxygen tox, smoke inhalation, reperfusion post PE); hematogenous lung injury (sepsis, pancreatitis, xfusion, IV drug use); elevated hydrostatic pressures (re-expansion, high altitude, neurogenic)

Treatment

- Target cause (eg, cardiogenic vs. noncardiogenic). Restoration of clinical euvolemia; avoid overuse of IV fluids. Consider echocardiogram to diagnose new/worsening cardiac fxn. Initial measures: Supplemental oxygen, positive pres ventilation. ↓ Preload w/ loop diuretics (furosemide), consider nitrates, morphine, ACEI (not in Preg), pt should be upright in bed if poss. Consider transition to intensive care.

Considerations in Pregnancy *(Anaesthesia 2012;67:646)*

- Increased incid 0.08–0.5%. Rapid appearance of flash pulm edema.
- Risk factors in Preg: Preeclampsia, preterm labor, sepsis, AFE, PE, β-adrenergic tocolytics, magnesium sulfate, corticosteroids, positive fluid balance, multifetal gest

INFLUENZA IN PREGNANCY

Pregnancy Considerations (NEJM 2014;370:2211–8)
- ↑ HR → ↑ SV + ↓ FRC → ↑ hypoxemia. 2009 H1N1: Pregnant pts ↑ risk of ICU admission, death. 3rd trimester riskiest in pregnancy

Vaccination and Prevention (Obstet Gynecol 2014;124:648–51)
- ACOG & the CDC's Advisory Committee on Immunization Practices recommend that all pregnant women be vaccinated against influenza, regardless of trimester (MMWR 2016;65(5);1–54) mat/fetal safety of influenza vaccination in Preg is well established (Am J Obstet Gynecol 2012;207(3 Suppl)). Antepartum vaccination → decreased stillbirth, neonat death, & premature deliv, w/ no ↑ in congen anomalies (Obstet Gynecol 2012;120:532).
- Mat vaccination provides passive immunity to the neonate through 6 mo of age (N Engl J Med 2008;359(15):1555). Pregnant women should receive the trivalent or quadrivalent inactivated (killed) injection vaccine only, & not the LAIV; FluMist.
- Pregnant/postpartum women do not need to avoid contact w/ those who have received LAIV. Postpartum/breastfeeding women can receive LAIV.
- Data do not support adverse effects attributable to preservative thimerosal (MMWR 2010;59(rr08)). Preservative eliminated or reduced in most preparations. Proven protection against serious dz outweighs theoretical concerns regarding preservative.

Prophylaxis and Treatment (MMWR 2016;65(5):1–54)
- Clinical dx is preferred (abrupt onset fever, cough, myalgia) to lab dx for rapid rx
- Oseltamivir & zanamivir are both Preg Category C. Oseltamivir preferred due to greater clinical experience in pregnancy. Most effective if ≤48 h of sx (Obstet Gynecol 2010;115(4):717).
- **For ppx** after exposure during Preg or up to 2 w postpartum:
  Zanamivir 10 mg (2 puffs inhaled) daily
  Oseltamivir 75 mg PO daily
  Duration: 10 d (household exposure), 14 d (hospital exposure), 7 d (other)
- **For rx** w/ onset of sx
  Zanamivir 10 mg (2 puffs inhaled) daily × 5 d
  Oseltamivir 75 mg PO twice daily × 5 d
  Can consider longer rx for severely ill pts

Additional Considerations
- Women w/ influenza hospitalized on labor & deliv wards should have respiratory precautions per hospital std for influenza
- Discuss the need for neonat antivirals or mat–neonat separation w/ pediatricians
- Postpartum, women w/ influenza should express breast milk, rather than breastfeed. Milk may still go to the infant, as oseltamivir is poorly excreted (Int J Infect Dis 2008;12:451).

ASTHMA AND PREGNANCY

(Obstet Gynecol 2008;111:457; and NIH Publication https://www.nhlbi.nih.gov/health-topics/guidelines-for-diagnosis-management-of-asthma)

Definitions/Pathophysiology
- Chronic airway inflammation w/ hyperresponsiveness to various stimuli & partially reversible airway obst
- Sev cases a/w increased prematurity, cesarean deliv, preeclampsia, growth restriction, & mat morbidity/mortality
- Mat–fetal pathology caused by mat hypoxia. Decreased FEV_1 → ↑ low birth weight/prematurity

Diagnosis
- Wheeze, cough, SOB, chest tightness; fluctuating; often worse at night; worse w/ known triggers (allergens, exercise, infections). Consider GERD, postnasal drip w/ cough, bronchitis in diff
- Airway obst on spirometry, reversible w/ bronchodilator therapy
- Document h/o hospitalization, ICU stay, intubation, & steroid rx. Preg may improve, worsen or have no effect on asthma severity (rule of 1⅓'s). Past pregnancies may better predict course of subseq pregnancies.

Asthma severity classification

Severity	Symptom freq	Night-time awakening	Interference w/ activity	FEV$_1$ or peak flow (% of best)
Mild intermittent	<2 d/w	<2×/mo	None	>80
Mild persistent	2–6 d/w	>2×/mo	Minor	>80
Mod persistent	Daily	>1×/w	Some	60–80
Sev persistent	All day	>4×/w	Extreme	<60

From Dombrowski MP, Schatz M, ACOG Committee on Practice Bulletins-Obstetrics. ACOG practice bulletin: Clinical management guidelines for obstetrician-gynecologists number 90, February 2008: Asthma in pregnancy. Obstet Gynecol. 2008;111(2 Pt 1):457–64.

Treatment

Asthma management, outpatient therapies

Severity	Mgmt
Mild intermittent	Short-acting β-agonist (albuterol) as needed
Mild persistent	**Add:** Low-dose inhaled Cort. Alternative: Cromolyn, leukotriene receptor antag (montelukast), or theophylline.
Mod persistent	**Add:** Long-acting β-agonist (salmeterol), OR change to medium-dose inhaled Cort ± salmeterol. Alternative: Low-dose or medium-dose inhaled Cort + leukotriene receptor antag or theophylline.
Sev persistent	**Change** to long-acting β-agonist + salmeterol ± oral Cort (prednisone). Alternative: High-dose inhaled Cort w/ theophylline ± oral Cort.

From Dombrowski MP, Schatz M, ACOG Committee on Practice Bulletins-Obstetrics. ACOG practice bulletin: Clinical management guidelines for obstetrician-gynecologists number 90, February 2008: Asthma in pregnancy. Obstet Gynecol. 2008;111 (2 Pt 1):457–64.

- **Rx for acute asthma exacerbation**
  Supplemental O$_2$ to maintain sat >95% (important for fetal oxygenation)
  Albuterol nebulizer q20min × 3, then q4h
  Consider inhaled ipratropium on presentation (0.5 mg neb/8 puffs MDI)
  Systemic corticosteroids; prednisone 40–80 mg PO × 5–10 d (until PEFR >70%)
- **Triage for acute presentation of asthma in Preg**
  FEV$_1$ or PEFR >70% after rx, no distress, reassuring fetal status → discharge
  FEV$_1$ or PEFR 50–70% after rx → individualize disposition
  FEV$_1$ or PEFR <50% after rx → hospitalize
  If poor resp/sev sx, drowsiness, confusion, pCO$_2$ >40 mmHg consider ICU admission ± intubation
- Arrange close outpatient follow-up

Surveillance During Pregnancy
- Assess asthma status w/ PEFR at each prenatal visit; adjust maint regimen
- Prepare Asthma Action Plan & instruct on use. Eg, www.nhlbi.nih.gov/health/public/lung/asthma/asthma_actplan.pdf
- Focus on avoidance of allergens/irritants (eg, tobacco smoke, GERD, mold, dust mites, dander, cockroaches)
- Albuterol & budesonide are preferred short-acting β-agonist/inhaled steroid in Preg. Consider weekly fetal testing (NST, AFI, or BPP) from 32–34 w if mod–sev asthma or poor control.

Intrapartum Considerations
- Maintain hydration, continue asthma meds, including systemic steroids
- Consider cesarean deliv if unstable asthma & mature fetus
- Avoid carboprost tromethamine (Hemabate)
- ASA, indocin, other NSAIDs can cause asthmatic bronchospasm
- No contraindication to breastfeeding postpartum for asthma meds above

ANAPHYLAXIS

Definition and Diagnosis (J Allergy Clin Immunol 2006;117(2):391)
- Sev, potentially fatal, systemic allergic (IgE mediated) rxn, occurring suddenly after exposure to an allergen. Dx requires **1** of the following:
  - Acute onset w/ involvement of the skin, mucosae, or both & compromise of respiratory, CV, or other end-organ fxn

- Acute onset of compromise of fxn of at least 2 organ systems (skin, GI, respiratory, CV) after exposure to likely allergen
- HoTN after exposure to known allergen
- Skin sx present in ≥80% of cases. Consider total tryptase level (drawn when pt symptomatic) to confirm dx.

Treatment
- Removal of potential allergen(s). Mobilize resources (EMS, ICU, or Code team)
- Prompt dosing of 0.3–0.5 mg (at 1:1000 dilution) epi intramuscularly. May rpt q5–15min.
- Position supine, apply oxygen, monit vital signs, obtain IV access w/ crystalloid support as needed. Consider albuterol, H2/H1 blockers, methylprednisolone (1–2 mg/kg q6h). Consider glucagon if refrac sx in pt on β-blocker.
- Consider observation for biphasic rxn (recurrence of sx w/i 72 h in 1–20% of cases)
- Ensure appropriate follow-up w/ allergist; discharge w/ >1 epi autoinjector if appropriate

Considerations in Obstetric and Gynecologic Populations
- Sx & rx in Preg are generally the same as for nonpregnant women. Consider amniotic fluid embolism (bronchospasm more likely w/ anaphylaxis, coagulopathy more likely w/ AFE), or preeclampsia-related airway/subcutaneous edema depending on clinical setting. Breastfeeding reported as a rare cause of anaphylaxis (*Obstet Gynecol* 2009;114(2 Pt 2):415).
- Monit fetal cardiac activity continuously, w/ deliv for persistent category III tracings despite aggressive mat intervention. Consider hospital exposures when anaphylaxis is diagnosed inpt (latex, perioperative Abx, oxytocin, laminaria, chemotherapeutic agents).

URINARY SYSTEM CHANGES IN PREGNANCY

- **Renal changes:** Kidney increases in size, 30% ↑ volume, dilation of renal collecting system (right > left) due to hormonal changes (progesterone, relaxin, endothelin) & mechanical obstruction more on right side (uterus is usually dextrorotated)
- **GFR:** Increased (50%), with even greater ↑ in plasma renal flow due to increased cardiac output & decreased renal vascular resistance. Renal plasma flow peaks in 1st trimester, decreases at the end of 3rd trimester. GFR 25% ↑ by 2 w after conception, 50% ↑ by 2nd trimester. Increased GFR → ↓ serum Cr (*J Am Soc Nephrol* 2009;20:14). In pregnancy, normal Cr range = 0.4–0.8 mg/dL.
- **Testing:** Due to altered Cr clearance in Preg, use 24-h urine Cr to estimate GFR
- **Other:** ↑ Proteinuria (up to 300 mg/d), ↓ serum bicarbonate due to respiratory alkalosis, ↑ glycosuria (decreased renal threshold <150 mg/dL), ↓ serum Na (HoNa)

ACUTE KIDNEY INJURY (AKI)

Definition and Epidemiology (*Crit Care* 2016;20:299)

- ↑ Serum Cr by 0.3 mg/dL (or 50% ↑ from baseline) in 48 h OR Urine volume <0.5 mL/kg/h for 6 h. This definition also applies in pregnancy.
- Incid 2/1000 overall. Pregnancy-associated AKI ~1/15,000 (*Cur Op Crit Care* 2011;17:548; *Crit Care Med* 2005;33:S372). See also Chap. 3 (periop oliguria).

Etiology and Pathophysiology

Etiology & pathophysiology of acute kidney injury			
Location		**Etiology**	**Pathophysiology**
Prerenal (decreased renal perfusion)		Hypovolemia Hypotension ↓ Cardiac output	↓ Mean arterial pressure → ↑ sympathetic neural tone → renal vasoconstriction → ↓ renal tissue perfusion
		NSAIDs	↓ Prostaglandin production → ↓ vasodilation renal afferent art
		ACE-inhibitors/ARB	↓ Angiotensin II production → ↓ vasoconstriction renal efferent art "contraindicated in Preg"
Intrarenal (damage to renal parenchyma)	Glomerular	Glomerulonephritis	Nonproliferative vs. proliferative (pathophysiology differs)
		Glomerular endotheliosis	↓ Glomerular size, increased cytoplasm in glomerular epithelial cells → ↓ capillary diameter → capillary occlusion "Pathognomonic for preeclampsia"
	Vascular	Antiphospholipid Ab syn	Microvascular thrombosis → ischemia
		Malig nephrosclerosis	
		TTP/HUS	
		Radiation nephritis	
		Scleroderma	
	Tubules/ Interstitium	ATN – acute tubular necrosis (sepsis, ischemia) AIN – acute interstitial nephritis (drugs, infection, systemic syndromes – lupus, sarcoid etc.)	Endothelial damage → microvascular thrombosis → free radical production, leukocyte migration/ adhesion → tubule damage Cytoskeletal tubule breakdown, apoptosis, tubular obst → inflammation, filtrate backleak across damaged tubular epithelium, tubular obst → cortical necrosis

Location		Etiology	Pathophysiology
	Nephrotoxins	Aminoglycosides	Filtered across glomerulus → accum in renal cortex → AKI seen after 5–7 d of rx
		Amphotericin B	Binds to tubular membrane cholesterol → pore introduction → polyuria, nonanion gap metabolic acidosis, hypomagnesemia, HypoCa
		Cisplatin/carboplatin	Accumulates in prox tubular cell → necrosis/apoptosis
		Ethylene glycol	Metabolite 2-HEAA → tubular injury
		Iodinated contrast	Renal outer medulla hypoxia from small vessel occlusion, cytotoxic tubular damage, tubule obst
		Rhabdo	Prox tubular tox, intrarenal vasoconstriction, distal nephron obst (myoglobin/hemoglobin + Tamm–Horsfall prot → precipitation)
		Tumor lysis syndrome	Cytotoxic therapy → uric acid release → uric acid precipitation in tubules
Postrenal (obst)		Bladder obst Bilateral ureteral obst	Impaired outflow → ↑ intratubular pressure → ↓ GFR Preg: Partial obst may lead to urinary distention
		GU injury	
		Nephrolithiasis	
		Retroperitoneal fibrosis	
Preg (Adv in Chronic Kidney Disease 2013;20(3): 215–22)		Preeclampsia/HELLP	AKI 1–2% preeclampsia, 3–15% HELLP. Glomeruloendotheliosis is pathognomonic
		Acute fatty liver	ATN, fatty infiltration of kidney
		Amniotic fluid embolism	DIC, cardiovascular dysfxn, hemorrhage → AKI
		TTP/HUS	AKI develops in 2/3 (microvascular thrombosis → ischemia

Clinical Findings and Exam
- Uremia, oliguria/anuria, hematuria
- **Prerenal:** tachycardia, dry mucous membranes, orthostatic hypotension
- **Intrarenal:** Pulm hemorrhage, palpable purpura → vasculitis + glomerulonephritis, livedo reticularis → atheroembolic dz, limb ischemia → rhabdo
- **Postrenal:** Flank pain which radiates to groin, suprapubic pain, ↑ post void residual volume

Diagnostic Workup

Study findings			
Study	Prerenal	Intrarenal	Postrenal
UA: Prot	0–trace	Mild–mod	0–trace
UA: Leukocyte esterase	0	±	±
UA: Bld	0	±	±
Microscopy	Hyaline casts	Cellular or granular casts	None
Urine Na (mEq/L)	<20	>40	Varies
FENa = (UNa/PNa)/(UCr/PCr)	<1	>2	
Urine Osmol (mOsm/kg)	>500	<350	

- **Imaging:** Renal ultrasound – 1st-line imaging study, sensitive for obstruction, ↑ parenchymal echogenicity can suggest intrarenal cause; CT Urogram – most accurate for evaluating for stone or underlying renal/abdominal abnormalities. Avoid contrast! MRI – useful when unable to get contrast with CT. Careful with gadolinium-enhancement → ↑ risk of nephrogenic systemic fibrosis
- **Renal bx:** Consider when etiology is unk and results will change mgmt. 5% complication rate (perirenal hematoma, gross hematuria). Preg: Consider pts <28 w w/AKI of uncertain etiology when results will change mgmt (Am J Perinatol 2008;25:385)

Treatment
- Correct underlying factors, remove renal toxins, adjust dosing of renally cleared meds. Prevent/treat infxn
- **Fluid mgmt:** Goal = adequate hydration to reverse preischemic change. See "Fluids and Electrolytes"
- Metabolic acidosis → sodium bicarbonate
- **Renal Replacement Therapy (RRT)** (JAMA 2008;299:793)
    For AKI refrac to medical mgmt, as evidenced by metabolic acidosis, hyperK, hypervolemia, uremia, intoxication, etc. Mode: IP, intermittent hemodialysis, continuous
    Continuous RRT: Slower solute clearance/min, continuous anticoagulation
    Use in Preg: Symptomatic uremia (changes in mental status, pericarditis, neuropathy), or + for other indications for RRT

CHRONIC KIDNEY DISEASE

Definition and Epidemiology (Am J Kidney Dis 2018;71(3)(suppl 1):Svii, S1)
- **CKD** = kidney damage (urine albumin excretion ≥30 mg/d) **or** decreased kidney function (GFR <60 mL/min/1.73 m^2) **for >3 mo**
- **CRF:** Irreversible nephron number reduction
- **ESRD:** GFR <15 mL/min per 1.73 m^2 OR need for dialysis &/or transplant
- **Prevalence of CKD in US:** 14% adults ≥20 y, increased prevalence w/ comorbidities such as DM (44%), HTN (28%)

Etiology
- **Glomerular:** Diabetes, systemic infection, autoimmune
- **Vascular:** HTN, ischemia, atherosclerosis, vasculitis, thromboembolic
- **Tubular/interstitial:** Urinary tract stones, infection, obstruction, nephrotoxins

Pathophysiology
- **Initiating mechanisms:** Specific to etiology of CKD
- **Progressive mechanisms:** Increased renal bld flow/pres → renin–angiotensin axis stimulation → nephron hyperfiltration & hypertrophy → glomerular distortion, sclerosis, permanent damage to nephrons → reduction in nephron number
- Failure of renal excretion → accum of toxins (including Cr, urea → uremic syn)
- Failure of other renal functions → anemia, abn metabolism, fluid/electrolyte imbalance, hormone regulation (glucagon, insulin, Vit D, sex hormones, parathyroid hormone). Progressive inflammation (elevated C reactive prot + acute phase reactants).

Clinical Manifestations
- Edema (from nephrotic syn), fatigue (from anemia), decreased appetite → malnut, inability to perform activities of daily living, altered mental status (uremic syn)
- **Preg** (CJASN 2011;6:2587): ↑ Complications: Proteinuria, decreased GFR, HTN
    Maternal complications: Gestational HTN, preeclampsia/eclampsia, nephrotic syn, maternal death (higher incid w/ lupus nephropathy)
    Fetal complications: Preterm birth, IUGR, IUFD, neonat death

Physical Exam
- Most pts are asymptomatic until moderate–severe renal failure develops
- Findings: Peripheral edema, pericardial friction rub (in presence of uremic syndrome), sensory neuropathy (evidence of end-organ damage)

Diagnostic Workup/Studies
- GFR (mL/min/1.73 m^2) = Creatinine Assay × [Serum Cr]$^{-1.154}$ × [Age]$^{-0.203}$ × [Sex] × [Race]
    Creatinine assay: Isotope dilution mass spectrometry (IDSM) = 175, Non–IDSM = 186; Sex: Females = 0.742, males = 1; Race: AA = 1.21, others = 1
- GFR peak = 120 mL/min/1.73 m^2 btw age 20 & 30 (lower for women)
- GFR then declines 1 mL/min/1.73 m^2 per year

Laboratory trends in CKD	
Test	**Result**
Serum phosphorus	Increased
Serum calcium	Decreased
Serum PTH	Increased
Bone alk phos	Increased
24-h urine total prot	>300 mg
Serum/urine prot electrophoresis	Bence Jones proteins (multimyeloma)

Stages of GFR (mL/min/1.73 m^2)
- G1: ≥90 + kidney damage (proteinuria, abn renal imaging)
- G2: 60–89
- G3a: 45–59
- G3b: 30–44
- G4: 15–29
- G5: <15

Stages of Albumin Excretion Rate (mg/d)
- A1: <30
- A2: 30–300
- A3: >300

CKD Staging
GFR and albuminuria stages plotted on grid to reflect risk of progression, frequency of monitoring needed (Ex. G1A1 = low, G5A3 = high)

Imaging
- Renal US (preferred modality in Preg)
  CKD: Small kidneys bilaterally
  Polycystic kidney dz: Cystic, enlarged kidneys
  >1 cm discrep in length: Developmental abnormality, arterial insufficiency which affects 1 kidney more
- **Voiding cystogram:** To evaluate for reflux nephropathy
- **CT, MRI:** Avoid IV dye if poss in Preg
- **Renal bx:** Should be avoided during Preg
- Serial renal fxn measurements (to differentiate acute vs. subacute vs. CKD)

Treatment and Medications
- Dietary adjustments – restrict Na (HTN), K (hyperK), protein; glycemic control in DM
- HTN control (*J Am Soc Neph 2016;epub*)
  Goal = 130/80 (125/75 in pts w/ diabetes & proteinuria >1 g/24 h)
  Reduce intraglomerular HTN to slow nephron injury progression
- **Potassium sparing meds:** ACE inhibitors, ARB, spironolactone, eplerenone, amiloride, triamterene
- **Renal replacement therapy:** IP vs. intermittent hemodialysis vs. continuous RRT. Initiate when GFR = 10 mL/min/1.73 m^2, or symptomatic CKD
- **Preg:** 24-h urine total prot in the 1st trimester + HTN control (β-blocker, Ca-channel blocker, hydralazine, clonidine) + Serial USs for fetal growth + antepartum testing: Initiate btw 28 & 32 w. *Avoid ACE inhibitors/ARBs.*

URINARY TRACT INFECTION (UTI)

Definitions (*Obstet Gynecol 2008;111:785*)
- **Asymptomatic bacteriuria:** ≥100,000 CFU/mL in 2 voided specimens with urine cultures isolating the same bacterial strain
  OR a single cath specimen with 1 bacterial species ≥100 CFU/mL. Screening recommended before GU procedures where mucosal bleeding anticipated
  (*Clin Inf Diseases 2005;643–54*)
- **UTI:** ≥1,000,000 CFU/mL in urine culture w/ or w/o sx
- **Uncomplicated:** Healthy female with normal urinary tract and function
- **Complicated:** UTI plus one of the following: Pregnancy, urologic abnormality, urinary calculi, catheter, recent GU surgery, DM, spinal cord injury, pyelonephritis, immunosuppression
- **Recurrent UTI:** 2 UTIs in 6 mo or 3 positive cx in preceding 12 mo (*Obstet Gynecol Clin North Am 2008;35*)

Epidemiology
- 50% ♀ will have a UTI in their lifetime; 10% ♀ will have a recurrent UTI by age 70
  (*Obstet Gynecol* 2008;111:785)
- Asymptomatic bacteriuria in Preg: 20–30× increased risk of pyelo

Etiology
- *Escherichia coli* = 75–95% (*NEJM* 2012;366:1028), Proteus (can cause renal calculi). Klebsiella, Enterobacter, Pseudomonas, *Staphylococcus saprophyticus* (common in young women)

Pathophysiology
- **Ascending infxn:** Vagina → urethra → bladder
- **E. coli:** Virulence factors P fimbria, S fimbria, Type 1 fimbria → ↑ uroepithelial/vaginal cell binding, ↑ resistance to host phagocytosis, ↑ resistance to bactericidal activity

Clinical Manifestations and Exam
- Dysuria, increased urgency, increased urinary frequency, suprapubic pain
- Suprapubic tenderness to palpation
- Pyuria, urethral tenderness (seen w/ urethritis)

Diagnostic Workup/Studies
- **UA:** Leukocyte esterase or nitrites: 75% sensitive, 82% specific (*NEJM* 2003;349:259); WBC ± RBC; bacteria on gram stain
- **Urine culture:** ≥100,000 CFU/mL
- Consider upper tract imaging and/or cystoscopy for recurrent UTI

Treatment

Medications for UTI				
Diagnosis	**Treatment**	**Dose**	**Duration**	**Comments**
Asymptomatic bacteriuria				Only treat in Preg. Rescreen each trimester
1st line (PO)	Nitrofurantoin monohydrate Data on nitrofuran or sulfonamide antibiotics and birth defects is mixed. Discuss pros/cons in 1st trimester especially. (*Obstet Gynecol* 2017;130:e150)	100 mg q12h	7 d	Nitrofuran and sulfonamides are contraindicated for G6PD deficiency
Alternative (PO)	Amoxicillin	500 mg q8h, 875 mg q12h	3–7 d	
	Cephalexin	500 mg q6h	3–7 d	
	Cefpodoxime	100 mg q12h	3–7 d	
	Fosfomycin	3 g once		Not therapeutic in kidney, avoid if pyelo
	TMP/SMX	160/800 mg q12h	3 d	Avoid in 1st trimester and 3rd trimester (kernicterus)
Uncomp UTI (Per IDSA Guidelines)				
1st line (PO)	Nitrofurantoin monohydrate	100 mg q12h	5 d	Avoid if early pyelo suspected
	TMP–SMX	160/800 mg q12h	3 d	Do not use if local resistance >20% or used for UTI in last 3 mo
	Fosfomycin trometamol	3 g	Single dose	

Diagnosis	Treatment	Dose	Duration	Comments
Alternative (PO)	Ofloxacin	200 mg q12h	3 d	Contraindicated in Preg
	Ciprofloxacin	250 mg q12h	3 d	
	Levofloxacin	250 mg daily	3 d	
	Amoxicillin–clavulanate	500 mg q12h	7 d	
	Cefdinir	300 mg q12h	3–7 d	
	Cefaclor	500 mg q12h	7 d	
	Cefpodoxime-proxetil	100 mg q12h	7 d	
Complicated UTI (outpt, PO therapy)				
	Ciprofloxacin	500 mg q12h	10–14 d	Contraindicated in Preg
	Ofloxacin	200–300 mg q12h	10–14 d	
	Lomefloxacin	400 mg daily	10–14 d	
	Levofloxacin	250 mg q12h	10–14 d	
Complicated UTI (inpt)				
Initial IV therapy	Ampicillin	500 mg q6h	Treat IV until afebrile, clinically improved	
	Gentamicin	1 mg/kg q8h		
	Ciprofloxacin	400 mg q12h		
	Levofloxacin	250 mg daily		
	Ceftriaxone	1–2 g daily		
	Ticarcillin/clavulanate	3.1 mg q4–6h		
	Aztreonam	1 g q8–12h		
	Imipenem–cilastatin	250–500 mg q6–8h		
Subseq PO therapy	TMP–SMX	160/800 mg q12h	10–21 d	
	Ciprofloxacin	500 mg q12h	10–21 d	
	Ofloxacin	200–300 mg q12h	10–21 d	
	Lomefloxacin	400 mg daily	10–21 d	
	Levofloxacin	250 mg q12h	10–21 d	
≥3 symptomatic UTIs/y				
Suppression (PO)	TMP/SMX	80/400 mg	Daily or 3×/w	
	Trimethoprim	100 mg	Daily or 3×/w	
	Nitrofurantoin	50 mg	Daily or 3×/w	
Preg: ≥2 UTIs or asymptomatic bacteriuria				
Suppression (PO)	Nitrofurantoin	100 mg	Daily	

PYELONEPHRITIS

Definition
- Infxn of renal pelvicalices/parenchyma from ascending bladder infxn or renal bacteriuria. Clinical syn defined by flank pain, fevers, chills.

Epidemiology
- 23/10,000 women ages 15–34 (NEJM 2012;366:1028)
- 1–2% of pregnancies, >50% present in the 2nd trimester (Obstet Gynecol 2005;106:1085)
- Untreated asymptomatic bacteriuria in Preg → 1/4 will develop pyelo

Etiology
- Same as for UTIs (above). Most are E. coli.

Pathophysiology
- **Risk factors:** Same as for UTI (see "UTI")
- **ARDS:** IV antibiotic therapy → endotoxin release 24–48 h later → damage to alveolar capillary membranes
- Preg complications
  Increased risk of preterm labor if pyelo is not aggressively treated

Pulm insufficiency: Increased risk if temperature >103°F, tachy >110 bpm, gestational age ≥20 w

Clinical Manifestations and Exam
- Chills, fever, flank pain, dysuria, urinary frequency/urgency
- Costovertebral angle tenderness

Diagnostic Workup/Studies
- Urinalysis
- Urine culture w/ susceptibilities
- If no response to initial therapy, consider blood cultures

Treatment and Medications
- Inpt admission is recommended for all women w/ pyelo during Preg *(Obstet Gynecol 2005;106:1085)*
- IV hydration to maintain adequate urine output
- **Acetaminophen:** Hyperthermia can be teratogenic in 1st trimester
- IV therapy 24–48 h (avoid fluoroquinolones), follow w/ oral therapy 10–14 d
- Suppression therapy for remainder of Preg: Nitrofurantoin 100 mg PO daily
- Rpt urine culture each trimester

Medications for pyelonephritis				
	Rx	**Dose**	**Duration**	**Comments**
Outpt PO therapy (IDSA Guidelines)	Ciprofloxacin	500 mg q12h	7 d	Can load w/ ciprofloxacin 400 mg IV Avoid ciprofloxacin if resistance >10%
	TMP–SMX	160/800 mg q12h	14 d	
	Ciprofloxacin	1000 mg ER daily	7 d	Fluoroquinolones not used in Preg
	Levofloxacin	750 mg daily	5 d	
	Amoxicillin–clavulanate	875/125 mg q12h	10–14 d	
Inpt IV therapy (if unable to tolerate PO, or if evid of sepsis)	Ciprofloxacin	400 mg q12h	Treat IV until afebrile for 24 h, follow w/ PO therapy	
	Ceftriaxone	1–2 g q12–24h		
	TMP–SMX	2 mg/kg q6h		
	Cefotaxime	1–2 g q8h		
	Levofloxacin	500 mg daily		
	Cefepime	2 g q8h		
	Cefotetan	2 g q12h		
Preg (inpt IV therapy)	Ampicillin	2 g q6h	24–48 h	Use in combination
	Gentamicin	3 mg–5 mg/kg/d	24–48 h	
	Ceftriaxone	1 g q24h	24–48 h	

NEPHROLITHIASIS

Definition and Epidemiology
- **Calcium-based:** Calcium oxalate, calcium phosphate (80%) *(NEJM 2010;363:954)*
- **Noncalcium-based:** Uric acid, cystine, struvite (may form staghorn calculi)
- 10% of the US population will have 1 kidney stone in lifetime *(J Urol 2012;188:130)*
- **Preg:** Btw 1/200 to 1/1500 women have symptomatic nephrolithiasis *(Cur Op Uro 2010;20:174)*

Pathophysiology
- Increased excretion rate or increased water conservation → supersaturation of urine w/ insoluble substances → crystal formation → crystal aggregation into stone(s)
- Stones become symptomatic when entering ureter or occluding ureteropelvic junction

Clinical Manifestations
- Flank pain (episodic, may radiate to abd), nausea, vomiting, hematuria, dysuria, frequency

Diagnostic Workup/Studies
- **CT w/o contrast** = imaging modality of choice
- **Renal US** – preferred modality in pregnancy
- **Abdominal radiograph (KUB):** Only + if radio-opaque stones

- **Recurrent symptomatic nephrolithiasis:** Evaluate possible etiologies
  Serum: Calcium, uric acid, electrolytes
  Urine: pH, vol, calcium, citrate, oxalate, 24-h urine collection (2 occasions), strain for stone, culture

Treatment and Medications
- **Conservative mgmt:** Hydration, pain control (most stones smaller than 5 mm pass spontaneously), antibiotics if UTI
- **Medical mgmt:** CCB or Alpha-1 blockers to ↑ ureteral relaxation, ↑ motility
- **Active intervention:** Persistent pain, progressive obst, solitary kidney obst, infection, AKI *(J Urol 2012;188:130)*
  Shock wave lithotripsy: May require multitreatments
  Semirigid ureteroscopy: Higher stone free rate after one rx, fewer retreatments needed. Improved success w/ distal ureteral stones.
  Percutaneous nephrolithotomy: Most invasive. Use for large stone burden, renal stones.
- **Pregnancy** *(Cur Op Uro 2010;20:174)*:
  Temporary drainage: Ureteral stent or percutaneous nephrostomy (risk of infxn, bacteriuria, migration/dislodgement)
  Definitive tx: Ureteroscopy is preferred
  Avoid shock wave lithotripsy in Preg (increased risk of miscarriage, congen malformations, abruption)

FLUIDS AND ELECTROLYTES

IV fluid composition									
IVF	**Na**	**Cl**	**K**	**Ca**	**Mg**	**Buffers**	**pH**	**Osmolality mOsm/L**	**Osmotic pres mmHg**
				mEq/L					
Plasma	140	103	4	5	2	Bicarb (25)	7.4	290	20–25
Crystalloid: 75% enters interstitial space									
0.9% NaCl	154	154					5.7	308	
7.5% NaCl								2465	
Lactated Ringer's	130	109	4	3		Lactate (28)	6.4	273	
5% dextrose (50 g dextrose/L)							4	278	
Colloid: 50–75% remains intravascular									
5% Albumin (50 g/L)									20
Hetastarch (6% in NS)	154	154							30
Hextend	143	125	3	5	0.9	Lactate (28)			

IVF	Comments
0.9% NaCl	Increased risk of hyperchloremic metabolic acidosis
7.5% NaCl (hypertonic saline)	Intracellular → extracellular shift is 5× amt infused; 2 fold ↑ in plasma vol
Lactated Ringer's	Calcium binds drugs (aminocaproic acid, amphotericin, ampicillin) Calcium binds bld products' citrated anticoagulant → increased clot formation
5% dextrose (50 g dextrose/L)	Can ↑ risk of hyperglycemia in critically ill pts <10% remains intravascular, 2/3 intracellular

IVF	Comments
5% albumin (50 g/L)	250 mL aliquots in isotonic saline 70% remains intravascular → lost in 12 h
25% albumin (250 g/L)	50 mL or 100 mL aliquots Increases plasma vol 3–4× amt infused Consider in hypovolemia due to fluid shift to interstitial space
Hetastarch (6% in NS)	High molecular weight (450,000 daltons) broken down by Amy → 50,000 daltons → kidney clearance (takes 2–3 w) Oncotic effect lasts 24 h Inhibits vWF, Factor VII, platelet adhesion → limit use to 1500 mL/24 h
Hextend	Contains 6% Hetastarch

Hyperkalemia

- **Definition:** Serum potassium (K^+) >5.0 mEq/L
- **Clinical manifestations:** Weakness, paresthesias, palpitations
  - **ECG changes:** Peaked T waves → ↑ PR interval → ↑ QRS width → loss of P wave → sine wave pattern → Vfib/PEA → asystole
- **Workup:** Rule out pseudohyperkalemia, transcellular shift (academia, DM, β-blocker, cellular necrosis, etc.). Assess GFR
  - Urine K^+: >30 mEq/L → transcellular shift; <30 mEq/L → impaired renal excretion
- **Treatment** (*J Int Care Med* 2005;20:272):
  - Continuous telemetry
  - **Sodium polystyrene sulfonate (Kayexalate):** Cation exchange resin binds K^+ → fecal excretion; **PO:** 15 g 1–4×/d; **Rectal:** 30–50 g q6h. Do not use in pts w/ bowel obst, ileus, bowel ischemia
  - If ECG changes are present
    - *Calcium gluconate:* 10 mL of 10% (1 ampule): IV push over 2 min. Rpt in 5 min.
    - *Calcium chloride:* 10 mL of 10% (1 ampule): Use in pts w/ circulatory compromise. 3× more calcium than calcium gluconate → improved cardiac contractility
    - *Insulin/gluc:* Give 10 U insulin & 25 g dextrose (1 amp of D_{50}). Hold D_{50} if bld gluc >250 mg/dL
    - *Albuterol:* 10–20 mg of 5 mg/mL nebulized solution
    - *Sodium bicarbonate:* Use only in pts w/ sev metabolic acidosis
  - Dialysis (hemodialysis faster at removing K^+ than peritoneal dialysis)
  - **Digitalis tox:** Magnesium sulfate 2 g IV bolus. Do NOT use calcium (can potentiate digitalis tox)

Hypokalemia

- **Definition:** Serum potassium (K^+) <3.5 mEq/L
- **Clinical manifestations:** Nausea, vomiting, weakness, rhabdo, polyuria
  - Nonspecific ECG changes: U wave (Amp >1 mm), Prolonged QT interval, flattened inv T waves, digitalis-induced arrhythmia
- **Dx:** Rule out transcellular shift (alkemia, insulin, catecholamines, hypothermia etc.)
- **Treatment:** Treat causes of transcellular K^+ shifts
  - **Replace K^+:** KCI 10–40 mEq IV. Infuse 20 mEq in 100 mL NS over 1 h
  - Replace serum magnesium

Hypernatremia

- **Definition:** Serum sodium (Na^+) >145 mEq/L
- **Clinical manifestations:** Altered mental status, Rhabdo, Absence of thirst vs. intense thirst, polyuria, diarrhea
- **Dx:** I/Os, volume status, serum osm, urine osm, urine electrolytes
- **Treatment** (*NEJM* 2000;342:1493):
  - Stop any continuing causes of HyperNa
  - **Correct serum sodium:** Give hypotonic fluid PO or parenterally
  - Calculate water deficit & daily water loss
    - Total body water = total body weight × 0.5 in women
    - Free water deficit = [(serum Na − 140)/140] × TBW
    - Free water clearance = (V[1 − (UNa + UK)])/PNa
      - V = urine vol; UNa = urine [Na^+]; UK = urine [K^+]; PNa = plasma [Na^+]
    - Insensible losses: 10 mL/kg/d
  - Replace daily water loss, correct water deficit
    - *Chronic HyperNa:* ↓ Serum Na^+ by 10 mmol/d
      - Avoid correcting too quickly to prevent cerebral edema
    - *Acute HyperNa:* ↓ Serum Na^+ by 1 mmol/L/h

Fluids: Give hypotonic fluids only (0.2% NaCl, 0.45% NaCl)
  The more hypotonic the fluid, the lower the rate of infusion
  Calculate change in serum Na$^+$ w/ 1 L infusion:
    [(infusion Na + infusion K) − serum Na$^+$]/(total body water + 1)
  Avoid: 0.9% NaCl, dextrose solutions (hyperglycemia → osmotic diuresis →
    worsening HyperNa

Hyponatremia
- **Definition:** Serum sodium (Na$^+$) <130 mEq/L
- **Clinical manifestations:** Altered mental status
- **Dx:** Volume status (hypovolemic vs. euvolemia vs. hypervolemia), serum osmolality,
  urine osmolality, urine electrolytes, FeNa
- **Treatment:**
  Stop any continuing causes of HypoNa. Asymptomatic – correct at rate ≤0.5 mEq/
  L/h. Symptomatic – rapid correction 2 mEq/L/h for 1st 2–3 h). Do not exceed
  correction >10–12 mEq/L/d to avoid osmotic demyelination syndrome

Hypercalcemia
- **Definition:** Total serum calcium >11 mg/dL, ionized calcium >3 mmol/L
- **Clinical manifestations** (seen when ionized calcium >3 mmol/L):
  GI: Constip, N/V, ileus, pancreatitis
  Renal: Polyuria, nephrocalcinosis, nephrogenic DI
  Neuro: Altered mental status, coma, ↓ DTRs
  Cardiovascular: HoTN, hypovolemia, ↓ QT interval, AV block
- **Treatment:**
  Correct hypovolemia: IV hydration w/ isotonic saline
  Furosemide: 40–80 mg IV q2h to maintain urine output of 100 mL/h
  Calcitonin: To ↓ bone resorption. 4 U/kg q12h SC or IM. Will ↓ serum calcium by
  0.5 mmol/L
  Hydrocortisone: 200 mg IV daily (divided 2–3 doses). Use w/ calcitonin.
  Bisphosphonates: Max resp seen in 4–10 d. Zoledronate 4 mg IV, infuse over
  15 min, Pamidronate 90 mg IV, infuse over 2 h

Hypocalcemia
- **Definition:** Total serum calcium <8.8 mg/dL, ionized calcium <2.1 mmol/L
- **Clinical manifestations:** Paresthesias, cramps, rickets, osteomalacia
- **Treatment:** Symptomatic: IV Ca gluconate (1–2 g IV over 20 min), calcitriol, vit D

Hypermagnesemia
- **Definition:** Serum Mg >4 mEq/L
- **Clinical manifestations:** Flushing, headache, ↓ DTR, lethargy, somnolence, muscle
  paralysis, resp failure, heart block, cardiac arrest
- **Treatment:** Normal renal function – stop magnesium therapy. Moderate renal
  impairment – IV fluids, furosemide. Severe renal impairment – dialysis, IV calcium

Hypomagnesemia
- **Definition:** Serum Mg <1.8 mg/dL
- **Clinical manifestations:** Tetany, arrhythmia, seizures
- **Treatment:** Symptomatic – 1–2 g IV magnesium over 5–60 min

Hyperphosphatemia
- **Definition:** Serum Ph >5 mg/dL
- **Clinical manifestations:** Mostly asymptomatic, can be life-threatening with
  symptomatic hypocalcemia
- **Treatment:** Symptomatic – IV fluids, hemodialysis if impaired renal function. Chronic –
  phosphate binders, low Ph diet

Hypophosphotemia
- **Definition:** Serum Ph <2 mg/dL
- **Clinical manifestations:** Muscle weakness, rhabdo, encephalopathy
- **Treatment:** Symptomatic – IV Ph repletion

Hyperchloremia
- **Definition:** Serum Cl >107 mEq/L
- **Clinical manifestations:** Due to free water loss, metabolic acidosis
- **Treatment:** Hydration, correct acidemia

Hypochloremia
- **Definition:** Serum Cl <97 mEq/L
- **Clinical manifestations:** Due to loss of gastric fluid, diuretic use
- **Treatment:** Stop underlying causes, correct metabolic alkalosis

GASTROINTESTINAL CHANGES IN PREGNANCY

- Decreased gut motility in pregnancy theorized to be due to progesterone effects
- GERD due to ↓ gastric emptying & ↓ lower esophageal sphincter tone
- N/V of pregnancy exacerbated by ↓ gut motility
- Constipation from both decreased transit time and nutrient absorption
- Enlarging uterine fundus also thought to impact early satiety, GERD, and constipation
- In normal pregnancy, most liver parameters are unchanged (size, hepatic blood flow, overall histology, PT, T Bili, AST, ALT, GGT), but synthetic function increases

Changes in proteins and enzymes in pregnancy		
Total serum prot concentration	↓	Due to fall in serum albumin
Coagulation factors (fibrinogen, factors VII, VIII, IX, X)	↑	Due to ↑ estrogen
Cytochrome P-450	↑	Due to ↑ progesterone
Total alkaline phosphatase	↑	Due to placental production
Binding globulins	↑	Due to hormonal stimulation of liver

CHOLELITHIASIS

Epidemiology
- 10–15% prevalence in adults overall; gallstone-related disease: <1% of pregnant women
- **Risk factors:** Pregnancy (↓ gallbladder motility, ↑ biliary sludge, & cholesterol synthesis); ↑ estrogen (gender [♀ 2× > ♂], obesity, rapid weight loss, pregnancy); ethnicity (75% of Native Americans); age (>40 y); drugs (OCPs, estrogen, clofibrate, octreotide, ceftriaxone, TPN); bile acid metabolism disorders; hyperlipidemia syndromes (↑ biliary cholesterol secretion & saturation of bile)

Pathophysiology
- Bile = pathway for elimination of excess cholesterol either as free cholesterol or as bile salts; cholesterol-saturated bile → crystal formation → bile stasis → aggregation
- Types of stones: Mixed; cholesterol (up to 80% of gallstones, up to 80% radiolucent); black pigments (unconjugated bilirubin + calcium, sterile; radiopaque); brown pigments (calcium soaps, infected ducts; radiolucent)

See Table for workup and management

CHOLECYSTITIS

Definition and Epidemiology
- **Inflammation of the gallbladder:** Acute (rapid onset, gallstone obstruction); chronic (transient obstruction → low-grade inflammation/fibrosis); acalculous (inflammation w/o obstruction)
- ♀ >> ♂ due to estrogen (↑ cholesterol secretion) & progesterone (↓ bile acid secretion & ↑ stasis)
- 1:1600 to 4/10,000 pregnancies; 2nd most common cause of surgery during pregnancy

Pathophysiology
- >90% due to cystic duct stone → inflammation
- Gallbladder stasis/ischemia → acalculous cholecystitis; in severe injury, major nonbiliary surgery, severe trauma, burns, sepsis, infection (CMV, cryptococcus, HIV), vasculitis (polyarteritis nodosa)

See Table for workup and management

PANCREATITIS

Acute Pancreatitis
- Inflammation of the pancreas; diagnosed by 2 of the following criteria: Characteristic abdominal pain, elevation of lipase greater than 3× upper limit of normal (amylase less specific), CT, MRI, or US evidence of acute pancreatitis

- Incidence ~0.1% in pregnancy
- **Consider:** Gallstones, EtOH use, medications, hypertriglyceridemia, post-ERCP, hypercalcemia, pancreatic neoplasm or trauma, infection (EBV), vasculitis. Consider if pain, N/V after upper abdominal procedures (eg, splenectomy).

Management: Initial – Fluids, nutrition, pain control, ERCP for choledocholithiasis
- Complications: Pancreatic necrosis, pseudocysts, SIRS, chronic pancreatitis

Chronic Pancreatitis
- Primary cause is alcoholism, less likely genetic causes, ductal obstruction, autoimmune
- Pathogenesis unclear. Fibroinflammatory process, permanent damage to pancreas with endocrine and exocrine dysfunction
- Primary clinical manifestations: Abdominal pain and pancreatic insufficiency
- Complications include diabetes, pseudocysts, splenic vein thrombosis, bile duct, or duodenal obstruction
- Treatment is supportive/symptomatic

See Table for workup and management

Differential diagnosis of upper abdominal pain			
Disease	**Clinical manifestations**	**Workup**	**Treatment**
Cholelithiasis	70–80% asymptomatic, biliary colic: Episodic RUQ/epigastric pain, resolves in hours, worse with fatty food & at night, ±nausea and vomiting, ±tenderness to palpation, no F	**Labs:** Normal LFTs, CBC, lipase **RUQ US:** Mobile echogenic focus with acoustic shadow Monitor for complications including cholecystitis, choledocholithiasis, ascending cholangitis, hepatic abscess, pancreatitis, obstructive jaundice, fistulae	• IV fluids, analgesia • Cholecystectomy: If fail medical management • Prophylactic cholecystectomy only if large stones or ↑ risk gallbladder cancer • Poor surgical candidates: Ursodiol, lithotripsy (contraindicated in pregnancy)
Acute cholecystitis	Persistent RUQ/epigastric pain, fever, nausea, vomiting, abdominal tenderness on exam (Murphy's sign), rebound/guarding Acalculous cholecystitis: Fever, RUQ pain within 2–4 w of major surgery, critically ill patients with prolonged NPO or multisystem organ failure	**Labs:** Mild ↑ WBC, LFTs (amylase if +V), ± Bilirubin **RUQ US:** Thickened GB wall, pericholecystic fluid, gallstones > MRI in pregnancy if nonconclusive **Abdominal x-ray:** 15% radiopaque stones **HIDA scan:** Most sensitive if bilirubin <5, can show obstructed cystic duct (not in pregnancy)	• NPO, IV fluids, analgesia, antibiotics (2/3 generation cephalosporin+ metronidazole) • Cholecystectomy within 2–4 d of admit • Surgery difficult in pregnancy but ↓ morbidity, safest in 2nd trimester • Poor surgical candidates: Cholecystostomy, percutaneous drainage
Choledocholithiasis with ascending cholangitis	RUQ pain, fever, jaundice (Charcot triad)	**Labs:** ↑ WBC, LFTs, draw blood cultures ×2 **RUQ US:** Dilated gallbladder, ± gallstones **ERCP:** Dilated gallbladder, ± gallstones	• NPO, IV fluids, correct BMP, antibiotics (80–90% respond) • 15% need decompression by ERCP with sphincterotomy (may be done in pregnancy) or percutaneous drainage

Disease	Clinical manifestations	Workup	Treatment
Acute pancreatitis	Epigastric pain radiating to the back, nausea, vomiting, fever, abd pain on exam, distention, guarding Severity assessed by APACHE II criteria	**Labs:** ↑ Lipase, WBC, CMP, TG **Abdominal US:** Enlarged non-homogeneous pancreas, peri-pancreatic inflammation	• NPO, IV fluids, correct BMP, analgesia • Consider tube feeds or TPN if prolonged • Cholecystectomy vs. ERCP if due to gallstones

RUQ, right upper quadrant.

APPENDICITIS

Definition and Epidemiology

- Inflammation of appendiceal wall → ischemia or perforation
- Most common nontraumatic surgical emergency during pregnancy; 1:1600 pregnancies; usually in 2nd trimester
- Peak incidence in 2nd & 3rd decades of life; rare at extremes of age
- Incidence much lower in developing countries & in lower socioeconomic groups
- Morbidity & mortality often higher in pregnancy due to delay in diagnosis (25% perforated at time of diagnosis)

Pathophysiology

- Appendiceal luminal obstruction (50–80%) usually by fecalith (accumulated/hardened fecal matter around vegetable fibers) → inflammation/distention/ulceration/rupture. Other causes: Lymphadenitis (viral infections), inspissated barium, parasites (eg, pinworm, *Ascaris, Taenia*), & tumors (eg, carcinoid or carcinoma).
- Visceral pain poorly localizes to periumbilical or epigastric region; spread of peritoneal inflammation eventually localizes to right lower quadrant

Clinical Manifestations

- Vague periumbilical or right lower quadrant pain, anorexia, nausea, vomiting, low-grade fever
- In pregnancy appendix displaced superiorly and laterally by gravid uterus → right upper quadrant pain possible
- Tender McBurney point = ⅓ distance from anterior–superior iliac spine & umbilicus; psoas sign = pain with right hip flexion; Rovsing sign = left lower quadrant palpation elicits right lower quadrant pain; referred rebound tenderness often absent early & in pregnancy (due to separation of abd wall from viscera)
- Temperature >38.3°C (101°F) & rigidity suggest perforation
- ↑ Abortion or PTL risk; no impact on fertility unless ruptured appendix w/ subsequent adhesive disease

Workup

- **Labs:** Moderate leukocytosis, neutrophilia (not helpful in pregnancy), elevated CRP/ESR
- Abdominal US (1st-line in pregnancy) = enlarged thick-walled appendix, periappendiceal fluid; useful to exclude ovarian cysts, ectopic pregnancy, or tubo-ovarian abscess (sensitivity 86%, specificity 81%)
- Contrast-enhanced or nonenhanced abdominal CT (gold standard in nonpregnant patients): Distended, noncontrast-filled appendix, thickened appendiceal wall with periappendiceal stranding & often the presence of a fecalith (PPV 95–97%, overall accuracy 90–98%).
- MRI preferred in pregnancy (sensitivity 100%, specificity 93%)

Treatment and Medications

- Electrolyte correction & IV fluids
- **Perioperative Antibiotics:** Broad coverage for gram-positive/negative & anaerobes (2nd generation cephalosporin + clindamycin or metronidazole). Conservative management with antibiotic alone may be successful in some nonpregnant patients (*BMJ* 2012;344:e2156).
- Immediate appendectomy (laparoscopic preferred, safe during all trimesters of pregnancy, safest in 2nd trimester)

IRRITABLE BOWEL SYNDROME (IBS)

Definitions
- Chronic relapsing functional bowel disorder characterized by abdominal pain or discomfort & altered bowel habits in the absence of any other detectable organic disease

Subtypes of IBS		
Subtype	% Bristol stool form 1 or 2	% Bristol stool form 6 or 7
IBS-C (with constipation)	≥25	<25
IBS-D (with diarrhea)	<25	≥25
IBS-M (mixed)	≥25	≥25
Unsubtyped IBS	Insuff to meet criteria for other subtypes	

From *Gastroenterology* 2016;150:1393–407.
The Bristol stool form is a classification for human stool, with 1 being the hardest/driest stool lumps and 7 is liquid stool without solids.

Epidemiology
- 7–21% adults & adolescents affected worldwide (US 12%), with female predominance (1.5–2× greater than male)
- Prevalence decreases with age, most present with first symptom before age 45

Pathophysiology (*JAMA* 2015;313(9):949–58)
- Pathogenesis likely due to interaction of multiple factors
- Environmental factors: Early life stressors, food intolerance, antibiotics, enteric infection
- Host factors: Altered pain perception, altered brain-gut interaction, dysbiosis, increased intestinal permeability, increased gut mucosal immune activation, visceral hypersensitivity to stimuli

Clinical Manifestations

Rome III and Rome IV IBS diagnostic criteria				
(J Neurogastroenterol Motil 2017;23(2):151)				
	Presentation	Frequency	Duration	Associated with 2 or more of these
Rome III (previous diagnostic criteria)	Recurrent abd pain or discomfort	≥3 d/mo	Within last 3 mo	• Improves with defecation • Onset associated w/ change in freq of stool • Onset associated w/ change in appearance of stool
Rome IV* (current)	Recurrent abd pain	On average ≥1 d/w	In the last 3 mo	• Related to defecation (increase or decrease) • Associated w/ change in frequency of stool • Associated w/ change in stool form or appearance

*Nonspecific term "discomfort" removed; frequency simplified; defecation does not have to improve symptoms; and association with stool frequency and appearance no longer needs to be onset.

- **Typical features** (not diagnostic): Defecation straining, urgency or tenesmus, passing mucus & bloating, dyspepsia, heartburn, nausea & vomiting, loose/frequent stools, constipation, bloating, abdominal cramping, discomfort, pain, symptoms brought on by food intake, symptomatic change over time (change in pain location, change in stool pattern), symptoms often improved by passage of stool or flatus

- **Red flags** (concern for organic disease): Diagnosis >50 yo, severe or worsening symptoms, unexplained weight loss, nocturnal diarrhea, family history of cancer, celiac or IBD, rectal bleeding, unexplained iron deficiency anemia

Diagnostic Workup/Studies
- Diagnosis based on Rome IV criteria (see above)
- Studies to rule out other etiologies dependent on patient symptoms & presentation
- Workup can include CBC, endoscopy, celiac testing, and stool specimens (giardia) for those with diarrhea

Differential diagnosis of presenting IBS symptoms	
Primary symptom	**Differential diagnoses**
Epigastric or periumbilical pain	Biliary tract disease, peptic ulcer disorders, intestinal ischemia, carcinoma of stomach & pancreas
Lower abdominal pain	Diverticular disease, IBD, colon cancer, pelvic disease (including structural, pelvic floor myalgia, PID)
Postprandial pain	Gastroparesis, intestinal obstruction, gallbladder disease
Diarrhea	Intestinal infection, lactase deficiency, laxative abuse, malabsorption, celiac sprue, hyperthyroidism
Constipation	Side effect of drugs, endocrinopathies, intermittent porphyria, lead poisoning

Treatment and Medications
- Avoid food precipitants (common triggers include coffee, disaccharides, legumes, cabbage, artificial sweeteners)
- High-fiber diets (low evidence); avoid FODMAP foods (highly fermentable carbs)
- Increased physical activity, stress reduction, & psychosocial therapy
- Diarrhea → antispasmodics (peppermint oil), loperamide as needed, probiotics (low evidence)
- Constipation → psyllium, methylcellulose, calcium polycarbophil, lactulose, polyethylene glycol, lubiprostone, magnesium hydroxide
- Prescriptions: TCA, SSRI, antispasmodics, prosecretory agents (linaclotide), rifaximin, serotonin antagonists

INFLAMMATORY BOWEL DISEASE

Definitions
- Immune-mediated, noninfectious, chronic intestinal inflammation
- **Ulcerative colitis (UC):** Idiopathic continuous inflammation of colonic mucosa
- **Crohns disease (CD):** Idiopathic granulomatous transmural inflammation of gastrointestinal tract, from mouth to anus, with skip lesions

Pathophysiology
- Multifactorial; theoretically a chronic state of dysregulated mucosal immune function that is further modified by specific environmental factors (eg, smoking)

IBD and Pregnancy (Obstet Gynecol 2015;126:401–12)
- Preconception: Effective birth control, achieve remission before conception (≥6 mo), check vitamins and minerals (CBC, B12, folate, iron, D), discontinue medications that are harmful to the fetus when possible
- Conception: Normal fertility unless has had pelvic surgery (Ileal pouch anal anastomosis); ↑ disease activity ↑ SAB, infertility
- Medications that must be stopped: Methotrexate (stop 3–6 mo prior to conception)
- Pregnancy: Active disease is more dangerous that most medications, don't discontinue maintenance medications except methotrexate, monitor by high-risk OB, serial growth scan >28 w. ↑ Risk of PTL, LBW, IUGR with ↑ disease activity. Pregnancy does not ↑ likelihood of IBD flare
- Delivery: If active perineal disease (anorectal & perirectal abscesses & fistulas) → cesarean, otherwise no recommendations for mode of delivery
- Postpartum: Most meds are safe for lactation, if infant exposed to biologics, no live vaccines ×6 mo, otherwise normal vaccine schedule

Features of Crohns disease and ulcerative colitis		
	Crohns disease	**Ulcerative colitis**
Epidemiology	Incidence: 0.03–15.6/100000 persons per year Prevalence: 3.6–214/100000 Bimodal peak age of onset: 15–30 yo, 60–80 yo Associated with female gender, smoking, OCPs, & genetic predisposition	1.2–20.3/100000 new diagnoses per year Prevalence: 7.6–246/100000 Bimodal peak age of onset: 15–30 yo, 60–80 yo Appendectomy prior to age 20 & tobacco use may be protective factors (*N Engl J Med* 2011;365:1713)
Pathology	Macroscopic: Transmural inflammation that can affect any portion of GI tract from mouth to anus. "Skip lesions," nonfriable mucosa, long ulcers & fissures with "cobblestone" appearance, perirectal fistulas, fissures, abscesses, & anal stenosis Microscopic: Loose aggregations of macrophages form noncaseating granulomas in all layers of bowel wall 30–40% small bowel only, 40–50% affects small & large bowel, 15–25% colon only	Mucosal inflammation, ulceration, & chronic mucosal damage of colon, begins at rectum & extends proximally in a continuous fashion Macroscopic: Granular, friable mucosa with diffuse ulceration, pseudopolyps Microscopic: Inflammation limited to mucosa & superficial submucosa, crypt abscesses 40–50% disease limited to rectum & rectosigmoid, 30–40% extends beyond sigmoid but not entire colon, 20% total colitis
Clinical Manifestations	Either fibrostenotic-obstructing pattern or a penetrating-fistulous pattern Chronic history of recurrent abdominal pain & nongrossly bloody diarrhea, fever, malaise, bowel obstruction Extraintestinal symptoms: Erythema nodosum (15%), periph arteritis (15–20%), ankylosing spondylitis (10%), sacroiliitis, uveitis, episcleritis, hepatic steatosis, cholelithiasis, nephrolithiasis, low bone mass, thromboembolic events	Chronic relapsing & remitting attacks of bloody mucoid diarrhea; often grossly bloody diarrhea Abdominal cramping, tenesmus, colicky lower abdominal pain relieved by defecation Fever, weight loss Fulminant disease can result in toxic megacolitis or megacolon Extraintestinal manifestations: Erythema nodosum (10%), pyoderma gangrenosum (1–12%), sacroiliitis, uveitis, hepatic steatosis, thromboembolic events
Diagnostic Workup/Studies	Elevated ESR, CRP Hypoalbuminemia, anemia, leukocytosis in severe disease Endoscopy reveals rectal sparing, aphthous ulcerations or strictures Barium enema shows filling defects CT enterography shows radiographic "string sign"; areas of circumferential inflammation & fibrosis resulting in luminal narrowing ASCAs in 60–70% Colorectal cancer risk similar to UC, same recommendations as UC regarding surveillance	Elevated CRP, Plts, ESR Decreased Hb, leukocytosis Negative stool culture for bacteria, *Clostridium difficile*, O&P Sigmoidoscopy with colonic biopsies to confirm diagnosis via histology Barium enema – fine mucosal granularity, "collar-button" ulcers, loss of haustra: "Lead pipe" appearance pANCAs in 60–70% Monitor for colon cancer with annual or biennial colonoscopy with multi biopsies if >8–10 y of pancolitis or 12–15 y left-sided colitis

Treatment and medications for IBD

	Drug/ Intervention	Dose	Notes/Preg risk level
Mild IBD	Diet & lifestyle		Not primary treatment, avoid aggravating foods
	Sulfasalazine	500 mg/d–6 g/d	Antibacterial (sulfapyridine) & anti-inflammatory (5-ASA) Low risk in pregnancy & breastfeeding Folate supplementation 2 mg/d
	5-ASA	Mesalamine oral, enema, or suppository	Low risk in pregnancy & breastfeeding
Mod IBD	Corticosteroids Prednisone Hydrocortisone Methylprednisolone	40 mg/d PO with taper 300 mg/d IV 60 mg/d IV	Use if not responsive to 5-ASA; not maintenance drug Moderate risk in pregnancy; animal studies show associated with cleft palate in 1st trimester, also PROM, AI, GDM, SAB
	Antibiotics Metronidazole	1–1.5 g/d PO, maint therapy 750 mg/d	Use for inflammatory, fistulous, & perianal CD (not in UC) Moderate risk in pregnancy: MSK dysfunction (ciprofloxacin)
	Immunosuppressives 6-mercaptopurine Azathioprine MTX	In collaboration with GI specialist	Treatment & maintenance of remission, steroid-sparing agents High risk in pregnancy and breastfeeding: MTX (teratogenic)
Sev IBD	Immunosuppressives Cyclosporine Tacrolimus Anti-TNF Ab	In collaboration with GI specialist	Use if refractory to IV steroids
	Surgery		50% UC patients undergo surgery within 1st 10 y, most CD patients require at least 1 surgery in their lifetime; Indications for surgery: Intractable disease, toxic megacolon, colonic perforation, massive hemorrhage, extracolonic disease, colonic obstruction, intestinal stricture & obstruction, fistula, abscess, colon cancer prophylaxis

Note: Determine CD & UC severity using disease activity calculator (www.gastrotraining.com/calculators/cdai)
Data from Rajapakse R, Korelitz BI. Inflammatory bowel disease during pregnancy. *Curr Treat Options Gastroenterol.* 2001;4(3):245–251 and Mahadevan U & Matro R. Care of pregnant pt with inflammatory bowel disease. *Obstetrics and Gynecology.* 2015;126:401–12.

VIRAL HEPATITIS

Clinical Manifestations
- **Symptoms of acute hepatitis:** Anorexia, nausea & vomiting, fatigue, malaise, arthralgias, myalgias, headache, photophobia, pharyngitis, cough, coryza 1–2 w prior to jaundice; low-grade fever more common in HAV & HEV
- Dark urine & clay-colored stools may occur 1–5 d prior to onset of jaundice
- Jaundice with enlarged & tender liver w/ right upper quadrant pain
- Splenomegaly & cervical adenopathy 10–20%
- During "recovery phase," constitutional symptoms resolve but liver enlargement & abnormal liver enzymes may persist for 2–12 w

Diagnostic Labs/Exams
- Elevated AST & ALT (40–4000 U/L). Elevated bilirubin (jaundice visible when serum bilirubin >2.5 mg/dL [typically 5–20 mg/dL]). Assess PT/PTT, albumin, glucose.

Hepatitis A

- Nonenveloped RNA picornavirus. Replication limited to liver, but virus present in liver, bile, stools, & blood.
- Prevalence increases as a function of age & decreasing socioeconomic status
- **Transmission:** Fecal–oral route. 15–45-d incubation period, mean 4 w
- **Dx:** Active infection = anti-HAV IgM (can persist for several months)
  Prior exposure = anti-HAV IgG, detectable indefinitely → protective
- **Rx:** Supportive, recovery within 4–6 w
- No evidence that HAV is teratogenic; transmission to fetus has not been reported

Hepatitis B

- Small, circular DNA hepadnavirus
- Prevalence increases with lower socioeconomic status, older age groups, & persons with risk for exposure to blood
- Acute HBV occur in 1–2/1000 pregnancies; chronic HBV occur in 5–15/1000 pregnancies
- **Transmission:** Blood, sexual, perinatal (especially in infants born to HBsAg carrier mothers or mothers with active infxn, transmission correlates with presence of HBeAg). 30–180-d incubation period, mean 8–12 w.
- 85–90% complete resolution of infection after acute phase, 10–15% chronic infection
- Chronic HBV may develop cirrhosis, fulminant liver failure, & increased risk for hepatocellular carcinoma
- **Diagnostic serology:**
  HBsAg: 1st detectable marker, before LFTs or symptoms, acute or chronic infection
  Anti-HBs: Detectable indefinitely after disappearance of HBsAg or after vaccine
  HBcAg: Not typically detectable in serum
  Anti-HBc: Present 1–2 w after HBsAg, may be only serologic marker during "window" period; anti-HBc IgM suggests acute infection
  HBeAg: Increases with infectivity

Diagnosis of Hepatitis B by serology					
Diagnosis	HBsAg	Anti-HBs	Anti-HBc	HBeAg	Anti-HBe
Acute hepatitis	+	−	IgM	+	−
Window period	−	−	IgM	±	±
Recovery	−	+	IgG	−	±
Immunization	−	+	−	−	−
Chronic hepatitis	+	−	IgG	±	−

- **Prevention:** 3-dose pre-exposure vaccinations (at 0, 1, 6 mo)
  HBIg postexposure prophylaxis (including sexual exposure, needle stick, newborns)
- **Treatment:** Acute HBV → supportive. Chronic HBV → IFN-α, lamivudine, adefovir dipivoxil, PEGylated IFN, entecavir
- **HBV in pregnancy**
  Routine screening at 1st prenatal visit
  Increased risk of PTL, transplacental infection uncommon, **not** teratogenic
  Most neonatal infection vertically transmitted by peripartum exposure
  High perinatal transmission rate. 30% in HBeAg (−) mothers; >85% in HBeAg (+) mothers (N Engl J Med 1975;292(15):771)
  Cesarean delivery & bottlefeeding does **not** lower risk of transmission

Hepatitis C

- RNA virus; in US 70% genotype 1 (& most common worldwide), 30% genotype 2 or 3
  ~20% chronic HCV leads to chronic active hepatitis or cirrhosis, increased risk of hepatocellular carcinoma
  1–5% prevalence in pregnancy, highest rates in urban populations
- **Transmission:** Blood exposure; 15–160-d incubation period, mean 7 w
- **Serology**
  HCV antigens not detectable in serum so difficult to diagnose acute HCV
  Anti-HCV (ELISA) positive in 6 w–6 mo, does not imply recovery
  If + Anti-HCV, use HCV RIBA or HCV RNA (via PCR) to confirm diagnosis

Diagnosis of Hepatitis C by serology			
Diagnosis	HCV RNA	Anti-HCV (ELISA)	Anti-HCV (RIBA)
No infection	–	–	–
False positive	–	+	–
Early acute hepatitis	+	–	–
Past infection	–	+	+
Chronic hepatitis (active/ongoing)	+	+	+

- **Treatment:** PEGylated IFN, ribavirin. Newer regimens very successful – eg, glecaprevir (Hep C NS3/4 protease inhibitor) and pibrentasvir (NS5A inhibitor) for genotypes 1 through 6.
- **HCV in pregnancy:**
  Prenatal screening in high-risk women (concurrent alcoholism, IVDU, coexisting HIV infection, prior blood transfusion, tattoos)
  May be associated with LBW, need for assisted ventilation, NICU admit (*Am J Obstet Gynecol* 2008;199(1):38.e1)
  Unclear effect of pregnancy on progression of hepatic fibrosis
  Vertical transmission 5–10%. 3× higher with HIV coinfection (*Lancet* 1995;345(8945):289)
  Risk for vertical transmission increases with viral load. Cesarean delivery does not ↓ risk of transmission. Prolonged rupture of membranes may ↑ transmission.
  Ribavirin contraindicated in pregnancy. Breastfeeding **not** contraindicated.

Hepatitis D
- Defective RNA virus that requires coinfection or superinfection with HBV for replication & expression. In nonendemic areas, HDV infection confined to persons exposed frequently to blood (IVDU, hemophiliacs). In endemic areas, HDV infection predominantly by nonpercutaneous means.
- **Transmission:** Blood, sexual. 30–180-d incubation period, mean 8–12 w
- **Diagnosis:** Anti-HDV, HDV RNA
  No screening indicated as counseling & treatment same as HBV
  May consider screening if with symptomatic HBV
- **Treatment:** Similar to HBV

Hepatitis E
- RNA virus common to India, Asia, Africa, & Central America
- **Transmission:** Fecal–oral, rarely secondary person-to-person spread
  14–60-d incubation period, mean 5–6 w
- **Diagnosis:** IgM anti-HEV
- **Treatment:** Supportive
- **HEV in pregnancy:** Fatality rate up to 10–20% in pregnant women (1–2% nonpregnant), can cause fetal/neonatal hepatitis

Prevention/Vaccinations
- HAV & HBV vaccines safe during pregnancy. Vaccinate high-risk patients (more than 1 sex partner during previous 6 mo, treated for an STI, recent or current IVDU, having had an HBsAG-positive sex partner). May be vaccinated during pregnancy.

INTRAHEPATIC CHOLESTASIS OF PREGNANCY (ICP)

Definitions and Epidemiology
- Disease of intrahepatic biliary tree or hepatocellular secretory system resulting in elevated bilirubin & other solutes eliminated in bile (bile salts & cholesterol) that occurs during pregnancy
- Incidence 2 per 10000 in North America, 20 per 10000 in Europe
- Chronic hepatitis C associated with 20-fold ↑ in incid of cholestasis

Pathophysiology
- Unknown but likely genetically susceptible alterations in steroid & bile acid metabolism
- HLA-B8 & HLA-BW16 & gene mutations in hepatocellular transport systems (MDR3)
- May be related to circulating estrogen levels (increased incidence in twin pregnancies)
- Bile acids incompletely cleared & accumulate in plasma with associated dyslipidemia
- ↑ Meconium & intrapartum fetal distress (22–41%), PTL (19–60%), & IUFD (0.75–1.6%); especially if bile acids >40 μmol/L (*Glantz Hepatology* 2004;467)

Clinical Manifestations and Physical Exam
- Generalized pruritus in 2nd or 3rd trimester especially on palms & soles of feet
- Jaundice (20–75%)
- No associated rash, but excoriations from scratching

Diagnostic Workup/Studies
- Pruritus precedes lab abnormalities by several weeks
  - Hyperbilirubinemia (rarely exceeds 4–5 mg/dL)
  - ↑ Serum bile acids (chenodeoxycholic acid, deoxycholic acid, cholic acid) >10 μmol/L
  - ↑ Alkaline phosphatase more than nml pregnancy
  - Normal to moderately ↑ AST/ALT but seldom >250 U/L
- Liver biopsy shows mild cholestasis with centrilobular dilation and bile plugs (rare to biopsy)
- Rule out preeclampsia, not likely in setting of normal BP & absence of proteinuria
- Can consider right upper quadrant US to rule out cholelithiasis & biliary obstruction, normal in ICP

Treatment and Medications
- Symptoms & labs normalize 2–4 w after delivery but likely to recur in subsequent pregnancies or with exogenous estrogen use
- Antihistamines & topical emollients for symptomatic relief of pruritus
- Ursodeoxycholic acid recommended, cholestyramine alternative
- Consider antepartum testing after diagnosis; consider delivery at 37–38 w

HELLP SYNDROME

Definition and Epidemiology
- Variant of severe preeclampsia characterized by any combination of microangiopathic hemolysis, elevated serum transaminases, & low platelet count. (Partial HELLP refers to condition with only some criteria.) See also Chaps. 11–12.
- 0.5–0.9% of all pregnancies. 10–20% of those with eclampsia. See Chap. 18.
- Increased risk for eclampsia, PTL, & perinatal mortality

Pathophysiology
- Microangiopathic hemolysis leading to elevation of serum lactate dehydrogenase level & fragmented red blood cells on peripheral smear. Same process as preeclampsia, but more severe.
- Decreased platelets due to increased consumption

Clinical Manifestations
- Signs & symptoms of preeclampsia (elevated BP, proteinuria, focal edema, headache, vision changes)
- Right upper quadrant abdominal or midepigastric pain, nausea, vomiting
- Severe complications: Spontaneous rupture of subcapsular liver hematoma, placental abruption, DIC

Physical Exam and Diagnostic Workup/Studies (ACOG. Hypertension in pregnancy. 2013. Pg 3 (Box E-1))
- **Preeclampsia with severe features diagnostic criteria (highlighted are HELLP syndrome):**
  SBP >160, DBP >110 on 2 occasions, >4 h apart
  Plts <100,000 cells/mm^3
  LFTs >2× ULN
  Severe persistent right upper quadrant pain not responsive to medication and not from other diagnosis
  Cr >1.1 mg/dL, or doubling of baseline serum Cr
  Pulmonary edema
  Persistent neurological sx (headache, visual disturbances) not responsive to medications
- Criteria in past also included hemolysis on peripheral smear, LDH >600 U/L, or total bilirubin >1.2 mg/dL (Sibai criteria) or LDH >600 U/L (Martin criteria)
- **Imaging:** Right upper quadrant US, MRI, CT to assess hepatic hemorrhage that may result in subcapsular hematoma ± rupture. Consider if ↑↑ elevation in transaminases or severe pain.

Treatment and Medications
- Treatment similar to that for severe preeclampsia: Antihypertensives, magnesium sulfate, delivery: <Viability: Immediate delivery; Viability – 33 w6d: Betamethasone then delivery

in 24–48 h if stable; >34 w0d: Immediate delivery (not necc CS unless for obstetric indications).

- Presence of HELLP → immediate delivery due to ↑ maternal death (1%) & increased maternal morbidity: Blood transfusion (25%), DIC (15%), wound disruption (14%), placental abruption (9%), pulmonary edema (8%), renal failure (3%), & intracranial hemorrhage (1.5%) (Obstet Gynecol 2004;103:983)
- Dexamethasone may improve severe thrombocytopenia, but probably does not improve outcomes (Cochrane Database Syst Rev 2010;(9):CD008148)
- Increased risk for recurrence of HELLP in subsequent pregnancies (5–25%); higher incidence of PTL, IUGR, placental abruption & cesarean delivery in subsequent deliveries even without recurrence of HELLP

ACUTE FATTY LIVER OF PREGNANCY (AFLP)

Definitions and Epidemiology
- Hepatic microvesicular steatosis associated with mitochondrial dysfunction that can result in acute liver failure
- 1/10000 pregnancies
- Associated with mitochondrial abnormalities of fatty acid oxidation from autosomal inherited mutation (ie, LCHAD deficiency: Most common mutation G1528C)
- Occurs more often with nulliparas, male fetus, preeclampsia, & multifetal gestations

Clinical Manifestations
- Presents late in 3rd trimester – often with PTL or decreased fetal movement
- Nonspecific symptoms including persistent nausea & vomiting, malaise, fatigue, anorexia, epigastric pain, progressive jaundice, low-grade fever
- 50% with symptoms concerning for preeclampsia including hypertension, proteinuria, edema
- If severe: Ascites, coagulopathy, & spontaneous bleeding, SOB due to pulmonary edema, stillbirth, hepatorenal syndrome, hepatic encephalopathy, renal failure

Diagnostic Workup/Studies
- **Labs:** LFTs – ↑ bilirubin (>10 mg/dL), ↑ AST/ALT (typically less than 1000 U/L), CBC (hemoconcentration, leukocytosis, thrombocytopenia), coagulopathies (hypofibrinogenemia, hypoalbuminemia, hypocholesterolemia, prolonged clotting times, prolonged PT), hypoglycemia, or hyperglycemia secondary to pancreatitis
- Mother should undergo testing for LCHAD; can be lifesaving for neonate and inform risk for future pregnancies
- **Imaging** – Right upper quadrant US shows increased echogenicity; CT & MRI demonstrate lower liver density
- Liver biopsy, standard for confirming diagnosis but rarely used in clinical practice, shows microvesicular steatosis

Differentiating between AFLP and HELLP		
Signs & symptoms	AFLP (%)	HELLP (%)
Hypertension	50	85
Proteinuria	30–50	90–95
Fever	25–32	Absent
Jaundice	40–90	5–10
Nausea & vomiting	50–80	40
Abdominal pain	35–50	60–80
Hypoglycemia	Present	Absent

From Obstet Gynecol 2007;109(4):956–66.

Treatment and Medications
- **Supportive care:** Glucose infusion, reverse coagulopathy, IV fluid resuscitation
- **Delivery recommended** when diagnosis confirmed; spontaneous resolution after delivery, typically takes 1 w postpartum for hepatic dysfunction to resolve. During recovery period, 25% with transient diabetes insipidus & 50% with acute pancreatitis.
- May recur in subsequent pregnancies, even if no LCHAD mutation in mother. Historically with 70% maternal mortality rate, improved with early diagnosis to <10%.
- Perinatal mortality 13% due to high rate of preterm delivery

TOTAL PARENTERAL NUTRITION (TPN)

Definition, Indications, and Contraindications

- **TPN:** Intravenous supplementary nutrition including protein, caloric fat & dextrose, electrolytes, vitamins, minerals, & fluids. Generally a *temporary* intervention for severely limited oral intake (eg, intractable vomiting/diarrhea, gastrointestinal ischemia, high output fistula) or conditions of severe bowel dysfunction (eg, bowel obstruction, protracted ileus).
- **Contraindications:** Hyperosmolality, severe hyperglycemia, severe electrolyte abnormalities, volume overload, sepsis. Not recommended in advanced cancer
  (*J Parenter Enteral Nutr* 2009;33(5):472).

Ordering TPN

- Parameters depend on specific dysfunction; **consult nutritionist for TPN regimen**
- TPN initiated with slow continuous feed, can be advanced to 12-h cycle if tolerated
- Daily requirements: Water 30–40 mL/kg/d, energy 20–35 kcal/kg/d (based on activity level)
- Modify formula based on disease: Heart or kidney failure > limit volume, renal insufficiency > reduce protein, respiratory insufficiency > increase lipids as calorie source to decrease carbon dioxide production by carbohydrate metabolism

Average adult daily requirements		
TPN component	**Nutrition goal**	**Notes**
Protein	0.8–2 g amino acids/kg/d	
Carbohydrate	~60–70% nonprotein calories	<7 g dextrose/kg/d to avoid complications
Fat	25–40% nonprotein calories, no less than 2–4% total kcal as fat	<2.5 g/kg/d to avoid complications
Electrolytes	1–2 mEq Na/kg/d 1–2 mEq K/kg/d 5–7.5 mEq Ca/kg/d 20–40 mmol PO_4/kg/d 4–10 mEq Mg/kg/d	
Vitamins & trace elements	<u>Vitamins</u>: 3 mg B1, 3.6 mg B2, 40 mg B3, 400 μg folate, 15 mg B5, 4 mg B6, 5 μg B12, 60 μg biotin, 100 mg C, 1 mg A, 5 μg D, 10 mg E, 1 mg K <u>Minerals</u>: 10–15 μg Cr, 0.3–0.5 mg Cu, 60–100 μg Mn, 20–60 μg Se, 2.5–5 μg Zn	• MVI, thiamine, & folate for chronic EtOH abuse • Add zinc to promote wound healing • Add folate ± prenatal vitamin for pregnancy • Add trace elements if desired

From *JPEN J Parenter Enteral Nutr* 2002;26:1SA–138SA (available at www.nutritioncare.org).

TPN Monitoring

- **Baseline:** Chemistry panel, LFTs, lipids, albumin, transferrin, prealbumin
- **Daily (while increasing feed rates):** CBC, BMP, weight, fluid balance, gluc ≥4×/d
- **Weekly:** TG, LFTs, albumin, transferrin, prealbumin, PT time, Ca, Mg, Phos, P&Uosm
- Insulin sliding scale initially & transition to insulin in TPN mix when feasible

Complications

- **Access related (5–10% pts):** Sepsis, line infection, pneumothorax, hemothorax, brachial plexus injury
- **Metabolic effects (90% pts):** Hyper/hypoglycemia, hepatic dysfunction (mostly from amino acids), hepatomegaly (fat accumulation from excess carbohydrates), hyperammonemia, electrolyte alterations (ie, hyperK), nutrient excess or deficiency, Wernicke encephalopathy, refeeding syndrome (hypoPhos, hypoK, hypoMg), volume overload, bone demineralization, adverse reaction to lipid emulsions, gallbladder complications (stones, sludge, infection)
- Fetal complications of material TPN uncommon; supplement Vit K for pregnant patients on TPN, & follow serial growth US (*Obstet Gynecol* 2003;101(5 Pt 2):1142)

HEMATOLOGIC CHANGES OF PREGNANCY

Plasma Volume
- ↑ By 40–50% of baseline plasma vol (1000 m–1500 mL)
- Plasma vol ↑ at ~6 w & ↑ until 30–34 w, normalizes by 6 w postpartum
- Dilutional anemia of pregnancy due to expansion of plasma compared to RBCs – Lowest Hgb noted 28–36 w

RBC Mass
- 20–30% ↑ in RBC mass during Preg beginning at ~8–10 w gestation
- ↑ 2,3 Bisphosphoglycerate in pregnancy causes lower maternal O_2 affinity, facilitates O_2 across placenta
- 1000 mg iron req for Preg (RBCs – 500 mg, fetus – 300 mg, bleeding – 200 mg)

Leukocytes
- Leukocytosis of pregnancy due to increased circulation of PMNs
- PMN increase ~8 w gest, WBC = 5000–15000/μL
- Physiologic leukocytosis in labor & puerperium, WBC = 14000–16000/μL

Coagulation System
- 5-fold increased relative risk of thromboembolic dz; absolute risk 1/1500 pregnancies
- ↑ Risk from venous stasis (uterine mass effect), vessel wall injury, hypercoagulable state (↑ procoagulants up to 200%; ↓ prot S; ↓ antithrombin; decreased fibrinolysis; increased thrombin cleavage)
- Coagulation parameters normalize 6–12 w postpartum (*N Engl J Med* 2014;370:1307–15)

Blood Loss with Delivery
- Avg Estimated Blood Loss (EBL): Vaginal delivery = 500 mL; Cesarean delivery = 1000 mL. Cesarean hysterectomy = 1500 mL (nonurgent) & 2500 mL (emergent)
- Majority of blood loss 1st h after delivery → ~80 mL lochia over next 72 h

ANEMIA

Definition
- **Gravid:** Hgb ≤11 g/dL in 1st and 3rd trimester; ≤10.5 g/dL in 2nd trimester
- **Nongravid:** ≤12 g/dL
- IOM recommends decreasing Hgb cutoff for anemia by 0.8 g/dL for AAs
- **Risks:** Non-Hispanic Black, malabsorption (eg, celiac sprue), gastric bypass, iron-poor diet, menorrhagia, teenage, minority, low socioeconomic status, short Preg interval

Pathogenesis of anemia by mechanism	
↓ RBC production	Iron deficiency, B_{12}/folate deficiency, GI dz, chronic dz, bone marrow suppression, hypothyroidism
↑ RBC destruction	*Extravascular:* Sickle cell dz, thalassemias, G6PD deficiency, spherocytosis, liver/spleen dz, infxn (malaria, babesia), autoimmune hemolysis (SLE) *Intravascular:* HELLP, TTP–HUS, DIC, transfusion rxn, infection
Blood loss	Trauma, Surg, GI bleed
Dilution	IV fluids, *Dilutional anemia of pregnancy*

Clinical Manifestations
- Fatigue, headache, IUGR, preterm delivery, perinatal mortality, pica, restless leg syn
- Hb <6 g/dL a/w NRFHT, oligohydramnios, fetal death, CHF (Hgb <4 g/dL)
- **Signs:** Pallor (conjunctiva), tachy, orthostatic HoTN, jaundice (hemolysis), splenomegaly (thal, sickle cell, spherocytosis), petechiae (TTP, HUS, DIC)

Diagnostic Evaluation
- **Screening:** CBC w/ indices at 1st OB visit & 24–28 w gest; (MCV, RDW, retic count)
- **Adjunct Tests:** Periph smear, differential, MCV, iron, iron sat, ferritin, TIBC, folate, B_{12}, Hb electrophoresis, LFTs, BUN/Cr, TFTs, hemolysis labs (↑ indirect bili, ↑ LDH, ↓ haptoglobin), Bone marrow aspirate/bx
- RI = [retic count × (pt's Hct/nml Hct)]/maturation factor
  Maturation factor dependent on Hct; Hct ≤15% = 2.5, >16% = 2, >26% = 1.5, >36% = 1 (Nml is 1–2% for healthy ♀. >2–3% = adequate retic for anemia. <2% = inadeq.)

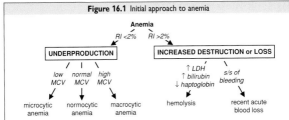

Figure 16.1 Initial approach to anemia

Anemia

RI <2% — RI >2%

UNDERPRODUCTION | INCREASED DESTRUCTION or LOSS

low MCV / normal MCV / high MCV

microcytic anemia | normocytic anemia | macrocytic anemia

↑ LDH
↑ bilirubin
↓ haptoglobin — s/s of bleeding

hemolysis — recent acute blood loss

(From: Sabatine MS. *Pocket Medicine*. 6th ed. Philadelphia, PA: Lippincott Williams & Wilkins; 2017.)

Normal iron indices		
Test	**Nml pregnant**	**Nml nonpregnant**
Serum iron level	40–175 μg/dL	60–150 μg/dL
TIBC	216–400 μg/dL	300–360 μg/dL
Transferrin sat	16–60%	20–50%
Serum ferritin level	>10 μg/dL	40–200 μg/dL

From *Obstet Gynecol* 2008;112(1):201–7.

Diagnosis of iron deficiency anemia		
Pathophysiology	**Lab profile**	**Additional testing**
Iron deficiency anemia	↓ Iron, ↑ TIBC, ↓ ferritin	↓ Transferrin sat Iron/TIBC <18%
Thal	Nml iron, TIBC, & ferritin	Periph smear – basophilic stippling Hb electrophoresis
Anemia of chronic dz	↓ Iron, ↓ TIBC, ↑ ferritin	↓ Transferrin sat Iron/TIBC >18%
Sideroblastic anemia	↑ Iron, ↓ TIBC, ↑ ferritin	Periph smear – basophilic stippling Bone marrow bx – ringed sideroblasts

Iron supplementation			
Form	**Preparation**	**Dose**	**Elemental iron**
PO	Ferrous gluconate	325 mg	34 mg/tablet
	Ferrous sulfate	325 mg	65 mg/tablet
	Ferrous fumarate	325 mg	106 mg/tablet
IV	Iron dextran (1% risk anaphylaxis)	Dose (mL) = 0.0042 (Desired Hb – Observed Hb) × LBW + (0.26 × LBW). Max 100 mg	50 mg/mL
	Iron sucrose	100 mg daily; max 10 d	20 mg/mL
	Sodium ferric gluconate	125 mg daily; max 8 d	12.5 mg/mL

Lean Body Weight (LBW) = (9270 × total body weight [kg])/(8780 + (244 × BMI)).
Data from Samuels P. Hematologic complications of pregnancy. In: Gabbe SG, et al. *Normal and Problem Pregnancies.* 6th ed. Churchill Livingstone; 2012:967–970 and ACOG Practice Bulletin No. 95: Anemia in Pregnancy. *Obstet Gynecol.* 2008;112(1):201–7.

Microcytic Anemia (MCV <80 fL)
- **Causes:** Iron deficiency, Thalassemia, chronic disease, copper/lead poisoning, most common anemia of pregnancy is iron deficiency
- **Eval:** Serum iron, TIBC (transferrin), ferritin (most sens/specific for iron def), transferrin sat
- ~30 mg/d of elemental iron req during Preg for prevention of anemia (in most PNV)
- **Rx:** Iron-rich foods (red meat, spinach, beans; Vit C rich foods for ↑ Absorp), iron supplements, IV iron, transfusion (for symptomatic anemia or Hb <6), erythropoietin

Normocytic Anemia (MCV 80–100 fL)

- DDx includes *acute blood loss, early iron deficiency*, bone marrow suppression (marrow invasion, RBC aplasia, aplastic anemia), chronic renal insufficiency, hypothyroidism, anemia of chronic dz, sideroblastic anemia

Macrocytic Anemia (MCV >100 fL)

- **Megaloblastic anemia:** Impaired DNA synthesis, *Hypersegmented neutrophils* are pathognomonic, tends to be highest in 3rd trimester

    Folate deficiency: Age, malnutrition (alcoholism), malabsorption (celiac sprue), meds (trimethoprim, methotrexate, nitrofurantoin), ↑ requirement (Preg, malig, dialysis)

    B_{12} deficiency: Causes – vegan diet, pernicious anemia, gastritis, bariatric Surg, malabsorption (Crohns, ileal resxn, tapeworm), meds (metformin, PPIs). May cause neurologic sx (eg, bilateral paresthesias and/or neuropathy)

- **Nonmegaloblastic anemia:** Causes include liver dz, alcoholism, reticulocytosis, hypothyroidism, myelodysplastic syn, medication (AZT, acyclovir, azathioprine)
- **Eval:** Serum B_{12}/folate, periph bld smear, homocysteine, methylmalonic acid, RBC folate (↑ Homocysteine in B_{12} & folate deficiency, ↓ methylmalonic acid in B_{12} deficiency only) Schilling test, anti-IF antibodies → positive in pernicious anemia
- MCV >115 fL almost exclusively in B_{12}/Folate def pts
- **Rx:** Folate deficiency – 1 mg PO QD, can precipitate neuro sx from B_{12}; B_{12} deficiency – 1 mg IM QD × q7d then weekly × 4 w then monthly as needed

Hemolytic Anemia

- **Eval:** ↑ Retic count (RI >2%), ↑ LDH, ↓ haptoglobin, ↑ indirect bilirubin
- Direct Coombs test, periph smear, Hb electrophoresis, osmotic fragility test

	Diagnosis of hemolytic anemia
Sickle cell anemia	Hb electrophoresis; sickled RBC/Howell–Jolly bodies on smear
Autoimmune	+ Warm AIHA: IgG; + direct Coombs
Microangiopathic	Schistocytes on smear, ↓ Plts; *DIC:* ↑ PT; *TTP–HUS:* ↑ Cr
HELLP	↑ LFTs; ↓ Plts; ↑ LDH; pregnancy; preeclampsia
Hereditary spherocytosis	+ Osmotic fragility test

HEMOGLOBINOPATHIES

Pathophysiology

- Genetic mutation of globin molecule: Qualitative (Sickle cell) or quantitative (Thalassemias)
- Adult Hb structure = 2 α-chains + 2 β-chains (HbA) or 2 δ-chains (HbA$_2$)
- Fetal Hb = 2 α-chains + 2 γ-chains (HbF) (12–24 w gest)

Thalassemias (Lancet 2012;379:373; Obstet Gynecol 2007;109:229)

- ↓ Synthesis of α- or β-chains → microcytic anemia
- **α-thal:** 4 α-chains (αα/αα) from 2 genes on chromo 16

    Gene mutation or deletion of ≥1 of 4 genes → abn Hb assembly → hemolysis & ↓ production

Types of alpha thalassemia		
Genes	**Description**	**Manifestations**
(α-/αα)	α-thal trait	Asymptomatic, Nml labs, At risk: Southeast Asian, African, W. Indian, & Mediterranean
(α-/α-) (αα/- -)	*Trans (diff chrom)* *Cis (same chrom)*	Mild, asymptomatic microcytic anemia; *Trans* = ↑ incid in African *Cis* = ↑ incid w/ Southeast Asian descent & ↑ risk HbH/Hb Bart in offspring
(α-/ – –)	HbH dz	Mild–mod hemolytic anemia, symptomatic at birth
(– –/– –)	Hb Bart's dz	Hydrops fetalis, IUFD; a/w preeclampsia

- **β-thal:** 2 β-chains from 1 gene on chrom 11

    At risk: Mediterranean, Asian, Middle Eastern, Hispanic, & West Indian

    1 β-chain mut → β-thal minor → mild anemia

    2 β-chain mutations → β-thal major (Cooley's anemia) → severe anemia, extramedullary hematopoiesis

    β-thal intermedia = 2 β-chain mutations w/ milder sx

- **Dx:** CBC (MCV <70), Hb electrophoresis, periph smear → basophilic stippling

- **Screening in Preg:** Pts in high-risk groups → CBC & iron indices → ↓ MCV & no iron deficiency → Hb electrophoresis. If Southeast Asian, DNA testing for α-thal
- Prenatal testing for α- & β-thal if mut/deletions in both parents via CVS, amnio, or PGD
- Preg in β-thal major recommended only if nml cardiac fxn & prolonged hypertransfusion → Hb >10 & w/ iron chelation
- **Rx:** Transfusion for anemia + iron chelation; splenectomy; hematopoietic xplant

Sickle Cell Disease (Lancet 2010;376:2018; Obstet Gynecol 2007;109(1):229)
- Autosomal recessive, β-chain mut (valine replaces glutamic acid at 6th amino acid) resulting in abn Hb structure (HbS replaces HbA)
- HbS (heterozygote) = sickle cell trait; HbSS (homozygote) = sickle cell anemia
- **Sickle cell variants:** HbC not a/w dz; HbSC same as HbSS but ↓ frequency; HbS + thal a/w varying severity of dz
- 1 in 12 AAs w/ trait, 1 in 500 w/ dz; ↑ risk in Mediterranean, Indian, Middle Eastern, Central/South American
- HgbSS: ↓ Oxygen tension → Hgb less soluble, RBC aggregate into sickles → hemolysis & microvascular occlusion
- Normocytic, normochromic anemia, ↑ Retic ct, ↓ haptoglobin, ↑ LDH
- **Microvascular occlusion and extravascular hemolysis → severe anemia, infection, pain crises**
    Hemolysis: Splenic sequestration, aplastic (parvovirus B19)
    Infarction: Painful crises, acute chest syn, CVA, multiorgan failure: Functional asplenia, kidneys (renal papillary necrosis), heart, & brain (CVA)
    Infection: Asplenia by adulthood, encapsulated organisms (Hib, S. pneumoniae, Meningococcus), osteomyelitis
    Acute chest = new lung infiltrate + respiratory symptoms + T >38.5 from vaso-occlusion of pulm vessels; 3% mortality (see below)
- **Dx:** Hb electrophoresis (gold standard); bld smear w/ sickled RBCs & Howell–Jolly bodies
- **Rx:** Hydroxyurea → ↑ HbF (more soluble) → ↓ frequency of pain crises, acute chest syn & need for transfusion (simple vs. exchange xfusion); iron chelation; hematopoietic stem cell xplant (selected pts w/ sev dz)
    Acute pain crisis → Opioids are mainstay, O₂ for oximetry <95%, IV hydration
    Infxn → vaccination against Hib, S. pneumoniae, N. meningitides outside pregnancy; influenza, & HBV inside pregnancy
    Acute chest syndrome: Simple versus exchange transfusion, broad spectrum antibiotics, supplemental O₂
- **HgbSS Preg:** ↑ Risk pain crises, acute chest syn, PROM, preeclampsia, pyelo, bld xfusion, alloimmunization, & infxn; ↑ fetal/neonat risk SAB (30%), IUFD, IUGR, PTD (25%), ↓ birth weight (20–40%). Prenatal diagnosis available
    Mgmt: Avoid hydroxyurea (teratogenic in animal studies, limited pregnancy data), 4 mg folate daily, avoid cold, exertion, dehydration to prevent pain crises. Goal: Hb ~10 g/dL & ≤40% HbS (Obstet Gynecol 2007;109(1):229)
    Serial growth US & antenatal testing at 32 w for fetal monitoring
    ↑ Risk of pyelo w/ asymptomatic bacteriuria. Consider urine cx each trimester and UTI ppx only for routine indications

THROMBOCYTOPENIA (Plt <150000/μL)

- Plt 50000–100000: ↑ Risk for bleeding w/ major trauma, thought to have minimal surgical risk, typically does not require transfusion
- Plt 20000–50000: ↑ Bleeding risk w/ minor trauma or surgery
- Plt <20000: ↑ Risk spont bleeding (<10000 ↑ risk of life-threatening bleeding)

	Etiology of thrombocytopenia by mechanism
↑ Destruction	ITP, infxn (HIV, HSV, HCV), SLE, APS, CVVH, meds (Heparin, quinidine, AZT, sulfonamides), DIC, TTP-HUS
↓ Production	Viral infxn, chemo, radiation, EtOH, folate/B₁₂ deficiency, MDS, leukemia, malig infiltrating bone marrow, myelofibrosis
Abn distribution	Splenic sequestration, dilution, hypothermia
Preg assoc	Gestational thrombocytopenia (66%), pregnancy-associated HTN (21%), HELLP syn, NAIT

Etiology (Obstet Gynecol 2016;128:43)

- **Gestational thrombocytopenia:** 8% of pregnancies; most common thrombocytopenia in preg (66%); 2nd–3rd trimester, Plt typically >75000/μL; Causes hemodilution, ↑ turnover, Asx, no h/o bleeding or prior thrombocytopenia, <1% incidence of neonatal thrombocytopenia, low bleeding risk, resolves 2–12 w postpartum
- ITP → IgG-mediated; persistent Plt <100000/μL; dx of exclusion (nml bld smear, no systemic dz); 15% of neonates have Plt <50000/μL (trans placental IgG)
- TTP–HUS → thrombocytopenia + microangiopathic hemolytic anemia ± renal failure ± fever ± Δ mental status; etiology: Meds (quinine, chemo, cyclosporine), Preg, Shiga toxin-producing *E. coli*, SLE, sev *ADAMTS13* deficiency
- DIC → etiology: Sepsis, Preg (abruption, HELLP, PPH, IUFD, septic AB, preE), Surg, hepatic failure, transfusion rxn (see section below)
- HELLP syndrome → See Chap. 15
- HIT → (see section below)

Evaluation

- **H&P:** PMHx, meds, infxns, splenomegaly, LAD, petechiae, mucosal bleeding
- **Labs:** CBC ± periph smear; retic count, LDH, haptoglobin, bilirubin, PT/aPTT, fibrinogen, D-dimer, Coombs, ANA, enzyme-immunoassay for HIT, HIV, HCV, Parvovirus, CMV, antiphospholipid antibodies, bone marrow bx

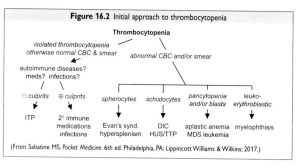

Figure 16.2 Initial approach to thrombocytopenia

(From Sabatine MS. *Pocket Medicine*. 6th ed. Philadelphia, PA: Lippincott Williams & Wilkins; 2017.)

Management of thrombocytopenia	
Gestational	Monthly to bimonthly CBC; check for resolution 1–3 mo postpartum to exclude ITP
ITP	Treatment indicated if sx bleeding, plts <30K, for procedures 1st line: PO corticosteroids, IVIG, Anti-RhD Ig (*Blood* 2010;115(2):169) 2nd line: Splenectomy, rituximab, immunosuppression, danazol
HIT	Stop heparin; consider alternate agent (lepirudin, argatroban, danaparoid) vs. no rx w/ screening for DVT
TTP–HUS	Plasma exchange ± glucocorticoids; FFP if delay in rx & bleeding
DIC	Rx underlying cause; Plts & FFP/cryoprecipitate (goal fibrinogen >100 mg/dL)

Neuraxial analgesia: No threshold predicts complications (eg, epidural hematoma); generally safe if Plt >100–80K; contraindicated for Plt <50K; may be safe for Plt less than 75K, requires consensus among OB, anesthesia, & pt, individualized decision
From *Anesthesiology* 2007;106(4):843–63.

Heparin-induced Thrombocytopenia (HIT)

- Plts <150K, ↓ plt >50%, venous/arterial thrombosis, necrotic skin lesion, systemic rxn after IV heparin bolus following new start or long-term LMWH or UFH use
- HIT Type I (Nonimmune) → ↓ plt w/in day 1–2 of heparin; not clinically significant, plts ~100K, can manage expectantly and continue heparin
- HIT Type II (Ab to heparin-PF4 complex), Plt 30–70K w/in 4–10d; ↑ risk thrombosis – venous (DVT, PE) & arterial (MI, CVA)
- **Dx:** Pts w/ intermediate or high 4T's pretest probability require confirmatory testing
- Ag assays (Anti-heparin/PF4 ELISA) vs. functional assays (serotonin release assay [gold std], heparin-induced Plt aggregation)

- **Rx:** Acute HIT — stop heparins & initiate parenteral direct thrombin inhibitor (argatroban or bivalirudin) or fondaparinux (SubQ) at therapeutic dosing; use danaparoid (1st line but not available in US) or fondaparinux (2nd line) for pregnant pts; after initial IV or SQ therapy transition to warfarin alone in nonpregnant pts when INR therapeutic (after bridging w/ nonheparin) AND Plt >150K

Incidence of HIT after ≥4 d of heparin exposure (% HIT)	
Postop pts	Prophylactic heparin (1–5%); therapeutic heparin (1–5%); prophylactic or therapeutic LMWH (0.1–1%)
Medical pts	Cancer pts (1%); prophylactic or therapeutic heparin (0.1–1%); prophylactic or therapeutic LMWH (0.6%); OB pts (<0.1%)

From Linkins LA, Dans AL, Moores LK, et al. Treatment and prevention of heparin-induced thrombocytopenia: Antithrombotic Therapy and Prevention of Thrombosis, 9th ed: American College of Chest Physicians Evidence-Based Clinical Practice Guidelines. *Chest.* 2012;141(2 suppl):e495S–530S.

Pretest probability of HIT for presumptive diagnosis			
4 "T's"	2 points	1 point	0 points
Thrombocytopenia	Plts fall >50% & nadir ≥20K	Plts fall 30–50% & nadir 10–19K	Plts fall <30% & nadir <10000
Timing of Plt count fall	Onset 5–10 d after heparin rx OR fall ≤1 d if heparin rx w/i last 30 d	Onset 5–10 d (but unclear) OR onset after day 10 OR fall ≤1 d if heparin rx w/i last 30–100 d	Onset <4 d w/o recent heparin rx
Thrombosis	Thrombosis, skin necrosis, or acute systemic rxn after heparin	Recurrent thrombosis on anticoagulation OR suspected thrombosis (awaiting confirmation) OR nonnecrotizing skin lesion	None
O**T**her causes	None likely	Poss	Probable (see "Etiology")

Probability (based on score) 0–3: Low (<1%); 4–5: Intermediate (~10%); 6–8: High (~33%)

From J Thromb Haemost 2006;4(4):759–65.

VENOUS THROMBOEMBOLIC DISEASE

Definition
- **DVT:** Most commonly in legs; Distal (calf vein) vs. Proximal (popliteal/femoral/iliac veins) Prox vein thrombosis → ↑ risk embolism, Calf vein thrombosis 80% spont resolve
- **PE:** Thrombus from venous system mobilizes to pulm arterial circulation
- **VTE:** Up to 600K pts affected annually causing up to 100K VTE-related deaths

Pathology
- Virchow's triad:
    1. *Endothelial injury* — Surg, tobacco use, trauma, atherosclerosis, age
    2. *Hypercoagulable state* — thrombophilia, hyperestrogenic (pregnancy, med), malig
    3. *Alterations to blood flow/stasis* — prolonged immobilization, cardiac dz, sickle cell

Clinical Manifestations
- **DVT:** Most asymptomatic, some have unilateral ext pain, lower-extremity edema (asymmetric), pain, erythema, palpable cord, (+) Homan's sign (calf pain on dorsiflexion in <5% of pts). Exam: >2 cm midleg diameter asymmetry (most sensitive), Homan's sign (pain in calf w/ ankle dorsiflexion; not sensitive)
- **PE:** Dyspnea, pleuritic chest pain, cough, syncope. Exam: Tachy, tachypnea, hypoxia, crackles, fever, Homan's sign, cyanosis, pleural rub, loud P₂, massive ↑ JVP

Diagnostic Evaluation (DVT)
- **Studies:** Mod/high sens D-dimer <500 ng/mL has NPV = 94% for absence of DVT (Not reliable in postop state or in Preg or if high pretest probability), compression ultrasonography (PPV = 94%), contrast venography, MRI

Pretest probability of DVT (Wells DVT Score)

Factors increasing score (1 point for each factor)

Active cancer	Entire leg swollen
Paralysis/paresis/immobilization	Calf swelling ≥3 cm c/w asymptomatic side
Bed rest ≥3 d or major Surg last 4 w	Pitting edema >in symptomatic leg
Localized tenderness along veins	Collateral superficial vein Prev documented DVT

Factor decreasing score (–2 points)

Alternate dx at least as likely as DVT (eg, muscle strain, lymphangitis, Baker's cyst)

Score: ≥3 → high probability; 1–2 → mod probability; ≤0 → low probability

From *Lancet* 1997;350(9094):1795–8.

Figure 16.3 Evaluation for DVT based on pretest probability (Wells DVT Score, see above)

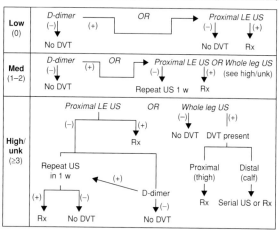

(From Bates SM, Jaeschke R, Stevens SM, et al. Diagnosis of DVT: Antithrombotic Therapy and Prevention of Thrombosis, 9th ed: American College of Chest Physicians Evidence-Based Clinical Practice Guidelines. *Chest.* 2012;141(2 suppl):e351S–e418S.)

Figure 16.4 Suspected DVT in pregnancy

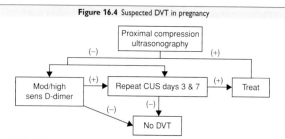

(From Bates SM, Jaeschke R, Stevens SM, et al. Diagnosis of DVT: Antithrombotic Therapy and Prevention of Thrombosis, 9th ed: American College of Chest Physicians Evidence-Based Clinical Practice Guidelines. *Chest.* 2012;141(2 suppl):e351S–e418S.)

Diagnostic Evaluation (PE)

• **D-dimer:** <500 ng/mL may exclude DVT/PE; may be difficult to interpret in Preg

- **Compression US/Doppler US (CUS):** Sufficient to rule in PE; 2% false (+) *(Ann Intern Med 1997;126(10):775)*
- **CTA:** Most common 1st-line test; sens 83% & spec 96% w/ MDCT & institutional experience; contraindications include renal dz, contrast allergy or prior rxn
- **V/Q:** Use for pts w/ contraindications to CTA, centers not experienced w/ CTA, or pregnant women w/ nml CXR & w/o leg sx. Abn CXR obscures findings.
- **Echocardiography:** ↑ RV size, ↓ RV fxn, tricuspid regurgitation, RV thrombus signs more likely w/ large PE; use in critically ill pts w/ high probability of PE
- **ABG:** Hypoxemia, hypocapnia, respiratory acidosis, ↑ A-a gradient; not routine screen
- **ECG:** Sinus tach, $S_1Q_3T_3$ or RBBB *(Am J Cardiol 1991;68(17):1723)*
- **CXR:** Atelectasis, effusion, ↑ hemidiaphragm, Hampton hump, Westermark sign; 1st study for PE workup in pregnant pts if no leg sx; not routine in nongravid pts for PE eval
- **MRA/MRV:** Sens 78% & spec 96% if technically adequate; 52% of studies inadeq; sens 100%, 84%, & 40% for lobar, segmental, & subsegmental PE, respectively
- **Pulm angiography:** Reserved for pts w/ consideration for endovascular rx of PE

VEN THR DISEASE 16-8

Pretest probability scoring of PE *(JAMA 2006;295:172)*	
Points	**Factors**
3 each	(1) Alternate dx less likely than PE, (2) clinical S/S of DVT
1.5 each	(1) Prior PE/DVT, (2) HR >100
1 each	(1) Surg w/i 4 w or bed rest ≥3 d, (2) hemoptysis, (3) cancer
Dichotomized Wells Score (use for CTA)	
Score ≤4: PE "unlikely"	Score >4: PE "likely"

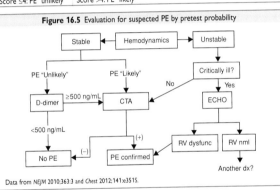

Figure 16.5 Evaluation for suspected PE by pretest probability

Data from *NEJM 2010;363:3* and *Chest 2012;141:e351S*.

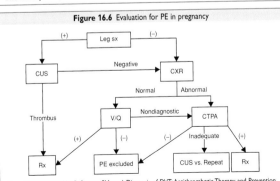

Figure 16.6 Evaluation for PE in pregnancy

(From Bates SM, Jaeschke R, Stevens SM, et al. Diagnosis of DVT: Antithrombotic Therapy and Prevention of Thrombosis, 9th ed: American College of Chest Physicians Evidence-Based Clinical Practice Guidelines. Chest. 2012;141(2 suppl):e351S–e418S.)

- If high clinical suspicion, treat immediately, do not wait for diagnostic testing. If hemodynamically unstable, consider thrombolysis.
- **Initial rx:** ≥5 d of UFH, LMWH, fondaparinux + warfarin, or thrombolysis/embolectomy
- **Long-term rx:** ≥3 of non-vitamin K oral anticoagulant (NOAC); also called direct oral anticoagulant (DOAC) dabigatran, rivaroxaban, apixaban, edoxaban over warfarin

Acute treatment of VTE	
LMWH	Preferred medication in setting of VTE associated with malignancy • Enoxaparin 1 mg/kg SQ q12h • Tinzaparin 175 U/kg SQ QD; contraindication if pt >70 yo w/ renal failure • Dalteparin 200 U/kg QD (max 18,000 U); Avoid if pt >90 kg
Non-Vitamin K oral anticoagulants (NOAC or DOAC)	• Dabigatran 150 mg PO BID • Rivaroxaban 15 mg PO BID × 3 w, then 20 mg PO QD × 6 mo • Apixaban 10 mg PO BID × 7 d, then 5 mg BID • Edoxaban: >60 kg 60 mg PO QD, <60 kg 30 mg PO QD
UFH	Target aPTT 1.5–2.5 times reference range; may use if renal dz • IV: Bolus 80 IU/kg or 5000 IU, then 18 IU/kg/h • SQ: 17500 U or 250 U/kg q12h
Factor Xa inhib	• Fondaparinux 5 mg (<50 kg), 7.5 mg (50–100 kg), & 10 mg (>100 kg) QD; use pts w/ current or prior PE; contraindication in renal failure
IVC filter	• Pts w/ contraindication to anticoagulation, failed anticoagulation, or complication w/ rx
Thrombolysis	• tPA reserved for acute PE w/ sev HoTN & no bleeding risk, Thrombolytics with relative contraindication in pregnancy
Embolectomy	• Unstable pts w/ failed or contraindication to thrombolysis
Long-term anticoagulation after VTE	
NOAC	• Rivaroxaban or apixaban can be initial monotherapy • Dabigatran or edoxaban require LMWH overlap
Warfarin	• Start after heparin, initial max 5 mg daily, titrate to goal INR 2–3

From Chest 2016;149(2):315–52.

Duration of anticoagulation	
Clinical scenario	**Duration**
1st DVT or PE due to provoked event	3 mo
1st unprovoked DVT or PE	≥3 mo
After 3 mo, reassess long-term need; if no contraindication → rx	Long-term rx
Recurrent DVT or PE or high-risk thrombophilia	Long-term rx
DVT or PE secondary to cancer (rx while cancer is "active")	>3–6 mo

From Lancet 2012;379(9828):1835–46.

Pregnancy Considerations (Obstet Gynecol 2011;118(3):717)
- Preg w/ 4–5-fold risk VTE; 0.5–2/1000 pregnancies, 80% = DVT, 20% = PE; increased risk across all trimesters, but 3rd trimester highest risk
- 50–60% DVT in preg occurs antepartum and 80% are left leg.
- Most important risk factor is personal history of VTE
- Thrombophilia present in 20–50% of women w/ VTE during Preg
- **D-dimer:** Levels ↑ during Preg & w/ preeclampsia, not for use as independent screen
- Warfarin contraindicated in Preg (except in setting of mechanical heart valve); crosses placenta, greatest risk of teratogenicity @ 6–12 WGA; fetal/neonatal hemorrhage in 3rd trimester; safe during lactation
- May use UFH or LMWH during Preg & lactation, use UFH after 36 w gest, do not cross placenta
- Stop anticoagulation at onset of labor. Delay neuraxial anesthesia for 10–12 h after prophylactic dose LMWH & 24 h after therapeutic dose LMWH.
- Resume UFH & LMWH usually 6–12 h after vaginal deliv or 12–24 h after C/S
- No data for novel oral anticoagulants in pregnancy or breastfeeding

THROMBOPHILIA EVALUATION

- **Coagulopathy:** Alteration in the ability of the blood to coagulate (↑ risk to bleed or to clot)
- **Thrombophilia:** Disease state that ↑ risk of thrombosis (acquired or inherited)

		Inherited thrombophilias			
	Prev (%)	VTE risk Preg (%) (no h/o VTE)	VTE risk Preg (%) (prior VTE)	Test reliable during preg?	Test reliable w/ thrombosis
FVL heterozygote	1–15	0.5–1.2	10	Yes	Yes
FVL homozygote	<1	4	17	Yes	Yes
PT gene heterozygote	2–5	<0.5	>10	Yes	Yes
PT gene homozygote	<1	2–4	>17	Yes	Yes
FVL/PT double heterozygote	0.01	4–5	>20	Yes	Yes
AT-III	0.02	3–7	40	Yes	No
Pro C deficiency	0.2–0.4	0.1–0.8	4–17	Yes	No
Pro S deficiency	0.03–0.13	0.1	0–22	No*	No

*May obtain free protein S antigen.
FVL, Factor V Leiden; PT, Prothrombin gene mutation; AT-III, Antithrombin III; Pro C, Protein C activity; Pro S, Protein S free antigen.
Data from *Obstet Gynecol* 2013;122:706 and *NEJM* 2001;344:1222.

Indications for Testing
- Personal h/o VTE
- 1st-degree relative w/ h/o high-risk thrombophilia, or VTE at <50 yo in absence of other risk factors (*Obstet Gynecol* 2011;118:718)
- See antiphospholipid antibody syndrome for acquired thromboembolic d/o

Diagnostic Evaluation
- **FVL:** Activated prot C resistance assay, if abn → DNA analysis
- **Prothrombin G20210A Mutation:** PCR DNA analysis
- **AT-III:** Antithrombin activity assay (<60% diagnostic)
- **Pro C & Pro S Deficiencies:** Functional assays for prot C & prot S (<50% diagnostic). Cannot detect in pregnancy due to risk of false negative.

Clinical Considerations
- No clear association between inherited thrombophilias & fetal loss, preeclampsia, IUGR, or abruption → screening not routinely recommended in these scenarios

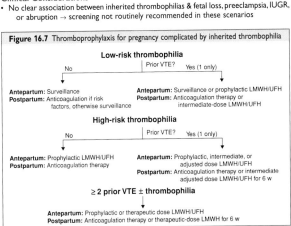

Figure 16.7 Thromboprophylaxis for pregnancy complicated by inherited thrombophilia

Low-risk thrombophilia

Prior VTE?

No → **Antepartum:** Surveillance
Postpartum: Anticoagulation if risk factors, otherwise surveillance

Yes (1 only) → **Antepartum:** Surveillance or prophylactic LMWH/UFH
Postpartum: Anticoagulation therapy or intermediate-dose LMWH/UFH

High-risk thrombophilia

Prior VTE?

No → **Antepartum:** Prophylactic LMWH/UFH
Postpartum: Anticoagulation therapy

Yes (1 only) → **Antepartum:** Prophylactic, intermediate, or adjusted dose LMWH/UFH
Postpartum: Anticoagulation therapy or intermediate adjusted dose LMWH/UFH for 6 w

≥ 2 prior VTE ± thrombophilia

Antepartum: Prophylactic or therapeutic dose LMWH/UFH
Postpartum: Anticoagulation therapy or therapeutic-dose LMWH for 6 w

- Avoid estrogen-containing contraceptives in pts w/ inherited thrombophilias
- **Low-risk thrombophilias:** Factor V Leiden heterozygous; prothrombin G20210A heterozygous; prot C or prot S deficiency
- **High-risk thrombophilias:** Antithrombin deficiency; double heterozygous for prothrombin G20210A mut & factor V Leiden; factor V Leiden homozygous or prothrombin G20210A mut homozygous

Anticoagulation regimens in pregnancy and postpartum*	
Prophylactic LMWH	Enoxaparin 40 mg SQ daily, dalteparin 5000 U SQ daily, or tinzaparin 4500 U SQ daily. NO MONITORING needed.
Therapeutic LMWH	Enoxaparin 1 mg/kg q12h, dalteparin 200 U/kg daily, or 100 U/kg q12h, tinzaparin 175 U/kg daily. Consider UFH at 36–37 w to permit neuraxial anesthesia.
Prophylactic UFH	1st trimester: UFH 5000–7500 U SQ q12h 2nd trimester: UFH 7500–10000 U SQ q12h 3rd trimester: UFH 10000 U SQ q12h, unless aPTT is elevated
Therapeutic UFH	UFH ≥10000 U SQ q12h to target therapeutic aPTT (1.5–2.5) 6 h after injection
Anticoagulation postpartum	Prophylactic LMWH/UFH for 4–6 w or warfarin 4–6 w w/ target INR 2–3 (need UFH or LMWH therapy until INR is 2 for ≥2 d)

*Warfarin, LMWH, and UFH can be continued in breastfeeding women; no data for novel oral anticoagulants.
From Obstet Gynecol 2013;122:706.

Monitoring Treatment
- Preg causes ↑ renal clearance which may ↑ heparin clearance & require ↑ dose; do not routinely monitor in pregnancy though can be considered in select situations
- UFH → check aPTT 6 h after injection (midinterval), goal 1.5–2.5× nml range, long-term rx check aPTT every 1–2 w; monitor for thrombocytopenia (see section on HIT)
- LMWH → reliable dose-dependent resp; may monitor rx w/ anti Xa level 4 h after injection, target 0.5–1 IU/mL; monitoring may be considered if CrCl <30 mL/min or obese pts

Anticoagulation Reversal
- UFH → Bleeding rapidly reversed by administration of protamine sulfate
- LMWH → Incomplete reversal of bleeding with protamine sulfate (aPTT slower to respond). Should be used if bleeding severe.
- Warfarin → Bleeding reversed with Vit K, FFP, 4-factor prothrombin complex concentrate

COAGULOPATHIES

Signs/Symptoms
- Mucocutaneous bleeds (ie, epistaxis, gingival bleeding), menorrhagia, bleeding w/ dental extraction, petechiae, ecchymoses, postop bleeding, PPH, hemarthrosis

Disseminated Intravascular Coagulation (DIC)
- **Pathogenesis:** Systemic activation of coagulation → thrombosis of small–mid-size vessels → depletion of coagulation factors → hemorrhage, thrombosis, multiorgan failure
- **Etiology:** Sepsis, trauma, shock, cancer, obstetric (abruption, AFE, IUFD)
- **Dx:** ↑ PT/aPTT, ↓ Plt (<100K), ↓ fibrinogen (<300 concerning in pregnancy, as fibrinogen is elevated in pregnancy above normal), ↓ haptoglobin, +schistocytes on peripheral smear
- **Rx:** Manage underlying condition; for bleeding or high risk of bleed, give platelet or FFP xfusion (Plt <20K or Plt <50K & bleeding; goal fibrinogen >100 mg/dL)

Von Willebrand's Disease (vWD) (AJOG 2010;203:194; Obstet Gynecol 2013;122:706)
- Most common bleeding d/o; send labs for patients with heavy menses since menarche, PPH, surgical or dental bleeding, or two or more sxs like epistaxis, gum bleeding, FH
- **Pathogenesis:** vWF forms bridge btw Plts/Plts & subendothelial surfaces; carrier of FVIII; deficiency → bleeding predisposition
- **Inherited:** Quantitative vs. qualitative deficiency
  - **Type 1:** ~80% of cases; partial quantitative deficiency; autosomal dominant
  - **Type 2:** Qualitative deficiency (4 subtypes); autosomal dominant
  - **Type 3:** Rare, autosomal recessive; sev quantitative deficiency; high risk of bleeding

- **Acq:** ↑ Clearance/inhibition of vWF (autoimmune dz), ↑ destruction of vWF (VSD, AS, pHTN), or medication (ie, ciprofloxacin, valproate)
- **Dx:** Isolated ↑ aPTT or nml w/ normal CBC; if ↑ aPTT, get mixing study to eval for FVIII inhib (PTT corrects with mixing study in vWD); confirm dx w/ ↓ vWF: Ag (vWF assay), ↓ vWF activity (ristocetin cofactor assay), ↓ factor VIII activity
- **Rx:** Trial of desmopressin (IV or intranasal) w/ Types 1 & 2 can ↑ vWF & FVIII → recheck vWF & FVIII levels for resp; risk for hyponatremia
  vWF replacement: For acute bleeding, risk bleeding, or planned Surg; FVIII concentrates (also contains vWF), cryoprecipitate, recombinant vWF
    Menorrhagia: OCP, levonorgestrel-IUD, endometrial ablation, tranexamic acid
- **Preg:** vWF/FVIII levels ↑ during Preg & fall postpartum, ↑ risk delayed PPH; check FVIII levels q trimester; maintain >50 IU/dL prior to procedures, intrapartum & 2 w postpartum; avoid operative vaginal deliveries or circumcision until fetal vWD status known; offer genetic counseling antepartum

Hemophilias (Lancet 2012;379:1447)
- X-linked recessive deficiency of factors VIII (hemophilia A) or IX (hemophilia B); wide phenotypic variation in heterozygous carriers → variable propensity to bleed in carriers
- **Severity:** Mild (5–25% nml factor activity), mod (1–5%), sev (<1%)
- **Dx:** ↑ aPTT that resolves w/ mixing study, nml PT & vWF, ↓ factor VIII or IX or XI
- **Mixing study for ↑ PT or aPTT:** Mix pt's plasma 1:1 w/ nml plasma & retest PT/aPTT PT/aPTT normalizes w/ mixing → factor deficiency; remains elevated → factor inhib
- **Rx:** Recombinant or A-purified factor replacement (factor VIII or IX); desmopressin (↑ FVIII for mild hemophilia A); antifibrinolytics, cryoprecipitate (FVIII only)
- **Hemophilia C:** Autosomal recessive deficiency of factor XI, less severe clinical presentation than A or B, treated with FFP or recombinant factor VIIa

Coagulation Factor Inhibitors
- Alloimmune antibodies directed against coagulation factors (FVIII inhib most common)
- **Etiology:** Repeated factor replacement in pts w/ hemophilia, autoimmune dz (ie, SLE), postpartum, malig
- **Dx:** ↑ aPTT (remains prolonged after mixing study; Bethesda coagulation assay titer)
- **Rx:** Acute bleed – FVIII concentrates for low titer; recombinant FVIIa or activated prothrombin complex for high titer; eliminating inhib – prednisone, rituximab, cyclophosphamide, plasma exchange

ANTIPHOSPHOLIPID ANTIBODY SYNDROME (APS)

Criteria for diagnosis of antiphospholipid antibody syndrome	
APS present if ≥1 clinical AND ≥1 laboratory criteria are met	
Clinical criteria	**Laboratory criteria**
Vascular thrombosis: ≥1 arterial, venous, or small vessel thrombosis in ANY organ	Lupus anticoagulant: Present in plasma on 2 tests ≥12 w apart*
Preg morbidity: ≥1 unexplained deaths of morphologically nml fetus (U/S or exam) at ≥10 w OR ≥1 premature births of morphologically nml neonat at ≤34 w due to (i) sev preeclampsia or eclampsia or (ii) placenta insufficiency OR ≥3 unexplained consecutive SABs <10 w	Anticardiolipin antibody: IgG &/or IgM in serum or plasma (>40 µg/mL [ie, >99th %ile]) on 2 tests ≥12 w apart Anti-β2 glycoprotein-I Ab: IgG &/or IgM in serum or plasma (>99th %ile) on 2 tests ≥12 w apart
*Patient cannot be anticoagulated during testing. From J Thromb Haemost 2006;4:295–306.	

Epidemiology
- 40% of SLE pts have APLA, of these, 40% have h/o thrombosis
- Antiphospholipid Abs present in 10–15% of pts w/ RPL

Pathophysiology
- Clinical manifestations result from impaired phospholipid-dependent steps in coagulation

Clinical Manifestations
- Arterial/venous thrombosis, thrombocytopenia (40–50%), nephropathy, hemolytic anemia, skin (livedo reticularis/ulcers), stroke/TIA/multi-infarct dementia, cardiac valvular dz
- **Pregnancy-specific:** ↑ Risk thrombosis (up to 25% w/o rx), IUGR (15–30%), IUFD, sev preeclampsia/eclampsia, recurrent Preg loss, preterm deliv

- **Catastrophic APS:** Requires (1) involvement of ≥3 organs, (2) dev in <1 w, (3) histo-pathology of small vessel occlusion, (4) presence of aPa; up to 50% mortality

Screening/Diagnosis
- **Indications:** Prior unexplained or pregnancy-associated arterial/venous thromboembolism, h/o 1 fetal loss, or ≥3 (ACOG) or ≥2 (ASRM) consecutive embryonic losses, unexplained prolonged aPTT (see "Recurrent pregnancy loss workup")
- Detection not poss if pt on UFH, & difficult w/ LMHW or Coumadin
- Preg c/b APS → consider serial US assessment of fetal growth in 3rd trimester

Management of APS	
Clinical scenario	**Rec**
Venous thrombosis	Indefinite therapeutic anticoagulation w/ INR 2–3 (warfarin not NOAC/DOAC still 1st line) (heparin if pregnant)
Arterial thrombosis	Indefinite anticoagulation w/ INR 3–4
SLE + LA	Hydroxychloroquine ± 81 mg daily ASA
APS + RPL (no prev thrombosis) + Preg	81 mg daily ASA ± UFH (5000–7500 IU SQ q12h) or prophylactic LMWH
APS + Preg + thrombosis	81 mg daily ASA + therapeutic UFH/LMWH
APS + h/o fetal death or prior PTD <34 w	If deliv due to sev preeclampsia or placenta insufficiency 81 mg daily ASA + prophylactic UFH or LMWH
Antiphospholipid Ab	Strict control of vascular risk factors (eg, smoking cessation)
Contraceptive counseling	Avoid estrogen-containing contraceptives
Surg	Adequate thromboprophylaxis

Adapted from *Lancet* 2010;376(9751):1498–509; *Obstet Gynecol* 2012;132.

ALLOIMMUNIZATION

Definition, Etiology, Epidemiology
- Mat antibodies to any fetal bld group factor inherited from father
- Mat antibodies can develop in pregnancy, from transfusion, or from sharing needles
- RhD Ag most commonly implicated; minor antigens include C, c, E, e, Kell (see below)
- Mat exposure to paternal Ag on fetal RBC in index pregnancy → IgM Ab formation → IgG Ab crosses placenta & directs immune-mediated destruction of fetal RBCs in next Preg
- 0.1 mL fetal bld may result in mat Ab formation; 2nd exposure → anamnestic immune resp
- 6.8/1000 live births affected by alloimmunization; 10% prior to routine testing/prevention
- Minor antigens present in ~2% of pregnancies

Clinical Manifestations
- Positive Ab screen on blood type
- Fetal anemia → hydrops fetalis (≥2 of the following: Ascites, pleural effusion, pericardial effusion, skin edema, polyhydramnios)
- Fetal complications (death, hemolytic dz of newborn)

Screening Diagnosis of Rh Alloimmunization (see also Chap. 11)
- **Screen for alloimmunization:** Mat bld type & Ab screen at 1st prenatal visit, 28 w, and delivery. If anti-D antibodies present, patient alloimmunized.
- **Determine risk to fetus:** If mat RhD neg & paternity known → obtain paternal bld type, if Rh+ → perform zygosity testing → homozygous father means fetus obligate Rh+, heterozygous 50% chance of affected fetus → cell free DNA testing for fetal RhD status (can test with amniocentesis, not necessarily recommended)
- **Monitor titers:** Anti-RhD Ab (+) → monthly indirect Coombs to test level of antibody in maternal blood; if rising titer test more frequently; Critical titer typically 1:8–1:32 (lab dependent based on association with fetal anemia at that institution). Prior affected Preg ↑ risk fetal anemia; Ab titers do not correlate w/ severity; risk of fetal anemia not correlated with titers for other minor antigens (Kell)
- **MCA Doppler:** 1–2 w assessment of fetal peak systolic velocity (PSV) in middle cerebral artery (MCA) PSV >1.5 multiple of median (MoMs) for GA predictive of mod–sev fetal anemia (*NEJM* 2000;342:9)

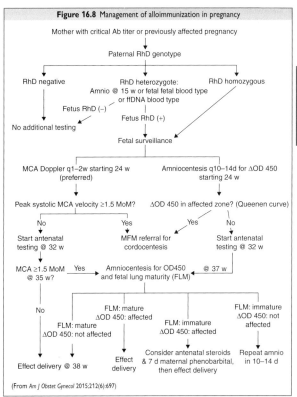

Figure 16.8 Management of alloimmunization in pregnancy

(From *Am J Obstet Gynecol* 2015;212(6):697)

Prevention and Treatment
- Anti-RhD Ig → 300 µg neutralizes 30 mL whole bld (15 mL fetal RBCs) after FMH
- Kleihauer–Betke (KB) test used to quantify fetal cells in mat circulation and guide dose
- 50 µg if <12 w gest; human serum-derived product; effect up to 12 w; max dose 1500 µg/24 h; give w/i 72 h of indication for *prevention* of alloimmunization
- Weak RhD pos (D^u) → treat as RhD pos, ppx not indicated
- Rx → deliv; intrauterine bld xfusion if remote from term

Indications for anti-RhD Ig in RhD (−)/antibody (−) patient		
Postdelivery (baby RhD +)	24–28 w gest	2nd/3rd trimester bleeding
Ectopic Preg	Amniocentesis	Chorionic villus sampling
Trauma	Threatened abortion*	Cordocentesis
External cephalic version	IUFD	Molar gestation

*No recommendation can be given at this time.
From *Obstet Gynecol* 2017;181.

Minor Antigens (Ag) (*Obstet Gynecol* 2006;108:457)
- Minor antigens present in ~2% of pregnancies, cause HDFN with varying severity
- Many may case RBC destruction; no prophylactic rx available; mgmt of sensitization is Ab dependent, but typically mirrors RhD
- Lewis & I most common → do not cause erythroblastosis fetalis

- Anti-Kell Ab → may cause sev anemia, follow w/ MCA Dopplers as antibody titers do not predict HDFN
- Anti-RhD Ig indicated in RhD neg pts w/ minor antigens but no RhD antibodies
- Management similar to RhD alloimmunization with paternal zygosity testing, monitoring of titers (if titers reliable for specific Ag) and MCA Dopplers

NEONATAL ALLOIMMUNE THROMBOCYTOPENIA (NAIT)

Epidemiology, Pathology, Etiology (Obstet Gynecol 2016;128:668)
- **Platelet** equivalent of Rh alloimmunization. ~0.01% of live births & can affect *first* pregnancy. Fetal/neonatal thrombocytopenia due to fetal platelet Ag (HPA-1a most commonly) inherited from father which the mother lacks. Maternal IgG antiplatelet antibodies → fetal thrombocytopenia. 100% of subsequent pregnancies affected if fetus has Ag

Clinical Manifestations
- Often presents in uncomplicated pregnancies as infant w/ signs of thrombocytopenia in utero (intracerebral hemorrhage [ICH]) or at birth (petechiae, ecchymosis over presenting part)
- Intracranial hemorrhage = most serious complication (15% of infants w/ plts <50k)

Diagnosis, Subsequent Workup
- ~50% of ICH able to be detected on US; 1st affected pregnancy often diagnosed at birth.
- Labs: HPA type and zygosity of both parents & confirm maternal Ab for paternal plts. Titers correlate poorly with severity of disease. Cordocentesis is the only direct means of dx but carries risk of fetal bleeding from cord puncture site if indeed thrombocytopenic.

Treatment (Obstet Gynecol 2011;118:1157)
- Aggressive intervention to prevent ICH, recommend not performing cordocentesis until 32 w and treating empirically. If not effective, plt transfusions with maternal plts to increase fetal plts can be necessary.
    High risk: Sibling with ICH dx at <28 w GA, start IVIG at 12 w, add Prednisone at 20 w. Deliver by CD at 35–36 w. Vaginal delivery only if plts >100k by cordo at 32 w
    Medium risk: Sibling with ICH dx at >28 w GA, start IVIG at 12 w, increase IVIG or add prednisone at 20 w. Delivery same as above.
    Standard risk: Sibling with thrombocytopenia but no ICH, start IVIG (± prednisone) at 20 w, give IVIG and prednisone at 32 w. Delivery by CD at 37–38 w. Vaginal delivery only if plts >100k by cordo at 32 w

BLOOD PRODUCTS FOR HEMORRHAGE AND CRITICAL CARE

Blood products	
pRBCs (240 mL)	Contains RBCs, WBCs, plasma; ↑ Hct 3% & ↑ Hb 1 g/dL Critically ill pts → Hb goal 7–9 g/dL; consider Hb 10–12 g/dL if coronary ischemia (NEJM 1999;340:409; 2001;345:1230)
Plts	Collection: Apheresis – single donor (predom method) Whole bld – multi donors. Contain: Plts, plasma, WBC/RBC 6 U Plt (whole bld) = 1 U Plt (apheresis) → ↑ Plt count by 25–30K Ind: Plt <10000/μL; Plt <20000/μL w/ bleeding risk or infxn; Plt <50000/μL w/ active bleed or preop; ABO match not essent Contraindication: HIT, HELLP, TTP–HUS *Refrac xfusion:* Plt ↑ <5000/μL; DIC, sepsis, splenomegaly, alloimmuni-zation. Serial CBCs → if refrac, give ABO matched Plts & screen plasma for HLA Abs. Consider HLA-matched Plts.
FFP (250 mL)	Contains all coagulation factors; ↑ fibrinogen 10 mg/dL Ind: (1) Fibrinogen <100 mg/dL, (2) INR >1.6 preop, (3) bleeding due to factor deficiency → inherited (ie, Factor XI deficiency) or Acq dz (ie, DIC, TTP–HUS, liver dz, warfarin tox), (4) Part of massive transfusion protocol (see below)
Cryoprecipitate (10–20 mL)	Contains fibrinogen, Factors VIII & XIII, vWF; ↑ fibrinogen 10 mg/dL Bleeding in factor deficiency (vWD or factor XIII) or fibrinogen <100 mg/dL

Leukoreduced	WBCs removed (>99%) from pRBCs; ↓ risk febrile nonhemolytic rxn, alloimmunization & infxn (esp CMV); "univ leukoreduction" at many centers, Ind: Prior xfusion rxn, frequent xfusions, risk for CMV infxn, bypass Surg
Irradiated	Destroys donor lymphocytes in pRBCs; reduces risk xfusion assoc GVHD; Ind: Immunodeficiency (ie, BMT, fetal/neonat xfusion, SCID, AIDS)
CMV negative	From CMV seronegative negative donors; use for xfusion of CMV seronegativity in Preg or immunodeficiency
Whole bld	Contains all bld components; use limited, use in neonat xfusion for hemolytic dz newborn, cardiac Surg, ECMO
Factor VIII	Human or recombinant; for bleeding a/w hemophilia A Preop → min Surg: 15–25 IU/kg bolus, then 20–25 IU/kg q8–12h Major Surg: 50 IU/kg until factor VIII level 100% then PRN 10–14 d
4 Factor prothrombin complex concentrate	• *Unactivated* (ie, Kcentra) Immediate reversal of Vitamin K antagonists. INR 2–3.9: 25 u/kg. INR 4–6: 35 u/kg. INR >6: 50 u/kg • *Activated* (ie, factor eight inhibitor bypassing activity [FEIBA]) Immediate reversal of noval oral anticoagulants (factor Xa inhibitors). 50–100 u/kg depending on severity of bleeding.
Autologous donation	↓ Risk infxn or xfusion rxn for elective procedures; need Hb >11 g/dL before donation; safe in Preg, but generally reserved for pts w/ rare Abs

Transfusion complications (# per unit transfused)	
For ALL reactions, stop transfusion & send remaining bld product to bld bank	
Febrile nonhemolytic (1:100)	S/S: Fever/rigors 0–6 h after xfusion (↑ 1°C w/i 2 h)
	Cause: Abs to donor WBCs; dx: R/o infxn & hemolysis
	Rx: Acetaminophen ± meperidine 25–50 mg IV/IM
Acute hemolytic (<1:250000)	S/S: Fever, ↓ BP, oliguria, flank/chest pain, DIC, may be fatal
	Cause: ABO incomp
	Rx: Maintain UOP w/ IVF & diuretics ± pressors
Delayed hemolytic (1:1000)	S/S: Same as acute (less sev); 5–7 d after xfusion
	Rx: Typically none req; follow Hct, Cr, LFTs, & coags
Allergic (1:100)	S/S: Mild – urticaria; sev – airway compromise, ↓↓ BP
	Rx: Antihistamines; sev: Epi ± glucocorticoids
Transfusion-related acute lung injury (TRALI) (1 per 5000)	S/S: Dyspnea, fever, hypoxia, pulm edema, HoTN
	Rx: Supportive respiratory care ± ICU admission/ vasopressors; intubation with mech vent similar to ARDS
Transfusion associated circulatory overload (TACO) (1 per 100)	S/S: Resp distress, HA, hypoxia, HTN, JVD
	Rx: Fluid mobilization, O₂, ventilation prn
Infections	
CMV: ~1:100 (leukocyte reduced)	HIV (1:1800000)
Hepatitis B (1:220000)	Hepatitis C (1:1600000)
Bacteria (1:500000 per U pRBC; 1:12000/U Plt)	

Data from Busch MP, Kleinman SH, Nemo GJ. Current and emerging infectious risks of blood transfusions. *JAMA.* 2003;289(8):959–62.

Massive Transfusion *(Transfusion 2007;47(9):1564; AJOG 2016;214:340)*
- **Red top tube test:** 5 mL bld in nonheparinized tube; nml = clot in 8–10 min; lack of clot or partial dissolution in 8–10 min is c/w fibrinogen <150 mg/dL
- Recombinant FVIIa → RCTs show no survival benefit, reserve for pts with hemophilia and bleeding refrac to intervention (pts should have plts >50, fibrinogen >50–100, T >32 & nl ionized Ca), ↑ risk thrombosis (including arterial)
- Core temp <30°C → ventricular arrhythmias, use bld warmer if ≥3 U pRBCs or cold RBCs/plasma infused @ >100 mL/min for 30 min to prevent hypothermia
- Periodic eval for ↓ Ca⁺⁺ & ↑ K⁺; risk citrate tox (↓ cardiac output/↓ SVR, met alkalosis). See also Chap. 11 for OB PPH.

Example Massive Transfusion Protocol for Obstetrics				
	PRBCs	**FFP**	**Platelets**	**Cryoprecipitate**
Round 1	6 U	6 U	6 U	10 U
Round 2	6 U	6 U	6 U	10 U
Round 3	Tranexamic acid 1 g IV over 10 min			
Round 4	6 U	6 U	6 U	

Consider activating the protocol when hemorrhage is expected to be massive (anticipated need to replace 50% or more of blood volume within 2 h), bleeding continues after the transfusion of 4 U of packed red blood cells within a short period of time (1–2 h), or systolic blood is pressure below 90 mmHg and heart rate is above 120 beats per minute in the presence of uncontrolled bleeding.

From *Am J Obstet Gynecol* 2016;214:340.

The Menstrual Cycle

- **Mean age of menarche:** 12.4 y. **Mean age of menopause:** 51 y.
  - 1st day of vaginal bleeding = day 1 of cycle; mean duration of menses is 4 ± 2 d; mean bld loss of 35 mL (10–80 mL); mean cycle length 21–34 d *(Clin Obstet Gynaecol 2010;2:157)*
- **Follicular phase:** Lasts 10–21 d, variable in duration, determines menstrual cycle length
- **Ovulation:** FSH stimulates estrogen production → LH surge → dominant follicle rupture/oocyte release
  - Follicle remnant → corpus luteum which secretes progesterone & maintains the endometrial lining *(Am J Hum Biol 2001;4:465)*. If fertilization occurs, the trophoblast cells synthesize hCG to maintain the corpus luteum.
- **Luteal phase:** Lasts 14 d, constant in duration. In the absence of preg, the corpus luteum regresses → E2/progesterone levels drop → uterine lining is shed & FSH (no longer suppressed) starts the next cycle

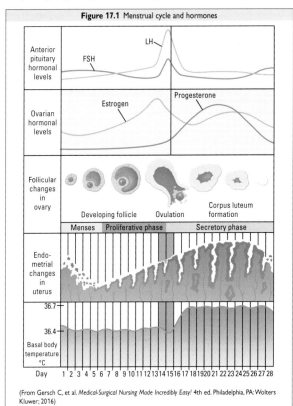

Figure 17.1 Menstrual cycle and hormones

(From Gersch C, et al. *Medical-Surgical Nursing Made Incredibly Easy!* 4th ed. Philadelphia, PA: Wolters Kluwer; 2016)

Hormones of Pregnancy

- **hCG** is secreted by placental trophoblast. Detected in the mother's bld 8 d after conception. Maintains corpus luteum progesterone production. Structurally similar to LH, FSH, & TSH (same alpha-subunit)

- **hPL** is produced by syncytiotrophoblasts. Detected 2–3 w after fertilization. Levels rise steadily until 34–36 w to a peak 5–10 μg/mL. Effects include maternal lipolysis → ↑ circulating free fatty acids to provide a source of energy for mother & fetus; anti-insulin action → increased maternal insulin levels → increased protein synthesis; angiogenic action → fetal vasculature formation
- **Progesterone** is mainly produced by the corpus luteum until 6–7 w gest when the placenta begins to produce. Maintains endometrial lining in early preg & uterine quiescence
- **Relaxin** is secreted by the corpus luteum → uterine relaxation, systemic vasodilation, & ↑ cardiac output (Am J Physiol Regul Integr Comp Physiol 2011:R267)

TYPE I DIABETES MELLITUS

Definition and Epidemiology (Diabetes Care 2012;35(suppl 1):S64)
- Gluc intolerance due to insulin insufficiency. Often caused by cell-mediated autoimmune pancreatic β-cell destruction. Only about 5% of all diabetes.
- Incidence increasing 1.8% (NEJM 2017;376(15):1419). Prevalence 1.93/1000 by age 19 (JAMA 2014;311(17):1778)
- A/w other autoimmune diseases (eg, Graves, Hashimoto, Addison dz) (Diabet Med 2011;28(8):896)

Etiology and Pathophysiology
- **Genetic:** 95% have either HLA-DR3 or HLA-DR4. Also positive for anti-GAD, anti-islet cell, & anti-insulin Abs.
- **Environmental:** Congenital rubella infxn, enterovirus, coxsackievirus B, CMV, adenovirus, & mumps (Diabetes Care 2012(suppl 1):S64)
- Lymphocytic infiltration, ↓ β-cell → insulin deficiency (Diabetes Metab Res Rev 2011;8:778)
- Hyperglycemia at ~80–90% β-cell loss

Clinical Manifestations
- Polyuria, polydipsia, polyphagia w/ weight loss, fatigue, weakness, muscle cramps, blurred vision, nausea, abdominal pain, changes in bowel mvmt
- Most present w/ acute sx of diabetes, markedly elevated bld gluc levels, DKA

Diagnostic Workup

Criteria for the diagnosis of diabetes in the nonpregnant patient*
Fasting glucose level (mg/dL) of 126 mg/dL or higher
OR
Glucose level 2 h after 75 g load (mg/dL) of >200 mg/dL or higher
OR
HbA1c of 6.5% or higher
OR
Random plasma glucose of 200 mg/dL or high in patient with classic symptoms of hyperglycemia or hyperglycemic crisis

*Same criteria for type 1 or type 2 DM; if pregnant, determine if GDM or pre-existing DM.
From ADA, Diabetes Care 2016:S13–22.

Treatment and Medications (JAMA 2003;289(17):2254)
- Lifelong insulin therapy is started w/ either multiple daily injection (MDI) therapy, or continuous subcutaneous insulin infusion (CSII).
- Gluc measurements in nonpregnant patients are fasting & preprandial, however pre- & postprandial shows greater improv in glycemic control in pregnancy (Clin Med 2011;2:154)
- **MDI nonphysiologic regimens** – do not mimic nml insulin secretion
  Once daily long-acting insulin (at bedtime)
  Twice daily intermediate-acting insulin (breakfast & dinner time)
- **MDI physiologic regimens** – attempt to mimic nml insulin secretion
  Twice daily intermediate-acting insulin w/ short-acting insulin (breakfast & dinner time)
  Once daily long-acting insulin (at bedtime) w/ mealtime rapid-acting insulin
  Twice daily intermediate-acting insulin (breakfast & bedtime) w/ rapid acting insulin w/ each meal
  Premixed insulin (70% NPH/30% regular) given twice daily
- **CSII** – Rapid-acting insulin preparation administered through a catheter that is inserted into the SQ tissue. There is a basal insulin infusion rate w/ patient-directed boluses given before meals.

- **Postpartum Goals:** Fasting gluc <110 mg/dL and 2-h postprandial levels <160 mg/dL
  (Obstet Gynecol Clin North Am 2007;34(2):335–49).
- **Nonpregnant goals:** HgbA1c <7%, fasting 70–130 mg/dL, postprandial <180 mg/dL
  (Diabetes Care 2015;38(Supp 1):S33).

Insulin types and pharmacodynamics			
	Onset (min)	Peak (h)	Duration (h)
Rapid-acting			
Lispro (Humalog)	15–30	0.5–2.5	3–6.5
Aspart (NovoLog)	10–20	1–3	3–5
Glulisine (Apidra)	10–15	1–1.5	3–5
Short-acting			
Regular (Humulin R, Novolin R)	30–60	1–5	6–10
Intermediate-acting			
Isophane insulin (NPH, Humulin N, Novolin N)	60–120	6–14	16–24
Insulin zinc (Lente, Humulin L, Novolin L)	120–240	4–12	12–18
Long-acting			
Glargine (Lantus)	66	—	Up to 24
Detemir (Levemir)	48–120	—	Up to 24
Insulin zinc extended (Ultralente, Humulin U)	360–600	10–16	18–24
Premixed			
BiAsp 70/30 (BIAsp 30)	10–20	1–4	Up to 24
Lispro 75/25 (Humalog Mix 75/25)	15–30	1–6.5	Up to 24
70% NPH/30% regular (Humulin 70/30)	30–60	2–16	Up to 18–24

Data from JAMA. 2003;289:2254 and Int J Clin Pract. 2010;64:305.

DIABETIC KETOACIDOSIS (DKA)

Definition
- Acute life-threatening complication due to insulin deficiency, w/ hyperglycemia, dehyd, & acidosis. Typically due to insulin noncompliance, acute illness/infxn, drugs, or new onset DM.
- Precipitating factors: Emesis, infxn, diabetic gastroparesis, poor compliance with therapy or insulin pump failure, use of β-sympathomimetic agents (for tocolysis) or corticosteroids, physician management errors (J Reprod Med 1991;36:797–800). Can occur more rapidly and at lower hyperglycemia level in pregnant patients.
- Occurs in 1–3% of all pregnancies w/ DM with associated morbidity of 9–35%

Pathophysiology (Clin Med 2011;2:154)
- Insulin deficiency → ↑ glucagon → ↑ hepatic gluconeogenesis & ↑ glycogenolysis → hyperglycemia → inability to use gluc → ↑ lipolysis → free fatty acids metabolized by liver (ketogenesis) as an alternative energy source → large quantities of ketones → acidosis

Clinical Manifestation (Hormones 2011;4:250)
- Nausea, vomiting, abdominal pain, confusion, Kussmaul respirations (deep labored breathing seen in metabolic acidosis)
- HHS can have similar presentation but with bld gluc much higher (eg, 1,000 mg/dL) >1,000 mg/dL and plasma osmolality >380 mOsmol/kg (see below)

Diagnostic Workup
- Bld gluc, bld gas (pH), Chemistry (bicarbonate, anion gap), serum ketones
  BG frequently 350–500 mg/dL; pregnant patients can have DKA w/ BS <200 mg/dL

Diagnostic criteria for DKA			
	Mild	Mod	Sev
Plasma gluc (mg/dL)	>250	>250	>250
Arterial pH	7.25–7.30	7–7.24	<7
Serum bicarbonate (mEq/L)	15–18	10–15	<10
Serum ketone	Positive	Positive	Positive
Anion gap	>10	>12	>12
Mental status	Alert	Alert/drowsy	Stupor/coma

From Endocrinol Metab Clin North Am 2006;35(4):725–51, viii.

Treatment
- Treat the underlying cause (eg, infxn). Inpatient admission.
- **Fluids:** 1 L NS 1st 1–2 h, then 250–500 mL/h. When gluc <250 mg/dL → change to 5% dextrose in ½ NS, and continue insulin till ketonemia resolved. Once gluc levels normalize, cont repletion until the fluid deficit is met (deficit: ~100 mL/kg body weight)
- **Insulin:** 0.1–0.4 U/kg IV bolus → 0.1 U/kg/h continuous infusion (or 2–10 U/h). Try for 50–70 mg/dL/h correction of serum gluc, or about 25% in 1st 2 h. When plasma gluc is ~200 mg/dL → ↓ insulin to 0.05 U/kg/h (or about 1–2 U/h) until urine ketones cleared. Adjust until gluc ~150–200 mg/dL. When pt can tolerate food, start her usual SQ insulin injection regimen.
- **Potassium:** K >5 mEq/L, no additional (Insulin drives K into cells w/ gluc → ↓ serum K)
  K 4–5 mEq/L → add 20 mEq/L to each liter of replacement fluid
  K 3–4 mEq/L → add 40 mEq/L to each liter of replacement fluid
  K <3 mEq/L → hold insulin, give 10–20 mEq/h until K >3.3, then 40 mEq/L in IVF
- **Bicarbonate:** Controversial
  If pH <6.9 → consider giving 100 mEq & 20 mEq of KCl in 400 mL of H_2O over 2 h; if pH 6.9–7 or bicarbonate <5 mEq → give 50 mEq in 200 mL of water over 1 h until pH ↑ to >7
  If pH >7, do not give bicarbonate
- **Phosphate:** If <1 mg/dL → give 20–30 mmol potassium phosphate over 24 h
- **Chloride:** If hyperchloremic, switch to more physiologic fluid (eg, PlasmaLyte)
- **Calcium/Magnesium:** Monitor serum Ca/Mag levels & replete prn
- **Fetal HR monitoring** for >24 w gest. Fetal loss 9–85% depending on severity of DKA

TYPE II DIABETES MELLITUS

Definition and Epidemiology (Diabetes Care 2012;35(suppl 1):S64)
- Insulin resistance ± inadeq insulin production (ie, inadeq production for the sensitivity of the target tissues). ~29 million people w/ DM, ~86 million prediabetes (Centers for Disease Control. At a Glance Reports 2016: Diabetes)

Pathophysiology
- Periph insulin resistance → ↑ insulin secretion → pancreas failure → defective insulin secretion in resp to ↑ gluc → increased liver gluconeogenesis → hyperglycemia

Clinical Manifestation
- **Classical sx:** Polyuria, polydipsia, polyphagia, fatigue, weakness, muscle cramps, blurred vision, nausea, abdominal pain, changes in bowel mvmt. Most are asymptomatic.

Diagnostic Workup
- Criteria for diagnosing T2DM outside of preg detailed above (Type 1 DM section)

Treatment and Medications
- Goal of rx is to achieve & maintain HbA1c levels of <7%. See also for preg, below.
- **At dx:** Lifestyle changes (weight loss, exercise) may ↓ HbA1c 1–2%
- Bariatric surg consideration for adults w/ T2DM & BMI >35 kg/m^2 w/ medical comorbidities

HYPEROSMOLAR HYPERGLYCEMIC STATE

Etiology and Pathophysiology (Emerg Med Clin North Am 2005;23:629)
- Extreme hyperglycemia + hyperosmolality, w/o ketoacidosis
- Infxn causing about 60% of cases: Physiologic stress → ↓ effectiveness of circulating insulin → ↑ counter regulatory hormones (glucagon, catecholamines, cortisol, GH) → ↑ periph resistance → gluconeogenesis → hyperglycemia → glycosuria → hypertonic osmotic diuresis (dehyd) → unable to maintain adequate fluid intake (2/2 acute illness) → sev hyperosmolality & intracellular dehyd, renal failure

Diagnostic Workup
- Plasma gluc level of ≥1000 mg/dL, serum osmolality of ≥320 mOsm/kg, ↑ serum urea nitrogen (BUN):Cr ratio, pH >7.3, small ketonuria, absent to low ketonemia, bicarbonate >15 mEq/L, neurologic abnormalities frequently seen (25–50%)

Treatment
- Treat the underlying cause. Mgmt very similar to DKA (above).
- 1st-line therapy is aggressive IV hydration, fluid deficit may be 8–12 L. Replace 1/2 of the fluid deficit in the 1st 12 h, & the remainder in the next 12–24 h w/ NS.
- Insulin infusion when potassium is ≥3.3 mEq/L. Regular insulin started at 0.1 U/kg/h w/ or w/o a 0.1 U/kg bolus.
- Once the serum gluc ≤300 mg/dL, D5 should be added & the insulin infusion ↓ to 0.05 U/kg/h
- If serum potassium level is <3.3 mEq/L → replete w/ KCl at a rate of up to 20–30 mEq/L/h until levels are above 3.3 mEq/L. 20–30 mEq/L KCl can then be added to each 1 L of IV fluid. Goal is to maintain nml serum K levels. Check K every 1–2 h.

DIABETES IN PREGNANCY

Epidemiology
- 6–9% of all pregnancies are complicated by pre-existing DM or GDM 90% of diabetes in pregnancy is GDM.

Clinical Manifestation
- Type I usually known prior to preg. Type II may have been unrecognized, but if gluc intolerance seen before 20 w, consider pregestational. Goal preconception HbA1c <6.5%. Consider hospital admission for very poor control during organogenesis.
- Fetal malformation rate in a nml preg is 2–3% vs. 6–12% in preg c/b diabetes (Obstet Gynecol 2003;102:857). Rate of fetal malformations w/ HbA1c 7–8.9% = 5–10%; HbA1c 9–10.9% = 10–20%, HbA1c >11% = >20%
- Most frequent defects include cardiac, renal, neural tube. Esp double outlet RV, truncus arteriosus, & caudal regression syn/sacral agenesis (considered pathognomonic).
- **Risks of DM in Preg:**
  Maternal: ↑ Progression of nephropathy/retinopathy/CV dz, ↑ preeclampsia, ↑ infection, ↑VTE, ↑ lacerations/poor wound healing
  Fetal: ↑ Malformations/IUGR, ↑ SAB/IUFD, ↑ polyhydramnios, ↑ labor dystocia/C/S deliv, ↑ macrosomia, ↑ shoulder dystocia/birth injury (clavicle/humerus fx, brachial plexus/facial nerve injury, cephalohematoma), ↑ neonat RDS/hypoglycemia/jaundice, ↑ mortality

White classification of diabetes mellitus			
Gestational class	DM existing only during Preg. Consider also unrecognized type II DM.		
A1	Diet controlled, no meds to control bld sugar		
A2	Requires medication (oral or injected insulin) for control		
Pregestational class	**Onset age (y)**	**Duration (y)**	**Complications**
B	≥20	<10	None
C	10–19	10–19	None
D	<10	>20	± Benign retinopathy, other vascular complications
F	Any	Any	Nephropathy
H	Any	Any	Heart
R	Any	Any	Proliferative retinopathy
T	Any	Any	Renal xplant

Screening for DM in Pregnancy
- **Univ GDM screening** at 24–28 w; early if risk factors (see below)
Screening tests:
- **1-h OGTT (50 g):** Serum gluc ≥130–140 mg/dL depending on institution
  Gluc >140 mg/dL identifies 80% GDM; ≥130 mg/dL identifies 90% GDM
  Positive screening test → 3-h OGTT (100 g) challenge test
- **2-h OGTT (75 g):** Alternative, less common approach, up to 18% of pregnant patients would screen positive using this method
  Fasting 92–125 mg/dL or 1 h >180 mg/dL or 2 h 153–199 mg/dL = GDM
  Fasting gluc >126 mg/dL or 2 h >200 mg/dL = overt DM

- **3-h OGTT (100 g):** Fasting plus 1-, 2-, 3-h post challenge bld gluc. 1 abn value = gluc intolerance (a/w fetal macrosomia), 2 or more abn values = GDM

Screening strategy for detecting pregestational diabetes or early GDM
Consider testing in all women with BMI >25 + one or more risk factors:
Physical inactivity
1st-degree relative with DM
High-risk face or ethnicity (AA, Latino, NA, Asian, Pacific Islander)
Previous GDM or previous ≥4000 g birth
Hypertension
HDL <35 mg/dL, triglycerides >250 mg/dL
Dx of PCOS
HbA1c >5.7%, impaired glucose tolerance, or impaired fasting glucose on previous testing
Preprep BMI >40
From *Obstet Gynecol* 2017;130(1):e17.

Criteria for diagnosis of gestational diabetes from oral glucose tolerance testing		
Time since 100-g glucose load (h)	**Modified O'Sullivan scale (mg/dL)**	**Carpenter and Coustan scale (mg/dL)**
Fasting	≥105	≥95
1	≥190	≥180
2	≥165	≥155
3	≥145	≥140
Data from O'Sullivan JB, Mahan CM. Criteria for the oral glucose tolerance test in pregnancy. *Diabetes.* 1964;13:278–285 and Carpenter MW, Coustan DR. Criteria for screening tests for gestational diabetes. *Am J Obstet Gynecol.* 1982;144:768–73.		

Management of DM in Pregnancy

- **GDM**
  Nutrition advice, diet/exercise, & 4×/d bld gluc testing (fasting + 2-h postprandial)
  If inadeq control → oral hypoglycemic agents (glyburide or metformin), if inadeq w/ max dose → insulin
  GDM-A1: Delivery by 41 w
  GDM-A2: Antenatal testing & delivery between 39 w0d and 39 w6d. If DM uncontrolled, may consider delivery between 37–39 w

Goals for glycemic control in pregnancy	
Goal blood sugar values (mg/dL)	
Fasting	60–90
Premeal	<100
1 h postprandial	<140
2 h postprandial	<120
Bedtime	<120
2–6 AM	60–90
Data from Metzger BE, et al. Summary and Recommendations of the Fifth International Workshop-Conference on Gestational Diabetes Mellitus. *Diabetes Care.* 2007;30(2):S251.	

- **Pregestational DM**
  Diet: 1800–2400 kcal daily, w/ 20% prot, 33–40% carbs (favor complex carbs), & 40% fat. ADA recommends insulin for pregnant women w/ type I or II DM. NPH & rapid-acting insulin combination used (see Table w/ insulin types, above). Type I DM usually ↑ insulin 50–100%. Type II DM often ↑ >200% in Preg.
  Antepartum: Consider baseline preeclampsia labs, thyroid testing (40% type I DM – thyroid d/o) in early Preg. Eye exam in 1st trimester, & baseline ECG (age >30 y or hypertensive). Consider ASA 81 mg after 12 w of gestation.
  Obtain early sonogram, confirm viability, offer mat serum AFP for NT defects, US for anatomy, serial growth US scans, and fetal echocardiography
  1–2×/w fetal NST/AFI starting at 32–34 w; if poor control, hx of DKA in current preg, or hx of vasculopathy/HTN, starting at 28 w
  Deliv: 39–40 w unless poor control, hx of vasculopathy, nephropathy, or prior stillbirth

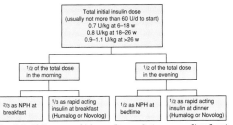

Figure 17.2 Calculation and dose distribution for initial insulin management in pregnancy

Adapted from Gabbe SG. Management of diabetes mellitus complicating pregnancy. *Obstet Gynecol* 2003;102(4):857.

Labor and Delivery for Diabetics
- Consider cesarean deliv for EFW >4500 g for pts w/ DM (>5000 g for nondiabetic)
- **Insulin mgmt during labor:** Usual intermediate insulin at bedtime. Morning dose insulin withheld. W/ active labor or gluc <70 mg/dL start D5NS IVF. Check fingerstick gluc hourly in labor. Usually pregestational DM → IV insulin drip & titrate. Tight gluc control in 2nd stage of labor to avoid neonat hypoglycemia.

Postpartum Management
- Usually insulin-dependent DM → resume prepregnancy regimen, or ½ of end of preg dose. GDM can stop rx, unless suspected T2DM. GDM resolves w/ deliv.
- Postpartum 75 g gluc tol test to identify nongestational DM for all GDM pts at 2–6 w postpartum visit.

Postpartum glucose tolerance test			
	No DM	**Impaired glucose tolerance**	**Overt DM**
8 h fasting	<100	100–125	≥126
2 h after 75 g glucose load	<140	140–199	≥200

Values are plasma glucose levels in mg/dL.
Data from Metzger BE, et al. Summary and Recommendations of the Fifth International Workshop-Conference on Gestational Diabetes Mellitus. *Diabetes Care.* 2007;30(2):S251 and American Diabetes Association Standards of Medical Care in Diabetes—2010. *Diabetes Care.* 2010;33:S11–S61.

GESTATIONAL DIABETES (GDM)

Definitions, Epidemiology, and Pathophysiology
- GDM is carbohydrate intolerance w/ onset or 1st recognition during Preg
- **Classification:** A1GDM is diet controlled; A2GDM requires pharmacologic intervention
- GDM in ~6–9% of pregnancies; 30–50% → recurrent GDM
- 70% of GDM pts will convert to DM within 22–28 y; 60% of Latina women within 5 y
- ↑ Human placental lactogen/cortisol/progesterone/estrogen → ↓ periph insulin sens → impaired gluc resp → hyperglycemia. Screening per above, under Diabetes in Pregnancy.

Treatment and Medications
- Treatment is considered if dietary mgmt cannot consistently achieve target glucose levels. Insulin is considered standard therapy for GDM, however oral hypoglycemic agents are increasingly being used.

Oral hypoglycemic agents		
Types	**Pharmacology**	**Dosing**
Sulfonylureas (ie, Glyburide)	• ↑ Insulin secretion, ↑ insulin sensitivity in periph tissues, ↓ hepatic insulin clearance • Peak conc 4 h • Duration of action 10 h	• 1.25 mg daily (<200 lb) or 2.5 mg daily (>200 lb) • If AM, 1 h before meal • For FBG control, use QHS • ↑ By 1.25–2.5 mg q3–7d until at goal • Max daily dose 20–30 mg

Types	Pharmacology	Dosing
Biguanides (ie, Metformin)	• Sensitizes insulin receptors to ↑ glucose uptake in liver and periph tissues • ↓ Gluconeogenesis • ↓ Hepatic glucose output • Peak conc 4 h • Half-life 2–5 h	• 500 mg 1–2×/daily with food • ↑ Dose by 50 mg q3–7d (2/2 GI side effects) • Max daily dose 2500 mg
α-Glucosidase inhibitors (ie, Acarbose)	• ↓ Postprandial glucose by slowing upper GI tract absorption • Inhibits metab of sucrose → glucose + fructose • Peak conc 1 h • Half-life 2 h	• 25 mg TID with meals • Max daily dose: 150 mg if <60 kg 300 mg if >60 kg

From *Clin Obstet Gynecol* 2013;56(4):827–36.

HYPOTHYROIDISM

Definition and Epidemiology
• Inadeq thyroid hormone to meet the requirements of periph tissues. Prevalence of 0.1–2% of the US pop (females > males)
• **Primary hypothyroidism:** Hashimoto's thyroiditis, surgical removal, radioactive ablation, infiltrative disease, postpartum hypothyroidism, iodine deficiency (95% of cases)
• **Secondary hypothyroidism:** Pituitary/hypothalamic neoplasm, trauma, ischemic necrosis (Sheehan's syn), infxn, inactivating mutations in TSH or TSH receptor
• **Subclinical hypothyroidism:** Chronic autoimmune thyroiditis, partial thyroidectomy, radioactive iodine therapy for rx of hyperthyroidism, infiltrative disorders, drugs impairing thyroid fxn, inadeq replacement therapy for overt hypothyroidism, iodine deficiency

Etiology
• In women, most common cause (95%) is autoimmune (Hashimoto's)
• **Hashimoto's thyroiditis:** Lymphocytic thyroid infiltration → gland atrophy & fibrosis
• **Subclinical hypothyroidism:** Elevated TSH w/o overt hypothyroidism or low T_3/T_4. Early, mild thyroid failure. ~60–80% have ⊕ antithyroid peroxidase or antithyroglobulin Abs. Progression to overt hypothyroidism in women is about 4%/y. No need to treat TSH <10 mU/L & asx. Often treated in infertility patients to optimize hormone status.

Clinical Manifestations and Diagnosis
• Weakness, dry skin, cold intolerance, hair loss, constip, weight gain, poor appetite, dyspnea, hoarse voice, menorrhagia, paresthesias, impaired hearing
• ↑ TSH, ↓ free T_4, ⊕ anti-TPO & other thyroid Abs. May also see hyponatremia, hypercholesterolemia, anemia, & elevated serum Cr kinase.

Treatment
• Daily levothyroxine 2 µg/kg body weight (typically 100–150 µg; start at 50–100 µg depending on severity). Adjust q4w 12.5–25 µg by TSH levels.

Hypothyroidism in Pregnancy (*Lancet* 2012;379(9821):1142)
• Similar causes as nonpregnant. Also postpartum (up to 1 y postpartum) thyroiditis (autoimmune inflammation) → thyrotoxicosis → hypothyroidism.
• Mat hypothyroidism can ↑ SAB, placental abruption, preterm deliv, preeclampsia, mat HTN, postpartum hemorrhage, low birth weight, stillbirth, & ↓ intellectual & psychomotor dev of the fetus.
• Difficult to assess in early preg: Physiologic ↑ in total T_3/T_4 due to hCG cross reaction and stim of TSH-R & ↑ TBG. In 1st tri total T_4 ↑ & TSH ↓, w/ no real hypo/ hyperthyroidism.
• No routine screening of asx pregnant pts. Screen if on therapy, goiter, nodularity, h/o thyroid d/o/neck irradiation, prior infant w/ thyroid dysfxn, type I DM, FHx. Order TSH with reflex to T_4 if TSH is high.
• Normal ranges in preg: 1st tri: 0.1–2.5 mIU/L; 2nd tri: 0.2–3.0 mIU/L; 3rd tri: 0.3–3.0 mIU/L
• Rx similar to nonpregnant pts but preg may ↑ thyroid hormone requirements

- Treat subclinical hypothyroid → improves obstetrical outcomes (but no changes in long-term neurologic dev in the fetus)

Thyroid function test results in pregnancy compared with nonpregnant hyperthyroid and hypothyroid conditions			
Test	**Normal pregnancy**	**Hyperthyroidism**	**Hypothyroidism**
Thyroid-stimulating hormone (TSH)	No change	↓	↑
Thyroxine-binding globulin (TBG)	↑	No change	No change
Total T_4 (T_4)	↑	↑	↓
Free T_4 (fT_4) or free T_4 index (FTI)	No change	↑	↓
Total triiodothyronine (T_3)	↑	↑ or no change	↓ or no change
Free T_3 (fT_3)	No change	↑ or no change	↓ or no change
T_3 resin uptake (T_3RU)	↓	↑	↓
Iodine uptake	↑	↑ or no change	↓ or no change

Data from American College of Obstetricians and Gynecologists. Thyroid disease in pregnancy. ACOG Practice Bulletin No. 148. Thyroid Disease in Pregnancy and Rashid M, Rashid MH. Obstetric management of thyroid disease. *Obstet Gynecol Surv.* 2007;62(10):680–8.

HYPERTHYROIDISM

Definition, Epidemiology, and Etiology (*Endocr Pract* 2011;17(3):456)
- Hyperthyroidism is caused by excess synthesis & secretion of thyroid hormone
- Prevalence 1.2% (0.5% overt & 0.7% subclinical), Ratio F:M of 5:1. More common in smokers.
- The most common causes are:

  Graves dz (80%): Autoimmune TRAbs → bind TSH-R → ↑ TSH. Accounts for 95% of hyperthyroidism in Preg.

  Thyroiditis (10%): Painless inflammation of thyroid due to viral infxn or postpartum inflammation → release of preformed thyroid hormone. May resolve and → hypothyroid.

  Toxic adenomas: Single or multinodular, autonomously functioning, secrete thyroid hormone. More common in setting of iodine deficiency.

  Other: Amiodarone, struma ovarii (ovarian dermoid), TSH secreting pituitary adenoma, gestational trophoblastic dz (hCG stimulates TSH receptor), follicular cell carcinoma, iodine-induced, thyrotoxicosis factitia

Clinical Manifestation and Physical Exam (*Lancet* 2003;362(9382):459)
- Nervousness, anxiety, heat intolerance, tremor, palps, weight loss, oligomenorrhea, tachy, exophthalmos, thyromegaly. Tachy (&/or arrhythmias), HTN, warm/moist/smooth skin, lid lag, goiter, tremors
- Thyrotoxicosis in 1 of 500 pregnancies → ↑ preeclampsia, thyroid storm, CHF, IUGR, preterm deliv, stillbirth
- **Thyroid storm:** Medical emergency, extreme hypermetabolism → seizures, arrhythmia, stupor, shock, coma. Do not delay therapy while fT_4, T_3, TSH pending. Tx includes β-blockers, thionamide, iodine, glucocorticoids, cholestyramine

Diagnostic Workup (*Endocr Pract* 2011;17(3):456)
- **Graves dz:** ↓TSH, ↑ fT_4, ↑ fT_3, ± antithyroid peroxidase Ab (TPO), ⊕ TSI, ⊕ TRAb, other antithyroid Abs poss

  When clinical presentation is not diagnostic, RAIU is performed (*J Fam Pract* 2011;60(7):388): Diffuse, homogeneous = Graves dz; diffuse, heterogeneous = toxic multinodular goiter; focal = adenoma; no uptake = thyroiditis. IgG crosses placenta → fetal Graves (characterized by fetal tachycardia and potentially hydrops)
- **Subclinical hyperthyroidism:** ↓TSH; nml fT_4 & fT_3. Asx.

Treatment (*Endocr Pract* 2011;17(3):456)
- **Symptom mgmt:** β-Blocker to control tachy (propranolol also blocks T_4 conversion to T_3)
- **ATDs:** PTU 1st-line during the 1st tri (blocks both iodide organification & periph T_4 → T_3 conversion); monit liver fxn. Methimazole in 2nd–3rd trimesters. Titrate meds to fT_4 q2–4w.

- **RAI:** Started for pts w/ contraind to ATD use. Pretreat w/ methimazole prior to RAI to prevent worsening of hyperthyroidism. Contraind in preg.
- **Surg:** For symptomatic compression, large goiter, low uptake, documented or suspected malig
- **Thyroid storm:** PTU 1000 mg PO load → 200 mg PO q6h; 1–2 h after PTU give sodium iodide, 500–1000 mg IV q8h, and dexamethasone 2 mg IV q6h for 4 doses (*Obstet Gynecol* 2015;125:996.)

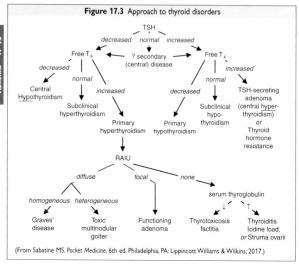

Figure 17.3 Approach to thyroid disorders

(From Sabatine MS. *Pocket Medicine.* 6th ed. Philadelphia, PA: Lippincott Williams & Wilkins; 2017.)

ADRENAL DISORDERS

Adrenal Hormones
- **Adrenal cortex:**
  Zona glomerulosa: Mineralocorticoids (aldosterone) → conserve sodium in nephron distal tubule & collecting duct → ↑ BP
  Zona fasciculata: Glucocorticoids (deoxycorticosterone, corticosterone, & cortisol) → ↑ blood glucose, suppress immune system, regulate metabolism
  Zona reticularis: Androgens (DHEA, DHEA-S, & androstenedione) → estrogen, androgens
- **Adrenal medulla:** Secretes catecholamines (epinephrine, norepinephrine, dopamine), in response to autonomic (sympathetic) nervous stimulation

Cushing Syndrome
- **Epidemiology:** 0.2–5.0 per 1 million annually, prevalence of 39–79 per million in various populations (*Lancet* 2015;386:913–27)
- **Etiology:** Cushing disease (benign pituitary adenoma, 65–70%), ectopic ACTH secretion by nonpituitary tumors (10–15%), adrenocortical tumors (18–20%), ectopic CRH secretion by nonhypothalamic tumors (<1%)

Disorders of cortisol production		
	↑ Cortisol	**↓ Cortisol**
↑ACTH	*Secondary hypercortisolism* Cushing disease (cortisol excess)	*Primary hypocortisolism* Addison's disease
↓ACTH	*Primary hypercortisolism* Cushing syndrome (adrenal adenoma)	*Secondary hypocortisolism* Sheehan's syndrome

- **Clinical manifestations:** Central obesity (extremity sparing), moon facies, buffalo hump, skin striae, easy bruising, hyperpigmentation (if ↑ ACTH), fungal infections, glucose intolerance, HTN, osteoporosis, hypokalemia, psychosis. ♀ → Menstrual irregularities (33% amenorrhea, 31% oligomenorrhea, 36% other) (*J Clin Endocrinol Metab* 1998;83:3083). Androgen excess → adrenal glands are the major source of androgens in ♀ → hirsutism, thinning scalp hair, oily skin, increased libido, infertility.

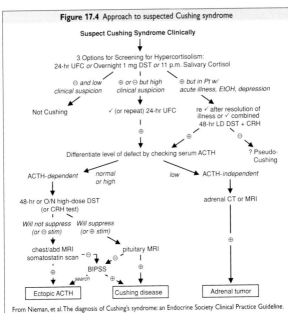

Figure 17.4 Approach to suspected Cushing syndrome

From Nieman, et al. The diagnosis of Cushing's syndrome: an Endocrine Society Clinical Practice Guideline. *J Clin Endocrinol Metab.* 2008 May;93(5):1526–40.

- **Rx:** Surgical resection of pituitary adenoma, adrenal tumor or ectopic ACTH-secreting tumor. Secondary options = pituitary XRT, bilateral adrenalectomy. Inhibitors for hypercortisolism if needed (ketoconazole, metyrapone, etomidate)

Adrenal Insufficiency (*Lancet* 2014;383:2152–67)
- **Definition:** Primary = adrenocortical insufficiency (Addison's). Secondary = ↓ ACTH. Tertiary = defect hypothalamus leading to ↓ secretion corticotropin
- **Epidemiology:** Primary: Incidence 4.4–6.0 cases per 1 million annually; Secondary: 150–280 cases per 1 million annually, women > men (*Lancet* 2014;383:2152–67)
- **Etiologies:** Autoimmune (most common in adults in industrialized nations, 80–90%; isolated vs. polyglandular autoimmune syn); infectious (most common in developing nations; TB, CMV, histoplasmosis); vascular (hemorrhage, thrombosis, trauma); drugs (ketoconazole, rifampin, anticonvulsants); deposition (hemochromatosis, amyloid, sarcoid); metastatic disease
  Primary or secondary hypopituitarism; rapidly terminated glucocorticoid therapy (≥2 w at ≥10 mg/d) → HPA suppression; Megestrol (progestin w/ glucocorticoid activity)
- **Clinical manifestations:** Fatigue, weakness, anorexia, orthostatic hypotension, nausea, vomiting, hypoNa, hyperK, hyperpigmentation (primary AI only). ± Manifestations of hypopituitarism. Consider adrenal insufficiency w/ sev hyperemesis gravidarum.
- **Adrenal crisis:** Above symptoms + severe abdominal or leg pain, syncope, dehyd, psychosis, seizures, lethargy, fever, hypoglycemia

- **Dx:**

  Early am cortisol <3 µg/dL = adrenal insufficiency. ≥18–20 µg/dL, AI ruled out.

  High-dose ACTH test: 1st-line test for most pts. Check serum cortisol → inject 250 µg cosyntropin (synthetic ACTH) → check cortisol at 60 min. Tests cortisol release.

  Low-dose (1 µg) ACTH test: Check serum cortisol → inject 1 µg cosyntropin → check cortisol at 30 min. Used if recent onset ACTH deficiency suspected.

  Serum ACTH: ↑ In primary, low–normal or ↓ in secondary

  Imaging if needed for pituitary or adrenal eval (MRI or CT)

- **Rx:**

  Acute adrenal insufficiency

  Rapid IV fluid hydration w/ isotonic saline

  4 mg dexamethasone IV q12h (dexamethasone does not interfere w/ serum cortisol level)

  Chronic adrenal insufficiency

  Hydrocortisone: 20–25 mg PO daily in BID or TID divided doses (eg, 10/5/2.5 mg), or prednisone 2.5–7.5 mg PO daily. ↑ Dose 2–3× for up to 3 d during acute illness.

  Fludrocortisone (only needed in primary adrenal insufficiency): 0.1 mg/d

  Consider adrenal androgen replacement in patients with impaired mood/wellbeing despite optimal replacement therapy. Start with dehydroepiandrosterone 25–50 mg single AM dose

  Preg: If adequately treated beforehand, most have uncomp preg, labor, & deliv. During labor, consider "stress dose steroids." Hydrate w/ IVFs & give hydrocortisone 25 mg IV q6h. At deliv, ↑ dose to 100 mg. After deliv, taper dose rapidly to maint dosing w/i 3 d. Only needed for >5 mg × >3 w of exogenous steroid.

Pheochromocytoma

- **Definition:** Rare catecholamine secreting chromaffin cell tumor originating from adrenal medulla (90%) & sympathetic ganglia (10%)
- **Epidemiology:** 0.8/100000 person y incid. <0.2% of pts w/ HTN. "Rule of 10's": 10% extra-adrenal, 10% in children, 10% multi/bilateral, 10% recurrence, 10% malig, 10% familial. If undiagnosed in preg, ~50% mat/fetal mortality. If diagnosed, mortality dec to <5 and 15%, respectively.
- **Etiology:** Approx 30% patients have disease as part of familial disorder. MEN 2A/2B (2A = pheo/MTC/parathyroid hyperplasia; 2B = pheo/MTC/mucosal neuromas), von Hippel–Lindau, neurofibromatosis-1, familial paraganglioma.
- **Clinical manifestations:** HTN most common (sustained or paroxysmal), HA, sweating, tachycardia, pallor. Can be triggered by stress, abdominal manipulation, maybe IV contrast. In Preg → paradoxical supine HTN
- **Dx:**

  High risk (familial syndromes, personal Hx): Plasma-free metanephrines (99% sens/89% spec)

  Low risk (all other): 24-h urine fractionated metanephrines & catecholamines (99% sens/98% spec). False + w/ sev illness, renal failure, OSA, labetalol, TCAs, sympathomimetics.

  Imaging after biochemical confirmation = CT Abd/pelvis preferred over MRI for imaging (98–100% sensitive). Consider MIBG scintigraphy if CT/MRI neg w/ + clinical/biochem. Genetic testing recommended (*J Clin Endocrinol Metab* 2014;99(6):1915–42).

- **Rx:** α-Adrenergic blockade (phenoxybenzamine) ± β blockade (propranolol) → Surg (laparoscopic if possible). In preg → same as above. Laparoscopic resxn after 10–14 d of medical optimization. If previable fetus, C/S + tumor resxn at deliv.

HYPERANDROGENISM

Hyperandrogenism:

Labs: Serum testosterone (>150 ng/dL in ♀ sugg ovarian/adrenal tumor), DHEA-S (>500 µg/dL in ♀ sugg adrenal tumor), 17-OHP (nml 100–300 ng/dL), prolactin (nml <20 ng/mL; prolactin acting on receptors in adrenal → ↑ DHEA-S), thyroid function tests, gluc tol testing (fasting +2-h OGTT). Fasting gluc:insulin ratio <4.5 sugg insulin resistance.

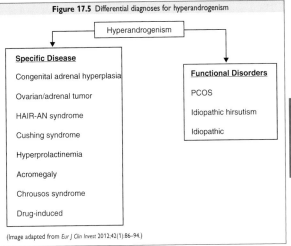

Figure 17.5 Differential diagnoses for hyperandrogenism

Hyperandrogenism

Specific Disease

Congenital adrenal hyperplasia

Ovarian/adrenal tumor

HAIR-AN syndrome

Cushing syndrome

Hyperprolactinemia

Acromegaly

Chrousos syndrome

Drug-induced

Functional Disorders

PCOS

Idiopathic hirsutism

Idiopathic

(Image adapted from *Eur J Clin Invest* 2012;42(1):86–94.)

Imaging: MRI or CT
- **Rx:** Depends on etiology; Surg recommended for ovarian/adrenal tumors

Polycystic Ovary Syndrome (See Chap. 8 [p. 8-2])
- **Definition:** Ovarian interstitial cells differentiate into islands of luteinized theca cells → ↑ steroid production. ↑ Periph conversion to estrogen → ↑ endometrial hyperplasia.
- **Dx:** Menstrual irregularities, obesity, hyperandrogenism. Serum testosterone >150 ng/dL, severe insulin resistance and hyperinsulinemia. Can be postmenopausal (unlike PCOS only in younger).
- **Rx:** Combination OCPs, weight loss, GnRH agonist (øLH secretion), surgical resxn
- **Other ovarian tumors:** See "Gynecologic Oncology" other sex hormone producing tumors (teratoma, gonadoblastoma, granulosa cell, Sertoli–Leydig cell).

HIRSUTISM

Definition, Pathophysiology, and Epidemiology
- Excess terminal hair that often occurs in male distribution in women
- 5α-reductase converts testosterone to DHT → increased sebum production, the differentiation of the hair follicle from vellus to coarser terminal hairs and the prolongation of the anagen phase resulting in longer thicker hairs
- Ethnicity-related trends in hair follicle conc/propensity toward hirsutism; distinguish hypertrichosis from hirsutism. Mediterranean descent > northern Europeans > Asians.
- Overall 5–8% of reproductive age ♀. Typical onset in adolescence to early 20's.

Etiology
- PCOS (72–82%), idiopathic hyperandrogenemia (6–15%), idiopathic hirsutism (4–7%), adrenal hyperplasia (2–4%), androgen-secreting tumors (0.2%). Rare causes: Meds (anabolic steroids, danazol, progestins, metoclopramide, methyldopa), acromegaly, Cushing syndrome, hyperprolactinoma, thyroid dysfunction

Clinical Presentation
- Terminal hair on lip, chin, chest, abd, arms, legs, back. Ferriman–Gallwey score evaluates 9 body areas on a 1–4 scale (>8 = mod hirsutism, >15 severe; 95% are nml w/ score <8).

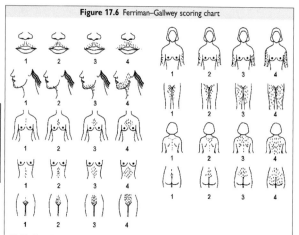

Figure 17.6 Ferriman–Gallwey scoring chart

Modified from Hatch, et al. Hirsutism: Implications, etiology, and management. *Am J Obstet Gynecol*. 1981; 140:815–30.

Diagnosis (See Chap. 8)

Treatment
- Combined OCPs 1st line (use lower androgenic progestin products), consider spironolactone (antiandrogen), finasteride, ketoconazole, eflornithine (facial hair only).
- Mechanical hair removal (shaving, waxing, laser). Currently there are no FDA-approved pharmacologic options for pregnant women with hirsutism.

PARATHYROID DISORDERS

Parathyroid Function
- **PTH:** Exclusively regulates serum ionized calcium through stimulation of renal tubular calcium reabsorption and bone resorption. PTH also stimulates the conversion of calcidiol (25-hydroxyvitamin D) to calcitriol in renal tubular cells, thereby stimulating intestinal calcium absorption.
  Regulated by negative feedback of serum ionized calcium. Secreted by chief cells.
- PTH → ↑ Ca release from bone, ↓ renal excretion, ↑ 1–25 Vit D → ↑ serum calcium
- PTH → ↑ renal PO_4 excretion by inhibiting proximal and distal reabsorption, ↑ intestinal PO_4 absorption (w/ Ca), ↑ release from bone (w/ Ca) → overall ↓ phosphorus
- **PTHrP** similar to PTH, synthesized in many tissues. Levels gradually ↑ in pregnancy & lactation. High conc in human breast milk. Pathologically ↑ in some cancers causing humoral HyperCa of malignancy (HHM, found in squamous cell lung cancer, non-Hodgkin's lymphoma)

Primary Hyperparathyroidism (PTH-related Hypercalcemia)
- ↑ PTH due excess glandular production. Usually age >60. ~85% adenoma, ~15% hyperplasia, 1% carcinoma, drugs (thiazides, lithium).
- **Epidemiology:** Varies by race, with significantly higher incidence among black individuals (92 per 100,000 in women and 46 per 100,000 in men) than in white individuals (81 per 100,000 in women and 29 per 100,000 in men). Other races have lower incidence, and incidence increases with age, more common postmenopausal women (*J Clin Endocrinol Metab* 2013;98(3):1122–9).
- **Dx:** HyperCa often found on routine biochemical testing. ↑ PTH or an inappropriately high-nml PTH in pt w/ ↑ Ca; exclude FHH (below).

- **Clinical manifestation:** Usually asymptomatic HyperCa (80%). Other symptoms include nausea, vomiting, constipation, abdominal pain, nephrolithiasis (sx of high Ca). Osteitis fibrosa cystica = demineralization of bone, subperiosteal resorption, bone cysts, osteoclastomas/"brown tumors," & pathologic fractures.
- **Dx:** ↑ Total & free serum Ca. ↓ PO_4. High serum PTH for Ca level. Consider: PTHrP, 25-OH Vit D, urinary calcium, SPEP, UPEP, ACE, CXR/CT, mammogram. Neck ultrasound or ^{99m}Tc-sestamibi scintigraphy to localize.
- **Rx:** Hyperparathyroidism has risk for mother & fetus: If Ca <12 mg/dL close monitoring, furosemide can be used for calciuresis. If Ca >12 mg/dL, parathyroidectomy recommended, ideally 2nd trimester. Surgery shown to be safe/eff in preg in limited case studies (*Gland Surg* 2014;3(3):158–64).
  – 50% of neonates of ♀ w/ hyperparathyroidism have low Ca/tetany; risk of IUGR, LBW, IUFD as a result of fetal PTH suppression.
  Nonpregnant → surgical mgmt for all symptomatic pts or for asx pts w/:
  Ca >1 mg/dL above the UL of nml (*J Clin Endocrinol Metab* 2013;98(3):1122–9)
  GFR <60 mL/min
  Bone T score <–2.5 &/or prev fragility fx
  Age <50 y

Secondary Hyperparathyroidism in Renal Disease
- ↑ PTH due to appropriate response to HypoCa
- When GFR <–40 mL/min → ↓ calcitriol & ↑ phosphorus → HypoCa & ↑ PTH
- Ca binds w/ PO_4 & can deposit in tissues
- Outside of Preg, treat w/ PO_4 binders, Vit D

Familial Hypocalciuric Hypercalcemia (FHH)
- Autosomal dominant mutation in Ca sensing receptor causes shift in set point for Ca
- Critical to differentiate from disorders of PTH, as a benign condition
- Ca ↑, but usually <12; PTH inappropriately nml or mildly ↑
- Urine Ca <200 mg/24 h, & Ca/CrCl <0.01 (24-h U_{ca} × S_{cr}/S_{ca} × 24-h U_{cr}) supports dx
- Treatment rarely indicated. ↑ Ca always recurs after surg unless total parathyroidectomy
- In preg, neonate at risk for HypoCa/tetany unless inherits gene & then asx
- Father w/ FHH → neonate at risk for HyperCa postpartum

Hypoparathyroidism
- **Acq:** Neck Surg w/ incidental removal of parathyroid glands (most commonly for hyperthyroidism), hypomagnesemia. Hereditary (rare): DiGeorge, polyglandular autoimmune type I. Dx is made w/ ↓ PTH in setting of ↓ Ca
- **Pseudohypoparathyroidism** (resistant to PTH due to mut) dx: ↑ PTH in setting of ↓ Ca
- **2° hypoparathyroidism** (appropriate ↓ PTH due to ↑ Ca) dx: ↓ PTH in setting of ↑ Ca
- **In preg:** Avoid mat HypoCa → precipitates neonat hyperparathyroidism → bone fractures
- **Postpartum:** May develop HyperCa, monit Ca postpartum & stop Vit D if develops
- **Rx:** Calcitriol + elemental Ca 1 g/d, titrate calcitriol weekly to low nml serum Ca level
- Treated pts are at risk for nephrolithiasis. If 24-h U_{ca} >300 mg/d → ↓ Vit D, can add thiazide diuretic to ↓ urinary calcium excretion

Hypocalcemia
- **Sx:** Many sx are nonspecific (anorexia, anxiety, dehydration, weakness). Also carpopedal spasm, oral paresthesias, Trousseau + Chvostek sign.
- **Dx:** Confirm w/ ionized Ca (preferred) or corrected calcium level for albumin. Corrected Ca (mg/dL) = measured total Ca (mg/dL) + 0.8 (4 – serum albumin [g/dL]).
- **Etiology:** Measure PTH, Vit D
  Low PTH: Postsurgical, genetic or autoimmune causes, HIV, infiltration
  Nml PTH: Calcium sensor defect
  High PTH: Vit D deficiency/resistance, renal disease, loss Ca from circulation (rhabdo, tumor lysis syn, pancreatitis), PTH resistance (pseudohyperparathyroidism), drugs (phenytoin, bisphosphonates, fluoride poisoning)
- **Rx:** Calcium (& treat hypomagnesemia)
  Asx or mild: Oral calcium 0.5–1 g elemental BID
  Sev: IV Ca-gluconate (preferred due to less tissue necrosis) or Ca-chloride. Vit D supplementation.

Hypercalcemia
- Confirm w/ ionized Ca (preferred) or corrected calcium level for albumin
- **Clinical manifestations:** Renal stones, abdominal pain, polyuria, depression, fatigue

- **Rx:** Indicated for pts w/ total calcium >14 mg/dL or mod/sev sx
  IV hydration with NS, bisphosphonate ± calcitonin
  Bisphosphonate onset of action is 1–2 d
  Calcitonin works in hours, but tachyphylaxis occurs after ~24 h
  Zoledronic acid more effective than pamidronate in malig (*J Clin Oncol* 2001;19(2):558)
  Denosumab has been shown effective in refractory malignant hyperCa (*J Clin Endocrinol Metab* 2014;99(9):3144–52)

PITUITARY DISORDERS

Definitions
- **Anterior pituitary:** GH, TSH, ACTH, Prolactin, LH, FSH, MSH
- **Posterior pituitary:** Oxytocin, ADH

Panhypopituitarism
- **Etiology:** Primary – Surgery, tumors, ischemia (Sheehan syn → postpartum pituitary necrosis due to hypovolemic shock after deliv, watershed effect), radiation, infection, autoimmune (lymphocytic hypophysitis). Secondary (hypothalamic) – Surg, tumors, infxn, trauma, autoimmune.
- **Clinical manifestations:** Based on specific hormones:
  ACTH: Hyponatremia (not due to salt wasting but rather ADH secretion d/t cortisol deficiency); possible postural hypotension/tachycardia. Less severe: Fatigue, anorexia, hypoglycemia, eosinophilia (**no** hyperpigmentation)
  TSH: Sx of hypothyroidism
  FSH/LH: Sx of menopause
  GH: Increased fat deposition, decreased BMD
  Prolactin: Inability to lactate after delivery (isolated prolactin def very rare)
- **Dx:** Pituitary hormone levels → low if chronic, normal if acute. Imaging w/MRI.
- **Rx:**
  ACTH deficiency: Hydrocortisone 15–25 mg/d – may also consider prednisone or dexamethasone
  Mineralocorticoid replacement not necessary (regulated by angiotensin II & potassium)
  LH/FSH deficiency: Estrogen/progest therapy to simulate nml physiology; estradiol on cycle days 1–25 + progesterone days 16–25. Ovulation induction w/ gonadotropins for fertility.
  GH deficiency: Recombinant hGH 2–5 μg/kg/d. Monit w/ serum IGF-1.

Hyperprolactinemia
- **Etiology:** 50% of adenomas cause hyperprolactinemia (prolactin → stimulates lactation → ↓ GnRH → ↓ FSH + LH → can ↓ menses); drugs (SSRIs, estrogen, methyldopa, verapamil, morphine, dopamine receptor agonists [metoclopramide, domperidone, haloperidol, risperidone]), pregnancy, hypothyroidism, chronic renal failure, stress
- **Epidemiology:** Pituitary adenomas account for 14% of primary intracranial and CNS tumors; overall prevalence in the general population (radiographic and autopsy) is estimated at 17% (*Neuro Oncol* 2012;14(Suppl 5):v1–49)
- **Clinical manifestations:** Amenorrhea, galactorrhea, infertility, ↓ libido, visual changes (bitemporal visual field losses w/ large adenomas)
- **Dx:** Serum prolactin (levels b/w 20–200 μg/L may be artificially low in large adenomas d/t "hook effect"). Brain MRI.
- **Rx:**
  Asx + microadenoma (≤10 mm) → follow w/ MRI. <2% progress to macroadenoma.
  Symptomatic ± microadenoma → dopamine agonist (bromocriptine 2.5 mg QD, or cabergoline 0.25 mg 2×/w). Side effects = N/V, orthostasis. Surgical: Transsphenoidal Surg. Radiation 3rd line
  In Preg, microadenoma unlikely to grow. Macroadenoma (>10 mm) = 23% w/ sign if enlargement during Preg if no prior Surg or radiation; 5% if prev Surg/radiation. Dopamine agonist recommended before Preg to shrink adenoma. Image at least q3mo. Serum prolactin <400 ng/mL reassuring. Consider MRI if visual changes or headaches. Breastfeeding does not ↑ growth
  Prolactinoma & fertility: Dopamine agonist → lower serum prolactin → ovulation

Galactorrhea
- **Definition:** Physiologic nipple discharge (milky white, brown or green, elicited after manual expression from milk ducts). Pathologic discharge is bloody, serous, spont.

Approx 50–80% women in their reproductive years can express one or more drops of fluid and 6.8% of women referred to surgeon d/t nipple discharge
- **Etiology:** Pregnancy, postpartum, nipple stimulation, pituitary adenoma (prolactinoma), hypothyroidism, craniopharyngioma, Cushing disease, acromegaly, neoplastic processes (breast, renal adenoCa, lymphoma), hydatidiform mole
- **Dx:** Occult blood testing & microscopy. Diagnostic mammography, mammary ductography. Breast exam to elicit nipple discharge & for mass. Multi ducts/expressed manually and bilateral → more likely physiologic.

Gigantism and Acromegaly

- **Definitions:** Gigantism → elevated GH & IGF-1 before fusion of the epiphyseal plates → extremely tall stature. Acromegaly (10% adenomas) → elevated GH + IGF-1 after fusion of the epiphyseal plates. May be seen in familial syndromes such as MEN-1 or 4, McCune–Albright syndrome, Carney Complex, X-linked acrogigantism.
- **Clinical manifestations:** Large hands & feet, coarsening facial features, macroglossia, HA, OSA, acanthosis nigricans, arthralgias, carpal tunnel, jaw enlargement, hoarseness, extremely tall stature (gigantism), may coexist w/ amenorrhea & or galactorrhea in adol girls
- **Dx:** Best single test: Serum IGF-1. If normal, acromegaly very unlikely. If high, oral GTT: Serum GH should be <1 ng/mL 2 h after ingesting 75 g gluc load. Inadequate suppression of GH after a glucose load confirms the diagnosis of acromegaly. If GH not suppressed → brain MRI to look for pituitary tumor.
- **Rx:** Transsphenoidal resxn for pituitary tumor. Octreotide (mimics somatostatin → more potent inhib of GH & insulin than natural hormone), bromocriptine (dopamine agonist), XRT (rarely used in children). In refractory cases and unable to receive GH receptor antagonist, a trial with estrogen compounds or SERMs could be an option, mainly in those with mild IGF-1 elevation.

Epidemiology (Headache 2006;46:365; Lancet Neurol 2013;12:175; Obstet Gynecol 2016;126:298, 301)
- HA prevalence is high in puerperium (~40%) but also outside of pregnancy (60–80%). Most are brief & do not prompt physician visit. Common neuro referral topic. ♀ > ♂, slightly. Decreases w/ age.
- 75% of primary HA will ↓ in Preg. But ~40% PP have HA, esp 1st w after delivery.

Pathogenesis
- 90% are tension-type, migraine, or cluster HA. In ♀, 70% are a/w menses, but <20% are pure menstrual migraine.
- Multifactorial initiation. Nociceptor activation/sensitization can → central sensitization, ↑ pain transmission, ↓ pain threshold. Minor role for genetics.

Differential Diagnosis
- **Primary (most common):** Migraine, tension-type HA, cluster, orgasmic HA (elevated estrogen, prolactin, oxytocin)
- **Secondary:** Ischemic stroke, hemorrhagic stroke (SAH, AVM, HTN), venous sinus thrombosis, carotid or vertebral artery dissection, vasculitides, reversible cerebral vasoconstriction syndromes (RCVS or Call–Fleming syn), PRES (posterior reversible encephalopathy syn)
- **Other:** Preeclampsia/eclampsia, benign intracranial HTN, sinusitis, overmedication, PDPH (postdural puncture headache), tumor, estrogen withdrawal, brain tumor
- **Primary care:** Meningitis, pseudotumor cerebri, trigeminal neuralgia, TMJ syn, temporal arteritis

Diagnostic Workup
- **Hx:** Age, aura, prodrome, frequency, intensity, duration, timing, quality, radiation, assoc sx, FHx, precipitating/relieving factors, changes w/ activity/food/EtOH, resp to rx, visual changes, h/o trauma, change in sleep pattern/exercise/weight/diet/contraceptives, environmental toxins/exposures, menstrual Hx
- **Warning signs:** Thunderclap HA, autonomic sx, 1st/worst HA of life, worsening, fever, change in mental status/personality, exercise assoc, very young or old age, h/o cancer/Lyme dz/HIV/Preg/PP, *focal neuro findings, *meningismus, *papilledema (*, obtain imaging)

Approach to HA by history			
Question	**Poss cause**	**Test to confirm/rx**	**Comments**
Postural? Tinnitus?	Dural puncture; can also see in women who have not had spinal anesthesia due to shearing forces when pushing	Typically by H&P only MRI + gadolinium for meningeal enhancement LP CT myelogram (most sensitive for leak) Analgesics, caffeine, bld patch	Worse when upright. Incid 10% in those with spinal epidural. Can occur days to weeks postproce-dure. Can be seen up to 1–7 d postpartum
H/o similar HA?	Migraine	Triptans or ergots	⅓–½ of ♀ w/ migraine Hx will have PP HA
Unilateral? Daily for limited time?	Cluster	100% oxygen CCBs, triptans, ergots, steroids	Assoc ipsilateral miosis, ptosis, conjunctival irritation, lacrimation
Sudden onset?	SAH Cerebral venous thrombosis	Plain CT, LP for hemorrhage If negative, MRI/MRA	Thunderclap HA
Elevated BPs, proteinuria, seizures?	Preeclampsia or eclampsia	Assess & monit for proteinuria, HTN, & hyperreflexia	HA can precede other signs of sev preeclampsia
Vasoconstrictive meds? Focal neuro deficits?	Reversible cerebral vasoconstrictive syndromes	See "sudden onset" category	Look for SSRIs, ergots, pseudoephedrine, bromocriptine PRES a/w cortical blind-ness & seizures

Data from Int J Obstet Anesth 2010;19:422; Can J Anaesth 2002;49:49; Lancet Neurol 2013;12:175; Curr Neurol Neurosci Rep 2016;16:40.

- **Physical exam:** BP, pulse, auscultation for bruits (neck, temporal), palpation (head, neck, spine), neuro exam w/ fundoscopy
- **Labs:** Usually not needed; TSH, ESR, CRP, toxicology screen, Lyme Ab, LP (if suspect SAH or infxn)
- **Imaging:** See warning signs. CT head/c-spine or MR ok. MRI/MRA head/neck if post fossa or vascular suspected.

Treatment and Medications
- **1st line:** Relaxation, ice packs, reassurance, acetaminophen, ibuprofen (not Preg). 2nd line: Add narcotics sparingly. 3rd line: Antiemetics (eg, chlorpromazine), IV magnesium. Avoid NSAIDs in 3rd trimester Preg (→ ductus arteriosus closure & oligohydramnios). Other treatments, see below.
- **Tension-type HAs:** Stress reduction, warm showers, massage, ice/heat packs, posture correction, physical therapy, prescription eyeglasses. NSAIDs, ASA, Tylenol, caffeine, muscle relaxants. Tricyclics for prevention.

MIGRAINE

Definition & Epidemiology (Curr Neurol Neurosci Rep 2016;16:40)
- Recurring synd of HA, nausea, vomiting, &/or other sx of neurologic dysfxn. Migraine w/ aura = visual sx occur/resolve w/ HA, risk factor for ischemic stroke.
- **Increases w/ age in ♀:** 22% at 20–24 yo; 28% at 25–29 yo; 33% at 30–34 yo; ~37% for 35–39 yo.; ½ of women have improvement during pregnancy, and greater than ¾ in later stages of pregnancy; 80% of women with migraine will experience one during pregnancy
- Risk for preeclampsia increased w/ HA (Am J Hypertension 2008;21(3):360). 2.4-fold ↑ w/ any HA Hx; 3.5-fold ↑ w/ migraine; 4-fold ↑ w/ migraines during Preg.
- **Status migrainosus:** >72 h → evaluate for secondary causes

Pathophysiology (Headache 2006;46:S49)
- Brain itself lacks pain receptors, but surrounding meningeal, muscle, skin, vessel, subcutaneous tissue, or mucous membrane inflammation/injury → HA pain
- Hormonal fluctuations in estrogen → menstrual migraine or PP migraine (withdrawal); ↓ estrogen → increased in serotonergic tone
- **Migraine phases:** Prodrome → ± aura → main migraine pain → resolution

Treatment (Neurology 2015;55:780–1, 86)
- See conservative measures above. Narcotics not 1st line; abortive therapy needed early. Acute therapies used more than 2 d weekly can lead to rebound HA.
- Avoid combined OCPs if h/o migraine w/ aura or age >35 yo & no aura. D/c combination hormonal contraception if severity/frequency of HA increases or in setting of new onset migraine w/ aura.
- Avoid triptans in patients with history of cardiovascular dz due to vasoconstriction; pts should be instructed to take triptans at onset of pain, rather than during aura
- Use of SSRIs/SNRIs with triptans is not a contraindication, but should be vigilant for serotonin syndrome

Acute migraine treatment strategies	
Severity	**Examples**
Mild–moderate	Acetaminophen (for milder attacks)
	ASA (after discussion of risks and benefits)
	Combination analgesics without opioids or barbiturates
	If not pregnant:
	Ibuprofen
	Diclofenac
	Naproxen
Nonresponsive moderate or severe	Sumatriptan
Refractory to above strategies	Steroids
	Combination analgesics without opioids or barbiturates
	Combination analgesics with opioids (not routine)
	If not pregnant:
	Triptan–NSAID combination
	Dihydroergotamine
	Dopamine antagonists

Severity	Examples

Patients with contraindications to vasoconstrictors	Combination analgesics without opioids or barbiturates
	Combination analgesics with opioids (not routine)
	If not pregnant:
	   NSAIDs
	   Dopamine antagonists

From Becker WJ. Acute Migraine Treatment in Adults. *Headache* 2015;55:778–93.

Acute therapy for migraine	
Class	**Examples**
Mild analgesic	Acetaminophen ASA Ibuprofen Naproxen Fioricet (butalbital, acetaminophen, caffeine) – (not currently standard of care)
Triptans[a]	Sumatriptan
Ergots[b]	Dihydroergotamine Ergotamine
BBs	Propranolol
Antidepressants	Amitriptyline Fluoxetine
CCBs	Verapamil, nifedipine

[a]Migraine ppx.
[b]Category X in Preg.
From *J Fam Plann Reprod Health Care* 2007;33(2):83–93.

SEIZURE DISORDERS

Definition/Epidemiology
- Abn discharge of neurons in the CNS; 5–10% of pop affected
- Epilepsy – recurrent seizures, 0.5–1% of pop; 41 cases per 100000 women
- **Generalized seizures:** Start in both cerebral hemispheres at onset
- **Tonic–clonic:** 10–20-s tonic phase (constant muscle contraction) followed by 30-s clonic phase (intermittent muscle contraction)
- **Absence:** Transient lapse of consciousness – no loss of posture, muscle tone
- **Myoclonic:** Brief contraction, sudden onset
- **Atonic:** Brief loss of complete muscle tone (also called "drop attacks")
- **Partial/focal seizures:** Limited to 1 area of 1 cerebral hemisphere at onset
- **Simple:** Motor, sensory, or autonomic; no impairment of consciousness
- **Complex:** Impairment of consciousness + automatisms

Differential Diagnosis (*Anaesth Crit Care Pain Med* 2016;16:S17–18)
- Syncope – no aura; motor manifestations <30 s; no postictal confusion; pt may have pallor & clamminess
- Psychogenic sz – asym limb movements, pelvic thrusting
- Other – metabolic (EtOH, hypoglycemia); migraine, TIA, thrombotic thrombocytopenic purpura/hemolytic-uremic syndrome (TTP-HUS)
- Eclampsia – generalized convulsions &/or coma in the setting of preeclampsia & w/o evid of other neurologic conditions. Preg assoc; pt often has elevated BPs, blurry vision, proteinuria, RUQ pain.
- Posterior reversible encephalopathic syndrome (PRES), reversible cerebral vasoconstriction syndrome (RCVS), cerebral venous sinus thrombosis, amniotic fluid embolism (AFE)

Pathophysiology/Etiology
- **A**lcohol withdrawal, illicit drugs, meds (β-lactams, antidepressants, clozapine)
- **B**rain tumor; BP (a/w preeclampsia/eclampsia)
- **C**erebrovascular dz (subdural hematoma, hypertensive encephalopathy)
- **D**egenerative disorders (Alzheimer's)
- **E**lectrolyte imbalance (HoNa, hypoglycemia)

Antiepileptic drugs, side effects, and effect on pregnancy				
Medication	Avg daily dose (max)	Systemic side effects	Preg side effects/ comments	FDA category
Phenytoin	300–400 mg (600 mg)	Gum hyperplasia, hypoCa, hyperK	Orofacial clefts, cardiac malformations, genitourinary effects (Neurol 2005;64:961)	D
Carbamazepine	400–600 mg (1600 mg)	Aplastic anemia, leukopenia, hepatotoxicity, HoNa	NTDs; avoid if FHx of NTDs	D
Valproic acid	10–15 mg/kg/d (60 mg/kg)	Hepatotoxicity, increased NH_3, thrombocytopenia	AVOID during Preg; if necessary, high plasma levels should be <70 µg/mL & drug should be given in divided doses TID–QID A/w NTDs, hypospadias, CV malformation, cleft lip/palate, ↓ in motor & mental developmental quotients – dose–resp relationship	D
Phenobarb	60–180 mg (300 mg)	Rash	Cardiac & orofacial malformations, genitourinary effects	D
Ethosuximide	20–30 mg/kg (1.5 g)	Rash, bone marrow suppression		C
Gabapentin	900–2400 mg (2400 mg)	GI upset	Limited data	C
Levetiracetam	1500–3000 mg (3000 mg)	GI upset (rare)	Rare findings of NTD, CV anomalies, and oral cleft	C
Lamotrigine	400 mg (600 mg)		A/w left palate &/or cleft lip in pts w/ 1st trimester exposure	C

Data from LaRoche SM, Helmers SL. The new antiepileptic drugs: Scientific review. *JAMA.* 2004;291(5):605–614 and Hernández-Díaz S, Smith CR, Shen A et al. Comparative safety of antiepileptic drugs during pregnancy. *Neurology.* 2012;78;1692.

Clinical Manifestations
- Aura – premonition, abn smells, tastes, oral automatism
- Postictal period – can last minutes to hours; slowly resolving period post sz. Pt may be confused, disoriented, lethargic.
- Status epilepticus – state of continuous seizures >30 min or repeated seizures w/o resolution of postictal periods. Assoc complications: Rhabdomyolysis, lactic acidosis, neuronal death.

Workup and Studies
- Obtain collateral Hx from witnesses as pt will often have amnesia of event
- Ask about loss of responsiveness, aura, unusual behavior, loss of autonomic control (urinary or fecal incontinence)
- Evaluate for etiology w/ h/o fever, illness, prev sz; in Preg, elevated BPs, prot in the urine, ext & facial swelling
- Exam to look for focal neurologic abnormalities or evid of injury from sz activity (oropharyngeal or musculoskeletal or secondary head injury & ecchymoses)
- **Labs:** CBC, CMP, LFTs, toxicology screen, medication levels
- **Preg:** Preeclampsia labs (CBC, LFTs, BUN/Cr, uric acid, LDH, proteinuria)

Pregnancy Care (Neurol 2006;66:354; Neurol 2009;73:143)
- 500000 WWE are of childbearing age; 3–5 births per 1000 will be to WWE (Neurol 2000;55:S21). Preg w/ AEDs → ↑ IUGR & hypertensive disorders, ↑ CS (Acta Obstet Gynecol Scan 2006;85:643). If sz free for 2 y, consider withdrawal of AEDs at least 6 mo prior to conception.

Management of WWE during pregnancy		
Antepartum	**Intrapartum**	**Postpartum**
Drug conc should be established during Preg Perform serum conc every trimester, monthly for pts w/ breakthrough seizures & in those taking lamotrigine Recommend folic acid supplementation	Pt should take AED during labor No water labor Intravenous lorazepam or diazepam should be given if sz starts NOTE: Minimal variability can be expected for FHRT for 1 h	Mat plasma levels of AEDs may fluctuate until 8th w PP AED requirement is likely to fall in the puerperium (particularly lamotrigine & oxcarbazepine) PP sz risk elevated, in the setting of sleep depriv Most AEDs compatible w/ breastfeeding Consider relationship btw AEDs & contraception when counseling for PP birth control Inadequate evidence regarding PP vitamin K supplementation to reduce hemorrhagic complications in neonate exposed to AEDs

Contraception
- **Anticonvulsants that ↓ steroid levels:** Phenobarbital, primidone, phenytoin, carbamazepine (and lesser extent w/ oxcarbazepine, felbamate, topiramate)
- If OCPs are deemed necessary, use 50 µg of estrogen component or extended cycle treatments (3 cycles followed by 4-d break)
- **Emergency contraception:** Levonorgestrel 1.5 mg separated by 12 h (doubled dose)
- **WHO recommends alternative form of contraception:** Levonorgestrel IUD, copper IUD, Depo-Provera (a/w decreased sz frequency)

ECLAMPSIA

Definition
- New onset seizures in a woman w/ preeclampsia, not attributable to other causes

Epidemiology
- Accounts for 12% of mat deaths, worldwide (developing countries > developed countries) (Semin Perinatol 2009;33:130). ~38% occur w/o preceding sx.
- 2% mortality; 23% will require ventilation; 35% have 1 major complication (pulm edema, renal failure, respiratory distress syn, dissem intravascular coagulation, stroke, cardiac arrest, acute respiratory distress syn)
- Seizures occur in 2–3% of pts w/ sev preeclampsia not receiving magnesium ppx; incid 1.6–10 cases per 10000 deliveries
- Distribution by GA:
  <20 w GA: Consider molar Preg or antiphospholipid Ab syn
  Antepartum: 38–55%
  Intrapartum: 13–16%
  Up to 48-h PP: 5–39%
  >48 h PP: 5–17%, think AVM, ruptured aneurysm, carotid artery dissection, or idiopathic sz d/o

Pathophysiology (Am J Obstet Gynecol 2004;190:714)
- Cerebral autoregulation in resp to high systemic BP → vasospasm of cerebral arteries, intracellular edema
- Loss of autoregulation of cerebral bld flow in resp to high systemic BP → hyperperfusion, endothelial damage, extracellular edema

Clinical Manifestations (Obstet Gynecol 2011;118:995)
- HA – cerebral edema, though poor sensitivity and specificity to predict adverse outcome (J Obstet Gynaecol Can 2011;33:803)
- Vision changes – vasospasm of cerebral & retinal vessels
- Neurologic sx – most common premonitory sx (rates vary from 50–90%)
- Full PIERS model – odds ratio of 2.92 for predicting adverse outcomes in preeclampsia; calculator at: piers.cfri.ca/PIERSCalculatorH.aspx (Lancet 2011;377:219)
- Note: Presence of HTN & proteinuria are poor predictors of eclampsia, rare event. See also Chaps. 11 and 12 for preeclampsia.

Treatment and Medication
- Drug of choice = magnesium sulfate (calcium channel antagonism) 4–6 g IV bolus then 1–2 g/h. If no IV → 5 g IM in each buttock (10 g total; rpt 3 g alternating buttock q4h). If seizing on magnesium, rebolus 2 g IV. Therapeutic level 4–6 mEq/L.
- **2nd line:** Phenytoin: Loading dose by weight (<50 kg = 1000 mg; 50–70 kg = 1250 mg; >70 kg = 1500 mg). Therapeutic level 12–20 µg/mL. Check 2 h after loading → subseq dose; if <10 µg/mL → 500 mg IV, if 10–12 µg/mL → 250 mg. Check level q12h.
- **3rd line:** Diazepam 5–10 mg IV bolus, rpt q10–15min prn, max 30 mg in 8 h
- Diazepam, phenytoin were a/w increased recurrence of seizures compared w/ magnesium sulfate (Br J Obstet Gynaecol 1998;105:300; N Engl J Med 1995;333)
- Fetal brady occurs during eclamptic sz. Stabilize mom; no need for urgent CS
- MagPIE trial: International RCT, >10000 ♀ w/ at least mild preeclampsia randomized to magnesium sulfate or placebo. Magnesium sulfate decreases relative risk of eclampsia by 58% (95% CI 40–71). No documented adverse effects on mom or baby in short-term or long-term period (Lancet 2002;359:1877; British J Obstet Gynecol 2006;114:300)

Magnesium toxicity (approx levels)			
	Serum magnesium level		
	mmol/L	mEq/L	mg/dL
↓ Patellar reflexes	4	8	10
Respiratory depression	6	12	14
Altered cardiac conduction	>7.5	>15	>18
Cardiac arrest	>12.5	>25	>30

Magnesium toxicity: Treat by stopping MgSO₄, give calcium gluconate 1 g IV, maintain airway, intubation if needed. Can use diuretics to remove excess magnesium.

STROKE IN PREGNANCY

Epidemiology and Pathophysiology
- Stroke in Preg = approx. 7% of maternal deaths in US (Am J Obstet Gynecol 2016;214:723.e1)
- Most common in 3rd trimester or puerperium, but also ↑ in PP (8.7× for ischemic stroke; 24× for hemorrhagic stroke)
- Most common cause of stroke in Preg is preeclampsia/eclampsia
- ↑ Due to hypercoagulable state of Preg; cerebral endothelial dysfxn
- Pregnant and PP women have favorable short-term outcomes (Am J Obstet Gynecol 2016;214:723.e1)

Diagnosis (Obstet Med 2011:4:2)
- **Acute:** Hx, PE (listen for murmurs, carotid & subclav bruits, & look for signs of periph emboli). Urgent CT, noncontrast, to rule out hemorrhage, followed by CT angio. MRI/MRA w/ gadolinium. Doppler scan of the LE → if negative, then MRV.
- **Risk factors:** Hypercoagulable state: Lupus anticoagulant, anticardiolipin antibodies, anti-β2 glycoprotein, Factor V Leiden, prothrombin, prot C & S, antithrombin III. Peripartum cardiomyopathy.

Postreversible Encephalopathy Syn (Mayo Clin Proc 2010;85:427; Lancet Neurol 2015;14:921)
- Related to cerebral autoregulation & endothelial dysfxn. Seen in preeclampsia and eclampsia (Am J Obstet Gynecol 2016;215:239.e1)
- New data suggests that certain types of PRES may have long-term neurocognitive outcomes and may not be reversible (Lancet Neurol 2015;14:921)
- **Features:** HA, altered consciousness, visual disturbances (hemianopia, visual hallucinations), seizures (often presenting manifestation)
- **Radiology:** Symmetrical white matter edema in the post cerebral hemispheres (but can include brain stem and spinal cord), rarely seen on CT, but better depicted on MRI; in rare circumstances, can have MRI-negative PRES if clinical features are present
- **Rx:** Lower BP, start AEDs if seizing; no recommended guidelines

Postpartum Cerebral Angiopathy (Am J Obstet Gynecol 2004;191:375)
- Reversible cerebral vasoconstriction syndromes
- **Timeline:** Few days post deliv. Features: Thunderclap HA, vomiting, seizures.
- **Radiology:** Multifocal segmental narrowing of cerebral arteries, resolution in 4–6 w
- CSF nml

Cerebral Aneurysm Rupture and SAH (N Engl J Med 1996;335:768)
- Relative risk of intracerebral hemorrhage during Preg & up to 6 w PP is 5.6 times that of the nonpregnant pt
- Surgical rx after SAH during Preg improves mat & fetal outcomes
- Favor vaginal deliv unless aneurysm is diagnosed at term or there has been neurosurgical intervention w/i the week before deliv

CEREBRAL VENOUS THROMBOSIS

Definition and Epidemiology (Stroke 2011;42:1158; Headache 2016;56:1380)
- Thrombosis of the venous sinuses, cerebral veins, or jugular veins
- Represents 2% of all Preg-related strokes; 1/10,000 deliveries; risk is highest during 3rd trimester & PP

Etiology/Pathophysiology
- Dehyd, puerperal & PP infxn, thrombophilia inherent to Preg
- Risk increased w/ use of OCPs (22.1-fold increased odds [95% CI 5.9–84.2%]); increased odds for pts w/ thrombophilia (eg, prothrombin gene mut)

Diagnostic Workup
- **Acute:** Brain CT &/or MRI, bubble study & vascular US of the venous sinuses, cerebral veins, or jugular veins–Best is MRI T2 + MRV – better visualization, good detection of brain parenchyma, no radiation. Can evaluate for both thrombosis & stroke (Stroke 2011;42:1158).
- A nml D-dimer, high negative predictive value, low probability of CVT
- Empty delta sign on contrast-enhanced CT (hyperdensity of cortical vein or dural sinus, filling defect) seen in 30% of cases; won't show for several days following onset of symptoms
- "Dense cord sign" seen on noncontrast CT (hyperdensity filling vein or sinus), seen in 33% of cases of CVT
- Venous infarction is flame-shaped
- If diagnosed, plan for repeat imaging in 3–6 mo. Postdiagnosis to see if vein has re-cannulized

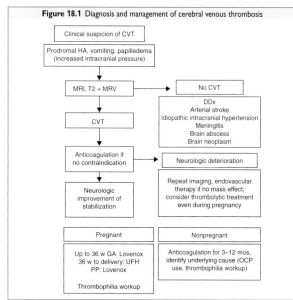

Figure 18.1 Diagnosis and management of cerebral venous thrombosis

MULTIPLE SCLEROSIS IN PREGNANCY

Definition/Epidemiology
- Immune-mediated demyelinating neurologic condition, characterized by inflamm lesions affecting the brain & spinal cord & resulting in neurologic disability
- Dz classification:
  Relapsing-remitting (RR): Manifestations develop in the context of clearly defined acute relapses followed by partial or complete recovery
  Secondary progressive: Following an initial RR course, manifestations worsen gradually w/ or w/o superimposed acute relapses
  Primary progressive: Manifestations gradually progress from onset w/o relapses
  Progressive relapsing: Manifestations gradually progress from onset w/ subseq superimposed relapses
- Occurs in 3:2 ratio of females to males; peak incid of 30 y of age
- Effect of Preg on MS activity *(PRIMS Study. N Engl J Med 1998;339:285; Brain 2004;127:1353)*
- 70% reduction in relapse risk in the 3rd trimester of Preg in RRMS pts
- 72% relapse in 1st 3 mo PP – a/w relapse in prepregnancy year, relapse during Preg, no association w/ breastfeeding or epidural placement *(Brain 2004;127:1353)*
- Long-term prog – increasing disability not related to Preg – fullterm Preg can lengthen time to secondarily progressive course *(N Engl J Med 1998;339:285)*

Diagnosis During Pregnancy and Postpartum
- Most common presenting sx are paresthesia in 1 or more ext, or 1 side of the face, weakness or clumsiness of leg or hand, or visual disturbances (eg, partial blindness, dimness of vision, or scotoma). Optic neuritis has been reported as the 1st symptom of MS in lactating women *(Obstet Gynecol 2001;98:902).*
- T2-weighted imaging remains the std tool for dx confirmation after 1st trimester

Rx During Preg
- **Acute flare:** 3–5-d course of high-dose corticosteroids administered IV
- Some corticosteroids cross the placenta. No association w/ prematurity, IUFD, or SABs
- DMT are offered to MS pt experiencing at least 1 relapse per year
- Interferon B – reduces relapse rates by ~30%; animal, human studies limited, but show no adverse fetal effects – not a/w increased risk of SAB *(Exp Cell Res 2011;317:1301; J Neurol 2010;257:2020; Neurol 2010;75:1794)*
- Natalizumab (monoclonal Ab against VCAM alpha-4-integrin) may be used for more aggressive dz; safety has not been established in Preg – pts should stop drug 3 mo prior to conception
- Fingolimod (modifies receptors involved in vascular genesis); no evid regarding safety in Preg – pts should stop drug 2 mo prior to conception
- IVIG – not licensed as std MS therapy, but beneficial effects reported w/ use during Preg

Treatment Postpartum
- 3–5-d course of high-dose corticosteroids (Solu Medrol 1000 mg QD) – protection from relapse for 4 w PP *(J Neurol 2004;251:1133)*
- DMT can be restarted but protective effects may be delayed for weeks
- Preliminary data suggests exclusive breastfeeding and menstrual suppression >4 mo. Reduces risk of postpartum relapse *(Arch Neurol 2009;66:961)*

NEUROPATHIES IN PREGNANCY

Bell's Palsy *(Otolaryngol Head Neck Surg 2007;137:858)*
- **Definition:** Paralysis of the facial nerve – involving V1, V2, V3
- **PE:** Asym facial expression & unilateral weakness of eye closure
- **Epidemiology:** 2–4-fold ↑ during Preg, esp 3rd trimester or in 1st-w PP
- **Pathophysiology:** Increased perineural edema, hypercoagulability (thrombus of vasa nervorum), relative immunosuppression in Preg
- Association w/ preeclampsia *(QJM 2002;95:359)*
- **Rx:** Cort taper; w/ exception of 1st 9 w of Preg

Meralgia Paresthetica
- **Definition:** Sensory neuropathy that occurs w/ compression of the lateral femoral cutaneous nerve as it penetrates the tensor fascia lata at the inguinal ligament

- **Pathophysiology:** Expanding abdominal wall & increased lumbar lordosis
- Rx rarely req

Postpartum Compression Neuropathies *(Obstet Gynecol 2003;101:279)*
- **Epidemiology:** Reported in 1–8/10000 deliveries
- **Femoral neuropathy:** Motor loss involving the quadriceps, w/ sparing of adduction; sensory loss involving the anter thigh & most of the medial thigh
- **Lateral femoral cutaneous neuropathy:** No motor fibers; lateral hip pain w/ paresthesias or hypesthesias over upper outer thigh
- **Peroneal neuropathy:** Foot drop caused by prolonged squatting sustained knee flexion, pres on the fibular head from stirrups or palmar pres during pushing
- **Obturator neuropathies:** Uncommon complication of deliv; pt p/w medial thigh pain & adductor weakness
- **Risk factors:** Fetal macrosomia, malpresentation, sensory blockade, prolonged lithotomy position, prolonged 2nd stage, improper use of leg stirrups & retractors

Definitions
- **Use:** Sporadic consump, no adverse effects
- **Abuse:** Maladaptive pattern or inappropriate use of a substance, adverse effects from use
- **Dependence:** Individual persists in substance use despite problems
  - **Physical:** Characterized by withdrawal sx if abrupt cessation of substance or antag administered
  - **Psychological:** Need for substance either for positive effects of use or to avoid negative effects of abstinence
- **Addiction:** Behaviors that include impaired control, compulsive use, use despite harm, & craving
- **Substance use disorder:** Pathologic pattern of behaviors related to the use of substances w/ impaired control, social impairment, risky use, tolerance, & withdrawal
- **At risk for alcohol use (for ♀):** ≥3 drinks on one occasion; &/or >7 drinks/w, &/or any amount of drinking for ♀ who are pregnant or at risk of pregnancy
- **Binge drinking (for ♀):** ≥4 drinks on one occasion
- **Prescription drug abuse:** Intentional use of a medication w/out a prescription, in a way other than prescribed, or for the experience or feeling it creates

Epidemiology (www.niaaa.nih.gov/alcohol-health/overview-alcohol-consumption/alcohol-facts-and-statistics)
- ♀ More likely to have rapid transition from use to abuse
- ♀ More likely to have dual dx (MDD, physical &/or sexual victimization, PTSD)
- ♀ More susceptible to liver disease & hepatitis than men who consume the same amount of EtOH
- EtOH related mortality rate is 50–100× greater for ♀
- Affects 10% of the general pop., 48% of 12th graders have reported using an illicit substance at some point
- EtOH: 140 million people worldwide are EtOH dependent. 30% of suicides relate to EtOH abuse. Accounts for up to 40% of hospital admissions.
- Tobacco: 15% of women >25 y are cigarette smokers, 50% decrease over past 30 y (varies widely by education level) (CDC, Health, US, 2016).
- Opioid epidemic (SAMHSA 2015; MMWR 2016;65:50–1; 1445, CDC): In the US, 12.5 million people misuse rx opioids; 2 million have a prescription opioid use disorder; 33,000 deaths/y from opioid overdose
  - In pregnancy (Obstet Gynecol 2016;128(1):4–10): 1 in 5 Medicaid patients filled an opioid rx while pregnant; rate of neonatal abstinence syndrome (NAS) has increased 5-fold from 2000-d12

Diagnostic Workup/Studies
- All patients should have routine screening for substance abuse, and all women before and in early pregnancy should also be screened
- **Single-item screening test:** 100% sens, 73% spec
  "How many times in the past year have you used an illegal drug or used a prescription med for nonmedical reasons?"

Substance abuse screening tools	
CAGE **CAGE-AID** (JAMA 1984;252:1905; Wis Med J 1995;94:135)	Screens for EtOH use (CAGE), or EtOH & drug use (CAGE-AID). Less sensitive for women & minorities Questions: 1. Have you ever felt you should **CUT** down on your drinking (&/or drug use)? 2. Have people **ANNOYED** you by criticizing your drinking (&/or drug use)? 3. Have you ever felt bad or **GUILTY** about your drinking (&/or drug use)? 4. Have you ever had a drink (or used drugs) first thing in the morning to steady your nerves or get rid of a hangover **(EYE-OPENER)**? Score: No = 1, Yes = 1. Score >2 warrants further evaluation
T-ACE (J Obstet Gynecol 1989;160:865)	Screening tool for EtOH use Questions 1. How many drinks does it take to make you feel high? **(TOLERANCE)**; ≤2 drinks = 1; >2 drinks = 2 2. Have people **ANNOYED** you by criticizing your drinking?; No = 0; Yes = 1 3. Have you felt you ought to **CUT DOWN** on your drinking?; No = 0; Yes = 1 4. Have you ever had a drink first thing in the morning to steady your nerves or to get rid of a hangover? **(EYE OPENER)**; No = 1; Yes = 1 Score: ≥2 indicates potential EtOH problem

- **Stages of change** (Am Psychol 1992;47:1102):

  Precontemplation: Lack of awareness of problem, no intention to change behavior

  Contemplation: Aware of problem, weighing pros & cons to solve problem, no commitment to change action but considering changing behavior in next 6 mo

  Preparation: Intend to take action in the next month, some reductions in problem behavior

  Action: Modification of behavior/experiences/environment to overcome problem

  Maintenance: Extends from 6 mo onward, working to prevent relapse & consolidate gains achieved in the action phase

- Screen for other comorbidities & address psychosocial needs and if patient needs treatment for withdrawal
- Counsel about risks of EtOH & drugs. Encourage cessation in pregnancy & breastfeeding
- 5 A's of smoking cessation: **ASK, ADVISE, ASSESS, ASSIST, ARRANGE** (Obstet Gynecol 2017;130:e200)
- Test for STIs, Hep B & C, TB. Repeat testing in the 3rd trimester for those who remain at risk
- Assess for fetal growth restriction in the 2nd half of pregnancy
- Perform antenatal fetal surveillance for standard OB indications or maternal withdrawal (substance use alone is not an indication for fetal monitoring)
- Consult anesthesia to develop a PP pain management plan
- Inform pediatrics team of the possibility of neonatal withdrawal

Drugs of abuse in pregnancy	
Tobacco (Obstet Gynecol 2017;130:e200)	Largest preventable cause of premature death & avoidable illness in ♀ in US. 13.2% of ♀ report tobacco use in preg Intoxication: Nausea/vomiting, ↑ HR, restlessness, diarrhea Withdrawal: HA, nausea, cough, insomnia, irritability Pregnancy: ↑ Risk of PTB, PPROM, IUGR, SGA infant, SIDS Tx: Most effective is counseling + meds (nicotine replacement, bupropion, or varenicline). Limited data in pregnancy for medical treatment. National Quit Line – 1-800-QUIT-NOW
Alcohol (Obstet Gynecol 2011;118:383)	10.8% of ♀ report EtOH use in preg Intoxication: Slurred speech, nystagmus, disinhibited behavior, uncoordinated, unsteady gait, stupor, coma Withdrawal: Insomnia, tremors, anxiety, HA, diaphoresis, palpitations, seizures, delirium tremens Pregnancy: Teratogen – fetal alcohol spectrum disorder (FASD): CNS abnormalities, growth defects, facial dysmorphism, behavioral disorders, & impaired intellectual development. **FASD is the most common nongenetic cause of mental retardation** Tx: Alcoholics may experience withdrawal. **Monitor with CIWA-Ar** (N/V, tremor, sweats, anxiety, tactile, auditory, &/or visual disturbances, HA, agitation, orientation. Score >10 = May need meds for withdrawal). Tx for withdrawal = benzodiazepines
Marijuana (Obstet Gynecol 2017;130:e205)	2–5% of ♀ report marijuana use in preg Intoxication: Dry mouth, red eyes, ↑ appetite, nystagmus, ataxia, slurred speech, ↑ HR, ↑ BP, ↓ reaction time Withdrawal: Irritability, anxiety, sleep disturbances Pregnancy: In animals crosses the placenta & may disrupt brain development & function. Limited data in humans but arrests development in adolescents and is lipophilic so concerns about deposition in fetal brain tissue exist. Tx: No specific tx. Limited data suggest that haloperidol is efficacious in cases of marijuana-related hyperemesis syndrome.
Methamphet-amine & Amphet-amines (Obstet Gynecol 2011;117:751)	0.4% of US residents (1.2 million) used meth in the last y Intoxication: ↑ HR, HTN, hyperthermia, diaphoresis, mydriasis, agitation, violent behavior, psychosis, seizures Withdrawal: Dysphoria, anhedonia, fatigue, ↑ sleep, vivid dreams, agitation, anxiety, ↑ appetite Pregnancy: ↑ Risk of SGA infant. Possible ↑ risk gHTN/preeclampsia, abruption, PTB Tx: Limited data suggest that bupropion may ↓ meth cravings (not well studied in pregnancy). Acute intoxication and psychosis may be treated with short-acting benzodiazepine.

Opioids (Obstet Gynecol 2017;130:e81; Obstet Gynecol 2015;125:1529; NEJM 2010:363:2320)	Most frequently abused prescription drugs. 23% of ♀ 18–34 y have ever illegally used prescription pain relievers, 1% of pregnant ♀ report nonmedical use of opioids Intoxication: Depressed mental status, ↓ respiratory rate, ↑ bowel sounds, miosis. Methadone can cause QTc prolongation & Torsades de Pointes. Overdose can cause respiratory depression & death Withdrawal: Anxiety, restlessness, GI distress, diaphoresis, ↑ HR, flu-like sx, fever, ↑ WBC count, muscle aches Pregnancy: Withdrawal in preg may now thought to be less life threatening to fetus than previously believed. Chronic untreated heroin use is associated with ↑ risk of SAB, PTL, PPROM, IUGR, placental abruption, fetal death, pre-E. Tx: Controlled opioid maintenance in preg is recommended to prevent relapse to illicit opioid use & opioid overdose or withdrawal. Prescribers require additional DEA licensure and training. **Methadone:** May require dosage adjustments to avoid withdrawal sx in preg. **Buprenorphine:** Acts on the same receptors as heroin & morphine. Single agent med (w/out naloxone) recommended in preg. Advantages: ↓ Risk of overdose, fewer drug interactions, can receive outpatient w/out daily visits, & less severe neonatal abstinence syndrome, but limited long-term data. PP may have ↑ pain scores. **In acute opioid poisoning: Airway support + naloxone, a short-acting opioid antagonist** (limited data in preg)
Cocaine (Am J Obstet Gynecol 2011;204:340)	0.6% of US residents (1.5 million) used cocaine in the last month Intoxication: ↑ Energy, ↓ appetite, paranoia, restlessness, psychosis, ↑ HR, pupil dilation, diaphoresis, nausea Withdrawal: Depression, anxiety, fatigue, difficulty concentrating, ↑ appetite, ↑ sleep, tremors, chills Pregnancy: Vasoconstrictive effects may cause HTN emergencies & placental abruption. Adrenergic effect causes ↑ HR, BP & vascular resistance, risk of **myocardial ischemia & infarction**, arrhythmias (↑ risk in pregnancy). ↑ Incidence of cranial defects, limb reduction defects, urogenital abnormalities, intestinal perforation, obstruction & atresia in exposed fetuses. Tx: **Beta-blocker rx is contraindicated** for mgmt of cocaine-induced HTN, b/c it leads to unopposed adrenergic stimulation, resulting in end-organ ischemia & coronary vasospasm. Acute intoxication and psychosis may be treated with short-acting benzodiazepine.
Sedatives & Tranquilizers (Obstet Gynecol 2017;130:e81)	7.6% of ♀ report ever illegally using tranquilizers, 2.4% report ever illegally using sedatives Intoxication: Slurred speech, ataxia, depressed mental status, depressed respiration, stupor, coma, death Withdrawal: Tremors, anxiety, perceptual disturbances, insomnia, dysphoria, psychosis, seizures Pregnancy: Abrupt withdrawal can cause seizures, acute heart conditions, & acute psychiatric conditions. Infants w/ prolonged exposure may have neonatal abstinence syndrome. Tx: Avoid withdrawal w/ use of benzos w/ long half-lives & very gradual tapering of dose. If withdrawal occurs, treat w/ a long-acting benzo (diazepam). These patients will need help with sleep as insomnia is one of the last withdrawal symptoms to resolve (zolpidem, antihistamines may help).

DEPRESSION

Definition
- **Major depression (MDD):** Depressed mood/anhedonia, <u>AND</u> 4+ of the following sx present <u>most of the day, nearly every day for 2 consecutive w:</u> weight loss or gain, insomnia or hypersomnia, psychomotor agitation or retardation, fatigue or loss of energy, feelings of worthlessness or excessive guilt, diminished ability to concentrate, recurrent thoughts of death or suicide (SIG E CAPS – **S**leep, **I**nterest, **G**uilt, **E**nergy, **C**oncentration, **A**ppetite, **P**sychomotor, **S**uicide)
- **Persistent depressive d/o (dysthymia):** Depressed mood for 2+ y

- **Adjustment d/o:** Depressed mood or impairment in response to identifiable stressor w/in 3 mo of onset of stressor, resolved w/in 6 mo
- **Postpartum "Blues":** Mild depressive symptoms, impaired concentration, & insomnia. Occurs within the first 2–3 d of delivery & *resolves within 2 w.*
- **MDD with Peripartum Onset (Postpartum Depression):** Dx criteria same as MDD. Typically occurs 1–6 w postpartum (but up to 12 mo).

Epidemiology *(Obstet Gynecol 2015;125:1268)*
- 17% lifetime prevalence of MDD. Women twice as likely as men to have depression. Highest rates in women ages 25–44
- 10–16% of preg women fulfill dx criteria for depression; 70% of preg women report sx of depression
- 40–80% of women have PP blues; 8–15% of women have PP depression
- Depression is often accompanied by comorbid anxiety

Clinical Manifestations *(Obstet Gynecol 2008;111:1001 and Obstet Gynecol 2015;125:1268)*
- See definitions above
- Preg & PP: ↑ Risk of LBW infant, ↓ fetal growth, postnatal complications, infant crying, & admission to NICU

Diagnostic Workup/Studies *(Psychiatry Res 2011;187:130; JAMA 2016;315:388)*
- Screen for depression in perinatal period & at 4–8 w PP. Screening shown to ↓ depressive sx in women w/ MDD & ↓ prevalence of MDD. If positive screen, always ask about suicidal ideation &/or intent, & homicidal ideation &/or intent
- **PHQ-9** – 9 questions (available free online)
- **Edinburgh postnatal depression scale (EPDS)** – 10 questions, validated for antepartum and postpartum use, exists in multiple languages. Is the recommended screening test for perinatal populations and is ideally administered at 2 pregnancy and 1 (or more) postpartum time points. (Available free online and at perinatology.com)

Treatment and Medications *(Obstet Gynecol 2009;114:703)*
- Screen for bipolar d/o & mania sx prior to initiating therapy
- **Psychotherapy:** Similar efficacy to pharmacotherapy
- **Pharmacotherapy (nonpregnant):** SSRIs, SNRIs, TCAs, MAOIs. SSRIs are 1st-line therapy. Start low dose, ↑ PRN. Evaluate pts q1–2 w in 1st 8 w of therapy. If no response on max clinical dose, switch to another antidepressant
- **Pharmacotherapy (pregnancy):** Mild or no sx for 6 mo, and patient desires, can taper → d/c meds. Recommend continued psychotherapy during pregnancy and the postpartum period at minimum as *high risk* for relapse postpartum.
- If severe, recurrent, or other psych comorbidity then continue meds and titrate dosing *upward* as needed
- If dx w/ depression during preg then psychotherapy &/or antidepressants depending on severity and patient's past psychiatric history. SSRIs have longest safety profile during pregnancy AND lactation. If a medication is working well for a woman during pregnancy there is no need to change to another medication of the same type during lactation.
- Available (free) resources for clinicians:
  - Maternal Mental Health Safety Bundle: www.safehealthcareforeverywoman.org
  - Massachusetts Child Psychiatry Access Program for Moms Toolkit, Massachusetts: www.mcpapformoms.org
- **Electroconvulsive therapy (ECT):** Safe in pregnancy. Use for those who have not responded to meds, or are psychotic, suicidal, or severely disabled.
- **Refer** if severe depression endangering the life of pt or others, failed response to initial rx, psychosis, or depression that is part of bipolar or schizoaffective d/o

ANXIETY DISORDERS

Definition and Epidemiology
- Includes GAD, panic d/o, social anxiety, & specific phobia
- Collectively, the most common psych d/o. Prevalence of 18.1%

Clinical Manifestations *(Obstet Gynecol 2008;111:1001)*
- **GAD:** Persistent, excessive worry that interferes w/ life
- **Panic d/o:** Maladaptive change in behavior or persistent worry over anticipated panic attacks (sudden periods of intense fear w/o cause)
- **Social anxiety:** Marked fear of social or performance situations

- **Specific phobia:** Strong irrational fear related to exposure to specific objects or situations
- **Preg:** ↑ Risk of prolonged or precipitous labor, fetal distress, PTB, & SAB ↓ developmental scores & slowed mental development at 2 yo in infant

Diagnostic Workup/Studies
- Hx including comorbid psychiatric & other medical conditions
- Consider CBC, BMP, TSH, Urine for toxicology to screen for drug use
- GAD-7: 7 question screening tool for GAD
- EPDS (as above) also designed to screen for comorbid anxiety (and suicidality)

Treatment and Medications
- **Psychotherapy**
- **Regular physical activity (150 minutes or more weekly)**
- **Help patient with regular sleep if there is co-existing sleep disturbance (common)**
- **Pharmacotherapy (nonpregnant):** Antidepressants 1st line (esp SSRIs), Benzodiazepines only for emergent rx (regular benzo use can worsen anxiety)
- **Pharmacotherapy (pregnancy):** Same as above. Avoid prolonged exposure to benzos if possible. However, short-acting *occasional* benzodiazepines are efficacious during pregnancy without major safety concerns.

BIPOLAR DISORDER

Definition
- Includes both manic (Bipolar I) or hypomanic episodes (Bipolar II). These are distinct periods of abnormally & persistently elevated, expansive, destructive, or irritable mood. More commonly have depressive episodes.

Epidemiology (Obstet Gynecol 2008:111:1001)
- 3.9–6.4% lifetime prevalence. Equal rates in men & women. Women more likely to have depressive episodes, rapid cycling, & mixed episodes.
- Rates of PP relapse are 32–67%. ↑ Risk of PP psychosis (up to 46%)

Clinical Manifestations
- See definitions above, main concerns during the PP period are psychosis and mania which have been reported to occur early (1–4 w PP). Anticipatory guidance about these concerns should be addressed during prenatal care.
- Preg: ↑ Risk of LBW, PTB, decreased fetal growth, postnatal complications, infant crying, and admit to NICU

Diagnostic Workup/Studies
- Hx including sx of depression, mania, hypomania, hospitalization, SI or suicide attempts, psychosis, comorbid psychiatric & other medical d/o
- CBC, BMP, TSH, Urine for toxicology to screen for drug use

Treatment and Medications (Am J Psychiatry 2004:161:608; JAMA 1994:271:146)
- **Psychotherapy should be included in treatment plan both during pregnancy and postpartum**
- **Careful attention to prevent sleep disturbances as much as possible**
- **Pharmacotherapy (nonpregnant):** Lithium, antipsychotics, anticonvulsants
- **Pharmacotherapy (pregnancy):** Same as above. Antipsychotics 1st line for mania. In pregnancy, if on lithium, will need co-management with psychiatry and MFM consultation. If severe episodes but mod. risk of relapse short term, consider a taper of lithium before conception and restart after organogenesis. If severe & frequent episodes, continue lithium all pregnancy. Maternal labs will need regular surveillance by psychiatrist. Lamotrigine is another evidence-based treatment for bipolar d/o with less pregnancy and postpartum concerns.
- **Electroconvulsive therapy (ECT):** Safe in pregnancy

PSYCHOSIS

Definition
- Syndrome of chronic or recurrent psychosis. Often disabling. May include positive sx, negative sx, cognitive impairment, mood & anxiety sx

Epidemiology
- Prevalence is 1%. Slightly more men than women affected.

Clinical Manifestations (Obstet Gynecol 2008;111:1001)
- See definition above
- Positive sx: Hallucinations, delusions, disorganization
- Negative sx: Flat affect, poverty of speech, etc. Tends to be more difficult to treat
- Preg: ↑ Risk of congenital malformations (esp cardiovascular system), ↑ risk of PTB, LBW, placental abnormalities, antenatal hemorrhage, postnatal death

Diagnostic Workup/Studies
- Dx of exclusion. Need to r/o medical causes of psychosis, substance use d/o, & other psych dx that may have psychotic component

Treatment and Medications
- **Pharmacotherapy (nonpregnant):** Antipsychotics
- **Pharmacotherapy (pregnancy):** Antipsychotics, collaboration with psychiatry

SCHIZOPHRENIA

Definition
- D/o with loss of contact with reality with psychotic sx
- Postpartum psychosis: Onset of psychotic symptoms PP, often in the 1st 2 w

Epidemiology (J Womens Health 2006;15:352)
- Psychotic disorders occur in 1–4% of the population
- Postpartum psychosis occurs in 0.1–0.2% of all deliveries
- Of women with PP psychosis, 0.2% commit suicide, 28–35% have delusions about their infant, 9% express thoughts of harming their infant
- Many women with PP psychosis have, or will later be diagnosed with, bipolar d/o

Clinical Manifestations
- See definition above. Psychotic sx includes hallucinations, delusions, confusion, disorganization of thought &/or behavior

Diagnostic Workup/Studies
- R/o medical causes of psychosis, substance use d/o, & other psych dx that may have psychotic component. Evaluate for suicidal or homicidal ideation.

Treatment and Medications
- Emergency psychiatric care, often requires **hospitalization**, esp if danger to self or others
- **Pharmacotherapy (nonpregnant):** Antipsychotics
- **Pharmacotherapy (pregnancy or PP):** Antipsychotics
- **If psychosis/agitation on L&D or inpatient postpartum, consider:** Lorazepam 2 mg IV/PO, diazepam 5–10 mg IV/PO, haloperidol 2 mg IV/PO, or risperidone 2 mg PO (takes longest time to act)
- Electroconvulsive therapy (ECT): Safe in pregnancy and the postpartum period
- Generally try to increase one med and optimize dosing in pregnancy (vs. starting 2nd med)
- **Online Resources:** Reprotox (http://www.reprotox.org) & TERIS (http://depts.washington.edu/terisweb).

Psychiatric medications in pregnancy & lactation	
Class	Birth defects, pregnancy considerations, neonatal risks, & lactation considerations
Benzodiazepines (Clonazepam, Lorazepam, Alprazolam)	Birth defects: Possible ↑ risk of cleft lip or palate Pregnancy: Detailed U/S for facial morphology Neonatal risks: Floppy infant syndrome; neonatal withdrawal syndrome Lactation: Infant sedation reported

Class	Birth defects, pregnancy considerations, neonatal risks, & lactation considerations
SSRIs (FLUOXETINE, SERTRALINE, PAROXETINE, Citalopram)	<u>Birth defects</u>: Possible ↑ risk of cardiac defects w/ paroxetine. Otherwise no consistent teratogenesis. <u>Pregnancy</u>: There will be ↓ serum concentrations of the meds so dosing often must be increased to improve symptoms. Consider fetal echo if paroxetine use. <u>Neonatal risks</u>: Postnatal adaptation syndrome. SSRI use before 20 w of gestation may ↑ risk of persistent pulmonary HTN (conflicting results and no higher risk than prematurity, GDM or African American race-related risks) <u>Lactation</u>: None. Continuance during lactation may lessen/eliminate neonatal symptoms.
SNRIs (Venlafaxine)	<u>Birth defects</u>: No consistent pattern of teratogenesis <u>Pregnancy</u>: There will be ↓ serum concentrations of the meds so dosing often must be increased to improve symptoms <u>Neonatal risks</u>: Minimal postnatal adaptation syndrome <u>Lactation</u>: None. Continuance during lactation may lessen/eliminate neonatal symptoms
TCAs (Nortriptyline)	<u>Birth defects</u>: None <u>Pregnancy</u>: Sedating – recommend night time dosing. May also help with chronic neuropathic pain and sleep. <u>Lactation</u>: None
Lithium	<u>Birth defects</u>: ↑ Risk of cardiac defects including Ebstein's anomaly although weaker association than previously believed <u>Pregnancy</u>: Do U/S &/or echo for cardiac development. There will be ↓ serum concentrations. Need to monitor levels. During labor there is an ↑ risk for lithium toxicity, ensure adequate hydration. <u>Neonatal risks</u>: Risk of lithium toxicity in infant <u>Lactation</u>: Monitor infant CBC, TSH, & lithium levels if desires breastfeeding. AAP discourages breastfeeding with lithium use.
Antiepileptic drugs/mood stabilizers (Valproate, Carbamazepine, Lamotrigine)	<u>Birth defects</u>: ↑ Risk of: *Valproate*: Neural tube defects, craniofacial anomalies, limb abnormalities, cardiovascular anomalies, fetal valproate syndrome (growth restriction, facial dysmorphism, limb & heart defects), cognitive impairment. *Contraindicated in pregnancy due to significant developmental delay in children exposed to valproate in utero* *Carbamazepine*: Fetal carbamazepine syndrome (facial dysmorphism & fingernail hypoplasia), possible neural tube defects, developmental delay *Lamotrigine*: None known (limited data, preferred in bipolar d/o) <u>Pregnancy</u>: Avoid valproate entirely. Avoid carbamazepine in 1st trimester if able. Serum concentrations followed with dose adjustments anticipated. Increase folate to 4 mg/d if on an antiepileptic. Give vitamin K 20 mg/d in the final month of pregnancy if on carbamazepine. <u>Neonatal risks</u>: Neonatal symptoms. Give vitamin K 1 mg IM if exposed to carbamazepine. <u>Lactation</u>: Monitor infant behavior. Can consider monitoring of infant CBC, LFTs, antiepileptic drug levels.
Antipsychotic drugs (Haloperidol)	<u>Birth defects</u>: None confirmed <u>Pregnancy</u>: May have ↑ risk of GDM (risperidone). Avoid anticholinergic meds for side effects. <u>Neonatal risks</u>: Possible risk of neuroleptic malignant syndrome & intestinal obstruction <u>Lactation</u>: None

Adapted from *Obstet Gynecol* 2008;111:1001 (Reaffirmed 2018).

Disease	Epidemiology	Clinical characteristics and physical exam	Treatment
Chloasma "Mask of Preg"	50–75% ↑ In Hispanics and those w/ dark complexions May fade w/i 1 y Persists in up to 30%	Onset in 1st–2nd trimester Hormone-assoc facial hyper-pigmentation in centrofacial distribution ± mandibular/ maxillary involvement Patchy, light, gray/brown, macular, facial hyperpigmentation	Avoid sun Sunscreen Bleaching; Hydro-quinone; azelaic acid Chemical peel
Polymorphic eruption of pregnancy "Pruritic Urticar-ial Papules and Plaques of Pregnancy (PUPPP)"	Common in up to 1/300 ↑ In multifetal gestations, nulliparas Caucasians	Onset in 3rd trimester, typically resolving 1–2 w postpartum Lesions may be target-like, wheals, or vesicles Intensely pruritic, urticarial papules and plaques w/i abdominal striae Thighs, arms, buttocks may be affected Face, palms, soles, periumbilical region usually spared	Symptom relief: Emollients; topical steroids; nonsedating antihistamines Oral steroids for sev cases
Pustular psoriasis of pregnancy "Impetigo herpetiformis"	Case reports only	Onset in 3rd trimester, resolves postpartum Nonpruritic sterile pustules surrounding erythematous plaques in flexures → periph spread. Trunk, extremities, mucous mem-branes involved with infec-tion risk. Bx w/ spongiform pustule of Kogoj (neutrophil-containing pustule) Complications: Constitutional sx; mat sepsis; and placen-tal insufficiency. ↑ WBC and ESR. ↓ Albumin and Ph.	Oral steroids Cyclosporine Abx if bact super-infxn occurs Fetal surveillance
Pemphigoid gestationis "Herpes gestationis"	1/1700–50000 May occur w/ ges-tational tro-phoblastic dz ↑ In Caucasian >50% are HLA-DR3 or DR4+	Onset 2nd–3rd trimester or postpartum Remits and recurs through-out preg, worsens in sub-seq preg; 75% flare at delivery; may recur with menses/OCPs Extreme pruritis Erythematous papules → vesicles, bullae Periumbilical → trunk + extremities; mucous membrane/facial sparing Neonat lesions in 10% Bx w/ immunofluorescent C3 deposition along the dermo-epidermal junction (distinguishes it from PUPPP) Risk of placental insufficiency, SGA, prematurity. Risk increases with diagnosis severity	High potency topical steroids Nonsedating antihistamine Often requires oral steroids Avoid oral contra-ceptive agents for 6 mo postpar-tum (can pre-cipitate flare in up to 50%) Fetal surveillance

Disease	Epidemiology	Clinical characteristics and physical exam	Treatment
Atopic eruption of pregnancy "Prurigo gestationis"	Up to 1/450	Onset 2nd–3rd trimester, resolving w/i 3 mo postpartum Atopic eczema component Pruritic papules or plaques on trunk and extensor surfaces of extremities Excoriated, "insect bite" appearance	Emollients Topical steroids Nonsedating antihistamine
Atopic eruption of pregnancy "Folliculitis"	Rare	Onset 2nd–3rd trimester Resolving w/i 2–3 w postpartum Sterile papules or pustules arise from follicles on trunk May spread to extremities	Topical steroids Benzoyl peroxide Nonsedating antihistamine

Data from *J Am Acad Dermatol* 2006;54:395; *Am Fam Physician* 2007;75:211; *J Clin Obstet Gynecol* 2015; 58:104. *Ann Dermatol* 2011;23: 265–75.

LICHEN SCLEROSUS

Epidemiology
- Prevalence unk: Often asymptomatic, underreported (*Obstet Gynecol Surv* 2012;67:55)
- Bimodal distribution: Prepubertal and postmenopausal females, w/ a mean age btw the 5th and 6th decade (*Obstet Gynecol* 2008;111:1243)
- Risk of malig transformation to squamous cell carcinoma 4–6% if untreated, rare otherwise (*Cancer Epi Biom Prev* 2016;25:1224)

Pathology
- Atrophic epidermis ± hyperkeratinization (typically due to persistent scratching), homogeneous collagen layer w/ underlying lymphocytic infiltrate, blunting of rete ridges

Etiology
- Autoimmune component and genetic predisposition suspected
- Hormonal influences (low estrogen) and local inflamm responses may also play a role

Clinical Characteristics
- Vulvar pruritis is most common symptom
  - May also present w/ vulvar irritation, pain, burning, dyspareunia
- Ddx: Lichen planus, postmenopausal atrophy, vitiligo. May have concomitant lichen simplex chronicus, cutaneous candidiasis, or bacterial infection

Physical Exam (*J Clin Obstet Gynecol* 2015;58:464)
- Vulva thinned w/ a pale plaque-like appearance, "cigarette paper," ± petechiae, purpura, fissures, and erosions
- "Figure-of-eight/hourglass" around the vaginal and anal openings
- Excoriations and lichenification may be present due to persistent scratching
- Labia majora and minora may eventually lose distinction and fuse
- Generally spares the vagina

Diagnostic Workup
- H&P
- Bx of affected area
- Rule out concurrent candidiasis/bacterial infection

Treatment (*Obstet Gynecol* 2008;111:1243; *J Clin Obstet Gynecol* 2015;58:464)
- Oral sedating antihistamines for symptom relief
- High-dose topical steroids: Clobetasol 0.05% ointment QHS for 6–12 w, followed by maint 1–3×/w (1 of many rx regimens). See steroid chart, below.
- Topical retinoids for sev cases
- Topical tacrolimus, 0.1% ointment BID, or pimecrolimus 1% cream BID (do not use for extended periods)

- Triamcinolone injections: 2nd-line agents, indicated for persistent dz
- Consider adjunctive therapy with intravaginal, topical estrogen in postmenopausal women
- Pts should return in 3-mo intervals during initial rx stages, until stable
- Lifetime surveillance in 6–12-mo intervals recommended

LICHEN SIMPLEX CHRONICUS

Epidemiology (Dermatol Clin 2010;28:669)
- Common cause of vulvar pruritis w/ unknown prevalence
- Personal and/or FHx of atopy is common

Pathophysiology (J Clin Obstet Gynecol 2015;58:464)
- Nonscarring process characterized by epidermal thickening secondary to repeated scratching/rubbing, triggered by vulvar irritation (heat, sweat, clothing, contact dermatitis, topical products, atopic conditions, infxn)
- Lichenification: Epidermal thickening and accentuation of skin markings

Clinical Manifestations
- Pruritis ± sleep disturbances often due to pruritis and intense scratching

Physical Exam (J Clin Obstet Gynecol 2015;58:464)
- Well-defined, erythematous, lichenified papules and plaques
- Vulvar skin may be hyper- or hypopigmented and appear "leathery or bark-like"
- Excoriations may be present

Diagnostic Workup/Studies
- Usually a clinical diagnosis based on history and physical examination
- Bx w/ chronic inflamm changes, hyperkeratinization, acanthosis (epidermal thickening)

Treatment (Obstet Gynecol 2005;105:1451; J Clin Obstet Gynecol 2015;58:464)
- Oral antipruritics such as hydroxyzine, doxepin, or oral sedating antihistamines
- Eliminate triggers by encouraging gentle skin care without irritants and allergens
- Avoid scratching: Gloves at night, barrier creams, occlusive dressing, cold pack
- Topical steroids (triamcinolone 1% applied to affected area QD for mild dz. betamethasone 0.05% or clobetasol 0.05% applied QD for mod–sev dz) followed by a gentle emollient (eg, white petrolatum)

LICHEN PLANUS

Epidemiology
- Affects 0.5–2% of the population, w/ vulvar lesions in up to 50% of affected women (Br J Dermatol 1996;135:89; Dermatol Ther 2010;23:251)
- Most common in the 5th–7th decade of life in females

Pathology
- Different morphologies: Papulosquamous, erosive (most common vulvar type), hypertrophic, and mixed
- Dev of squamous cell carcinoma is uncommon (1–2.5%)

Etiology
- Unknown, but presumed autoimmune process against basal keratinocytes mediated by T-cell activation → chronic inflammation (Arch Dermatol 2008;144:1432)

Clinical Manifestations (J Clin Obstet Gynecol 2015;58:464)
- Skin: "P's" – Planar, Purple, Pruritic, Polygonal, Papules, and Plaques
- Mucosa: "P's" – Bright red, eroded, desquamated, ± green/yellow discharge
- Vulvar pain and burning are the most common symptoms
- May also present w/ vulvar or vaginal irritation, pain, burning, dyspareunia, discharge refrac to conventional rx
- Chronic inflamm changes, band-like dermal lymphocytic infiltrate, basal layer liquefactive necrosis, colloid bodies, acanthosis, and hyperkeratinization, primary affecting skin/nails. Erosive subtype affects mucous membranes (mouth and vagina)

Physical Exam (Obstet Gynecol 2008;111:1243; J Clin Obstet Gynecol 2015;58:464)
- Desquamation, ulcerations, and loss of architecture
- Wickham striae: White, lacy formation overlying papular lesions

- Bullae, ulceration, erosion in sev cases
- Scar tissue, adhesions, synechiae, and total obliteration may be seen in the vagina
- Oral and nongenital cutaneous lesions often coincide

Diagnostic Workup
- H&P
- Bx of affected area not diagnostic, but may help rule out other conditions

Treatment (Obstet Gynecol Surv 2012;67:55)
- Symptom relief: Sitz baths, vulvar hygiene, barrier creams or petroleum jelly
- High-dose topical steroids: Clobetasol 0.05% ointment applied QHS for 6–12 w (treats external labia), followed by maint 1–3×/w. Vaginal mucosa treated with hydrocortisone 25 mg suppositories or compounded preparations (monitor for adrenal suppression)
- Topical tacrolimus, 0.1% ointment BID
- Triamcinolone injections for recalcitrant, thick lesions
- Oral steroids for sev erosive dz: Prednisone 40 mg po daily × 1 w → taper
- Immune mediators (after failure of other methods): Methotrexate, azathioprine, cyclosporine, hydroxychloroquine
- Surgical procedures for adhesions or synechiae: Indicated when other treatments have failed
- Chronic condition, w/ relapsing-remitting course depending on resp to rx
- Routine yearly surveillance, as dev of squamous cell carcinoma is rare but poss

Topical corticosteroids		
Classification	**Steroid (brand name)**	**Strength (%)**
Class I (Super-high potency)	Clobetasol propionate (Temovate)	0.05
	Betamethasone dipropionate (Diprolene)	0.05
	Halobetasol propionate (Ultravate)	0.05
Class II (High potency)	Amcinonide (Amcort, Cyclocort)	0.1
	Desoximetasone (Topicort)	0.25
	Triamcinolone acetonide (Kenalog)	0.5
	Halcinonide (Halog)	0.1
	Fluocinonide (Lidex)	0.05
	Diflorasone diacetate (ApexiCon)	0.05
Class III (High potency)	Fluticasone propionate (Cutivate)	0.005
	Betamethasone valerate (Valisone)	0.1
	Triamcinolone acetonide (Kenalog, Triderm)	0.5
	Mometasone furoate (Elocon)	0.1
	Diflorasone diacetate (Florone)	0.05
Class IV (Mid potency)	Flurandrenolide (Cordran)	0.05
	Fluocinolone acetonide (Synalar)	0.025
Class V (Low–mid potency)	Prednicarbate (Dermatop)	0.1
	Desonide (DesOwen, Desonate)	0.05
	Hydrocortisone butyrate (Locoid, Cortizone-10)	0.1
	Hydrocortisone probutate (Pandel)	0.1
	Hydrocortisone valerate (Westcort)	0.2
	Triamcinolone acetonide (Kenalog)	0.025
Class VI (Low potency)	Betamethasone valerate (Beta-Val)	0.1
	Alclometasone dipropionate (Aclovate)	0.05
Class VII (Lowest potency)	Hydrocortisone (many brand names and OTC preparations)	0.5–2.5

PSORIASIS

Epidemiology (Clin Obstet Gynecol 2015;58:464)
- 1–2% of overall population have psoriasis. 2–5% of those have isolated genital psoriasis
- 15% of pts w cutaneous psoriasis → inflammatory dz w/ arthritis/enthesitis

Clinical Characteristics and Physical Exam
- Pruritis is common

- Well-demarcated, pink plaques. For vulvar psoriasis, extension to the perianal skin or labia majora/mons pubis/medial thighs
- Classic, silvery scales are often absent due to the moist environment

Diagnostic Workup
- H&P, examining for psoriasis elsewhere on the body
- Bx of affected area to establish the diagnosis, or if no response with rx

Treatment (J Clin Obstet Gynecol 2015;58:464)
- Gentle skin care regimen. Low to medium dose topical corticosteroids (eg, hydrocortisone 2.5%). Adjunctive topical vit D analogues or calcineurin inhibitors decrease the risk of skin atrophy, bruising, striae, and telangiectasias that may result from chronic topical steroid admin. Oral antihistamines for severe pruritis

HIDRADENITIS SUPPURATIVA

Epidemiology (NEJM 2012;366:158)
- Prevalence 1–4%
- Most common in the 2nd–3rd decades of life
- 3× more common in women
- Familial inheritance with identified mutations has been reported in some cases

Etiology
- Often related to hormonal changes (hyperandrogenism), obesity, smoking, and meds

Pathophysiology
- Abn shedding of keratinocytes → terminal follicles in areas w/ apocrine glands become occluded and rupture → chronic inflammation, abscesses, sinus tract formation

Clinical Characteristics and Physical Exam (NEJM 2012;366:158)
- P/w erythematous, painful, nodular lesions, hyperhidrosis, odor
- Axilla and perineal regions most common, in addition to inguinal, perianal, and vulvar regions
- Less commonly p/w strictures, fistulae, lymphedema, osteomyelitis
- Nodular lesions form abscesses → resultant drainage causes sinus tracts and scarring
- Depression, decreased quality of life
- Hurley staging: Stage 1 – localized nodules or abscesses w/o scarring or tract formation, Stage 2 – recurrent nodules or abscesses w/ scarring or tract formation, Stage 3 – widespread nodules or abscesses w/ scarring and tracts

Treatment (J Eur Acad Dermatol Venereol 2015;29:619)
- General measures: Proper hygiene, use of neutral soaps, warm compresses, bandages, lightweight loose-fitting clothing, weight loss, smoking cessation, psychosocial support
- Topical exfoliants and peels
- Topical abx (clindamycin), systemic abx for more sev cases (tetracycline, clindamycin-rifampin)
- Anti-inflamm corticosteroids (intralesional or systemic)
- Antiandrogens (spironolactone, drospirenone, finasteride)
- Retinoids (isotretinoin)
- Immune mediators (infliximab, adalimumab, cyclosporin)
- Surgical treatments: Incision and drainage, wide local excision, laser excision, unroofing or debridement. Usually reserved for widespread and sev dz

APOCRINE MILIARIA

Epidemiology
- **"Fox–Fordyce disease"**
- Not prevalent (<1%). Most common in 2nd–4th decade of life.
- Female to male ratio 9:1

Etiology
- Keratotic occlusion of apocrine glands → gland rupture and papular eruption → pruritis and chronic inflammation
- Apocrine gland involvement is necessary for dx
- Often related to humidity, obesity, hormones, stress

Clinical Characteristics

- Multiple, small, darkened or flesh-colored, 2–3-mm papules
- Affects areas with multiple apocrine glands (axilla, areolar, perineum, and pubic regions)
- Most often p/w intense pruritis (but may be asymptomatic) → potential for lichenification
- May be associated with anhidrosis and acanthosis

Treatment (*J Pediatr Adolesc Gyn* 2011;24:108)

- Topical low-potency corticosteroids
- Topical abx (clindamycin)
- Topical calcineurin inhibitors (pimecrolimus or tacrolimus)
- 2nd-line therapy: Topical retinoids, intralesional corticosteroids
- Refractory cases may benefit from combination OCPs, oral retinoids, or botulinum toxin
- Severe cases: Surg excision of apocrine glands, liposuction curettage, or fractional laser

GYN-DERM CYSTS

Vaginal and perineal cysts			
Cyst type	**Clinical characteristics**	**Physical exam**	**Treatment**
Epidermoid cyst Epidermal proliferation due to disruption of dermis Lined by keratinized epidermal cells	Commonly asymptomatic, may cause discomfort, altered cosmetic appearance, discharge	Mobile cyst commonly filled w/ white or clear fluid upon incision Located at vulva and perineum	Observation Excision
Gartner duct cyst Remnant of mesonephric duct	Dyspareunia, difficulty inserting tampons, feeling a bulge/mass	Cystic mass commonly found in the posterolateral vagina	Marsupialization Excision
Skene duct cyst Obst of Skene duct Lined by squamous epithelial cells	Commonly asymptomatic, dyspareunia, pain, urethral obst, UTI	Cystic mass in inferolateral periurethral region	Observation Excision
Bartholin gland cyst Obst of Bartholin gland	Dyspareunia, pain, drainage, may form abscess	Cystic mass in medial labia majora (at 5 or 7 o'clock, relative to the introitus)	Incision and drainage Word catheter placement Marsupialization Excision (Chap. 5)
Sebaceous gland cyst Obst of sebaceous gland	Commonly asymptomatic; may cause discomfort, altered cosmetic appearance	Mobile cyst filled w/ thick yellow material upon incision, often multi cysts Located at vulva and perineum	Observation Excision

Data from Hoffman BL, Schorge JO, Schaffer JI, et al. Benign disorders of the lower reproductive tract. In: Hoffman BL, Schorge JO, Schaffer JI, et al, eds. *Williams Gynecology*. 2nd ed. New York, NY: McGraw-Hill; 2012; Black M, Mckay M, Braude P, et al., eds. *Obstetric and Gynecologic Dermatology*. 2nd ed. Philadelphia, PA: Mosby; 2002.

COMMON DERMATOLOGIC MANIFESTATIONS OF SYSTEMIC DISEASE

Crohns Disease

- Approximately 30% of pts w/ Crohns dz have gyn-derm complications. See Chap. 15
    Findings: Vulvar edema, ulcerations, inflammation, granulomas, "knife cut" lesions or fissures. Inflammation, granulomas of the ovary and fallopian tube. Sinus tracts, enteric fistulae to the female reproductive tract
    Rx: Topical steroids, topical metronidazole, intralesional steroid injections, surgical correction of fistulae.

Autoimmune Disorders
- Thyroid dz, vitiligo, pernicious anemia, SLE, atopic dermatitis, and alopecia areata are seen in patients with lichen simplex chronicus, lichen sclerosus, and lichen planus

Behçet Disease
- Diagnostic criteria: Recurrent oral ulcers *and* 2 or more of the following: Recurrent genital ulceration, ocular lesions (uveitis), skin lesions, or positive pathergy testing
- Rule out infxn as source of ulceration, such as HSV, syphilis, HIV, chancroid
- Rx: Topical or intralesional steroids; may require systemic rx

Stevens–Johnson Syndrome
- Systemic hypersensitivity rxn causing edema, sloughing, and/or necrosis of mucous membranes, including lower genital tract
- Usually caused by meds; can also be secondary to infxn
- Rx: D/c medication, supportive care, Abx, wound care; systemic steroids and IVIG may be helpful

Fixed Drug Reaction
- Small, hyperpigmented lesions, erythematous plaques or bullae
- Genital, oral, and facial lesions are most common
- Local rxn to systemic or local administration of some meds, most commonly: Tetracycline, phenolphthalein, sulfa medications, NSAIDs, and ASA
- Resolves w/ discontinuation of the drug

Erythema Multiforme
- Small, cutaneous target-like lesions
- Bullae and erosions of the genital, oral, and ocular mucous membranes
- May be a/w infxn (HSV most common) or due to drug rxn
- Rule out infectious source (ie, HSV, syphilis, mycoplasma PNA)
- Rx: Withdrawal of causative agent, oral antihistamines, topical steroids, wound care, rx of infxn if present

HIV/AIDS IN WOMEN

Definition and Epidemiology
- **AIDS:** HIV infxn w/ or w/o sx + CD4 count <200/mm^3 CD4% <14% of lymphs or AIDS-indicator condition (OI or AIDS-related malig)
- Caused by infxn w/ HIV-1 or HIV-2 retroviruses. Female infxn in US = 19% of new cases; 85% from sexual transmission (*HIV Surveillance Report. Atlanta (GA): CDC;2015*). Risk factors: Minority ethnicity (AA = 10× ↑ infxn, & 5th leading cause of death for AA ♀ 25–54 yo); low socioeconomic status; urban location (*National Vital Statistics Report 2016;65(5)*).

Pathophysiology
- HIV RNA virus targets CD4 receptor on T-lymphocytes
- Destruction & impairment of CD4 cells → immunodeficiency → OIs
- Monitor dz progression & response to rx w/ CD4 count & viral RNA-load
- Potentiation of transmission by other STIs. Infxn w/ STI (HSV, BV, trichomonas, gonorrhea/chlamydia & HPV) ↑ HIV risk 2–5× due to ↑ viral shedding, genital mucosal disruption, & local recruitment of inflamm cells (*Curr Opin HIV/AIDS 2010;5:305*)

Testing and Screening (*Ann Intern Med 2013;30*)
- HIV screening recommended for (1) those between age 15 and 64 once, (2) all pregnant women, and (3) at more frequent intervals for those with risk factors: IVDU, bisexual, multiple sexual partners, exchange sex for drugs
- 1st-step screening by ELISA → Western blot for band specific confirmation

Gynecologic Care of HIV+ Patient (*Obstet Gynecol 2016;128:e89–110*)
- Combination antiretroviral therapy (cART [≥2 drugs from 2 classes] = HAART = ART, all similar terms) recommended for all HIV-infected individuals, indep. of viral load
  - Avoid efavirenz without neg preg test (teratogen in 1st trimester) or in patients planning pregnancy
- Double coverage (condoms + other agent) recommended for HIV+ patient. All contraception options are considered safe.
- ↓ OCP efficacy w/ some PIs & NNRTIs from cP450 metabolism (see CDC MEC for guidelines). Depo provera and LARC are safe & effective.
- HIV+ ♀ 6× greater odds of ↓ bone mineral density & 4× ↑ odds of osteoporosis
- Cervical cancer screening: ↑ Atypia and ↑ rates of progression, 48% with atypia on initial screen and 7% progression to high grade lesions and 5% to cancer (*J Infect Dis 2003;188*). HPV driven dysplasia cART with CD4 count >350 reduces this (*JAMA 2012;308(4):362–9*)
  - Start with 1st sexual activity or within 1 y of HIV diagnosis
  - <30 y annual pap, NO HPV co-screen
  - >30 y can do cotest, can space to q3y after 3 neg cytology results or 1 neg cotest
  - ASCUS or greater → colpo
  - Should still get HPV vaccine if eligible
- VIN, VAIN, & AIN also ↑ in HIV+ women (*Obstet Gynecol 2006;107:1023*)
- Additional screening includes: Annual syphilis, annual GC/CT and trichomonas, Hep C at initial diagnosis
- STI clinical course differs and is ↑ duration and severity w/ HIV coinfection. HSV → ↑ frequency, pain, duration; use HSV suppression ppx. Syphilis → ↑ neurosyphilis & rx failure; re-evaluate clinically & w/ serologic titers at 3, 6, 9, 12, & 24 mo after therapy (*CDC MMWR 2010;59:No.RR-12*)

Transmission
- Latex condoms are the only contraceptive that reduce HIV transmission (80% ↓); spermicides do NOT reduce transmission
- HIV+ should be on cART to decrease transmission in serodiscordant partners
- Pre-exposure prophylaxis PrEP has been shown to ↓ risk of transmission up to 83% (*NEJM 2012;367(5):399–410*), rec for HIV-partner, rec for attempting pregnancy
  - Tenofovir disoproxil fumarate and emtricitabine PO QD

HIV in Pregnancy (http://aidsinfo.nih.gov/guidelines)
- **Univ routine testing (opt-out)** for all pregnant women at initial prenatal visit. Women who present in labor w/o prenatal care should get rapid HIV test; intrapartum AZT ↓ perinatal transmission. HIV a/w SGA, preterm deliv.
- Due to Preg plasma vol changes, CD4 count ↓ but no change on CD4 percentage. Preg does not change dz progression Preg (*J infect Dis 1992;165:1116*)
- HIV+ women should get pneumococcal, influenza, hepatitis A (if noninmune), & hepatitis B vaccines + other standard Preg vaccination. Screen for hepatitis C, given high rates of coinfection (*MMWR Recomm Rep 2009;58:1*).

- Transmission can occur transplacentally (related to mat viral load), during deliv, & w/ breastfeeding (N Engl J Med 1999;341:1698). cART can ↓ perinatal transmission to <1% (untreated 15–25%) (N Engl J Med 1994;331:1173). Start cART during Preg to suppress viral load, continue ppx at deliv, & provide neonat ppx to the infant.
- **Transmission prevention:**
  - **Antepartum:** All women should receive cART during Preg – should cont prev meds if good viral control. If needs to be started then generally a combination from at least 2 classes of drugs. Recommended regimen is: Zidovudine/ Lamivudine/Ritonavir/Lopinavir. Efavirenz (NNRTI) category D: A/w increased neural tube defects.
  - **Intrapartum AZT mgmt:** AZT at onset of labor 2 mg/kg loading dose followed by 1 mg/kg/h until deliv. Optional for women on cART w/ HIV viral load <1,000 copies/mL. Continue oral cART intrapartum. Avoid artificial rupture of membranes & instrumentation (scalp electrodes, operative deliv) if poss. Methergine not as effective if cART uses nevirapine, efavirenz, or etravirine
  - **Postpartum:** Infants should receive AZT for 6 w can consider 4w Rx with moms with good suppression. Infants born to mothers not on cART should receive 3 doses of nevirapine. Mat cART continuation is essent given high rates of non-adherence & subseq mortality postpartum.
  - **Mode of deliv:** CD ↓ transmission rates in women NOT receiving HAART & zid-ovudine monotherapy (2–4×). No signif difference in transmission rates btw CD & VD in women on cART. CD indicated if viral load >1000 copies/mL. 3 h of AZT should be administered prior to operation if poss. Duration of ROM a/w transmission in women w/ unsuppressed viral load → best to perform CD prior to ROM or active labor.
  - **Breastfeeding** not recommended in developed countries even when mother on cART, due to postnatal transmission risk (MMWR Morb Mortal Wkly Rep 1985;34:721). Rate of HIV transmission ~10% from breastfeeding, but varies based on mat CD4 count, HIV viral load, & cART use. In developing world, do recommend breastfeeding b/c infant mortality from HIV offset by increased diarrheal & PNA illness in formula-fed infants (JAMA 2006;296:794).

TORCH INFECTIONS

- **T**-oxoplasmosis, **O**-ther (Syphilis, Varicella, Parvo), **R**-ubella, **C**-ytomegalovirus, **H**-erpes simplex virus
- Infections classically transmitted transplacentally or during deliv = vertical transmission
- **General rule:** ↑ Gestational age @ time of infxn = ↑ transmission rate
- Rubella & syphilis routinely screened in Preg, others if indicated by Hx/risk factors
- Most carry risk of IUFD, prematurity, growth restriction in addition to congen defects

Toxoplasmosis (Clin Infect Dis 1994;18:853; Clin Infect Dis 2008;47:554)
- **Epidemiology:** ~38% of women have immunity. Incident infxn during Preg is 0.2–1%. Congen infxn due to re-infection rare. Congen toxoplasmosis incid 1–2 cases out of 100000.
- **Microbiology:** Toxoplasmosis gondii: A ubiquitous protozoan parasite. Life cycle: Cat (definitive host of parasite) intestines produce oocysts which produce sporozoites → passed in feces → animals eat sporozoites → cysts form in bone & muscle → humans eat raw, undercooked meat, consume the tissue → infxn. OR, humans ingest oocysts while handling cat litter or soil.
- Maternal–fetal transmission occurs during **active phase of new infxn**. Transmission rate btw around 30%. Likelihood of **transmission ↑ w/ gestational age – 15% at 13 w, 44% at 26 w, 71% at 36 w**. Severity of congen infections peaks during transmission around 24–30 w.
- **Clinical manifestations:** Mat usually subclinical or nonspecific (fever, malaise, LAD, myalgia). Fetal classic triad of **chorioretinitis, hydrocephalus, intracranial calcifications**. Also seizures, jaundice, HSM, anemia. Late manifestations, ocular, & neurologic (developmental delay). Subclinical dz more common – only 10% show signs of congen infxn.
- **Dx/screening:** No univ screening. Dx by mat serology. A **single bld test does not distinguish btw acute & chronic infxn**. Nor does IgM vs. IgG distinguish, as both persist in chronic infxn. Rising titers demonstrate new infxn → 4× ↑ or greater done at least 2 w apart (stable titers = chronic infxn which poses no risk to fetus).

Once new infxn documented: PCR of amniotic fluid. US surveillance of fetal dev & manifestations of infxn.
- **Rx** (*Lancet* 2004;363:1965): **Spiramycin** (1 g TID) or **pyrimethamine & sulfadiazine w/ leucovorin** (teratogenic risk in 1st trimester w/ latter combo). Rx reduces serious neurologic sequelae. Unclear if rx prevents transmission & ocular sequelae.
- **Prevention:** Hand hygiene, avoiding un- & under-cooked meats, cats, unfiltered water, & travel to less developed countries

Syphilis (see below)

Varicella Virus (VZV) (*BJOG* 2011;118:1155)
- **Epidemiology: Prior to vaccination** 90% of women were infected (had chickenpox) before adulthood. From 1995, vaccination common. VZV incid in Preg ~5/10000.
- **Microbiology:** Herpes virus responsible for 1° infxn known as **VZV (chickenpox) w/ subseq reactivations known as zoster**. Mat zoster (shingles) rarely a/w congen VZV syn.
- Clinical manifestations (*Obstet Gynecol* 1987;69:214): Mat VZV infxn can be sev. VZV PNA = common complication (10–20%) w/ 20–40% mortality w/o antiviral therapy. Congen syn rare <2%. Transplacental transmission <20 w gestation characterized by limb hypoplasia, cutaneous scars, neurologic abnormalities, ocular abnormalities, high mortality. After 20 w transmission, infxn w/i 5 d of deliv has neonat mortality as high as 30%. Infxn >5 d from deliv, mat Ab xfer → more benign neonat infxn.
- **Dx/screening:** Mother: Characteristic vesicular papules in different stages of progression. Culture or immunofluorescence studies. Serology early in infxn can confirm mat nonimmunity. PCR testing of amniotic fluid + US to detect fetal infxn.
- **Rx:** 1° chickenpox: Antiviral therapy w/i 24 h of rash appearance. Acyclovir 800 mg 5× daily or Valacyclovir 1 g TID for 7 d. VZV zoster secondary infxn: Ig w/i 72 h of exposure. May be effective up to 10 d after exposure. Pregnant women w/ varicella PNA should be admitted & treated w/ IV acyclovir.
  Post exp: Exposed & VZV IgG negative with no hx of chickenpox can give VariZIG

Parvovirus (*N Engl J Med* 1987;316:183; *Prenat Diagn* 2011;31:419)
- **Epidemiology:** Incid of acute parvovirus in Preg = 3%. By adulthood 30–60% of women have had infxn.
- **Microbiology** (*Rev Med Virol* 2003;13:347): Risk of vertical transmission to fetus ~33%. Virus affects fetal erythroid progenitor cells.
- **Clinical manifestations:** Children & adults → erythema infectiosum: Lace-like rash often on face "slapped check," arthropathy, aplastic anemia. Fetal infxn: **Hydrops & stillborn <24 w;** >24 w, persistent risk of hydrops, but ↓ likelihood of sev infxn & death. Hydrops from anemia (BM failure) → reduced survival of fetal red cells → high-output CHF.
- **Dx/screening:** Exposed women should be tested w/ serology: **+ IgM w/o IgG** = acute infxn. PCR amniotic fluid + US to confirm dx
- **Rx:** W/ confirmed infxn → **surveillance for** up to 12 w. **Weekly US & MCA Doppler** to look for fetal anemia. Intrauterine xfusion can be done to correct fetal anemia & ↓ fetal mortality.

Rubella (*Lancet* 1982;2:781; *Glob Libr Women's Med* 2012)
- **Epidemiology:** Rare in the US given immunization programs. ~90% of pop immune
- Congen rubella extremely rare → <1 case/y in US recently
- **Microbiology:** Self-limited viral infxn transmitted in droplets or nasopharyngeal secretions from infected persons, commonly from contact w/ infected child. Congen infxn occurs via hematogenous spread across placenta. **Earlier transmission = higher likelihood of sev defects.**
- **Clinical manifestations:** Mat often subclinical: Fever, maculopapular rash, LAD (postauricular), URI-like, nonspecific sx. Infxn in 1st trimester usually results in miscarriage. Infxn **after 20 w unlikely to result in neonat manifestations.** Classic fetal syn: Growth restriction, cataracts, cardiac defects, hearing defects, hepatosplenomegaly. "Blueberry muffin rash." Late manifestations: DM, thyroid disorders, panencephalitis.
- **Dx/screening:** Univ screening at initial prenatal visit → nonimmune pts vaccinated postpartum. Dx by serology titer immediately following exposure. If Ab+ → woman likely immune, no risk to fetus. Conversion of (–)Ab or 4× ↑ titer indicates acute infxn (rpt titers 2–4 w apart). Confirm by IgM or direct PCR of fetal bld.
- **Rx/prevention:** Mat supportive measures. No rx exists for preventing transmission or for fetal infxn. Nonimmune mothers should be vaccinated postpartum. MMR vaccine should not be administered to pregnant women b/c of theoretical risk of transmission from live virus. Advised to avoid conception for 1 mo following vaccine

Cytomegalovirus (CMV) (Infect Dis Obstet Gynecol 2011;2011:1)
- **Epidemiology:** Most common congen infxn. Birth prevalence ~0.5%. Seropositivity in childbearing women ~58% in US. Risk factors: Low socioeconomic status (near 100%), non-White, multiparous. Most common infectious cause of sensorineural hearing loss.
- **Microbiology:** Herpes virus family, latent in numerous organs following infxn. Transmitted by close interpersonal contact including sexual contact & breastfeeding.
- **Transmission** (Obstet Gynecol Surv 2010;65:736): Congen CMV: Transplacental transmission. Peripartum transmission does not harm dev of neonate. 1° mat infxn, ~35% transmission. More likely to cause fetal infxn & sequelae. Reactivation of latent virus: 1–2% transmission rate. Reinfection w/ different strain poss.
- **Clinical manifestations:** 1° CMV – asx or a/w a mononucleosis-like syn. Fetal infxn & sequelae more common at <20 w gestation. 90% are asx; 5–10% overtly symptomatic w/ 5% mortality or w/ 50–60% w/ sever neurologic morbidity: **Microcephaly, ventriculomegaly, chorioretinitis, HSM, sensorineural hearing loss.** Late infxns a/w hepatitis, PNA, purpura, & thrombocytopenia.
- **Dx/screening:** Routine screening not currently recommended in US. Dx by seroconversion during Preg. IgM helpful for reactivated infxn. Low IgG avidity Indicative of primary infxn. Viral culture can be performed, but does not distinguish btw new & recurrent. US screening for anomalies should be performed in suspected case. If CMV infxn present → amniocentesis after 20 w to detect fetal infxn.
- **Prevention:** Hygienic precautions: Washing hands, avoidance of close contact
- **Rx:** High-titer CMV Ig may ↓ transmission & fetal/neonat morbidity

Herpes Simplex Virus (HSV) (N Engl J Med 1997;337:509)
- **Epidemiology:** HSV-1 or HSV-2 seroprevalence in pregnant females up to 72%. Congen HSV very rare, 1 in 5000–20000. Seroconversion during Preg = 3.7% in women seronegative to both types.
- **Microbiology:** 50–70% of genital HSV caused by HSV-2. Genital HSV-1 ↑ due to oral–genital practices. Transmission can occur transplacentally (rare) or through contact w/ mother's genital tract during labor/deliv. Mat 1° infxn **(0.1% incid)** a/w **higher transmission rates at deliv** than recurrent infxn (mat antibodies are protective).
- **Clinical manifestations:** 1° infxn: Fever, malaise, dysuria, tender inguinal LAD, painful genital ulcers. Many pts have mild or **subclinical presentation. Vesicles** → crusting ulcers. Recurrent episodes vary in frequency, usually milder & shorter than 1° episode. Latency: Dorsal nerve roots btw episodes. Neonat HSV: Mucocutaneous involvement (~45%), CNS dz assoc. with ~15% mortality (~33%), dissem dz w/ multiorgan involvement assoc. with ~50% mortality (~25%). Congen infxn extremely rare, can cause systemic dz w/ mortality >50%. Late trimester mat infections correlated w/ increased rates of preterm labor, preterm birth, & IUGR.
- **Dx/screening:** Univ screening not recommended. Dx by culture or PCR if lesion present. Serology can distinguish HSV type; IgM indicative of acute infxn.
- **Rx** (MMWR Recomm Rep 2010;59:1): 1° infxn: **Acyclovir** 400 mg TID × 7–10 d or Valacyclovir 1 g BID × 7–10 d. Recurrent infxn: Acyclovir 400 mg TID × 5 d or Valacyclovir 500 mg BID × 3 d. Suppressive therapy recommended for women w/ **recurrent** genital HSV from 36 w until deliv: Acyclovir 400 mg TID or Valacyclovir 500 mg BID. At time of deliv, **careful exam of woman's genital tract** should be performed. Women w/ active lesions of vulva, vagina, or cervix **should be offered CD.** Lesions on buttocks, mons, thighs, or anus can be covered during deliv.

OTHER INFECTIONS IN PREGNANCY

Zika (NEJM 2016;115:717) (https://www.acog.org/Clinical-Guidance-and-Publications/Practice-Advisories/Practice-Advisory-Interim-Guidance-for-Care-of-Obstetric-Patients-During-a-Zika-Virus-Outbreak)
- **Epidemiology:** Outbreaks in Brazil and Central America in 2015, previously in French Polynesia (Lancet 2016;(16):00651–6)
- **Microbiology:** Caused by a flavivirus (similar to dengue) with neurotropism, 3–14 d incubation period
- **Transmission:** Classically by mosquito (Aedes aegypti and Aedes albopictus) but also **sexual transmission, transplacental and exposure to body fluids**
- **Clinical manifestations:** 20% asymptomatic, fever, arthralgia, malaise, conjunctivitis, Preg → risk of pregnancy loss and fetal anomalies, increases Guillain–Barré syndrome

- Risk of fetal anomalies "Congenital Zika Syndrome" in approximately 10–15% of infected pregnant women: **Microcephaly**, cataracts, brain development, developmental delay, growth retardation, and IUFD. Risk greater with infxn in 1st tri
- Diagnosis: Diagnosed by antibody testing and nucleic acid testing (PCR), can test from sx onset – 12 w. Can also do serum testing alone but cross reactive to other flavivirus and req confirmation with plaque reduction neutralization test (PRNT)
- Travel restrictions – pregnant women are advised to avoid areas where Zika transmission is a risk (Latin America, Puerto Rico, etc.)
- Conception – women infected with Zika should wait at least 8 w before attempting pregnancy; if partner is infected, use barrier contraception for 6 mo before attempting pregnancy
- Zika diagnosis and treatment advice changes frequently. Visit the CDC website for the most up to date information: www.cdc.gov/zika/pregnancy/index.html

Influenza (Obstet Gynecol 2010;115:717) (See also Chap. 13 [p. 13-6])
- **Epidemiology:** During flu pandemics (including 2009 H1N1), pregnant women ↑ hospitalization, ↑ ICU admission, & ↑ mortality rate
- **Clinical manifestations:** Fever, tachycardia, respiratory, GI sx. Physiologic changes of Preg → **less cardiopulmonary reserve & altered immune system.** Transplacental transmission rare & insig. Mat illness may lead to premature deliv.
- **Dx/screening:** Rapid flu testing available in ≤15 min, sensitivity poor ~63%. In pregnant & recently (<2 w) postpartum women, **rx should be administered empirically. Do not await diagnostic results.**
- **Rx:** Neuraminidase inhibitors. Ppx for exposed: Oseltamivir 75 mg daily × 10 d or Zanamivir 10 mg daily × 10 d. Rx: Oseltamivir 75 mg BID × 5 d or Zanamivir 10 mg BID × 5 d.
- **Prevention:** All pregnant women should receive inactivated influenza vaccination regardless of gestational age, & preferably by the beginning of flu season

Hepatitis B Virus (HBV) (See Chap. 15 [p.15-7])
- **Epidemiology:** Prevalence ~1% US & 15–20% endemic areas (SE Asia, China, sub-Saharan Africa). Major source of morbidity from hepatitis is from chronic infxn assoc with cirrhosis, & HCC. 5–10% of acutely infected will become chronic carriers. In endemic areas, perinatal/vertical is primary form of transmission.
- **Microbiology** (JAMA 1985;253:1740): Maternal–fetal transmission primarily during deliv. Transmission 40–90% w/o prev treatment, higher if HBeAg+. CD does not prevent transmission. Breastfeeding does NOT ↑ rate of transmission (Obstet Gynecol 2002;99:1049).
- **Clinical manifestations:** Mat 1° infxn: Abdominal pain, fever, N/V, jaundice. Almost all infected infants become chronic carriers, although infxn generally asx. Infected newborns have approx. 25% risk of premature death from liver dz later in life.
- **Dx/screening:** Dx by + surface Ag (HBsAg). Immunity is indicative of loss of HBsAg & appearance of HBsAb (Ab). IgM anti-HBc is indicative of primary infxn; sometimes only sign of infxn btw loss of HbsAg & rise of HBsAb. HBeAg a marker of high infectivity, carries high vertical transmission rates. Chronic infxn is determined by persistence of HBsAg >6 mo. ACOG recommends univ screening by checking HBsAg in prenatal panel.
- **Rx:** Vaccination universally recommended if serologically negative. Lamivudine during 3rd trimester may ↓ rate of transmission (Obstet Gynecol 2010;116:147). HepBIg & HBV vaccine recommended as ppx for neonates of HbsAg+ women. ↓ Rate of transmission by almost 90% (JAMA 1985;253:1740).

Hepatitis C Virus (HCV) (Hepatology 2001;34:223; Am Fam Physician 2010;82:1225) (see Chap. 15)
- **Epidemiology:** 1.8% of noninstitutionalized persons carry HCV antibodies
- **Microbiology:** Vertical transmission ~2% – primarily during deliv. Risk factors for increased transmission include increased viral load, HIV coinfection, mat drug use, prolonged ROM, procedures during labor (fetal scalp electrode, operative vaginal deliv). CD does not appear to ↓ transmission (Arch Gynecol Obstet 2011;283:255). Breastfeeding does not to appear to ↑ transmission. Infected infants are generally asx, sometimes w/ temporary transaminitis.
- **Dx/screening:** Hepatitis C screening based on risk factors. HCV Ab + → obtain viral load, genotype. HCV by RIBA if concern for false-positive.
- **Rx:** No meds during pregnancy. Vaccinate for HBV if not infected or immune. Rx with Sofosbuvir and Velpatasvir, highly effective but response vary with genotype (N Engl J Med 2015;373:2599–607)

Tuberculosis (TB) (Chest 1992;101:1114)
- **Epidemiology:** Same in Preg as general pop. 5–10% of reproductive women have reactive tuberculin skin test. Worldwide TB = **leading infectious dz cause of**

mat mortality. Risk factors in US: Low socioeconomic status, urban area, IV drug use, homelessness, immigrant from underdeveloped country, & incarceration.

- **Clinical manifestations:** 3–4% develop active TB during 1st year. 5–15% will later develop an active infxn. Active TB: **Cough, fever, hemoptysis, weight loss, fatigue, night sweats.** Untreated active infxn has a 50% mortality rate at 5 y. Active TB → congen infxn through transplacental transmission. This is extremely rare & a/w miliary TB.
- **Dx/screening:** Screening should occur in women w/ risk of progression from latent to active. **TST or interferon gamma release assay.** Those w/ positive testing should undergo CXR.

Classification of TST reaction	
TST size (mm)	**Group in which this is considered positive**
≥5	HIV+, close contact w/ cases, abn CXR, immunosuppression (chemo, glucocorticoids)
≥10	Persons at risk of reactivation, chronic renal failure, DM, malignancies, children <4 yo, foreign born from TB prevalent countries, residents & employees of high-risk settings
≥15	Healthy individuals w/ low likelihood of true TB infxn

From *MMWR Recomm Rep* 2005;54(RR-17):1–141.

- **Rx** (*MMWR* 2000;49:1):
    Latent TB: 9 mo INH 5 mg/kg/d. Can delay rx of latent TB until 2–3 mo PP unless high risk of progression to active dz (HIV+, recent contacts)
    Active TB: RIPE: Rifampin, INH, ethambutol ± pyrazinamide × 9 mo minimum. Streptomycin should be avoided in Preg (congen deafness). Breastfeeding not contraindicated during rx. Infant should be given pyridoxine (B6) if mother is on INH.

HUMAN PAPILLOMA VIRUS (HPV)

Epidemiology
- Most common sexually transmitted virus worldwide
- Most common viral cause of cancer worldwide (5% of all cancers)
- Worldwide prevalence around 10% although 80% of sexually active adults will acquire an HPV infxn in their lifetime (*Am J Epidemiology* 2000;151:1158)
- Prevalence highest in teenagers & young women shortly after sexual debut (*JAMA* 2007;297:813)
- **Risk factors:** Young age, early age at 1st intercourse, number of sexual partners, other STIs (HIV, HSV, chlamydia), smoking, low education, minority race

Microbiology
- DsDNA virus. ~40 strains of HPV infect the anogenital tract & can be a/w anogenital warts & cancer including **cervical, vaginal, vulvar, oropharyngeal, anorectal, & penile.** High-risk HPV types cause cancer: HPV16, 18, 31, 33, 35, 39, 45, 51, 52, 56, 58, 59, 66, 68. Types 16 & 18 account for 70% of cancer cases (*N Engl J Med* 2003;348:518). Low-risk HPV types cause warts: HPV6, 11, 42, 43, 44.
- Transmission usually through intercourse, but can occur through close personal contact.
- Warts esp contagious → 60% infectivity with contact. Vertical transmission may be as high as 55% during vaginal deliv. Infxn generally **transient** → 90% cleared by 24 mo (*Vaccine* 2006;24:S42).
- Risk factors for persistence/progression of HPV to precancerous lesions: Older age, immunosuppression, cigarette smoking, high-risk genotypes (*Vaccine* 2006;24:42).
- HPV's carcinogenic potential related to (*J Virol* 1989;63:4417)
    E6 gene a/w inactivation of p53 (tumor suppressor prot)
    E7 gene a/w inactivation of the Rb apoptotic pathway

Clinical Manifestations
- Based on strain & site of infxn. Include genital & nongenital warts (condyloma acuminatum), Bowen's dz (squamous carcinoma in situ), giant condyloma, & intraepithelial neoplasia.
- **Cervical dysplasia:** HPV infxn leading to cellular atypia & progression from low-grade to high-grade histology is the basis for cervical cancer (*J Pathol* 1999;189:12). See also Chaps. 1 and 22.

- **Genital warts (condylomata acuminata):** Caused by low-risk HPV6 & 11 (90%) (*MMWR Recomm Rep* 2010;59:1). Usually asx papillomatous growths, commonly appear around introitus. Vary in appearance: Hyperpigmented, papilliform, flat, papular, pedunculated (in contrast to **condylomata lata** of syphilis which is flat & velvety). Regression occurs ~20–50% of cases. Persistence a/w immunocomp status & dev of squamous cell carcinoma. Lesions a/w HPV6 & 11 are almost 100% benign. 30% of flat condylomas a/w high-risk types & have oncogenic potential.

Diagnostic Studies
- **HPV testing:** Current testing exists in either a binary (± high-risk HPV) form or specific genotyping that can detect presence of specific strains (HPV16, HPV18). See Chaps. 1 and 22.
- **Genital warts:** Dx of **condyloma** made by inspection. 5% acetic acid solution → causes acetowhite change for easier identification. Bx considered if dx uncertain, lesion does not respond to rx or worsens w/ therapy, pt immunocomp, warts are pigmented, indurated, fixed, bleeding, or ulcerated.

Treatment (*MMWR Recomm Rep* 2010;59:1)
- Rx goal for **genital warts** is amelioration of sx & cosmetic improv
- CDC recommended regimens:
  - Patient-applied:
    - Podofilox 0.5% gel applied BID × 3 d followed by 4 d off, up to 4 cycles
    - Imiquimod 5% cream applied QHS 3× a week for up to 16 w
    - Sinecatechins 15% ointment TID for up to 16 w
    - 5-fluorouracil 5% cream applied BID × 5 d followed by 9 d off, up to 4 cycles
    - (Safety of all of these therapies in Preg is unk & should not be used)
  - **Provider-administered:** Cryotherapy, trichloroacetic acid 85%, surgical removal (excision, laser, electrosurgery, infrared coagulation)
- Ppx (*CDC-ACIP* 2011) (*Obstet Gynecol* 2017;129:e173)
  - Bivalent (*Cervarix*), quadrivalent (*Gardasil*), and 9-vlalent (Gardasil-9) vaccine. 9-Valent includes HPV6, 11, 18, 31, 33, 45, 52, 58; Quadrivalent includes HPV16, 18 as well "low-risk" strains HPV6, 11. Bivalent effective against HPV16, 18. Vaccination recommended in females & males 11–26 yo. Very effective with decreasing HPV disease >90% but uptake is poor.

SYPHILIS

Epidemiology (www.cdc.gov/std/stats16/default.htm)
- Once highly prevalent dz now uncommon
- 2013–2016 with 35% ↑ in women with assoc ↑ 28% in congenital syphilis 1.5/10,000 births, has led to concern for rising epidemic

Microbiology
- **Caused by the spirochete: Treponema pallidum.** Sexually transmitted through microabrasions of intercourse or vertical transmission. Following infxn, the organisms invade tiss/ul to disseminate to other organs.
- Sexual transmission occurs during both primary & secondary infxn. Rate ~30%. Requires open lesions w/ organisms present

Clinical Manifestations
- Primary syphilis
  - **Chancre** at site of inoculation. Ulcer is usually single, **painless,** indurated, a/w LAD. Most common location in women: Labia majora + minora, fourchette, cervix, perineum. Generally heal w/o rx secondary to natural immune resp.
- Secondary syphilis
  - Weeks to months after primary infxn. ~25% develop systemic illness.
  - **Rash** (typically palms & soles), up to 90% of pts. 0.5–2 cm in diameter often referred to as copper pennies.
  - **Condyloma lata:** 10–15% pts. Large raised white lesions usually near chancre Highly infectious – not to be confused w/ condyloma acuminatum (HPV/warts)!
  - **Systemic sx:** Fever, HA, malaise, LAD.
  - Immunocomp can develop ocular dz, ulcerative lesions
- Latent syphilis
  - **Asx w/ + serologic testing.** If pt never had sx = latent of unk duration. Early/late distinction is <1 y (**early latent**) vs. >1 y (**late latent**) from sx. Pts >1 y from sx are relatively noninfectious.

- Tertiary syphilis (late)

    Develops after latent period of 1–30 y after primary infxn. Most common manifestations: CNS (neurosyphilis), CV (aortitis), Gummatous (on skin & bones)

    Neurosyphilis: Syphilitic meningitis (syphilis in CSF), meningovascular syphilis (ischemia/infarction of CNS), parenchymal syphilis (tabes dorsalis, general paresis)

- Congen syphilis

    Preg does not change course of mat dz. Fetal manifestations depend on time of transmission. Early infxn → high rates of SAB. Late infxn → placental involvement, hydrops, IUGR, stillbirth. **Transmission ↑ w/ GA, but severity ↓.**

    Vertical transmission highest w/ 1° or 2° syphilis (50%). Rx lowers risk of transmission to 1–2%. Congen syphilis is classified as **early** or **late. Early: Sx prior to 2 yo:** Rhinitis (snuffles), rash, PNA, HSM, osteochondritis (similar to adults). **Late: Sx after 2 yo:** Saddle nose, Hutchinson's teeth (peg-shaped incisors), keratitis, deafness, gumma, skeletal & CNS malformations

Diagnostic Studies

- Organism cannot be cultured. Definitive dx made by direct visualization of organisms w/ either dark field microscopy (gold std), direct fluorescent Ab, or PCR.
- **Serologic testing:** Nontreponemal (VDRL, RPR) vs. treponemal (FTA-ABS, TPA)

    Nontreponemal tests – used for pop screening (Preg, MSM). Low cost, widely available. Use titers to monit resp to rx. 4-Fold decrease in titer necessary to demonstrate resp to rx. False positives a/w Preg, autoimmune dz, IV drug use, TB, rickettsial infxn, hepatitis, malig. Sensitivities can be poor esp during primary & late stages (70–80%).

    Treponemal tests – more specific, generally used for confirmatory testing. Cannot be used alone to diagnose rpt infxn as antibodies may stay positive following successful rx. False positives a/w lupus, Lyme's, leptospirosis.

- **Preg:** Screening at the 1st prenatal visit w/ nontreponemal test followed by rpt testing in 3rd trimester & at deliv if pt is high risk
- Lumbar puncture w/ signs of tertiary/neurosyphilis, or HIV+ & latent syphilis

Treatment

Treatment regimens for syphilis		
Adult recommended regimens	**PCN G**	**PCN allergic**
Primary or secondary syphilis	2.4 million units IM in single dose	Doxycycline 100 mg BID × 14 d + Tetracycline 500 mg QID × 14 d
Early latent syphilis	2.4 million units IM in single dose	Doxycycline 100 mg BID × 28 d + Tetracycline 500 mg QID × 28 d
Late latent or latent of unk duration	2.4 million units IM QW × 3 doses	Doxycycline 100 mg BID × 28 d + Tetracycline 500 mg QID × 28 d
Tertiary syphilis	2.4 million units IM QW × 3 doses	Consult ID
Neurosyphilis	Aqueous crystalline PCN G 18–24 U IV daily × 10–14 d OR PCN 2.4 IM daily + Probenecid 500 mg QID × 10–14 d	CTX 2 g IM or IV daily × 10–14 d OR Consult ID
Pregnant women	PCN G per stage of infxn	No proven alternatives. Desensitization.

- **Jarisch–Herxheimer rxn:** Febrile rxn w/i 24 h of rx → release of inflamm proteins from dead or dying organisms. Can induce preterm labor or cause fetal distress in pregnant women.
- Eval should be made at 6 & 12 mo after rx (24 if latent dz or worse). Serologic testing should show decline by 4 fold. Failure of decline = re-evaluation for HIV, CSF exam should be considered. Retreatment involves 2.4 million units IM QW for 3 w.
- Partners exposed w/i 90 d of dx & partners of pts w/ syphilis of unk duration & high nontreponemal titers (>1:32) should be treated presumptively (*MMWR Recomm Rep 2010;59:1*).

MOLLUSCUM CONTAGIOSUM

Epidemiology (J Am Acad Dermatol 2006;54:47)
- Common worldwide. A/w childhood, immunodeficiency (including HIV) & atopic dermatitis. Seropositivity up to 25% in general pop.

Microbiology
- **Pox virus** spread through direct skin-to-skin contact or through fomites
- Considered a sexually transmitted infxn when found in genital region

Clinical Manifestations
- Firm dome-shaped papules on skin w/ shiny surface & central umbilication
  Appear anywhere except palms & soles, but generally localized. Commonly in skin folds – axilla, popliteal folds. Sexually transmitted areas include groin, genitals, thighs, & lower abd. Dermatitis can occur around the lesion – erythema & pruritus.
- Widespread, large >15 mm lesions should raise suspicion for HIV+
- Natural Hx in immunocompetent person: Spont resolution in months
  Lesions can last years (Int J Dermatol 2006;45:93)

Diagnosis
- Clinical – based on appearance of lesion. Histology: H&E reveals **Henderson–Patterson Bodies:** Keratinocytes w/ cytoplasmic inclusion bodies

Treatment
- No clear evid for rx given lesions are self-limiting. Rx of sexually transmitted lesions indicated to avoid transmission of dz. **Perform comprehensive body exam** to locate all lesions for rx.
- **Cryotherapy:** Liquid nitrogen applied 6–10 s (can cause hypopigmentation)
- **Other 1st-line options:** Curettage, cantharidin, podophyllotoxin (Cochrane Database Syst Rev 2009)

CHANCROID

Epidemiology
- Uncommon in US & developed countries. Major cause of genital ulcers in developing countries. In US: Minority pop, female prostitutes, drug users. **Up to 10% have concurrent syphilis infxn.**

Microbiology
- **Haemophilus ducreyi** – Gram-negative rod (school of fish appearance). Extremely infectious. Incubation 3–10 d, reliant on break in skin. Cytotoxin secreted causes cellular damage & ulcer dev.

Clinical Manifestations
- **Erythematous papule**, 1–2 cm diameter → pustular & ulcerates. Distinguished from syphilis as it is painful, sometimes purulent & base is red & granular. Typically found on fourchette, vestibule, clitoris & labia (Clin Infect Dis 1997;25(2):292). Often single lesion but can be multi & bleeds.
- LAD present in ½ cases & can become fluctuant & painful

Diagnosis (MMWR Recomm Rep 1990;39:1)
- Difficult lab dx due to need for culture on special media (sens <20%)
  Special PCR test exists by private clinical labs. "Probable" dx based on clinical sx & negative testing for syphilis & HSV.

Treatment (MMWR Recomm Rep 2010;59:1)
- **CDC recommendation:** Azithromycin 1 g PO or CTX 250 mg IM or Ciprofloxacin 500 mg PO BID × 3 d. Ciprofloxacin contraindicated in pregnant & lactating women.
- Pt should be re-examined at 3–7 d after initiation of therapy. Lack of clinical improv w/i 7 d, consider incorrect dx, coinfection, HIV+, nonadherence, drugs resistance. Healing is slower for immunocompromised (HIV), uncirc men. LAD might require needle aspiration or drainage

PUBIC LICE

Epidemiology
- Generally transmitted sexually. Less commonly transmitted by fomites on clothing & bedding. Most commonly affected are teens, young adults.

Etiology
- **Phthirus pubis or "crab louse"** is primary organism. Crab-like claws attach to human hair, feeding on human bld, laying eggs. Eggs incubate for 6–8 d before hatching.

Clinical Manifestations
- **Pruritus** from attachment & biting
- **Maculopapular lesion may develop** (lower abd, prox thighs, buttocks)
- Manifestations can occur in any hairy area, but pubic area is often involved

Diagnostic Studies
- Demonstration of louse or nits (eggs) under microscopic exam
- Dx should trigger eval of family members, sexual contacts, & for other STIs

Treatment (MMWR Recomm Rep 2010;59(RR-12):1)
- Pediculicides kill both lice & eggs
- **CDC rec: Permethrin 1%** cream or Pyrethrins w/ piperonyl butoxide (washed off after 10 min). Alternative: Malathion 0.5% (8–12 h) or Ivermectin (250 ug/kg) (for rx failure). Permethrin, Pyrethrin safe in pregnant & lactating women.
- Re-evaluate after 7–10 d of rx. Bedding or clothing should be bagged or washed. Lice will die 48 h after removal from host or temperature >125°C.

GENITAL ULCERS

	Ulcerative lesions of the genital tract				
	Syphilis	**Herpes**	**Chancroid**	**Lympho-granuloma venereum**	**Granuloma inguinale/ Donovanosis**
Organism	Treponema pallidum	Herpes simplex I or II	Haemophilus ducreyi	Chlamydia trachomatis Serovars L1, L2, L3. More prevalent in Africa, India, SE Asia, Caribbean	Klebsiella granulomatis (gram neg encapsulated bacterium). Needs rpt exposure, long incubation.
Lesion characteristic	Single painless indurated ulcer w/ rolled edges	Painful fluid-filled vesicles w/ erythematous base	One or more painful ulcers varying in size	Single ulcer or papule; can be painful or painless. Infected lymph tissue → necrosis in nodes → abscess	Painless nodules → ulcerative lesions that bleed easily on contact; can become sclerotic & very large. Usually on genitalia, cervix. Resemble keloids.

	Syphilis	Herpes	Chancroid	Lympho-granuloma venereum	Granuloma inguinale/ Donovanosis
LAD	Bilateral, non-tender	Uni- or bilateral, tender	Unilateral, tender, suppurative, often fluctuant	Unilateral tender, can suppurate or mat together. Stages: Ulcer → healed → LAD → fibrosis/ strictures (*Clin Infect Dis* 2006;42:186).	None
Dx	Dark-field microscopy, serology w/ treponemal test confirmation	Culture or PCR of lesions	Culture or special PCR testing	Chlamydia serology correlated w/ presentation, PCR testing. IgG >1:64. Low success w/ cx. PCR testing exists.	Donovan bodies on microscopy (safety pin appearance) on Wright–Giemsa stain.
Rx	Benzathine PCN G. See section for algorithm based on stage of presentation.	Acyclovir or Val-acyclovir. See section for specific dosing.	Azithromycin 1 g PO or CTX 250 mg IM or Ciprofloxacin 500 mg PO BID × 3 d or Erythromycin 500 mg PO TID × 7 d	Doxycycline 100 mg PO BID × 3 w (nonpregnant) Alt: Erythromycin 500 mg QID × 3 w or Azithromycin 1 g weekly × 3 w. Aspirate bubo to prevent rupture. Check & treat <60 d sexual contacts. (*MMWR Recomm Rep* 2010;59:1)	Doxycycline 100 mg BID × 3+ weeks & resolution of lesions Alt: Azithromycin 1 g weekly; Ciprofloxacin 750 mg BID; Erythromycin 500 mg QID (preferred for Preg) or Bactrim BID, all × 3+ weeks & resolution of lesions Add aminoglycoside if no resp.

Data from Workowski KA, Berman S. Sexually transmitted diseases treatment guidelines, 2010. *MMWR Recomm Rep.* 2010;59(RR-12):1–110 and Holmes K, Sparling P, Stamm W. *Sexually Transmitted Diseases.* 4th ed. New York, NY: McGraw-Hill; 2008.

Hysterectomy Type Classification

- **Piver–Rutledge–Smith classification (1974):** 5 classes of hysterectomy (I–V)

  I: Simple extrafascial hysterectomy: Only uterus (& cervix) removed. For nonmalignant diagnoses or stage IA1 cervical cancer and uterus-confined endometrial cancer

  II: Modified radical hysterectomy (Wertheim): Uterus, cervix, prox vagina (1/3), parametrium/paracervix & uterine artery transected medial to ureter

  III: Radical hysterectomy (Meigs–Wertheim): Uterus, cervix, prox vagina (1/3), uterine artery ligated at origin

  IV: Extended radical hysterectomy: Uterus, cervix, 3/4 of vagina, superior vesical artery

  V: Partial exenteration w/ removal of distal ureter &/or bladder

Radical Hysterectomy

- Uterus removed en bloc w/ parametrium (round, broad, cardinal, & uterosacral ligaments) & upper vagina. Ovaries can be preserved; bilateral pelvic lymph node dissection (LND) usually included. For cervical cancer greater than stage IA1 or endometrial cancer involving cervix.
- Complications of radical hysterectomy (Gynecol Oncol 2009;114:75): Bladder/bowel dysfunction (up to 85%); lymphocyst requiring drainage (3%); vesicovaginal (1%) or ureterovaginal (2%) fistula; PE or deep vein thrombosis (1–3%); intra- or postoperative bleeding/hemorrhage

Querleu–Morrow classification of radical hysterectomy			
4 types of radical hysterectomy (A–D, below) based on lateral extent of resection.			
Type	**Description**	**Surgical considerations**	**Indication**
A	Minimal resxn of paracervix	Paracervix transected medial to ureter but lateral to cervix. Uterosacral & cardinal ligaments transected close to uterus. Vaginal resxn (<10 mm).	Early invasive cervical cancer (<2 cm), advanced cervical cancer after chemoradiation
B	Transection of paracervix at level of ureter	Partial resxn of uterosacral & cardinal ligaments. Ureter unroofed & mobilized laterally. Vaginal resxn (10 mm).	Early cervical cancer (stage 1A)
C1	Transection of paracervix at junction w/ internal iliac artery (w/ nerve preservation)	Uterosacral ligament transected at rectum, cardinal ligament transected at bladder. Ureter mobilized. 15–20 mm of vagina resected. Hypogastric nerves identified, preserved.	Stages IB–IIA cervical cancer
C2	Transection of paracervix at junction w/ internal iliac artery (w/o nerve preservation)	Paracervix completely transected. Hypogastric nerves not isolated or preserved.	Stages IB–IIA cervical cancer
D1	Laterally extended endopelvic resxn	Resxn of entire paracervix (at pelvic sidewall) & hypogastric vessels	Pelvic exenteration
D2	Laterally extended endopelvic resxn	D1 + resxn of entire paracervix, hypogastric vessels, & adj fascial or musc structures	Pelvic exenteration
From Lancet Oncol 2008;9(3):297–303. doi:10.1016/S1470-2045(08)70074-3.			

CERVICAL CANCER

Epidemiology *(Lancet 2017;398:847)*
- 4th most common GYN cancer worldwide; in some countries most common female cancer
- **Mean age at dx:** 40–59 y; bimodal distribution peaks 35–39 y & 60–64 y
- HPV vaccination expected to decrease rates globally

Pathology *(J Clin Pathol 1998;51:96)*
- **Squamous cell carcinoma:** 80% of invasive cervical cancer
- **AdenoCa:** 20–25% of invasive cervical cancer. In 15%, lesion located w/i endocervical canal, increasing in frequency
  Mucinous adenoCa: Most common type (well differentiated)
  Endometrioid carcinoma: 30% of cervical adenocarcinomas
  Clear cell carcinoma: 4% of adenocarcinomas. DES exposure ↑ risk
- **Adenosquamous carcinoma:** Benign & malig glandular & squamous elements. More aggressive than adenoCa.
- **Small cell carcinoma:** Neuroendocrine tumors. Clinically aggressive; ↑ propensity for metastases; a/w HPV18; CD56 marker often positive

Etiology *(Int J Cancer 2007;120:885)*
- Risk factors
  Lack of cervical cancer screening. Cigarette smoking: 2–3 fold ↑ risk in current & former smokers (squamous only). Multi sexual partners (more than 6 partners significantly ↑ risk). HPV infxn.
  H/o STIs. Early age of sexual activity. ↑ Parity. Long-term combined OCP use (higher hormone levels make cells vulnerable to mut). Immunosuppression (esp HIV/ transplant). Low socioeconomic status. DES exposure in utero. No known racial predilection but mortality Black > White.

Role of HPV *(J Pathol 1999;189:12)*
- HPV detected in 99% of cervical cancer
- HPV types 16, 18, 31, 33, & 45 = high-risk types. Most common HPV 16 & 18.
  E1–E7 (early oncoproteins in cervical cancer) expressed in HPV positive cases (E1 & E2 → viral replication; E6 & E7 → viral transformation). E6 & E7 form complexes w/ p53 & pRB (tumor suppressor genes); E6 inactivates p53; E7 inactivates Rb.
- **CIN:** Precursor lesion. Cervical cancer may take >10 y.
  CIN 1: 57% spontaneously regress; 1% progress to carcinoma
  CIN 2: 43% spontaneously regress; 5% progress to carcinoma
  CIN 3: 30% spontaneously regress; 12% progress to carcinoma

Clinical Manifestations
- Abn uterine bleeding or postcoital bleeding. Vaginal discharge (serosanguinous or yellow, foul smelling). Hematometra: Pelvic pain, difficulty w/ urination or defecation. Metastatic dz: Back pain, leg swelling (usually unilateral), & neuropathic pain.
- **Exam:** Firm barrel-shaped cervix; necrotic or friable lesion on cervix, poss extension into parametrium, vagina pelvic sidewall, & uterosacral ligament, can appear nml in adenoca

Diagnostic Workup and Staging (see Table)
- Cervical Cytology Screening Guidelines (American Society for Colposcopy and Cervical Pathology [ASCCP], American Cancer Society [ACS])
- Clinically staged. Advanced imaging does not influence staging dx but can affect treatment
- Inspection, palpation, CXR, colposcopy, cystoscopy, proctoscopy, IVP, lesions; cervical conization
- Preoperative imaging may guide mgmt. PET CT & MRI for imaging: PET − sens = 75%, spec 98% *(CMAJ 2008;178:855)*

Treatment (see Table) *(Gynecol Oncol 1980;9:90; 1980;32:135)*
- **Surg:** An option for stages IIA or less
- **Chemo & RT:** An option for stages IA2–IVB
- Adjuvant therapy: For intermediate risk factors, per Sedlis criteria (see table) RT decreases risk of recurrence for intermediate risk patients, although increased toxicity. High-risk patients (+ margin, + LN, + parametrium) chemoRT recommended
- **Recurrent cervical carcinoma:** Evaluated w/ PET scan to exclude distant metastases
  Localized recurrence after Surg → RT, chemotherapy, chemoradiation or Surg
  Central recurrences after definitive Surg or adjuvant RT: Pelvic exenteration. Rpt RT considered in selected pts.

- **Fertility sparing Surg:**
  - Radical trachelectomy (pts w/ up to stage IB1; tumor size <2 cm) similar recurrence rates to radical hysterectomy in carefully selected pts
  - Cervical conization in stage IA1 cancers w/o LVSI

Posttreatment Surveillance
- Cancer detected w/i the 1st 6 mo after rx = persistent cancer
- F/u exam q3–6mo for 1st year w/ pap yearly

International Federation of Gynecology and Obstetrics (FIGO) staging for cervical cancer, 2009	
Stage I	
IA1	Stromal invasion of ≤3 mm in depth, extension of ≤7 mm
IA2	Stromal invasion of >3 mm but ≤5 mm, extension ≤7 mm
IB1	Lesion ≤4 cm in greatest dimension
IB2	Lesion >4 cm in greatest dimension
Stage II	
IIA1	Upper 2/3 vagina, lesion ≤4 cm in greatest dimension
IIA2	Upper 2/3 vagina, lesion >4 cm in greatest dimension
IIB	Obvious parametrial invasion – no pelvic sidewall involvement
Stage III	
IIIA	Tumor invades lower 1/3 vagina, no extension to pelvic sidewall
IIIB	Tumor extends to pelvic sidewall &/or causes hydronephrosis
Stage IV	
IVA	Spread to adj organs, involving mucosa of bladder/rectum
IVB	Spread to distant organs

From *Int J Gynecol Obstet* 2009;105(1):3–4.

Management of cervical cancer by stage	
Stage IA1 – (fertility conservation desired)	Cold knife conization Postconization f/u: Pap smear, per ASCCP guidelines AIS: 25% risk of residual dz in hysterectomy specimens after cervical conization w/ negative margins, 50% w/ positive margins
Stage IA1 – (fertility not desired)	Simple hysterectomy
Stages IA2–IB1	Radical hysterectomy & pelvic LND Primary chemoradiation therapy (RT) equivalent to Surg (esp in medically unfit pts)
Stages IB2–IVA	Chemoradiation (*NEJM* 1999;340:1137) Cisplatin = agent of choice for chemoradiation: Radiosensitizer, ↓ risk of progression of dz & local recurrence
Stage IVB	Cisplatin, paclitaxel, and bevacizumab. Cisplatin resp rate: 20–25%. Combination chemo may have ↑ resp rates. Local radiation may be combined w/ chemo, palliative care

Postoperative radiation for intermediate risk patients "Sedlis criteria"		
(*Gynecol Oncol* 1999;73:177)		
LVSI	**Stromal Invasion**	**Tumor Size**
Positive	Deep 1/3	Any
Positive	Middle 1/3	≥2 cm
Positive	Superficial 1/3	≥5 cm
Negative	Deep or Middle 1/3	≥4 cm

Cervical Carcinoma in Pregnancy (*Best Pract Res Clin Obstet Gynaecol* 2005;19:611)
- **Stage IA1:** Conization vs. follow w/ colposcopy each trimester; surgical rx after vaginal deliv if invasion ≤3 mm & no LVSI. Risk of hemorrhage at deliv ↑. Or C-section + simple hysterectomy (stage IA1) if childbearing complete.
- **Stage IA2** (Tumors >3–5-mm invasion): Can be followed until term; modified radical hysterectomy + pelvic lymphadenectomy at deliv or 6 w postpartum. Vaginal deliv acceptable; C-section necessary for stage IB1 & above.

- **Stages IB1–IIA dz:** Delay of rx can impact survival; if dx made after 20 w, rx can be postponed → classical C-section; modified radical hysterectomy + pelvic/para-aortic LND. RT is as effective as Surg.
- If at or near term, immediate deliv & definitive rx is recommended. At gestational age <20 w, termination & definitive rx is an option. Consider lymphadenectomy 1st, early 2nd trimester, if node neg treatment based on stage (*Int J Cancer* 2014;24:364)
- Neoadjuvant chemo in preg may be an option for stages IB2–IIB

UTERINE CANCER

Epidemiology (*CA Cancer J Clin* 2016;66:7; *J Natl Med Assoc* 2006;98:1930; *Cancer Control* 2009;16:53)
- Most common gynecologic malig; 4th most common cancer in females in US
- 8th leading cause of cancer-related death among women in US
- **Lifetime incid:** 2.8%; White > Black > Hispanic > Asian. Mortality: Black > White
- **Median age at dx:** 62 y (5% <40 y; 90% >50 y)
- Tumors confined to the uterus in >60% of cases

Endometrial Hyperplasia (EH) (*Cancer* 1985;56:403)
- Precursor lesion of endometrioid EC. From continuous estrogen stimulation & relative progestin deficiency. Classification based on architecture (simple vs. complex) & cytologic features.

  Simple EH (w/o atypia): ↑ Gland proliferation; abundant stroma; no nuclear atypia
  Complex EH (w/o atypia): ↑ Gland:stroma ratio; crowded irreg glands; no nuclear atypia
  Simple EH w/ atypia: ↑ Gland:stroma ratio; simple appearing glands; glands lined by atypical nuclei
  Complex EH w/ atypia: Markedly ↑ gland:stroma ratio, severely crowded glands; nuclear atypia
- D&C rec prior to rx to rule out occult carcinoma. 43% have EC diagnosed at the time of hysterectomy for hyperplasia (*Cancer* 2006;106:1012)

	Outcomes by type of endometrial hyperplasia		
Pathology	**Progression to cancer (%)**	**Regression (%)**	**Persistence (%)**
Simple EH, w/o atypia	1	80	19
Complex EH, w/o atypia	3	80	17
Simple EH w/ atypia	8	69	23
Complex EH w/ atypia	29	57	14

Data from *Cancer*. 1985;56:403; *Hum Reprod.* 1999;14:479.

- **Rx of EH w/o atypia:**
  Progestins (cyclic or continuous); eg, MDPA 10 mg/d for 12–14 d for 3–6 mo or local progestogen (LNG IUD) or OCPs. Postmenopausal women: MDPA; D&C for f/u
  F/u: Rpt endometrial sampling if abn bleeding recurs
- **Rx of EH w/ atypia:**
  Hysterectomy. For fertility preservation or poor surgical candidates: LNG IUD or continuous progestins: Megestrol acetate (40–60 mg 2–4×/d for 6 mo) → 94% regression rate.
  F/u: Endometrial bx or D&C q3mo for at least 1 y; if regression does not occur, progesterone dosage should be increased or hysterectomy considered.

Pathology (*J Clin Oncol* 2006;24:4783; *Am J Surg Pathol* 1994;18:687)
- **Grading:** Based on degree of solid components, nuclear features, & architectural pattern
  Grade 1: 5% or less nonsquamous or nonmorular solid growth pattern
  Grade 2: 6–50% nonsquamous or nonmorular solid growth pattern
  Grade 3: >50% nonsquamous or nonmorular solid growth pattern
- **Epithelial tumors**
  Endometrioid adenoCa: 75–80% of EC; most common
  UPSC: 10% of EC; closely resembles tumors of the ovary and fallopian tube. More than 50% of pts w/ clinically early stage have extrauterine dz. Poor prog; high risk of recurrence. EIC: Poss precursor of UPSC.
  Clear cell: 3–4% of EC. Poor prog; 20–65% 5-y survival
  Others: *Mucinous, secretory, squamous*
- **Mesenchymal tumors (sarcomas):** 2–5% of uterine cancers

Epithelial endometrial cancer types

Type I (80–90%)	Type II (~10%)
Grade 1 or 2	Grade 3 endometroid
Endometrioid histology; background of EH	Papillary serous, clear cell, mucinous, squamous, transitional histology, usually no precursor lesion
Estrogen-associated	Atrophic background/polyps
Good prog, younger age	Worse prog, early metastasis
PTEN, K-ras, DNA mismatch repair mutations	P53 mutations

Data from *Gynecol Oncol. 1983;15:10* and *Cancer Causes Control 2010;21:1851.*

Etiology (*Obstet Gynecol 2005;104:413*)
- ↑ Unopposed estrogen → EH → EC
- **Microsatellite instability:** Germ-line mut in DNA mismatch repair genes (MLH1, MSH2, MSH6, PMS2) → Lynch syn: 2–5% of all EC; 40–60% lifetime risk of EC
- **Risk factors for EC:** Prolonged unopposed estrogen (RR 2–10); chronic anovulation (eg, PCOS); BMI >30 (RR 2–4); diabetes & HTN (independent risk factors); Tamoxifen (RR 2; older age (RR 2–3); nulliparity (RR 2); early menarche, late menopause, granulosa cell tumor, Lynch syndrome
- **Protective factors for EC:** Smoking (RR 0.5); OCPs ↓ EC risk by 30%, risk reduction increases with duration of use

Clinical Manifestations and Physical Exam (*Obstet Gynecol 2005;106:413*)
- **Presentation:** Abn uterine bleeding (10% postmenopausal bleeding is EC); chronic anovulation; abn pap smear 30–50%; asymptomatic 5%; leukorrhea 10%; hematometra due to cervical stenosis
- **Ddx:** Atrophic vaginitis, fibroids, endometrial polyps, cervical carcinoma, CIN

Diagnostic Workup
- **Office endometrial sampling:** Least invasive approach
- **Pelvic US** (not diagnostic but may help triage pts): ET <5 mm = 99% NPV (*NEJM 1997;227:1792*)
- **Fractional D&C:** Office endometrial bx results correlate well w/ uterine curettage & ET up to 6 mm (*Acta Obst Gynecol Scand 2001;80:959*)
- Consider cervical conization if cervical involvement suspected to rule out primary cervical carcinoma
- **CA-125:** Elevated in women w/ advanced stage dz & UPSC. Not routinely performed.
- **Chest radiograph, CT/MRI:** If extrauterine dz suspected or CA-125 elevated

FIGO staging for endometrial cancer, 2010

		5-y survival (%)
Stage I	Tumor confined to uterus	
IA	No or <50% myometrial invasion	IA: 90
IB	≥50% myometrial invasion	IB: 78
Stage II	Tumor invades the cervical stroma	II: 74
Stage III	Local &/or regional spread	
IIIA	Invasion of uterine serosa ± adnexa	IIIA: 56
IIIB	Vaginal ± parametrial invasion	IIIB: 36
IIIC	Metastasis to pelvic ± para-aortic nodes	IIIC: 49–57
IIIC1	Positive pelvic nodes	
IIIC2	Positive para-aortic nodes ± positive pelvic nodes	
Stage IV	Tumor invades the bladder ± bowel ± distant metastases	
IVA	Invasion of bladder or bowel mucosa	IVA: 22
IVB	Distant metastases including intra-abdominal ± inguinal nodes	IVB: 21

Data from AJCC: Corpus Uteri, In: AJCC Staging Manual. 7th ed, New York, New York: Springer; 403 and *Obstet Gynecol 2010;116:1141.*

Management (*Obstet Gynecol 2005;106:413; Int J Gynaecol Obstet 2000;70:209*)
- Surg depends on stage:
  All stages: Hysterectomy & BSO (std rx)
  All stages: LND (pelvic & para-aortic) & staging→ allows assessment of the extent of dz to tailor adjuvant therapy. Therapeutic value in stage I dz is unk (*Obstet Gynecol 2012;120:383*), sentinel nodes may be up to 93% sensitive (*Gyn Oncol 2011;123:522*) and minimize lymphedema risk

Stage II → radical hysterectomy & lymphadenectomy + adjuvant therapy based on pathology

Stages III–IV → optimal cytoreductive Surg

Laparoscopic or robotic Surg not inferior to open Surg *(Lancet Oncol 2010;11:763)*

Fertility preservation for grade 1/2, without evidence of myometrial invasion, non-high-risk subtype → progestin therapy with frequent surveillance followed by hysterectomy when childbearing complete or no treatment response. 48% response rate with 35% recurrence *(Gynecol Oncol 2012;125:477)*

High–intermediate risk patients: Deep myometrial invasion, gr 2 or 3, LVSI, age >70 with 1 risk factor, age 50–69 with 2, equal to or > 18 with 3 factors → adjuvant RT

Serous and clear cell → adjuvant chemo ±RT

- **Radiation therapy (RT):**
  PORTEC trial → pelvic radiation decreases locoregional recurrence (4.2% vs. 13.7%) but overall survival unchanged

  Vaginal brachytherapy → for risk for recurrence or pts who have vaginal recurrence → 60–75% survival

  In poor surgical candidates, *primary RT* may be considered

  Survival rate for pts treated w/ *primary RT* w/o Surg: 50% at 5 y

- **Adjuvant chemo:**
  Rx of choice in pts w/ metastatic or recurrent endometrial cancer

  Combination chemo (carboplatin & paclitaxel) GOG 209

  Serous & clear cell cancers: Carboplatin & paclitaxel = resp rate 60–70%

Posttreatment Surveillance

- Exam q3–6mo × 2 y, then q6mo for 2 y, then annually. If CA-125 elevated at the time of dx, it can be followed at each visit. Most recurrences diagnosed w/i the 1st 2 y; 10% recur >5 y after original dx. Routine chest radiographs or pap smears do NOT improve survival

Uterine Sarcomas *(Pathology 2007;39:55; Oncol 1993;50:105)*

- Uncommon (3–9% of all uterine tumors), arise from uterine mesenchyme (stroma)
  Carcinosarcoma (previously called MMMT [malignant mixed mullerian tumor], has epithelial component)
  Present w/ postmenopausal bleeding, prolapsing mass, pain and enlarging uterus; median age 65 y; h/o exposure to radiation; more common in AA women; lymphatic route of spread; ↑ potential for extrauterine metastasis, staged as endometrial carcinoma (see table) carbo/tax or tax/ifosfamide for chemotherapy

  Adenosarcoma: Benign epithelial with malignant stromal component
  Variable in size. Locally invasive

  Endometrial stromal sarcoma: Low grade
  Abn uterine bleeding or asymptomatic uterine enlargement. Indolent course, may recur late. 70% are stage I or stage II at dx. Can treat with hormonal therapy.

  Leiomyosarcoma
  Median age at dx: 55 y. Menorrhagia & pelvic mass. Hematogenous route of spread. **Primary sites of recurrence:** Lung (41%), pelvis (13%). Aggressive, stage I and stage II with 5-y OS of 51% and 25%, respectively *(Histopath 2009;54:355)*. Treat with gemcitabine/docetaxel.

FIGO staging for uterine sarcomas, 2009	
Stage I	Tumor confined to uterus
IA	Tumor 5 cm or less in greatest dimension
IB	Tumor more than 5 cm
Stage II	Tumor extends beyond the uterus within pelvic
IIA	Tumor invades adnexa
IIB	Tumor involves other pelvic tissue
Stage III	Tumor infiltrates abdominal tissues
IIIA	1 site of involvement (abdominal)
IIIB	More than 1 site of involvement
Stage IV	
IVA	Tumor invades bladder or rectum
IVB	Distant metastasis

From *Int J Gynaecol Obstet* 2009;104(3):177–8.

EPITHELIAL OVARIAN CANCER (EOC)

Definitions and Epidemiology (https://seer.cancer.gov/explorer/application.php)
- EOC is derived from surface epithelium of ovary. Incidence >22,000 women/y in US
- 5th leading cause of cancer death in US. 90% of all ovarian cancers.
- Lifetime risk: 1.5%. 5-y survival: 46%. Median age at dx: 63
- **Presentation red flag sx:** Vague abdominal discomfort, abdominal distension, loss of appetite, constipation, nausea/emesis, unintentional weight loss

Pathology (Human Pathology 2009;40:1213)
- **Serous tumors:** Low & high grade
- 40–50% of EOC; most common type of EOC. 60% bilateral. Psammoma bodies seen in low-grade tumors. Most common histological subtype in BRCA carriers & Lynch syn
- **Mucinous tumors** (Int J Gynecol Cancer 2008;18:209)
- 10% of EOC. 8–10% bilateral
- **Endometrioid adenoCa**
- 10% of all ovarian cancers. 28% bilateral. 42% a/w endometriosis; 15–20% a/w endometrial carcinoma
- **Clear cell cystadenocarcinoma**
- 10% of all ovarian cancers. 40% bilateral. A/w endometriosis & HyperCa.
- **Brenner/transitional cell carcinoma**
- Rare, poorly differentiated similar to high-grade transitional cell carcinoma of bladder
- **Carcinosarcoma**
- 1–4% of all ovarian neoplasms. Carcinomatous & sarcomatous elements. Often stage III or stage IV at dx. Poor overall survival.
- **Metastatic tumors**
- Signet ring cell, GI tumor (Krukenberg tumor). Colonic adenoCa. Pancr adenoCa. Breast cancer: Accounts for 6–40% of metastatic tumors to ovary; often bilateral. Renal cell carcinoma. Burkitt's lymphoma. Low malig potential (borderline) tumor: Mucinous or serous.

Etiology (Int J Gyn & Ob 2015;131)
- **Risk factors:** Nulliparity, FHx, early menarche, late menopause, White race, increasing age, residence in North America or Northern Europe, personal h/o breast cancer, European Jewish, Icelandic or Hispanic ethnicity, talc exposure
- **Protective factors:** Long-term OCP use, tubal ligation, hysterectomy, breastfeeding
- **Hypothesis of etiology:** Incessant ovulation, gonadotropin/hormone/inflammation stimulation
- **Hereditary breast & ovarian cancer** (See Chap. 1, screening)
- 10% of all ovarian cancers. BRCA1, BRCA2, & Lynch syn. Earlier onset
- Lifetime risk: **BRCA 1–2:** 28–44%; higher w/ BRCA1. **Lynch:** 12%

Diagnostic Workup
- **Pelvic US:** Complex adnexal mass (septations &/or solid components, size, wall loculation, papillary projections)
- **Abdominopelvic CT or MRI:** Complex adnexal mass, omental caking, ascites, peritoneal studding, perihepatic diaphragmatic implants, CA-125 ↑ esp w/ serous tumors
- Refer to gynecologic oncologist if complex adnexal mass, elevated CA-125, ascites, significantly elevated CA-125 in premenopausal (>200 U/mL) or postmenopausal (>35 U/mL) women, FHx of breast or ovarian cancer in 1st-degree relative (Obstet Gynecol 2016;128:e210)

Management (www.nccn.org/patients/guidelines/ovarian/files/assets/common/downloads/files/ovarian.pdf)
- Prevention for BRCA1/BRCA2 carriers: Risk-reducing BSO by age 40 or completion of child bearing. BRIP1/Lynch mutations/RAD51C&D risk-reducing BSO by age 45–50
- **Surgery**
  Stage I: TAH, BSO, omentectomy, peritoneal biopsies, pelvic & para-aortic LND, pelvic washings
  Stage I w/ desired fertility: Fertility sparing Surg w/ unilateral salpingo-oophorectomy, peritoneal biopsies, omentectomy, pelvic & para-aortic LND, pelvic washings
  Stages II–IV: TAH, BSO, omentectomy, debulking of gross dz; optimal reduction to residual dz <1 cm
- **Adjuvant chemo:** ≥Stage IC or high grade: Postsurgical systemic chemo w/ platinum & paclitaxel
- **Neoadjuvant chemo:** Used for pts who are not initial surgical candidates. Adjuvant RT not recommended. Typically 3 cycles prior to initial cytoreductive surgery

- **Recurrent/persistent dz**
  - Platinum sensitive dz (recurrence >6 mo from tx completion)-carboplatin + paclitaxel (platinum doublet) consider secondary cytoreductive surgery
  - Plat resistant dx (recurrence <6 mo) or plat refractory (progression during tx): Single-agent rx w/ alternative chemo agent (eg, topotecan, paclitaxel, bevacizumab, gemcitabine), targeted single agent (bevacizumab or PARP inhibitor) or clinical trial

Posttreatment Surveillance (https://www.nccn.org/patients/guidelines/ovarian/files/assets/common/downloads/files/ovarian.pdf)
- Exam ± CA-125 q3mo for 2 y, then q3–6mo for 3 y, then annually
- CT &/or PET, CA-125 if recurrence suspected

FIGO staging for ovarian cancer, 2014	
Stage I	Tumor confined to ovaries
IA	1 ovary; capsule intact; no surface tumor, neg washings
IB	Both ovaries; otherwise like IA
IC	Tumor limited to 1 or both ovaries
IC1	Surgical spill
IC2	Capsule rupture before surgery or tumor on ovarian surface
IC3	Malignant cells in the ascites or peritoneal washings
Stage II	Tumor in 1 or both ovaries w/ extension to pelvis, or PPC
IIA	Extension to uterus or fallopian tubes
IIB	Extension to other pelvic tissues
Stage III	Peritoneal implants outside pelvis or + pelvic LNs
IIIA	Tumor limited to pelvis w/ negative LNs, but microscopic peritoneal mets beyond pelvis
IIIA1	+ Retroperitoneal nodes only
IIIA1 (i)	Mets ≤10 mm
IIIA1 (ii)	Mets >10 mm
IIIA2	Micro extrapelvic mets; ± pos retroperitoneal LNs
IIIB	Macro extrapelvic mets ≤2 cm; ± pos pelvic LNs. Includes implants on capsule of liver/spleen
IIIC	Peritoneal extrapelvic mets >2 cm in diameter; ± pos LNs
Stage IV	Distant mets excluding peritoneal implants
IVA	Pleural effusion w + cytology
IVB	Hepatic/splenic parenchymal mets, mets to organs outside of abdomen (including LNs)

From *Int J Gynaecol Obstet* 2009;105:3.

GERM CELL TUMORS

Definitions and Epidemiology (*Cancer Treat Rev* 2008;34:427)
- Cancer derived from primordial germ cells. 1–2% of all ovarian malignancies
- 58% of all ovarian tumors in women <20 yo. Incid: 0.41/100000 women/y

Pathology (*Int J Gynecol Path* 2006;25:305)
- **Dysgerminomas (+LDH)**
  1–2% all of ovarian tumors; 32% of malig germ cell tumors. Adolescents/young adults. 10–15% bilateral. Monophasic proliferation of primitive germ cells w/ infiltrating T cells. Testicular seminoma equivalent; OCT4 positive & CD30 positive staining, "fried egg" cellular appearance
  Lymphatic spread common; humoral HyperCa common; rapid enlargement
  High cure rate w/ rx (88.6%)
- **Endodermal sinus tumor (yolk sac tumor) (+AFP, +LDH)**
  14–20% of malig germ cell tumors. Young girls/young women; 1/3 premenarchal
  Schiller–Duval bodies (microscopic feature w/ central capillary surrounded by flat-tened parietal cells). AFP, cytokeratin, & PLAP positive staining.
  Unilateral, aggressive tumor
  Early hematogenous spread to distant sites. Relatively chemoresistant.
- **Mixed germ cell tumor (variable tumor marker expression)**
  5% of all malig germ cell tumors. 2 or more malig germ cell elements w/ at least 1 primitive. Dysgerminoma most common component.
- **Immature (malignant) teratoma (variable tumor marker expression)**
  Embryonic tissue; predominantly neuroepithelial. Grades 1, 2, or 3 based on quantity of neuroepithelial tissue. Unilateral.

- **Mature teratoma**
  Solid, cystic (dermoid, 95%), or fetiform. Composed of fetal or adult structures, no embryonal components. Most common ovarian tumor. 46XX karyotype.
  Only 1–2% malig; most common malignancy is squamous cell carcinoma. 0.2–2% malignant transformation
- **Monodermal teratomas**
  Struma ovarii, carcinoid, central nervous center tumor, carcinoma group, sarcoma group, sebaceous tumor, pituitary-type tumor, retinal anlage tumor, others.
- **Rare subtypes**
  - **Embryonal carcinoma (+AFP, +LDH, +hCG, +E2)**
    4% of malig germ cell tumors. Avg age: 15 yo.
    Cohesive groups of large primitive cells w/ overlapping nuclei, indistinct borders, syncytiotrophoblastic giant cells. hCG production leads to isosexual pseudoprecocity. Staining positive for OCT3, OCT4, & CD30.
  - **Polyembryoma**
    Young girls. Numerous embryoid bodies resembling presomite embryos. hCG/AFP may be elevated. Often associated w/ immature teratoma
  - **Nongestational choriocarcinoma (+hCG)**
    2% of malig germ cell tumors. Cytotrophoblasts & intermediate trophoblasts capped w/ syncytiotrophoblasts in plexiform pattern. hPL, inhibin, & cytokeratin positive.

Clinical Manifestations
- Abdominal pain (55–80%), abdominal/pelvic mass, abdominal enlargement, fever (10–25%), ascites, ovarian torsion or rupture; abdominal distension (35%), vaginal bleeding (10%)
- Short duration of sx (2–4 w)
- 60–70% present at stage I or stage II, 20–30% stage III, stage IV uncommon. Metastasis by peritoneal or lymphatic spread; hematogenous spread more common than EOC.
- Dysgerminoma a/w primary amenorrhea/gonadal dysgenesis

Diagnostic Workup
- **Chest radiograph:** Eval for metastasis
- **Pelvic US:** Cystic lesion w/ densely echogenic tubercle (Rokitansky nodule for mature teratoma). CA-125 not useful.
- **Abdominal/pelvic CT:** Complex mass; fat attenuation in mature teratomas; calcification; speckled calcification in dysgerminomas (Radiographics 1998;18:1525)
- Karyotype if dysgerminoma suspected & h/o primary amenorrhea
- Staging same as for EOSs, above

Germ cell serum tumor markers

	AFP	hCG	LDH	E2	Inhibin	Testosterone	Androgen	DHEA
Dysgerminoma	−	±	+	±	−	−	−	−
Yolk sac	±	+	±	±	−	−	−	−
Immature teratoma	±	−	±	±	−	−	−	±
Choriocarcinoma	−	+	±	−	−	−	−	−
Endodermal sinus	+	−	+	−	−	−	−	−
Polyembryoma	±	+	−	−	−	−	−	−
Mixed germ cell	±	±	±	−	−	−	−	−

Inhibin + for granulosa cell, and ± for Sertoli–Leydig and gonadoblastoma. Testosterone/androgen + for Sertoli–Leydig and ± for gonadoblastoma. See sex cord stromal tumors, below.
From Pectasides D, Pectasides E, Kassanos D. Germ cell tumors of the ovary. Cancer Treat Rev. 2008;34(5):427–41.

Management
- **Surg:** TAH, BSO, omentectomy, peritoneal biopsies, pelvic washings, pelvic & para-aortic LND (8–28% risk of met depending on histology), surgical debulking if not sparing fertility. Fertility sparing Surg poss if contralateral ovary appears nml; cystectomy may be poss. Bx contralateral ovary if dysgerminoma or if appears abn.
  2nd-look Surg if residual mass postchemotherapy or residual teratoma
- **Adjuvant chemo:**
  BEP (bleomycin, etoposide, cisplatin) is gold std
  Recurrence treated w/ chemo again
- **Primary surveillance:** stage IA gr1, Immature teratoma and IA, IB dysgerminoma
- **Adjuvant radiation (RT):** Alternative therapy for dysgerminomas who are not candidates for chemo/surg

Posttreatment Surveillance (Am J Obstet Gynecol 2011;204:466)
- Exam & tumor marker(s) q2–4mo for 2 y, then yearly. Imaging w/ surveillance if no reliable tumor marker. CT & tumor marker(s) if recurrence suspected
- Overall prog based on stage, residual dz, histologic type, preop AFP & bhCG elevation; age not a factor

SEX CORD-STROMAL TUMORS

Epidemiology (Gyn Oncol 2005;97:519)
- 1.2% of all primary ovarian cancer. Indolent course w/ favorable prog, rare lymph node met, average age at diagnosis 50 y

Pathology (J Clin Oncol 2007;25:294)
- **Granulosa cell tumor (GCT):**
  70% of malig sex cord-stromal tumors. Incid: 0.4–1.7/100,000 women. More common in nonwhite, obese women.
  Adult type-estrogen product, w/ abn bleeding in 66%; EH 25–50%; endometrial ca 5%
  Juvenile type (5%): 90% in prepubertal girls; 95% unilateral; excellent prog
  Call–Exner bodies w/ eosinophilic material & nuclear debris, coffee bean nuclei. 95% unilateral. 78–91% stage I at dx; good prog. 5–10% coexisting endoCa, therefore endoBx
- **Sertoli–Leydig cell tumors:**
  0.2% of all ovarian neoplasms. 98% unilateral. Avg age 20–30 y.
  90% stage I; 70–90% 5-y survival; may recur soon after dx/rx
  Tubules of epithelial cells are steroid secreting → virilization 30% pt, crystals of Reinke seen pathologically
- **Thecoma:**
  Benign. Postmenopausal women. Estrogen → EH (15%).
  Luteinized thecomas → virilization. Abundant lipid cytoplasm; solid, yellowish tumors.
- **Fibroma:**
  Benign. Most common sex cord-stromal tumor; 4% ovarian neoplasms.
  4–8% bilateral. Postmenopausal women. Whorled bundles of spindle-shaped fibroblasts & collagen. A/w Meigs syn & basal nevus syn.
- **Steroid cell tumors:** 0.1–0.2% of all ovarian tumors. Stromal luteomas, Leydig (hilus) cell tumor, & steroid cell tumor not otherwise specified.
- **Others:** Sclerosing stromal tumors, sex cord tumor w/ annular tubules, gynandroblastomas

Clinical Manifestations
- **Presentation:** Abn bleeding, abdominal distension, abdominal pain. Isosexual precocious puberty w/ juvenile GCTs. Virilization from androgens in Sertoli–Leydig. Meigs syn (fibroma, ascites, pleural effusions).

Diagnostic Workup (Radiographics 1998;18:1525)
- **Pelvic US/Pelvic CT:** Large, unilateral, multicystic w/ solid components; rare calcifications; carcinomatosis in GCTs (rare); well-defined hypoechoic mass for Sertoli–Leydig cell tumors; lack of papillary projections
- **Pelvic MRI:** High signal intensity due to tumor hemorrhage; GCTs w/ sponge-like appearance; Sertoli–Leydig cell tumors as solid mass; fibrothecomas w/ low signal intensity on T2
  Staging same as for EOCs, above

Sex cord-stromal tumor markers						
Testosterone	**Androgen**	**E2**	**Inhibin**	**Testosterone**	**Androgen**	**DHEA**
–		±		–	–	–
±	–	±		–	–	–
±	±	±		–	–	±

From Pectasides D, Pectasides E, Kassanos D. Germ cell tumors of the ovary. *Cancer Treat Rev.* 2008;34(5): 427–41.

Management
- **Surg:** See table

Posttreatment Surveillance (Am J Obstet Gynecol 2011;204:466)
- Exam & tumor marker(s) q2–4mo for 2 y, then q6mo for 3 y, then yearly
- CT & tumor marker(s) if recurrence suspected

Treatment of germ cell tumors	
Stage IA	TAH, BSO, & staging (omentectomy, peritoneal biopsies, pelvic & para-aortic LND, pelvic washings). Fertility sparing Surg & staging if future fertility desired. Adjuvant chemo not indicated.
Stage IC, malig ascites, high mitotic activity, or Stage >1	TAH, BSO, staging, debulking Fertility sparing Surg & staging if future fertility desired Adjuvant chemo (BEP or platinum/taxane)
Recurrent dz or pelvic/ intra-abdominal dz	Secondary debulking Surg when feasible Postoperative therapy based upon prev treatments: Platinum-based chemo, radiation for localized dz, or hormone therapy
Distant recurrence	Platinum-based chemo, or hormonal rx in selected pts

VAGINAL CANCER

Epidemiology
- 2–3% of all gynecologic malignancies. Incid of VAIN: 0.2/100,000 women
- **Mean age:** 70–90 y. 80% are squamous histology

Pathology (Curr Opin Obstet Gynecol 2005;17:71)
- **VAIN** is precursor lesion. Upper 3rd of vagina most common. A/w CIN. Risk of transformation to invasive vaginal carcinoma 9–10%.
- **Squamous cell carcinoma**
  85% of vaginal cancer. Superficial spread, then invasion to paravaginal tissue. Metastasis to liver/lung.
- **AdenoCa:**
  15% of cases. Metastasis to lung, supraclavicular & pelvic LNs. Metastasis from other sites is more common than primary vaginal adenoCa.
- **Clear cell adenoCa:** DES exposure. Coexists w/ vaginal adenosis.
- **Melanoma:** <1–3% of vaginal malignancies. Pigmented or nonpigmented.
- **Sarcoma botryoides:** Multicentric; anter wall; grape like. More common in children.
- **Adenosquamous carcinoma:** 1–2% of vaginal cancer. Aggressive.
- **Secondary carcinomas:** Extension from cervix, endometrial metastasis, bowel/bladder local extension, gestational trophoblastic dz.

Etiology
- HPV 16 & 18 found in invasive cancer & VAIN. DES exposure. Endometriosis linked w/ adenoCa. Radiation exposure.

Clinical Manifestations
- Vaginal bleeding or bloody discharge usually indicates advanced lesions. Urinary sx.

Diagnostic Workup
- Bx for tissue disease; view by colposcopy w/ Lugol's solution (localized or diffuse/ multifocal disease). Biopsy cervix & vulva as well.

Management
- **VAIN I:** Observation
- **VAIN II or III:** Wide local excision, partial or total vaginectomy, intravag 5-FU, trichloroacetic acid, 5% imiquimod, laser therapy (J Low Genit Tract Dis 2012;16:00)
- **Stage I SCC:** <0.5 cm thick: Intracavitary radiation, wide local excision, or total vaginectomy; >0.5 cm thick: Radical vaginectomy w/ pelvic LND & inguinal LND (if lower 3rd), radiation if lower 3rd to pelvic/inguinal LNs or poorly differentiated/infiltrating
- **Stage I adenoCa:** Total radical vaginectomy, hysterectomy, LND, vaginal reconstruction ± intracavitary/interstitial radiation
- **Stage II SCC/adenoCa:** Brachytherapy/EBRT or radical vaginectomy or pelvic exenteration ± radiation
- **Stages III & IVA SCC/adenoCa:** Interstitial, intracavitary, & EBRT
- **Stage IVB SCC/adenoCa:** Radiation and/or chemo
- **Melanoma:** Wide local excision, radical excision w/ inguinofemoral LND, pelvic exenteration, radiation, chemo, or immunotherapy (Int J Gynecol Cancer 2004;14:687)
- **Local recurrence:** Pelvic exenteration or radiation
- **Distant recurrence:** Chemo
- **Prog:** 70% 5-y survival for stage I; 50% survival for advanced stage

FIGO staging for vaginal cancer, 2009	
Stage I	Tumor limited to vaginal wall
Stage II	Tumor involves the subvaginal tissue; not extended to the pelvic sidewall
Stage III	Tumor extends to the pelvic sidewall
Stage IV	Tumor extends beyond the true pelvis or has involved the mucosa of the bladder or rectum
IVA	Tumor invades bladder &/or rectal mucosa &/or direct extension beyond pelvis
IVB	Distant spread

From *Int J Gynaecol Obstet* 2009;105(1):3–4.

Posttreatment Surveillance *(Am J Obstet Gynecol 2011;204:466)*
- Exam (if low risk) q6mo × 2 y then yearly × 2 y; (if high risk) q3mo × 2 y, then q6mo × 2 y, then annually. Consider cytology. CT or PET if recurrence.

VULVAR CANCER

Definitions and Epidemiology *(Hematol Oncol Clin N Am 2012;26:45)*
- **VIN:** Dysplasia confined to epithelium (VIN II-III)
- **Vulvar carcinoma:** Lesion invading through basement membrane
- **Incid:** Vulvar cancer 2.3/100,000 women/y; VIN: 1.2–2.1/100,000 women
- 4–7% of all gynecologic malignancies. Median age at dx: 68 y.
- **Lifetime risk:** 0.27%

Pathology
- **VIN usual type:** Warty, basaloid, mixed. HPV related.
- **VIN differentiated type:** A/w lichen sclerosus, squamous cell hyperplasia. NOT HPV related. Risk of developing keratinizing squamous cell carcinoma.
- **SCC:** 92% of vulvar cancer. Warty & basaloid type; keratinizing, nonkeratinizing, basaloid, verrucous, warty, & acantholytic type; invasive or superficial invasion. Most common sites: Labia majora (50%), labia minora (15–20%). HPV16 & 18; 40% of invasive cancers are HPV positive; 80% of VIN are HPV positive; vaccination may prevent.
- **Basal cell carcinoma:** 2–4% of vulvar malignancies. Infiltrating tumor w/ basal cells of the epidermis. Labia majora is the most common site. Basosquamous or metatypical basal cell carcinoma: Malig squamous component, found in 3–5% of basal cell carcinomas (treat as squamous carcinoma).
- **Bartholin's gland carcinoma:** 40% adenoCa; 40% squamous carcinoma; 15% adenoid cystic carcinoma. Bx any Bartholin's gland abscess in woman >35 y.
- **Sarcoma:** 1–2% vulvar malignancies. Leiomyosarcoma, liposarcoma, fibrosarcoma, neurofibrosarcoma, rhabdomyosarcoma, malig schwannoma, angiosarcoma, epithelioid sarcoma.
- **Verrucous carcinoma:** Rare. Cauliflower-like appearance. Slow growing & locally invasive (will even invade bone).
- **Malig melanoma:** 2nd most common vulvar malig. Labia minora or clitoris most common sites. Arise de novo; pigmented lesion, asymptomatic.
- **Paget dz of vulva:** <1% of vulvar neoplasms. Concurrent w/ underlying adenoCa in 4–20%. 12% invasive; 35% recurrence rate. Large pale cells (Paget cells). Raised, velvety appearance. A/w adenoCa of other location (breast/colon): 30%.

Clinical Manifestations
- **Presentation:** Vulvar itching & irritation, burning, pain, dysuria. Pigmented lesions, ulcerations, papules, nodules, or scar-like lesions. Persistent condyloma (30% w/ VIN 3).

Diagnostic Workup
- Bx flat, elevated, or pigmented lesions; bx genital warts in postmenopausal women or women who fail topical therapy. Colposcopy.

Management *(J Natl Compr Canc Netw 2017;15:92)*
- **VIN:** Wide local excision (low risk of recurrence if negative margins); laser ablation if cancer not suspected (colposcopy to delineate margins); topical 5% imiquimod
- **Vulvar squamous carcinoma**
    Stage I: Wide local excision if microinvasive (<1 mm invasion), or, radical local excision w/ complete unilateral sentinel LND (bilateral LND if lesion >2 cm from midline)

Stage II: Modified radical vulvectomy w/ bilateral inguinal LND & femoral LND: Radiation if margins <8 mm, lymphovascular invasion, or >5 mm thick

Stage III: Modified radical vulvectomy w/ bilateral inguinal/femoral LND w/ radiation

Stage IV: Radical vulvectomy followed by radiation

Recurrence: Depending on location & extent of recurrence, options include re-excision, radical vulvectomy, pelvic exenteration, radiation, chemo

- **Basal cell carcinoma:** Radical local excision
- **Bartholin's gland carcinoma:** Radical local excision or hemivulvectomy, consider ipsilateral inguinal LND
- **Sarcoma:** Radical local excision
- **Verrucous carcinoma:** Radical local excision; radiation contraindicated (induces anaplastic transformation which may lead to metastasis)
- **Malig melanoma:** Radical local excision if <1 mm invasion; consider ipsilateral inguinal LND if >1 mm invasion
- **Paget's dz of vulva:** Wide local excision; modified radical vulvectomy if underlying adenoCa
- **Prog:** 5-y survival 72.7%; based on stage at dx; ↑ LN+ is most important determinant of survival. Improved if adequate surg margins (1–2 cm) at primary surgery.

Posttreatment Surveillance (*J Natl Compr Canc Netw* 2017;15:92)

- Exam q3–6mo × 2 y, then q12–6mo × 3–5 y, then annually CT &/or PET if recurrence suspected. VIN surveillance: q6mo for 1 y, then annually; recurrence high (30–50%).

	Clark, Breslow, and Chung staging for melanoma (see also Chap. 1)		
	Clark	**Breslow**	**Chung**
I	Confined to epithelium	0.75 mm or less	Confined to epithelium
II	Penetrate basement membrane; extend into papillary dermis	0.76–1.50 mm	Penetrates basement membrane; extends to 1 mm or less from granular layer
III	Fills papillary dermis	1.51–2.25 mm	Penetrates btw 1.1 and 2 mm from granular layer
IV	Invades deep reticular dermis	2.26–3 mm	Invades beyond 2 mm from granular layer
V	Invades subcutaneous adipose tissue	>3 mm	Invades into subcutaneous adipose tissue

Data from Jahnke A, Makovitzky J, Briese V. Primary melanoma of the female genital system: A report of 10 cases and review of the literature. *Anticancer Res.* 2005;25(3A):1567–74.

	FIGO staging for vulvar cancer, 2009
Stage I	Tumor limited to the vulva
IA	Lesion ≤2 cm in size, confined to the vulva or perineum & w/ stromal invasion ≤1 mm; no nodal metastasis
IB	Lesion >2 cm in size or w/ stromal invasion >1 mm; confined to perineum, w/ negative nodes
Stage II	Tumor of any size w/ extension to adj perineal structures (1/3 lower urethra, 1/3 lower vagina, anus) w/ negative nodes
Stage III	Tumor of any size w/ or w/o extension to adj perineal structures w/ positive inguinofemoral LNs
IIIA	(i) 1 LN metastasis ≥5 mm (ii) 1–2 LN metastases <5 mm
IIIB	(i) 2 or more LN metastases ≥5 mm (ii) 3 or more LN metastases <5 mm
IIIC	Positive nodes w/ extracapsular spread
Stage IV	Tumor invades other regional structures (2/3 upper urethra, 2/3 upper vagina) or distant structures
IVA	(i) Tumor invades urethral &/or vaginal mucosa &/or bladder mucosa &/or rectal mucosa; fixed to pelvic bone (ii) Ulcerated or fixed inguinofemoral LNs
IVB	Distant metastasis including pelvic LNs

From *Int J Gynaecol Obstet* 2009;105(1):3–4.

GESTATIONAL TROPHOBLASTIC NEOPLASIA

Definition and Epidemiology
- Originates from abn proliferation of placental trophoblasts. Incid varies by geography (2/1000 in Japan, 0.6–1.1/1000 in Europe/North America) *(NEJM 1996;335:1740)*
- GTD includes 4 types of related diseases: Complete & partial hydatidiform mole, invasive mole, placental site trophoblastic tumor, & choriocarcinoma. Invasive GTN usually follows molar Preg, but can follow any gest.

Molar Pregnancy

Features of complete and partial hydatidiform moles		
Feature	**Complete mole**	**Partial mole**
Karyotype	46XX (90%), 46XY (10%)	69 XXY (90–93%), 69 XXX (7%)
Fetal or embryonic tissue	Absent	Present
Hydatidiform swelling of chorionic villi	Diffuse	Focal
Trophoblastic hyperplasia	Diffuse, variable	Focal
Scalloping of chorionic villi	Absent	Present
Trophoblastic stromal inclusions	Absent	Present
Implantation-site trophoblast	Diffuse, marked atypia	Focal, mild atypia
P57Kip2 immunostaining	Negative	Positive
Risks	Low dietary carotene. Vit A deficiency. Extremes of maternal age. Prev SAB.	Prev SAB. Irreg menses. OCP use >4 y.
Risk of GTN	15%	1–4%

From *N Engl J Med* 1996;33:1740; *J Repro Med* 2004;49:527.

- **Clinical presentation – most diagnosed now on US by 12 w GA, classic presentations** *(NEJM 1996;335:1740)*:
  Complete hydatidiform mole: Vaginal bleeding (89–97%); enlarged uterus for gestational age (38–51%); Theca lutein ovarian cysts (26–46%); hyperemesis gravidarum (20–26%); preeclampsia (12–27%); hyperthyroidism; respiratory distress (2–27%)
  Partial hydatidiform mole: Signs & sx of incomplete or missed abortion; SGA or IUGR; less likely to present w/ medical complications
  Diagnostic w/u pelvic US, serum hCG level, CBC, PT/PTT, renal & liver fxn studies, type & screen, pre-evacuation chest radiograph, if exhibiting sx of hyperthyroidism → TSH, T3/T4; hyperemesis → chemistry

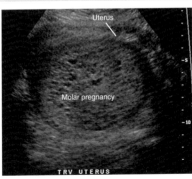

Figure 22.1 Transverse uterus ultrasound image of a molar pregnancy with characteristic snowstorm pattern

Courtesy of Patricia Johnson, University of Virginia.

- **Rx**
  - Suction curettage followed by sharp curettage if pt desires future fertility. Rh immune globulin for RhD-negative women. Hysterectomy an option if pt does not desire future childbearing.
  - Prophylactic chemo following molar Preg (Obstet Gynecol 1986;67:690) is controversial. Decreases postmolar GTN from 47–14% in high risk complete moles (WHO >6; see below).
- **Post rx surveillance** (Obstet Gynecol 2004;103:1365)
  - Serum hCG level w/i 48 h of evacuation
  - Serum hCG levels every 1–2 w until normalized (<5)
  - Serum hCG level monthly for 6 mo once negative
  - Use of reliable hormonal contraception needed during surveillance

Invasive Mole (Chemo Research and Practice 2011;2011:1; Obstet Gynecol 2004;103:1365)
- Diagnosed if:
  - ≥4 hCG values plateau (±10%) over at least 3 w
  - ≥10% rise in hCG for ≥3 values over at least 2 w
  - Presence of histologic choriocarcinoma
  - Persistence of hCG 6 mo after molar evacuation (& rule out new Preg)
- Metastatic GTN seen in 4% after evacuation for complete mole (Chemo Research and Practice 2011;2011:1)
  - Most common sites for metastases: Lung (80%), vagina (30%), (do NOT biopsy) brain (10%), & liver (10%)

Choriocarcinoma (Obstet Gynecol 2004;103:1365)
- Arises from cytotrophoblasts & syncytiotrophoblasts. Does not contain chorionic villi. 50% arise from complete hydatidiform mole, 25% from nml pregnancies, 25% from spont abortion/ectopic Preg. Most aggressive. ~14% mortality (Gynecol Oncol 2006;103:698)

Placental Site Trophoblastic Disease
- Uncommon variant of choriocarcinoma. Predominantly composed of intermediate cytotrophoblasts. Tumor marker, HPL.
- Secrete small amounts of bhCG → tumor burden may be large before hCG levels detectable
- Most often after nonmolar pregnancy/abortion, can occur mo to y later

Survival after GTN
- Prog depends on age, interval btw gest & dz, serum bhCG
- Subseq Preg after GTN (NEJM 1996;335:1740)
- 1% subseq pregnancies result in molar gest; women w/ GTN in remission have nml Preg rates following GTN; no ↑ incid of spont abortion, congenital anomalies, C-section
- **Low risk:** 84% stage I GTN & 87% low-risk stages II–III → complete remission w/ single-agent chemo (J Reprod Med 2006;51:835; Semin Oncol 1995;22:166; J Reprod Med 1992;37:461; Obstet Gynecol 1987;9:390; Gynecol Oncol 1994;54:76)
- **High risk:** 80% pts w/ stage IV dz achieve remission w/ multiagent therapy
- **Risk of relapse:** 2% nonmetastatic GTN; 4% low-risk metastatic GTN; 13% pts high-risk metastatic GTN (Cancer 1996;66:978). Median time to relapse: 6.5 mo. Survival rate for relapsed GTN: 77.8% (J Reprod Med 2006;51:829).

FIGO staging of GTN, 2009	
Stage I	Dz confined to uterus
Stage II	GTN extends outside uterus but limited to genital structures (adnexae, vagina, broad ligament)
Stage III	GTN extends to lungs, w/ or w/o known genital tract involvement
Stage IV	All other metastatic sites (brain, liver)

From Int J Gynaecol Obstet 2009;105(1):3–4.

Modified WHO prognostic scoring system as adapted by FIGO				
Low risk, WHO score of 0–6; high risk, WHO score of ≥7				
Score	0	1	2	4
Age (y)	<40	≥40	–	–
Antecedent Preg	Mole	Abortion	Term	–
Interval months from index Preg	<4	4–6	7–12	≥12
Pretreatment serum bhCG	$<10^3$	$10^3–<10^4$	$10^4–<10^5$	$≥10^5$
Largest tumor size	–	3–<4 cm	≥5 cm	–
Site of metastases	Lung	Spleen, kidney	GI	Liver, brain
Number of metastases	–	1–4	5–8	>8
Prev failed chemo drugs	–	–	1	≥2

Treatment regimens for GTN	
Protocol for low-risk GTN (stage I or low-risk stage II/III & WHO score ≤6)	
Initial therapy	Methotrexate or actinomycin D Hysterectomy if finished w/ childbearing (w/ adjunctive single-agent chemo)
Resistant therapy	EMACO Hysterectomy (w/ adjunctive multiagent chemo) Local uterine resxn (to preserve fertility)
F/u	12 consecutive months of undetectable hCG levels Contraception for 12 mo
Protocol for high-risk GTN (stage II or stage III & WHO score ≥7)	
Initial therapy	EMACO or EMAEP (etoposide, methotrexate, act D, carboplatin)
Resistant therapy	VBP Surg, as indicated
F/u	12 consecutive months of undetectable hCG levels Contraception for 12 mo
Protocol for Stage IV GTN	
Initial therapy	EMACO; w/ brain mets → radiation/dexamethasone, craniotomy for periph lesions; w/ liver mets → embolization, resxn to manage complications
Resistant therapy	EMAEP; VBP; experimental protocols; Surg, as indicated; hepatic artery infusion or embolization
F/u	Weekly hCG levels until undetectable for 3 w, then monthly hCG × 24 mo Contraception × 24 mo

Data from May T, Goldstein DP, Berkowitz RS. Current chemotherapeutic management of patients with gestational trophoblastic neoplasia. *Chemother Res Pract.* 2011;2011:806256.

CHEMOTHERAPY

Tumor Biology (*Principles and Practice of Gynecologic Oncology.* 5th ed. Philadelphia, PA: Lippincott Williams & Wilkins; 2009:381)

- 3 types of nml tissue growth explain chemo side effects
   Static: Well-differentiated cells, rare division (neurons, oocytes)
   Expanding: Normally quiescent, proliferate w/ stress (hepatocytes, vascular endothelium)
   Renewing: Continuous proliferation (bone marrow, GI epithelium, epidermis)
- **Gompertzian growth:** Tumor growth exponential during initial division followed by exponential growth retardation → as tumor mass ↑, time to double tumor size also ↑; metastasis doubling time is faster than primary lesion. Rapidly proliferating cells have short G1 → these cells are the most chemosensitive.
- Prolonged survival & cure achieved when cell pop ↓ to $10^1–10^4$ cells, which is microscopic dz → basis for adjuvant chemo following upfront surgical debulking

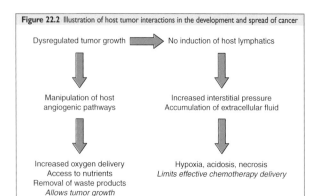

Figure 22.2 Illustration of host tumor interactions in the development and spread of cancer

Dysregulated tumor growth → No induction of host lymphatics

Manipulation of host angiogenic pathways

Increased interstitial pressure
Accumulation of extracellular fluid

Increased oxygen delivery
Access to nutrients
Removal of waste products
Allows tumor growth

Hypoxia, acidosis, necrosis
Limits effective chemotherapy delivery

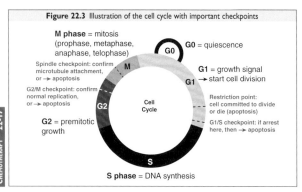

Figure 22.3 Illustration of the cell cycle with important checkpoints

M phase = mitosis (prophase, metaphase, anaphase, telophase)

G0 = quiescence

Spindle checkpoint: confirm microtubule attachment, or → apoptosis

G1 = growth signal → start cell division

G2/M checkpoint: confirm normal replication, or → apoptosis

Cell Cycle

Restriction point: cell committed to divide or die (apoptosis)

G2 = premitotic growth

G1/S checkpoint: if arrest here, then → apoptosis

S phase = DNA synthesis

Types of Chemotherapy
- **Neoadjuvant chemo:** Prior to Surg or RT
- **Adjuvant chemo:** Following Surg or RT
- **Concurrent chemo:** Administered w/ radiation to sensitize tumor to radiation effects

Common Chemotherapies for Gynecologic Cancers
- Platinum/taxane: Carboplatinum and paclitaxel are most common 1st-line regimen for ovarian, primary peritoneal, fallopian tube, endometrial cancers
- Cisplatin used for radiosensitization in cervical cancers
- Agents for recurrence:
    - Options include platinum/taxane (if plat. sensitive), PEGylated liposomal doxorubicin, gemcitabine, topotecan, etoposide, docetaxel
    - Hormonal agents: Increasing use of aromatase inhibitors in some histological subtypes of recurrent endometrial and ovarian cancers, still experimental
    - Novel biologics: Used for maintenance or recurrence, include antiangiogenesis (bevacizumab), PARP inhibitors (olaparib, pazopanib), immunotherapy (nivolumab)

Common Toxicities
- Graded using common terminology criteria for adverse events → Graded 1–4
- **Bone marrow tox**
    Most common dose limiting side effect
    Neutropenia → most common bone marrow tox. Occurs 7–14 d after rx.
    Use of G-CSF & PEG-filgrastim does not improve long-term survival compared to dose reduction

- **GI**
  N/V most common
  Anticipatory nausea: Occurs prior to administration of chemo
  Acute onset nausea: Occurs w/i 1 h of chemo, lasts <24 h
  Delayed onset nausea: Occurs >1 d following chemo & persists for several days
  Cisplatin: Most emetogenic tx used in gyn cancer
- **Alopecia**
  Important psychological side effect, almost always reversible
- **Skin tox**
  Allergic/hypersens rxn
  Skin hyperpigmentation
  Photosensitivity
  PPE
  Local extravasation necrosis
- **Neurotoxicity**
  Periph neuropathy → most common
  Highest rates seen w/ cisplatin, paclitaxel, docetaxel
  Paresthesias → loss of vibratory & position sense → functional impairment
- **GU**
  Cisplatin → renal tox from metabolites (carboplatin has little renal tox)
  Ifosfamide & cyclophosphamide → hemorrhagic cystitis due to byproduct, acrolein
    Mesna administered to bind & neutralize acrolein in the bladder
- **Hypersensitivity rxns**
  Early rxn → paclitaxel
    Occurs due to rxn to Cremophor EL (in which paclitaxel is compounded)
    80% reactions occur w/ 1st or 2nd cycle
  Late rxn → carboplatin
    Most common during 2nd course of chemo for recurrence (cycles 7–13)
    Thought to be due to Ag recall

RADIATION THERAPY

External Beam Radiation Therapy (EBRT)
- 3-dimensional conformal RT
  CT used to guide geometry of radiation rx → std of care for gynecologic cancers
  (Gynecol Oncol 1997;66:351)
  Intensity-modulated radiation therapy (Int J Radiat Oncol Biol Phys 2002;52(5):1330)
  Specialized 3-dimensional conformal RT
  Allows dose modulation w/i each beam & dose escalation for tumor site w/ decreased
    dose to nml tissue (may be useful in extended field EBRT)
  Proton therapy – high energy proton EBRT, increased precision
- **Definitions in EBRT**
  Borders of std pelvic fields
    Superior → S1–L5 interspace (early dz) or L4–5 (advanced dz)
    AP-PA field 15 × 15 cm w/ lateral width of 8–9 cm
  Extended field EBRT → includes para-aortic nodes in radiation field (T12–L1)
    Useful in cervical cancer w/ para-aortic nodal dz, but ↑ side effects given inclusion
    of more nml tissue (bowel, kidneys)
  Midline block → used to block tissue adj to planned brachytherapy during EBRT
  Parametrial boost → given to pts w/ parametrial/sidewall involvement following
    EBRT
  Fractions → total dose delivered in fractions (1.8–2 Gy) daily
    Decreases dose to healthy tissue by allowing for sublethal DNA damage repair
- **Side effects:** Acute (≤3 mo after rx) or late onset (>3 mo after rx)
  Skin → ulceration, necrosis; GI → diarrhea, fistula, perforation; GU → cystitis, fistula
  Reproductive organs → premature menopause; bone marrow/ pelvic bones → transient
    lymphopenia, fractures

Brachytherapy
- Highly concentrated radiation dose to immediately surrounding tissue
- **Interstitial brachytherapy** (vaginal/vulvar cancer): Radioactive sources temporarily
  loaded into hollow needles imbedded in tumor bed

- **Intracavitary brachytherapy** (cervical & endometrial cancer): Radioactive sources placed in body cavities (Barakat RR, Berchuck A, Markman M, et al. *Principles and Practice of Gynecologic Oncology.* 5th ed. Philadelphia, PA: Lippincott Williams & Wilkins; 2009:381)
  Low-dose rate → uses Iridium or Cesium
    40–100 cGy/h
    Requires 1–2 treatments that last 48–72 h each
    Requires inpt hospitalization
  High-dose rate → uses Iridium
    20–250 cGy/min
    Requires 3–5 outpt treatments following insertion
  Similar efficacy & late complications w/ HDR & LDR (Cochrane Database Syst Rev 2010;7:CD007563)
- **Anatomic landmarks for brachytherapy**
  Point A → 2 cm superior & 2 cm lateral to the external cervical os (point of crossing of ureter & uterine artery)
  Point B → 3 cm lateral to point A (location of obturator LNs)

Radiation treatment for gynecologic cancers	
Cancer	**Radiation type**
Cervical (stages 1B–IV)	Definitive whole pelvic (± extended field) EBRT w/ cisplatin chemo-sensitization, ± parametral boost, brachytherapy (LDR or HDR)
Endometrial	Adjuvant whole pelvic EBRT, adjuvant vaginal cuff brachytherapy as indicated
Vulvar (following resxn)	Adjuvant whole pelvic EBRT
Advanced dz	Chemo + EBRT, palliative treatment
Vaginal	Whole pelvic EBRT ± boost, brachytherapy (Int J Radiat Oncol Biol Phys 2005;62:138)

Figure APP-1-1 The female bony pelvis

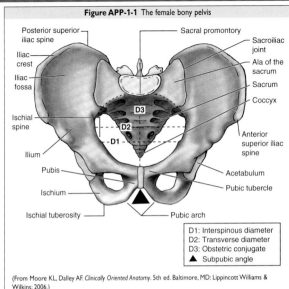

Posterior superior iliac spine
Iliac crest
Iliac fossa
Ischial spine
Ilium
Pubis
Ischium
Ischial tuberosity

Sacral promontory
Sacroiliac joint
Ala of the sacrum
Sacrum
Coccyx
Anterior superior iliac spine
Acetabulum
Pubic tubercle
Pubic arch

D1: Interspinous diameter
D2: Transverse diameter
D3: Obstetric conjugate
▲ Subpubic angle

(From Moore KL, Dalley AF. *Clinically Oriented Anatomy.* 5th ed. Baltimore, MD: Lippincott Williams & Wilkins; 2006.)

Figure APP-1-2 Internal female reproductive organs, posterior view

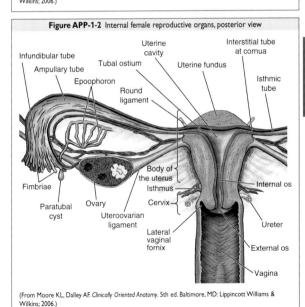

Infundibular tube
Ampullary tube
Epoophoron
Round ligament
Fimbriae
Paratubal cyst
Ovary
Uteroovarian ligament

Uterine cavity
Tubal ostium
Uterine fundus
Interstitial tube at cornua
Isthmic tube

Body of the uterus
Isthmus
Cervix
Lateral vaginal fornix
Internal os
Ureter
External os
Vagina

ANATOMY PRIMER 23-1

(From Moore KL, Dalley AF. *Clinically Oriented Anatomy.* 5th ed. Baltimore, MD: Lippincott Williams & Wilkins; 2006.)

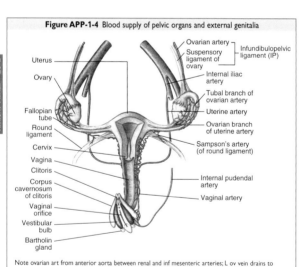

Figure APP-1-3 The course of the ureter and relationship to the sites of vulnerability

Pubovesical lig.

Bladder

Obturator a.

Arcuate tendon

Vesicovaginal space

Uterine a.

Right ureter

Sup. vesical a.

Vagina

Uterosacral lig.

Left ureter

Ovarian a. (infundibulopelvic lig.)

Rectum

☆ Most common places for ureter injury

(From Berek DL. *Berek & Novak's Gynecology.* 15th ed. Baltimore, MD: Lippincott Williams & Wilkins; 2012.)

Figure APP-1-4 Blood supply of pelvic organs and external genitalia

Ovarian artery

Suspensory ligament of ovary

Infundibulopelvic ligament (IP)

Uterus

Internal iliac artery

Ovary

Tubal branch of ovarian artery

Fallopian tube

Uterine artery

Round ligament

Ovarian branch of uterine artery

Cervix

Sampson's artery (of round ligament)

Vagina

Clitoris

Internal pudendal artery

Corpus cavernosum of clitoris

Vaginal artery

Vaginal orifice

Vestibular bulb

Bartholin gland

Note ovarian art from anterior aorta between renal and inf mesenteric arteries; L ov vein drains to L renal V; R ov vein drains to inf vena cava; vaginal blood supply is uterine artery + int iliac ant di; vaginal venous plexus drains to internal iliac veins.

(From Rohen JW, Yokochi C, Lutjen-Drecoll. *Color Atlas of Anatomy.* 7th ed. Baltimore, MD: Lippincott Williams & Wilkins; 2011.)

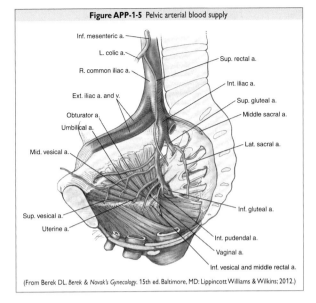

Figure APP-1-5 Pelvic arterial blood supply

Inf. mesenteric a.
L. colic a.
R. common iliac a.
Ext. iliac a. and v.
Obturator a.
Umbilical a.
Mid. vesical a.
Sup. vesical a.
Uterine a.

Sup. rectal a.
Int. iliac a.
Sup. gluteal a.
Middle sacral a.
Lat. sacral a.
Inf. gluteal a.
Int. pudendal a.
Vaginal a.
Inf. vesical and middle rectal a.

(From Berek DL. *Berek & Novak's Gynecology*. 15th ed. Baltimore, MD: Lippincott Williams & Wilkins; 2012.)

Pelvic arterial blood supply, considerations		
Artery	**Branches**	**Surgical significance**
Common iliac	1. Internal iliac artery 2. External iliac artery	Ureter crosses bifurcation at the pelvic brim
External iliac	1. Inferior epigastric artery 2. Deep circumflex iliac artery 3. Femoral artery (origin of superficial epigastric artery)	IEA may be injured during laparoscopic entry; can give accessory obturator branch

Internal iliac	1. Anterior division:
	   Obturator artery
	   Umbilical → superior vesical → obliterated
	   Uterine artery
	   Vaginal artery
	   Inferior vesical artery
	   Middle rectal artery
	   Internal pudendal artery
	   Inferior gluteal artery
		Ligation of the anter division may be done to control uterine hemorrhage

	2. Posterior division:
	   Iliolumbar artery (iliac & lumbar branches)
	   Lateral sacral arteries
	   Superior gluteal artery
		Ligation → gluteal necrosis

Internal pudendal	1. Inferior rectal 2. Perineal artery 3. Post labial branches 4. Artery of the bulb of the vestibule 5. Dorsal artery of the clitoris 6. Deep artery of the clitoris	Exits pelvis through greater sciatic foramen to gluteal region → curves around the sacrospinous ligament to enter perineum through the lesser sciatic foramen (through the pudendal canal w/ vein & nerve)

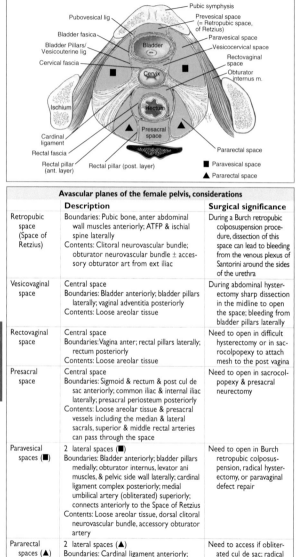

Figure APP-1-6 Avascular planes of the female pelvis

- Pubic symphysis
- Pubovesical lig
- Prevesical space (= Retropubic space, of Retzius)
- Paravesical space
- Bladder fascia
- Bladder Pillars/Vesicouterine lig
- Vesicocervical space
- Cervical fascia
- Rectovaginal space
- Obturator internus m.
- Cardinal ligament
- Rectal fascia
- Presacral space
- Pararectal space
- Rectal pillar (ant. layer)
- Rectal pillar (post. layer)
- Ischium
- Bladder
- Cervix
- Rectum

■ Paravesical space
▲ Pararectal space

Avascular planes of the female pelvis, considerations			
	Description		**Surgical significance**
Retropubic space (Space of Retzius)	Boundaries: Pubic bone, anter abdominal wall muscles anteriorly; ATFP & ischial spine laterally Contents: Clitoral neurovascular bundle; obturator neurovascular bundle ± accessory obturator art from ext iliac		During a Burch retropubic colposuspension procedure, dissection of this space can lead to bleeding from the venous plexus of Santorini around the sides of the urethra
Vesicovaginal space	Central space Boundaries: Bladder anteriorly; bladder pillars laterally; vaginal adventitia posteriorly Contents: Loose areolar tissue		During abdominal hysterectomy sharp dissection in the midline to open the space; bleeding from bladder pillars laterally
Rectovaginal space	Central space Boundaries: Vagina anter; rectal pillars laterally; rectum posteriorly Contents: Loose areolar tissue		Need to open in difficult hysterectomy or in sacrocolpopexy to attach mesh to the post vagina
Presacral space	Central space Boundaries: Sigmoid & rectum & post cul de sac anteriorly; common iliac & internal iliac laterally; presacral periosteum posteriorly Contents: Loose areolar tissue & presacral vessels including the median & lateral sacrals, superior & middle rectal arteries can pass through the space		Need to open in sacrocolpopexy & presacral neurectomy
Paravesical spaces (■)	2 lateral spaces (■) Boundaries: Bladder anteriorly; bladder pillars medially; obturator internus, levator ani muscles, & pelvic side wall laterally; cardinal ligament complex posteriorly; medial umbilical artery (obliterated) superiorly; connects anteriorly to the Space of Retzius Contents: Loose areolar tissue, dorsal clitoral neurovascular bundle, accessory obturator artery		Need to open in Burch retropubic colposuspension, radical hysterectomy, or paravaginal defect repair
Pararectal spaces (▲)	2 lateral spaces (▲) Boundaries: Cardinal ligament anteriorly; rectum medially; sacrum posteriorly; internal iliac & pelvic side wall laterally Contents: Loose areolar tissue		Need to access if obliterated cul de sac; radical hysterectomy, & sacrospinous fixation Ureterolysis is a prerequisite

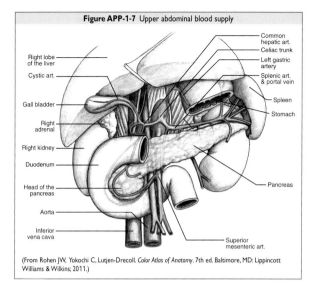

Figure APP-1-7 Upper abdominal blood supply

Right lobe of the liver

Cystic art.

Gall bladder

Right adrenal

Right kidney

Duodenum

Head of the pancreas

Aorta

Inferior vena cava

Common hepatic art.

Celiac trunk

Left gastric artery

Splenic art. & portal vein

Spleen

Stomach

Pancreas

Superior mesenteric art.

(From Rohen JW, Yokochi C, Lutjen-Drecoll. *Color Atlas of Anatomy*. 7th ed. Baltimore, MD: Lippincott Williams & Wilkins; 2011.)

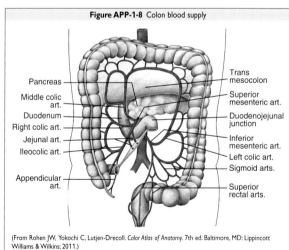

Figure APP-1-8 Colon blood supply

Pancreas

Middle colic art.

Duodenum

Right colic art.

Jejunal art.

Ileocolic art.

Appendicular art.

Trans mesocolon

Superior mesenteric art.

Duodenojejunal junction

Inferior mesenteric art.

Left colic art.

Sigmoid arts.

Superior rectal arts.

(From Rohen JW, Yokochi C, Lutjen-Drecoll. *Color Atlas of Anatomy*. 7th ed. Baltimore, MD: Lippincott Williams & Wilkins; 2011.)

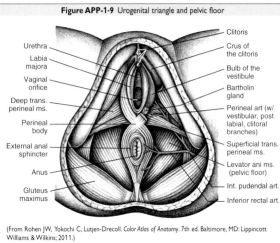

Figure APP-1-9 Urogenital triangle and pelvic floor

Clitoris

Crus of the clitoris

Bulb of the vestibule

Bartholin gland

Perineal art (w/ vestibular, post labial, clitoral branches)

Superficial trans. perineal ms.

Levator ani ms. (pelvic floor)

Int. pudendal art.

Inferior rectal art.

Urethra

Labia majora

Vaginal orifice

Deep trans. perineal ms.

Perineal body

External anal sphincter

Anus

Gluteus maximus

(From Rohen JW, Yokochi C, Lutjen-Drecoll. *Color Atlas of Anatomy.* 7th ed. Baltimore, MD: Lippincott Williams & Wilkins; 2011.)

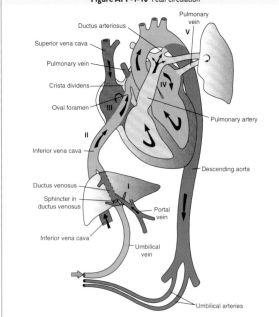

Figure APP-1-10 Fetal circulation

Ductus arteriosus

Pulmonary vein V

Superior vena cava

Pulmonary vein

Crista dividens

Oval foramen

IV

III

Pulmonary artery

II

Descending aorta

Inferior vena cava

Ductus venosus

Sphincter in ductus venosus

I

Portal vein

Inferior vena cava

Umbilical vein

Umbilical arteries

Arrows, blood flow. Oxygenated and deoxygenated blood mix in liver (I), inferior vena cava (II), right atrium (III), left atrium (IV), and confluence of ductus arteriosus and descending aorta (V).
(From Sadler TW. *Langman's Medical Embryology.* 12th ed. Baltimore, MD: Lippincott Williams & Wilkins; 2012.)

INTRAUTERINE DEVICE INSERTION (IUD)

Levonorgestrel Intrauterine System (LNG-IUS) (Adapted from Bayer HealthCare Pharmaceuticals Inc., physician insert, 2009)

- **Timing:** Insert after pregnancy ruled out, after termination of pregnancy, or postpartum
- **Preparation:**
   Informed consent, bimanual exam, urine hCG, consider pre-procedure NSAID.
- **Procedure (sterile):**
   Consider paracervical block
   Cleanse cervix w/ an antiseptic solution
   Place tenaculum on anterior lip of cervix
   Sound uterine cavity
   See http://www.mirena-us.com/hcp/placement-&-removal/precise-placement.jsp
   Ensure slider on inserter is advanced all the way toward the device. Ensure arms are parallel to slider. Set flange to depth measured by uterine sound.
   Hold the slider firmly. Apply gentle countertraction w/ tenaculum. Gently advance the insertion tube into the uterus until flange is 1.5–2 cm from external cervical os. While holding inserter, release device by pulling slider back until top of slider reaches mark. Advance inserter until flange touches cervix.
   Release LNG-IUS by pulling the slider down all the way
   Cut threads to 2–3 cm visible outside cervix
   Consider US to verify position. Remove if not positioned appropriately. Do not reinsert same device.
   Consider IUD check ~4–6 w after placement of IUD

ParaGard (Copper T 380A IUD) (Adapted from Teva Women's Health, Inc., physician insert, 2010)

- **Timing:** Same as LNG-IUS. Can be used as emergency contraception within 5 d of unprotected intercourse.
- **Preparation:** Same as LNG-IUS
- **Procedure:**
   Consider paracervical block
   Cleanse cervix w/ an antiseptic solution
   Place tenaculum on anterior lip of cervix
   Sound uterine cavity
   See http://www.paragard.com/Pdf/ParaGard-PI.pdf
   Using sterile technique, load IUD into insertion tube by folding the 2 horizontal arms against the stem, & push tips of the arms securely into the inserter tube (<5 min from insertion)
   Introduce white rod into the insertion tube until it touches the end of the IUD without dislodging the IUD
   Adjust the blue flange to the uterus cavity length. Advance insertion tube to uterine fundus (blue flange should be at external os).
   Hold white rod steady & withdraw the insertion tube 1 cm to release IUD
   Advance insertion tube to fundus. Hold the tube steady & withdraw rod
   Withdraw tube completely. Trim threads to 3–4 cm.
   Consider US to verify position. Remove if not positioned appropriately. Do not reinsert same device.
   Consider IUD check ~4–6 w after placement of IUD

SUBDERMAL DEVICE INSERTION

Etonogestrel Implant (Nexplanon) Insertion (Adapted from Merck & Co Inc., physician insert, 2016)

- **Timing:** Same as LNG-IUS
- **Preparation:** Informed consent
- **Procedure (sterile)**
   Position arm flexed at the elbow & externally rotated so that wrist is parallel to ear or hand is positioned next to head
   Identify insertion site on inner side of nondominant upper arm about 8–10 cm above the medial epicondyle of the humerus, avoiding the groove between biceps and triceps muscles.
   Mark the spot where implant will be inserted. Mark a spot a few centimeters proximal to the 1st mark as a direction guide.
   Insert just under skin to avoid deeper large blood vessels & nerves.

Clean insertion site w/ an antiseptic solution, consider anesthetic with epinephrine to decrease bleeding; anesthetize area along insertion path.

Remove implant applicator from package. Ensure implant needle & rod are sterile and implant is visible in device.

Hold the applicator just above needle at textured surface; remove transparent needle cap (slide horizontally, follow arrow away from needle)

DO NOT touch purple slider until fully inserted subdermally

Stretch skin around insertion site with thumb/index finger of free hand; puncture skin with tip of needle slightly angled <30°

Lower applicator to horizontal position. While lifting skin with needle, slide needle to full length toward proximal mark on skin along anesthetized path.

Keep applicator in same position and push purple slider slightly back; then move fully back into it stops. Remove applicator.

Verify presence of implant by palpation; have patient palpate it.

Apply pressure dressing for 24 h.

Figure APP-2-1 Nexplanon insertion

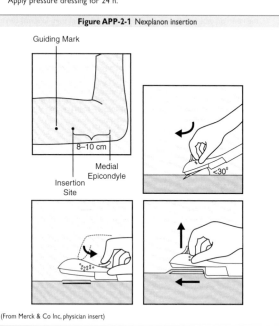

(From Merck & Co Inc, physician insert)

BARTHOLIN ABSCESS INCISION AND DRAINAGE

- **Indication:** For tx of cystic enlargement or abscess formation. Will not prevent recurrence.
- **Preoperatively:**
  Identify incision point (inner surface of abscess. INSIDE hymenal ring).
  Informed consent (risk of recurrence & possible need for additional procedures)
- **Steps:**
  Infiltrate skin w/ local anesthesia
  Incise using a scalpel w/ a no. 11 blade
  Explore the inside of the cyst/abscess & open any loculations
  A Word catheter can be used to reduce recurrence. Insert the deflated Word catheter into the cyst cavity & inject 2–3 mL of sterile saline through the catheter to inflate the balloon. Tuck end of Word catheter into the vagina.
  Leave in place for 4–6 w to allow for epithelialization of the new drainage tract

Figure APP-2-2 Word Catheter Insertion and Marsupialization procedure

Word Catheter Placement

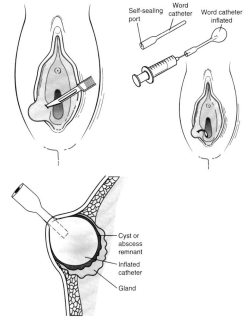

After local anesthesia and preparation, use a stab incision to create a 1–1.5-cm deep opening in the cyst. Insert the tip of a Word catheter, and inflate the bulb with water or lubricating gel. Keep the catheter in place for 4 w.

Bartholin Marsupialization

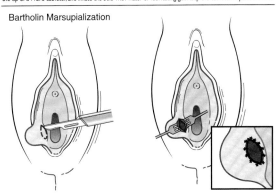

Make a fusiform incision adjacent to the hymenal ring. Remove an oval wedge of vulvar skin and the underlying cyst wall. Suture the cyst wall to the adjacent vestibular skin.

(From Zuber TJ, Mayeaux EJ. *Atlas of Primary Care Procedures.* Philadelphia, PA: Lippincott Williams & Wilkins; 2004.)

Bartholin Cyst Marsupialization With or Without Excision
- **Indication:** Recurrent cyst formation. Objective is to open a new ductal orifice.
- **Preoperatively:** Obtain informed consent, preoperative medical clearance if necessary
- **Steps:**
    Start w/ 2–4-cm fusiform incision 1 cm lateral & parallel to hymenal ring near medial edge of labium minus
    Incise the cyst wall & use Allis clamps to grasp the skin & cyst wall edges
    Drain the cyst completely; open any loculations
    Use interrupted stitches to suture the cyst wall to the adjacent skin edge
    Consider cyst wall excision/bx for repeated recurrences or if high risk for malignancy

LOOP ELECTROSURGICAL EXCISION PROCEDURE (LEEP)

- **Indication:** To better characterize glandular or squamous lesions after unsatisfactory initial workup by excising the transformation zone of the cervix
- **Preoperatively:**
    Exclude pregnancy (unless high suspicion of invasion)
    Informed consent
    Review cervical cytology and colposcopic pathology
- **Steps:**
    Ground pt, insert insulated speculum w/ smoke evacuation tubing. Select appropriately sized loop to excise entire transformation zone.
    Use iodine or acetic acid to identify lesions.
    Consider paracervical and/or intracervical block.
    Introduce loop 3–5 mm lateral to os at 90° angle to cervix. Activate current (cutting) prior to tissue contact.
    Draw loop parallel to surface until opposite side of os is reached. Withdraw at 90° angle. Stop electrical current.
    Perform an endocervical curettage or "top hat" excision.
    Obtain hemostasis using electrocautery or Monsel solution. Apply pressure.
    Tag specimen for orientation; send to pathology.

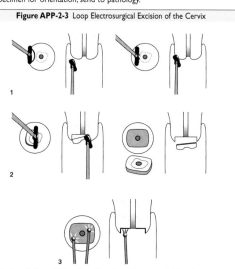

Figure APP-2-3 Loop Electrosurgical Excision of the Cervix

(1) To excise tissue, the loop is held just above the surface of the cervix and 2–5 mm lateral to the lesion, and current is applied before the loop contacts the cervix. (2) Draw the loop slowly through the tissue until the loop is 2–5 mm past the edge of the transformation zone on the opposite side. (3) Superficial fulguration is usually applied to the entire crater and to any spots of point hemorrhage.
(From Zuber TJ, Mayeaux EJ. *Atlas of Primary Care Procedures.* Philadelphia, PA: Lippincott Williams & Wilkins; 2004.)

ENDOMETRIAL BIOPSY

- **Indications:**
  Used to exclude endometrial cancer in high-risk pts w/ abn uterine bleeding (>45 y, obese, FHx, PCOS, etc.), as part of w/u for glandular abnormality on Pap smears, or f/u after conservative mgmt of endometrial hyperplasia
  Req before endometrial ablation and often before hysterectomy
- **Preoperatively:** Exclude pregnancy, obtain informed consent
- **Steps:**
  Perform speculum exam.
  Clean the cervix w/ an antiseptic solution. Consider tenaculum placement.
  Advance pipelle through the cervical canal to the uterine fundus.
  Withdraw the stylet to apply suction; use rotation or back and forth motion to obtain adequate tissue. Repeat if necessary.

AMNIOCENTESIS

- **Indications:**
  Detection of lung maturity, genetic diagnosis, exclusion of infection
  Confirm rupture of membranes using amnio-dye test ("tampon test")
  Relieve pressure symptoms in symptomatic polyhydramnios
- **Preoperatively:** Obtain informed consent
- **Steps:**
  Use US to identify large amniotic fluid pocket away from the fetus
  Cleanse skin with antiseptic solution over proposed site of needle insertion
  Consider local anesthetic injection at sampling site
  Advance spinal needle into amniotic fluid under sonographic guidance
  Withdraw stylet, attach syringe, draw back to obtain a fluid sample

DILATATION AND CURETTAGE (EVACUATION)

- **Indications:** Before endometrial ablation, definitive sampling of endometrium, termination of pregnancy, removal of retained products of conception
- **Preoperatively:**
  Exclude pregnancy (unless for termination)
  Informed consent, preoperative medical clearance if necessary
  Consider cervical softening w/ misoprostol
- **Steps:**
  EUA for uterine position/size. Consider catheterization to empty bladder.
  Insert a speculum, cleanse cervix with antiseptic solution, apply tenaculum to anterior lip of cervix
  Ensure adequate anesthesia (general, regional, or local)
  Using sterile technique, advance dilators through internal cervical os to gradually open the cervix. Optimal dilation depends on procedure.
  May perform curettage w/ suction device, or w/ a sharp curette. For suction curettage, the curette size usually corresponds to the gestational age/uterine size.
  Introduce the curette to fundus & sample all walls & fundus
  Consider forceps to remove larger tissue fragments, or US guidance for difficult procedures
  Ensure hemostasis at tenaculum sites after procedure end – may require prolonged pressure, silver nitrate, or suturing

COLD KNIFE CONIZATION (CKC)

- **Indication:**
  To better characterize glandular or squamous lesions after unsatisfactory initial workup by excising the transformation zone of the cervix
  Generally reserved for more difficult cases & pts w/ recurrence after LEEP
  A/w more obstetric complications compared to LEEP & laser conization

- **Preoperatively:**
  Exclude pregnancy (unless high suspicion for invasion)
  Informed consent; preoperative medical clearance if necessary
  Review cervical cytology and colposcopic pathology
- **Steps:**
  Ensure adequate anesthesia, catheterize to empty bladder
  Use iodine or acetic acid for identification of the lesions
  Inject vasopressin or dilute epi circumferentially into cervical stroma, lateral to line of resection
  Place "stay" sutures at 3 & 9 o'clock to manipulate the cervix
  Make an incision that creates a 2–3-mm border around lesion and transformation zone. Ensure inclusion of the endocervical canal by maintaining appropriate angle of scalpel. Consider placement of uterine sound or dilator in cervix to direct biopsy along endocervical canal
  Perform endocervical curettage
  Hemostasis w/ Monsel solution or electrocautery

OPERATIVE HYSTEROSCOPY

- **Indications:**
  Eval & tx of polyps, myomata, adhesions, septa. Also tubal sterilization, removal of retained IUD or foreign body.
- **Preoperatively:**
  Informed consent, exclude pregnancy. Preoperative medical clearance if necessary.
  In premenopausal women, consider performing during the early proliferative phase of the menstrual cycle, or treating w/ progestins to induce endometrial atrophy
  In postmenopausal women, consider misoprostol for stenotic cervix
- **Steps:**
  Ensure adequate anesthesia, catheterize to empty bladder
  Perform EUA to determine uterine position/size
  Insert speculum, cleanse cervix with antiseptic solution, apply tenaculum to anterior lip of cervix
  Using sterile technique, advance dilators through internal os to gradually open the cervix. Dilate to diameter of hysteroscope.
  Introduce the hysteroscope into the uterine cavity, survey cavity
  Distention media include isotonic electrolyte (LR, NS) & nonelectrolyte (glycine, mannitol). Infusion pressure should be ~45–80 mmHg depending on the patient's mean arterial pressure (MAP)
  Perform the indicated procedure
  Monitor fluid deficit. Plan completion of the case if the deficit reaches 750 cc; stop if 1500 cc (nonelectrolyte), or 2500 cc (electrolyte).

ENDOMETRIAL ABLATION

- **Indications:** Heavy menstrual bleeding
- **Preoperatively:**
  Informed consent; exclude pregnancy. Preoperative medical clearance if necessary.
  Exclude malignancy & hyperplasia prior to procedure with uterine sampling (eg, endometrial biopsy)
  Plan postablation contraception
- **Steps:**
  Ensure adequate anesthesia. Catheterize to empty bladder. Bimanual exam.
  Insert a speculum, cleanse cervix with antiseptic solution, apply a tenaculum to anterior lip of cervix
  Sound the uterus
  Using sterile technique, advance dilators through internal os to gradually open the cervix. Dilate to diameter of ablative device.
  Consider hysteroscopic eval if concern for cavitary abnormalities (polyps, etc.)
  Perform indicated procedure (variations include resectoscope, rollerball, thermal balloon, hydrothermal, radiofrequency, microwave, & cryoablation)
  Monitor fluid deficit if distending medium is used

HYSTEROSCOPIC TUBAL LIGATION

- **Indications:** Undesired fertility
- **Preoperatively:**
  Informed consent; preoperative medical clearance if necessary. Exclude pregnancy
  Best done during the early proliferative phase of the cycle, or after rx w/ OCPs, DMPA, etc. to induce endometrial atrophy for visualization
- **Steps:**
  Ensure adequate anesthesia. Catheterize to empty bladder. Bimanual exam.
  Insert a speculum, cleanse cervix with antiseptic solution, apply tenaculum to anterior lip of cervix, sound the uterus
  Using sterile technique, advance dilators through internal os to gradually open the cervix. Dilate to diameter of hysteroscope.
  Currently, only approved system is the microinsert (Essure)
  Cannulate each tubal ostium w/ Essure device. Follow package insert to deploy insert.
  Pt must use contraception until tubal occlusion is documented by HSG (at 3 mo)

OPERATIVE LAPAROSCOPY

- **Indications:** Minimally invasive access to abdomen
- **Preoperatively:**
  Informed consent, preoperative medical clearance if indicated
  Position patient in dorsal lithotomy. Consider tucking arms.
  Decide entry point (eg, umbilical, LUQ) & method of entry (eg, Veress, open)
- **Steps:**
  General anesthesia w/ neuromuscular blockade, OG tube, Foley catheter, EUA
  Consider inserting a uterine manipulator
  Use scalpel to make skin incision large enough to accommodate laparoscopic trocar
  Abdominal trocars can be inserted in several ways:
  - Introduce the Veress needle into the abdominal cavity w/ the abdominal wall elevated. 2 "pops" can be felt as the needle passes through the fascia & peritoneum. Abdominal entry is confirmed by "saline drop test" or by measurement of entry pressure; initial pressure of <5 mmHg is reassuring. Insufflate abd w/ CO_2 to max pressure of 10–12 mmHg. Remove Veress needle. A trocar can then be inserted into the peritoneal cavity.
  - Direct trocar insertion – insert trocar directly w/o insufflation, w/ elevated abdominal wall
  - Optical access trocar entry – direct visualization of abdominal wall through trocar during insertion
  - Open entry (Hasson technique) – A 1–2-cm incision is made below the umbilicus. Dissect tissue to fascia, incise fascia, open peritoneum, & insert blunt trocar. Tie in place with "stay sutures" at lateral aspects of fascial incision
  Systematically inspect the abdomen & pelvis; look for injury from entry
  Perform procedure (hysterectomy, cystectomy, oophorectomy, tubal ligation, etc.)
  Desufflate abd, close fascia for incisions 10 mm or greater. Close skin.

TOTAL ABDOMINAL HYSTERECTOMY

- **Indications:** Heavy uterine bleeding, symptomatic fibroids, pelvic organ prolapse, endometriosis, gyn malignancies
- **Preoperatively:**
  Informed consent, preoperative medical clearance if necessary
  Endometrial biopsy (in setting of abnormal uterine bleeding), Pap smear
  Position in either dorsal supine or dorsal lithotomy position
- **Steps:**
  General anesthesia, preoperative antibiotic, EUA, Foley catheter
  Abdominal entry through appropriate incision (midline, Pfannenstiel, etc.)
  Consider abdominal wall retractor & abdominal packing for bowel retraction

Grasp the round ligaments, uteroovarian ligaments, & fallopian tubes w/ curved Kelly clamps to elevate the uterus & provide traction

Divide the round ligament between 2 transfixion sutures (or with bipolar cautery) & extend the incision down to the broad ligament with monopolar energy or scissors

Dissect the broad ligament into anterior & posterior leaves

Identify ureter

Carry anterior broad ligament incision inferomedially to the level of the vesicouterine fold. Open the post leaf toward the uterosacral ligaments.

For oophorectomy: Identify ureter. Open a window in the broad ligament to isolate the IP ligament. Clamp IP w/ 2 Heaney or Zeppelin clamps & transect between them. Suture ligate the distal pedicle w/ a free tie & transfixion suture; ligate the prox pedicle w/ a single free tie. Can also use bipolar energy for transection/ligation.

To preserve the ovaries: Open an avascular window in the broad ligament to isolate the fallopian tube & the uteroovarian ligament. Clamp across these 2 structures; cut, & suture ligate.

Rpt above steps on opposite side of uterus

Dissect the vesicouterine peritoneum off the anterior uterus & cervix

Identify the uterine arteries & carefully dissect off the surrounding connective tissue. Use Heaney or Zeppelin clamps to come across the uterine vessels on either side at 90° to the vessel; incorporate the vessel, not adj uterine or cervical tissue. Cut the vessels & doubly ligate. Consider back clamp on the specimen side to decrease back bleeding

Clamp cardinal ligament; transect, & doubly ligate

Pull uterus upward & clamp across uterosacral ligaments. Cut ligaments close to the uterus (avoiding ureters) & suture ligate.

Place 2, curved clamps immediately below the cervix. Cut above these clamps to remove the uterus & cervix.

Close vaginal cuff w/ figure-of-eight stitches. Incorporate uterosacral & cardinal ligaments into cuff repair for additional support.

Ensure hemostasis, irrigate, & close the abdomen

VAGINAL HYSTERECTOMY

- **Indications:** See above, consider this route especially in patients with prolapse
- **Preoperatively:** Same as abdominal hysterectomy
- **Steps:**

Adequate anesthesia, antibiotic. EUA, Foley catheter w/ pt in dorsal lithotomy.

Place weighted speculum & use Deaver retractors to expose the cervix

Grasp the anterior & posterior lips of the cervix using 2 tenacula or thyroid clamps

Inject vasopressin or lidocaine/epi around the cervicovaginal junction

Make an incision with Bovie or scalpel around cervix at cervicovaginal junction

With downward traction, dissect bladder off cervix until anterior peritoneum visible

Open the anterior peritoneum with Metz scissors & slide retractor in along cervix

Using upward traction, open the post peritoneum into the Pouch of Douglas with scissors

Pull the uterus outward & identify the uterosacral ligaments. Clamp ligaments; cut, & suture ligate.

Clamp, cut, & suture ligate the cardinal ligaments, uterine arteries, uteroovarian ligaments & round ligaments. If oophorectomy is performed, the IP ligaments are identified, clamped, cut, & suture ligated in place of the uteroovarian ligaments.

Ensure hemostasis. Close vaginal cuff using interrupted or running sutures.

Incorporate uterosacral & cardinal ligaments into cuff repair for additional support.

CESAREAN SECTION

- **Indication:** Malpresentation, arrest of dilation/descent, nonreassuring fetal heart tracing, failed induction, placenta previa, prior Cesarean
- **Preoperatively:**

Informed consent. Determine if tubal ligation possible/desired.

Awareness of fetal presentation, placental location, preoperative hemoglobin.

Position in dorsal supine position with left lateral tilt. Consider lithotomy if arrest of descent.
- **Steps:**
  Test for adequate anesthesia (general, neuraxial, etc.)
  Abdominal entry: Pfannenstiel vs. midline vertical
  Pfannenstiel (most common) – 2 fingerbreadths above the pubic symphysis & slightly curved upward. Fascia is incised transversely & dissected off underlying rectus muscles laterally, inferiorly, and superiorly with Mayo scissors vs. Bovie. Rectus muscles separated in the midline. Peritoneum entered and extended with Metzenbaum scissors or bluntly with finger.
  Other abdominal entries: Maylard incision – 3–8 cm above the symphysis. Fascia incised transversely, inferior epigastric vessels are ligated, rectus muscles are divided transversely.
  Cohen incision – 3–4 cm above the symphysis. Fascia incised in the midline, extension of the fascial incision, separation of rectus, & entry to peritoneum done bluntly.
  Consider a bladder flap by incising the vesicouterine peritoneum in the midline with Metzenbaum scissors & extending the incision bilaterally. Use blunt or sharp dissection to expose the lower uterine segment and place bladder retractor.
  Hysterotomy: Generally transverse in lower uterine segment, above the bladder margin. Extend bluntly (cephalad/caudad) or w/ bandage scissors. Consider high transverse or classical incision depending on adhesions/access, fetal position, gestational age, etc.
  Delivery:
  Vertex presentation – slide hand below fetal head and elevate to level of incision with care not to torque hand inferiorly. Have assistant apply fundal pressure to facilitate delivery once the fetal vertex is at the level of the hysterotomy and flexed.
  Breech/transverse presentation – Identify and deliver either fetal legs to level of breech, or fetal breech. Deliver breech with fingers on ASIS and thumbs on sacrum. Wrap fetus in moist towel and deliver to level of scapula. Rotate and sweep arms to deliver shoulders. Flex head with fingers on maxillary bones (Mauriceau–Smellie–Veit maneuver) to deliver head.
  Deliver placenta w/ uterine massage or manually. Consider uterine exteriorization.
  Clear uterus of clot or remaining placental tissue with dry lap sponge.
  Close hysterotomy in 1 or 2 layers. The 1st layer closure is performed w/ a running, locking stitch. An imbricating, running stitch may then be used.
  Perform tubal ligation if indicated/preoperatively determined.
  Reapproximate fascia w/ a running, delayed-absorbable or permanent suture.
  Close subcutaneous layer if >2 cm thick; close skin w/ subcuticular suture or staples.

POSTPARTUM TUBAL LIGATION

- **Indication:** Undesired fertility
- **Preoperatively:** Informed consent including reversible contraception
- **Steps:**
  General, spinal, or epidural anesthesia, Foley catheter
  Make small (2–4 cm), transverse, infraumbilical skin incision
  Carry down to the fascia, incise fascia transversely, & enter peritoneum
  Immediately postpartum, the uterine fundus sits just below the umbilicus. Identify fallopian tubes & follow out to fimbriated ends.
  Ligate tubes via one of the following methods:
  Modified Pomeroy: Grasp isthmic portion of the tube ~4 cm from the cornua w/ Babcock clamp to elevate loop of the tube. Ligate the base of the loop w/ plain catgut. Divide the mesosalpinx in the center of the loop. Excise knuckle of tube within ligated loop.
  Parkland method: Use Babcock clamp to hold a segment of the tube about 3–4 cm from the cornua. Create a window in an avascular area of the underlying mesosalpinx. Doubly ligate the tube proximally and distally. Excise segment of tube.
  Irving method: Perform all steps of the Parkland method. Then, bury the prox end of the tube into a pocket created in the myometrium.
  Uchida method: Dissect mesosalpinx off the fallopian tube & excise a segment of the tube. Suture mesosalpinx closed; bury the prox stump of the fallopian tube w/i mesosalpinx. The distal stump is left exteriorized.

Alternatively, total salpingectomy can be performed
Ensure hemostasis
Close the fascia, subcutaneous layer if >2-cm thick, & skin
Similar techniques can be performed at the time of cesarean delivery

CERVICAL CERCLAGE

- **Indication:** History indicated, exam indicated, or ultrasound indicated
- **Preoperatively:** Obtain informed consent, confirm viability, confirm intact membranes, rule out intra-amniotic infection, discuss genetic screening with patient prior to placement
- **Steps:**
  General, spinal, or epidural anesthesia
  Empty bladder, position in lithotomy, place speculum and/or retractors to expose cervix
  Grasp the cervix w/ ring forceps
  Use Mersilene tape, Prolene, Ticron, or Ethibond suture
  McDonald cerclage: W/ the suture, make a bite in the cervix from 12–10 o'clock as close to the junction w/ the rugated vaginal epithelium as poss. The next bites go from 8–6 o'clock, from 6–4, & from 2–12. Cinch tightly & tie. Leave a 2–3-cm tail so the stitch can be removed. Consider placement of more than one stitch
  Shirodkar cerclage: Open the vesicocervical space by making a small incision at the cervicovaginal junction. Push the bladder up w/ careful dissection. Open the posterior rectovaginal space similarly. Hydrodissection before incision is sometimes useful. Use right angle allis clamps to pull the vessels lateral. Suture through cervix anterior–posterior in U-shaped fashion (two bites). Consider closing the mucosal incision.
  Ensure hemostasis
  Reconfirm fetal heart tones
  Consider postprocedure cervical length measurement

REPAIR OF OBSTETRICAL LACERATION

- **Preoperatively:** Ensure proper lighting, instruments, and anesthesia (neuraxial or local). If unable to fully visualize the laceration or source of bleeding, move pt to the OR.
- **Steps:**
  Examine the cervix, vagina, labia, & periurethral area
  Rectal exam to evaluate for 3rd- & 4th-degree lacerations
  Examine the cervix systematically. Use ring forceps for assistance in visualization. Repair w/ interrupted absorbable sutures.
  Hemostatic 1st-degree lacerations do not require repair
  For 2nd-degree lacerations, anchor suture 1–2 cm above the apex. Close the laceration w/ a running, locked stitch until the hymenal ring. Ensure closure of the "dead space" beneath the vaginal epithelium
  Pass the suture under the vaginal mucosa to the muscle layer of the perineal body ("crown stitch")
  Close the muscle layer w/ a running stitch
  Close the skin using subcuticular or interrupted sutures
  Perform a rectal exam to ensure no suture material is in the rectum

PUDENDAL NERVE BLOCK (SEE FIGURE 4.3)

- **Indication:**
  To obtain analgesia necessary for delivery or repair of perineal lacerations
- **Preoperatively:**
  Appropriate equipment and lighting
- **Steps:**
  Use an Iowa trumpet & 20G needle
  Prepare 10 cc of 1% lidocaine w/o epi
  Identify the spinous process of the ischium
  Inject 2.5 cc above & below the spinous process on each side
  Check for the anal reflex

MALE CIRCUMCISION

- **Indication:** Elective surgical procedure based on parental request
- **Preoperatively:**
  Informed consent
  Examine the infant and ensure: Adequate shaft length (>1 cm), no congenital anom-alies, no bleeding diathesis, normal median raphe
- **Steps:** The 3 major methods employ the GOMCO clamp, Hollister Plastibell, & Mogen clamp. The GOMCO clamp is the most widely used, & is a/w the fewest complications.
  Provide local anesthesia & prep the skin.
  Determine the size of the bell that will be needed (edge of bell should reach the frenulum & minimally extended over the corona).
  Apply 2 hemostats at 3 & 9 o'clock on the foreskin.
  Use a 3rd hemostat to open the space btw the glans & the foreskin, avoiding the 5 & 7 o'clock positions.
  The hemostat is then used to create a crush line on the dorsal aspect of the foreskin (>1 cm away from the coronal sulcus). Cut the crushed skin & retract the foreskin.
  Place the bell over the glans, inside the foreskin.
  Inspect to make sure that the remaining shaft skin is symmetrical, & not under tension.
  Tighten clamp, cut foreskin, & remove residual tissues.
  Wait for 5 min before opening the clamp.
  Inspect for bleeding & apply pressure if needed.
  Use petroleum-soaked gauze around the edges of the foreskin.
  Ensure infant is able to urinate before discharge home.
  Dressing should remain for 12–24 h.

COMMON SURGICAL INSTRUMENTS

Scissors:
  Mayo (straight/curved) – used for cutting heavier tissue such as fascia, adhesions
  Metzenbaum – used for dissection and cutting peritoneal tissue. Fine scissors
  Bandage – heavy duty, commonly used for extending hysterotomy in Cesarean
  Jorgenson – heavy duty sharply angled scissors, commonly used for cutting cervix from vagina in hysterectomy

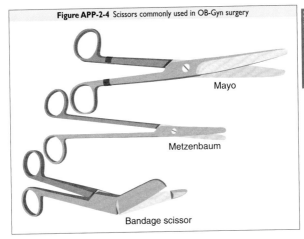

Figure APP-2-4 Scissors commonly used in OB-Gyn surgery

Mayo

Metzenbaum

Bandage scissor

Forceps:
  DeBakey – used for grasping vessels in order to arc electrocautery for sealing
  Ferris-Smith – heavyweight forceps used to grasp avascular tissue such as fascia
  Russian – large grasping surface, often used for hysterotomy closure in Cesarean
  Adson – used for grasping skin, often during closure
  Rat-tooth – used to grasp avascular tissue such as fascia

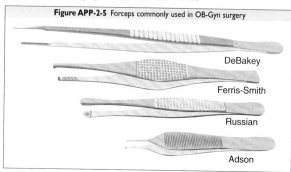

Figure APP-2-5 Forceps commonly used in OB-Gyn surgery

DeBakey

Ferris-Smith

Russian

Adson

Clamps:
  Ochsner/Kocher – heavy-duty and toothed to grasp large tissue such as fascia or
    vaginal cuff
  Allis – firmly grasps tissue, less traumatic than Ochsner/Kochers
  Babcock – atraumatic, used for grasping tubular structures such as fallopian tube
  Kelly (straight/curved) – firmly grasps tissue, used for clamping vascular pedicles or for
    traction

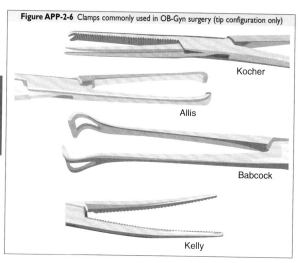

Figure APP-2-6 Clamps commonly used in OB-Gyn surgery (tip configuration only)

Kocher

Allis

Babcock

Kelly

Analgesics, and see page 4-7

Acetaminophen (Tylenol)	Unk	B Compatible	Analgesic, antipyretic	325–500 mg q8h, not to exceed 4000 mg daily	Hepatic dysfxn
ASA	Inhibits prostaglandin synthesis (cyclooxygenase inhib); inhibits platelet aggregation	D Signif effects on some infants, use w/ caution	Analgesic, antiplatelet	81–325 mg PO daily	Allergy to NSAID, GI upset, CI w/ GI ulcers
Ibuprofen (Advil, Morrin)	NSAID, inhibits prostaglandin synthesis	C – 1st & 2nd trimester, D – 3rd trimester Compatible	Analgesic, anti-inflammatory	200–800 mg PO q6–8h	Allergy to NSAID, GI upset, CI w/ GI ulcers, caution w/ HTN Not used in pregnancy
Fentanyl (Sublimaze)	Opioid receptor agonist	C Compatible	Analgesic (narcotic)	Dosage varies based on form: IV, transdermal, pt-controlled IV pump	N/V, respiratory depression, constip, pruritis
Hydromorphone (Dilaudid)	Opioid receptor agonist	C Compatible	Analgesic (narcotic)	Dosage varies based on form: IV, IM, PO, pt-controlled IV pump	N/V, respiratory depression, constip, pruritis
Morphine	Opioid receptor agonist	C Compatible	Analgesic (narcotic)	Dosage varies based on form: IV, IM, PO, pt-controlled IV pump	N/V, respiratory depression, pruritis, CI w/ renal insufficiency
Oxycodone (Roxicodone, Percocet)	Opioid receptor agonist	B Compatible	Analgesic	5–15 mg PO q4–8h	N/V, constip, respiratory depression
Hydrocodone (Vicodin)	Central acting analgesic	C Compatible	Analgesic, antitussive	5–10 mg PO q4–8h	N/V, constip, respiratory depression

Anesthetics, local see page 4-1

Antibiotic prophylaxis for ob-gyn surgery see page 3-7

Antibiotics (selected; see also specific topics, and for UTI/pyelo see page 14-5)

Drug	Mechanism of action	Pregnancy class (FDA) Breastfeeding (AAP/ Thompson)	Standard indication	Typical regimen	Adverse effects and contraindications
Ampicillin	β-lactam – inhibits cell wall synthesis	B Compatible	GBS ppx	2 g IV then 1 g IV q4h	N/V, diarrhea, hives
			Chorio (w/ gentamicin)	2 g IV q6h	
			Latency Abx (PPROM)	2 g IV q6h × 48 h, followed by amoxicillin	
Amoxicillin	β-lactam – inhibits cell wall synthesis	B Compatible	UTI (Preg), otitis media, respiratory tract infxn	500–875 mg q12h × 7–10 d	N/V, diarrhea, hives
			Latency Abx (PPROM)	250 mg TID × 5 d (s/p IV ampicillin course)	
Cefazolin (Ancef)	Cephalosporin (1st generation, β-lactam) – inhibits cell wall synthesis	B Compatible	Preop ppx	2 g IV × 1	N/V, diarrhea
			GBS ppx alternative	2 g IV × 1 then 1 g q6h	
Gentamicin	Aminoglycoside – inhibits protein synthesis by binding 30S ribosomal subunit	D Compatible	Chorio	1.5 mg/kg IV q8h OR	Renal dysfxn requires dose adjustment, ototoxicity
			Endometritis	5 mg/kg IV q24h	
Clindamycin	Inhibits protein synthesis by binding 50S ribosomal subunit	B Compatible (Avoid if possible, monitor infant)	Preop ppx	600 or 900 mg IV × 1	C. Difficile colitis, N/V
			GBS ppx alternative (PCN allergic, test for resistance)	900 mg q8h	
			Endometritis (w/ gentamicin) Wound cellulitis, incl MRSA	300–450 mg PO q6h × 7–14 d	

Ciprofloxacin (Cipro)	Fluoroquinolone – interferes w/ DNA synthesis	C (Avoid in pregnancy) Compatible (Avoid if possible, monitor infant)	UTI, GI tract infxn, respiratory tract infxn	400 mg IV/PO for 7–14 d	Rash, diarrhea, C. difficile colitis, N/V Avoid in pregnancy due to fetal musculoskeletal effects
Trimethoprim-sulfamethoxazole (Bactrim)	Trimethoprim – interferes w/ tetra-hydrofolic acid production & DNA formation Sulfonamide – blocks bact synthesis of dihydrofolic acid	D Infant risk minimal	UTI, cellulitis (incl MRSA)	160/800 mg BID PO × 3 d (7–14 d for complicated UTI)	Rash, N/V, diarrhea, hepatic dysfxn, CI w/ sulfa allergy Avoid in 1st & 3rd trimester of pregnancy if possible
Nitrofurantoin (Macrobid)	Inhibits prot synthesis	B Compatible	UTI (Preg)	100 mg BID PO × 5–7 d	N/V, hepatic dysfxn CI during labor/delivery, or when labor is imminent
Ceftriaxone (Rocephin)	Cephalosporin (3rd generation, β-lactam)	B Compatible	Pyelo Gonorrhea/PID	1 g IV q24h 250 mg IM × 1 dose	Allergy/anaphylaxis, N/V, diarrhea
Piperacillin/tazobactam (Zosyn)	β-lactam + β-lactamase inhib	B Compatible	PID Bacteremia PNA	3.375–4.5 g IV q6h × 7–10 d	Rash, GI upset, leukopenia
Erythro	Macrolide – inhibits prot synthesis by binding 50S ribosomal subunit	B Compatible	Chlamydia Latency Abx (PPROM)	500 mg PO q4h 250 mg IV q6h × 48 h, then PO TID × 5 d	GI upset, rash
Azithro (Zithromax)	Macrolide – inhibits prot synthesis by binding 50S ribosomal subunit	B Infant risk minimal	Chlamydia Community acquired pneumonia Latency Abx (PPROM)	1 g PO × 1 dose 500 mg PO daily × 3–5 d (Also IV)	GI upset, hepatic dysfxn
Fosfomycin	Inhibits bact cell wall synthesis	B Infant risk cannot be ruled out	UTI (avoid if suspect Pyelo)	3 g PO × 1	GI upset, HA Avoid in pregnancy due to limited safety data

Drug	Mechanism of action	Standard indication	Pregnancy class (FDA) (AAP/Thompson) Breastfeeding	Typical regimen	Adverse effects and contraindications
Vanco	Inhibits bact cell wall synthesis	MRSA skin infxn. bacteremia	C Infant risk cannot be ruled out	15–20 mg/kg IV q12h	Red man syn. caution w/ renal dysfxn. Check serum trough levels.
		GBS ppx (if PCN allergy)		1 g IV q12h during labor	
		C. difficile infxn		125 mg PO QID × 10–14 d	
PCN	β-lactam	GBS ppx	B Compatible	5 million units × 1 IV, then 2.5 million units q4h IV	Allergy/anaphylaxis, N/V, diarrhea
Cephalexin (Keflex)	Cephalosporin (1st generation, β-lactam) – inhibits cell wall synthesis	Soft tissue infxn. cellulitis UTI	B Compatible	500 mg PO BID × 7–14 d	Allergy/anaphylaxis, N/V, diarrhea
Metronidazole (Flagyl)	Bact enzyme deactivation	Bact vaginosis	B Infant risk cannot be ruled out, avoid if possible	500 mg PO BID × 7 d	N/V, rash, antabuse-type rxn w/ EtOH. Avoid in 1st trimester of pregnancy
		Trichomonas vaginalis		2 g PO × 1 dose	
		PID		500 mg PO BID × 14 d	
		C. difficile colitis		500 mg PO TID × 10–14 d	
Doxycycline	Tetracycline – inhibits prot synthesis	Chlamydia	D Avoid in breastfeeding	100 mg BID × 7 d	N/V, photosensitivity, CI throughout pregnancy
		PID		100 mg BID × 14 d	

Anticoagulants

Enoxaparin (Lovenox)	Antifactor Xa. antithrombin (LMWH)	DVT ppx DVT rx	B Compatible	40 mg SQ daily or BID 1 mg/kg q12	HIT, hypersensitivity Sev bld loss, CI w/ epidural anesthesia if <12–24 hours from last dose
Heparin	Activates antithrombin III	Same	C Compatible	5000 U SQ q8h IV infusion 5000–10000 BID	Same as LMWH CI w/ epidural anesthesia if <6 hours from last dose
Warfarin (Coumadin)	Inhibits synthesis of Vit K dependent clotting factors (2, 7, 9, 10, prot C&S)	Same	X Compatible	Varies – target INR 2–3	Bleeding. Do not give in pregnancy. CI w/ epidural anesthesia until INR normalizes

Antiemetics

	MOA				
Vitamin B6 (pyridoxine)	MOA unknown	N/V	A Compatible	10–25 mg q6h	Neuropathy at very high doses
Doxylamine succinate	Non-specific anti-histamine	N/V	C May decrease breastmilk supply	12.5 mg daily or BID	Sedation
Prochlorperazine (Compazine)	Depresses chemoreceptor trigger zone	N/V	C Infant risk cannot be ruled out	5–10 mg PO/PR q6–8h	Prolonged QT, tardive dyskinesia
Metoclopramide (Reglan)	Promotes GI motility; inhibits dopamine receptors	N/V	B Infant risk cannot be ruled out	10–20 mg PO/IV q8h	Tardive dyskinesia, neuroleptic malig syn
Ondansetron (Zofran)	Selective 5HT-3 receptor antag	N/V	B Infant risk cannot be ruled out	4–8 mg PO/IV q4–8h	Constipation, prolonged QT
Promethazine HCl (Phenergan)	H1 receptor blocker	N/V	C Compatible	12.5–25 mg PO/PR/IV q6h	Sedation, IV dosing can cause tissue necrosis

Anti seizure medications see page 18-5

Chemotherapy for Gynecologic Malignancy

Carboplatin	Alkylating agent	Ovarian cancer Endometrial cancer	BSA based	Myelosuppression (thrombocytopenia) Hypersensitivity, N/V, Electrolyte disturbances, alopecia
Cisplatin	Alkylating agent	Ovarian Cancer (IP therapy) Cervical cancer Germ cell tumors GTN	BSA based	Neuropathy, ototoxicity Nephrotoxicity, N/V, anemia, leukopenia, thrombocytopenia
Paclitaxel (Taxol)	Stabilizes microtubules	Ovarian cancer Carcinosarcoma Endometrial cancer Breast cancer	BSA based	Alopecia, N/V, neuropathy, hypersensitivity rxn, myelosuppression

DRUG INDEX 25-6

Drug	Mechanism	Indication	Dosing	Side Effects
Docetaxel (Taxotere)	Stabilizes microtubules	Recurrent ovarian cancer	BSA based	Alopecia, edema, nail/skin changes, N/V, diarrhea, mucositis
Bevacizumab (Avastin)	Monoclonal IgG Ab binds VEGF → inhibition of angiogenesis	Ovarian cancer; Cervical cancer (recurrent, metastatic)	Weight based	HTN, GI hemorrhage/perforation, proteinuria, arterial thromboembolism
Olaprib	PARP inhibitor	Recurrent ovarian cancer with known BRCA mutation	400 mg PO BID	Rash, N/V, Pancytopenia, arthralgia
Topotecan (Hycamtin)	Inhibits topoisomerase I	Recurrent ovarian cancer	BSA based	Alopecia, myelosuppression, N/V, fatigue
Gemcitabine (Gemzar)	Nucleoside analogue that inhibits DNA synthesis	Recurrent ovarian cancer	BSA based	N/V, myelosuppression, rash, stomatitis
Doxorubicin (Adriamycin, Doxil)	Inhibits topoisomerase I	Breast cancer; Ovarian cancer (Doxil = liposomal form)	BSA based	PPE, alopecia, myelosuppression (leukopenia), N/V, cardiotoxicity (requires MUGA before starting), mucositis
Bleomycin	Induces DNA strand breaks	GTN, germ cell tumors	BSA based	Pulm fibrosis, alopecia, hyperkeratosis, stomatitis, PPE
Etoposide	Inhibits topoisomerase II	GTN, germ cell tumors, recurrent Ovarian	BSA based	Alopecia, N/V, diarrhea, fever/malaise, AML, myelosuppression (leukopenia)
Methotrexate	Inhibits dihydrofolate reductase → decreased purine synthesis	GTN; Ectopic Preg	15–30 mg PO/IM × 5 d; 50 mg/m² IM	N/V, hepatotoxicity, photosensitivity, stomatitis, pulm fibrosis
Actinomycin D	Binds to DNA, intercalating btw base pairs	GTN	Weight based	N/V, diarrhea, esophagitis, agranulocytosis
Ifosfamide	Alkylating agent	Recurrent cervical cancer, high-grade endometrial stromal sarcoma	BSA based	N/V, hemorrhagic cystitis (give w/ Mesna), encephalopathy, myelosuppression (leukopenia)
Cyclophosphamide (Cytoxan)	Alkylating agent	GTN, Recurrent ovarian cancer	Weight based	N/V, pulm fibrosis, cardiotoxicity, myeloid leukemia
Fluorouracil (5-FU)	Inhibits thymidylate synthetase	Cervical cancer, vaginal dysplasia	5% cream topically as directed	N/V, diarrhea, myelosuppression, coronary artery spasm

Cholesterol medications see page 1-10

Constipation therapies and Stool softeners see page 9-7

Contraception

Medroxyprogesterone (Depo-Provera)	Suppresses ovulation, decreases tubal motility, causes endometrial atrophy, & thickens cervical mucus	X Compatible	Contraception, menorrhagia	150 mg IM every 3 mo	May cause irreg bleeding, weight gain, breast tenderness, HAs, reversible loss of bone density, delayed fertility. CI w/ sev HTN, stroke, liver dz, or breast cancer.
Mirena IUS (Levonorgestrel-releasing intrauterine system)	Thickens cervical mucus, thins the endometrium, decreases tubal motility, may suppress ovulation	X Compatible	Contraception, menorrhagia	Intrauterine device effective for 5 y	Risk of ectopic Preg if Preg does occur, irreg bleeding, uterine perforation/malposition, expulsion. Do not insert if active cervical/uterine infxn or h/o infxn in last 3 mo. No need to remove if IUD in place >1 month and new diagnosis of PID, just treat
Paragard IUD (Intrauterine Copper contraceptive)	Creates spermicidal environment	X Compatible	Contraception	Intrauterine device effective for 10 y	See above. May worsen dysmenorrhea or menorrhagia. CI w/ Wilson dz.
Subdermal Implant (Etonogestrel implant)	Suppresses ovulation, decreases tubal motility, thins the endometrium, & thickens cervical mucus	X Compatible	Contraception	Subdermal implant effective for 3 y	Unpredictable bleeding. CI w/ sev HTN, stroke, liver dz, or breast cancer.
Norethindrone (Micronor)	Thickens cervical mucus, prevents ovulation (~50% of the time), decreases tubal motility, & thins endometrium	X Compatible	Contraception, menorrhagia	5 mg PO daily	CI w/ sev HTN, stroke, liver dz, or breast cancer

Combined OCPs Low-dose (Alesse, Loestrin) Mid dose (Orthocyclen) High dose (Ovral) Multiphasic (Ortho Tri-Cyclen) Extended cycle (Seasonale, Seasonique)	Suppresses ovulation, thickens cervical mucus, decreases tubal motility, & thins endometrium. Increases circulating steroid hormone binding globulin (reduces acne/androgenic signaling)	Contraception, menorrhagia, irreg menses, dysmenorrhea, acne	X Usually compatible	Low-dose: 20 mcg ethinyl estradiol Mid-dose: 30–35 mcg ethinyl estradiol High-dose: 50 mcg ethinyl estradiol Multi progest forms	May cause breast tenderness, HAs, nausea, breakthrough bleeding. Increased risk of thrombotic events (but lower risk than in Preg). CI if h/o DVT, vascular dz, breast cancer, migraines w/ aura, stroke, poorly controlled DM or HTN, smoker >35 yo, liver or gallbladder dz, or SLE
Nuva-Ring (Ethinyl estradiol/ etonogestrel vaginal ring)	See above	Contraception, menorrhagia, irreg menses	X Usually compatible	1 ring placed vaginally for 3 w, remove for 1 w, rpt w/ new ring	See above. May cause vaginal irritation or discomfort.
Ortho Evra Patch (Norelgestomin/ethinyl estradiol transdermal system)	See above	Contraception, menorrhagia, irreg menses	X Usually compatible	Apply to lower abd, buttocks, upper torso (not breasts), or upper outer arm. Exchange weekly × 3 w & then leave off × 1 w.	See above. May cause skin irritation. Use w/ caution if wt >198 lbs

Diabetes Medications, and see insulin page 17-3

Metformin (Glucophage)	Suppresses hepatic gluconeogenesis, increases insulin sens, enhances periph gluc uptake	DM II PCOS	B Compatible	500 mg BID, titrated up to 2000 mg daily	GI upset, lactic acidosis, CI in renal insufficiency. Do not use w/ renal contrast
Sulfonylureas (glyburide, glipizide, glimepiride)	Closes K_{ATP} channels on β-cell plasma membranes → increased insulin secretion	DM II GDM A2 (glyburide)	B Infant risk cannot be ruled out	Varies based on drug Glyburide: Maximum daily dose 20 mg	Weight gain, hypoglycemia, CI Sulfa allergy
Thiazolidinediones (pioglitazone, rosiglitazone)	Activates nuclear transcription factor PPAR-g	DM II	C Infant risk cannot be ruled out	Pioglitazone: 15–30 mg PO daily Rosiglitazone: 4–8 mg PO daily	Edema, weight gain, CI in heart failure Not used in pregnancy

Insulin (multi forms)	Insulin receptor agonist Onset/peak/duration	B Compatible	DM I, DM II, GDM	Varies (SQ administration) Also IV insulin drip (regular)	Hypoglycemia
• Lispro (Humalog) • Regular (Novalin R) • NPH (Novalin N) • Lantus (Glargine)	15 min/30–90 min/3–5 h 30–60 min/50–120 min/5–8 h 1–3 h/8 h/20 h 1 h/no peak/24 h				

Diabetes oral hypoglycemic agents see page 17-7

Diarrhea medications see page 9-8

Epilepsy treatments see page 18-5

Hormone Replacement (Postmenopausal)

Estrogen • Oral (CEE, Premarin) • Patch (17β-Estradiol, Climara)	Systemic HRT	Menopausal/vasomotor sx	Oral: 0.3, 0.45, 0.65, 0.9, or 1.25 mg daily Patch: 0.0375, 0.5, 0.075, 0.1 mg/d, apply weekly	Increased risk of stroke, VTE, breast cancer. CI w/ h/o breast cancer, coagulopathy, smokers. Estrogen only preparations CI if pt has uterus (risk of endometrial hyperplasia).
Estrogen-progesterone • Oral (CEE + medroxyprogesterone acetate, Prempro) • Patch (17β-Estradiol + norethindrone acetate, Combipatch)	Systemic HRT	Menopausal/vasomotor sx in pts w/ uterus	0.3–0.625 mg CEE + 1.5 mg MDPA daily 0.05 mg/d E_2 + 0.14–0.25 mg/d NETA, apply patch twice weekly	Increased risk of stroke, VTE, breast cancer. CI w/ h/o breast cancer, coagulopathy, smokers.
Vaginal estrogen • CEE, Premarin • 17β-Estradiol, Estrace	Local HRT	Vaginal atrophy	0.5 g vaginally daily for 2 w, then twice weekly 2 g vaginally daily for 2 w, then twice weekly	CI w/ h/o endometrial or breast cancer

Hypertension and Preeclampsia Medications for Preeclampsia (and see page 12-4)

Alphamethyldopa (Aldomet)	Mechanism of action uncertain, central α2 agonist → inhibits sympathetic NS	B Compatible	HTN	250–500 mg PO TID	CI if concurrent MAOI therapy, caution w/ CHF
Hydralazine	Unknown MOA. Vasodilator	C Compatible	HTN	10–25 mg PO QID 5–20 mg IV q20' for acute BP control	Tachycardia
Labetalol	Non-selective adrenergic blocker; Blocks β1, β2 and α1	C Compatible	HTN (incl preeclampsia, hypertensive urgency)	HTN: 200 mg PO q12 up to 2400 mg daily HTN urgency: 20 mg IV, followed by 40 IV followed by 80 IV (max 300 mg in 24 hours)	Bradycardia, Use care in severe asthmatics
Magnesium sulfate	Nonspecific calcium channel blockade	A Compatible	Sz ppx in preeclampsia Eclamptic sz rx	4 g IV bolus, then 2 g/h 5 g IM into each buttock if no IV access	CI: myasthenia gravis; Flushing, HA, blurry vision, drowsiness Magnesium tox: Hyporeflexia, somnolence, pulm edema, resp depression, cardiac arrhythmia
Nifedipine (Procardia)	CCB	C Compatible	HTN	Extended release formula: Maximum 120 mg daily Immediate release: 10 mg, 20 mg, 20 mg q20 for acute BP control	Theoretical risk of hypotension with concurrent Mag sulfate use; HoTN Caution w/ hepatic dysfxn

Hypertension treatment see page 12-4
Incontinence Medications see page 7-5

Infertility medications

Clomiphene citrate (Clomid)	Interrupts estrogen's central negative feedback, increases FSH secretion → maturation of ovarian follicles	Ovulation induction	X Contraindicated	50 mg PO daily for 5 d (typically starting on cycle day 5), can ↑ by 50 mg increments to 250 mg	Hot flashes, mood swings, ovarian cysts, increased risk of multi gest
Letrozole (Femara)	Aromatase inhib, suppresses ovarian estradiol secretion, increases FSH secretion → maturation of ovarian follicles	Ovulation induction (Superior to clomid for PCOS)	X Contraindicated	2.5–5 mg PO daily for 5 d	Hot flashes, mood swings, joint pains, fatigue, increased risk of multi gest
Gonadotropins (Follstim, Fertinex, Gonal-f)	FSH/LH preparations	Stimulates ovarian follicle maturation	X Contraindicated	Start at 50–75 IU/d IM (protocols vary)	Ovarian hyperstimulation syn, increased risk of multi gest

Insulin, types and characteristics see page 17-3

Iron supplements and formulations see page 16-2

Lipid medications see page 1-10

Migraine therapies see page 18-4

Osteoporosis medications

Bisphosphonates • Alendronate (Fosamax) • Risedronate (Actonel) • Ibandronate (Boniva)	Inhibition of osteoclasts	Osteoporosis (rx & ppx), HyperCa of malig		Alendronate: 35 mg PO once weekly Risedronate: 35 mg PO once weekly Ibandronate: 150 mg PO monthly, 3 mg IV every 3 mo	Erosive esophagitis, osteonecrosis – caution w/ dental Surg, infxn. CI if renal dz.
SERM • Raloxifene	Binds to estrogen receptors (both activating & deactivating), reduces bone Absorp	Osteoporosis (rx & prevention), Breast cancer		60 mg PO daily	Stroke, VTE, CI in Preg, caution w/ coronary heart dz
Calcitonin	Reduces osteoclast number, increases osteoblast activity	HyperCa Osteoporosis		4 µ/kg subq or IM every 12 h 200 units intranasal daily	May cause hypocalcemic tetany

Psychiatric/Substance Abuse Medications (selected)

Drug	Mechanism	Preg. cat. / Breastfeeding	Indication	Dose	Side effects
Zolpidem (Ambien)	Non-BZD GABA receptor agonist	C / Caution with breast feeding	Sleep aid	5–10 mg nightly	Sedation
Buprenorphine (Butrans)	Opioid receptor agonist/antag	C / Compatible, monitor infant	Opioid dependence	10–30 mcg/h transdermal patch	Rash, GI upset
Bupropion (Wellbutrin)	Dopamine/norepi reuptake inhib	C / Compatible	Depression, smoking cessation	IR: 100 mg PO BID–TID, XR: 150–300 mg PO daily	HTN, constip, N/V, lower sz threshold
Citalopram (Celexa)	SSRI	C / Compatible, but alternative preferred	Depression, anxiety	20–40 mg PO daily	GI upset, sexual dysfxn, prolonged QT
Disulfiram (Antabuse)	Inhibits aldehyde dehydrogenase (enzyme that metabolizes EtOH)	C / May be of concern	Alcoholism	500 mg PO daily	Dermatitis. Can have fatal EtOH withdrawal rxn.
Fluoxetine (Prozac)	SSRI	C / Compatible	Depression, anxiety	20–80 mg PO daily	GI upset, HA, dizziness, fatigue, sexual dysfxn, serotonin syn, prolonged QT
Lithium	Unk	D / Effects on newborns – use w/ caution	Bipolar d/o	Varies by formulation	Hypothyroidism, tox, renal dysfxn, GI upset, CV effects. Fetal CV defects.
Methadone	Opioid receptor agonist	C / Compatible	Opioid dependence	80–120 mg PO daily for maint therapy	Cardiac dysrhythmia, prolonged QT, constip, dizziness
Sertraline (Zoloft)	SSRI	C / Compatible	Depression, anxiety	25–100 mg PO daily	GI upset, HA, dizziness, fatigue, sexual dysfxn, serotonin syn
Trazodone	Serotonin reuptake inhib & receptor antag	C / Compatible	Sleep aid, depression	50–150 mg PO nightly/daily	GI upset, drowsiness, prolonged QT, postural HoTN
Lorazepam (Ativan)	Benzodiazepine (binds GABA receptor)	D / Compatible	Anxiety, sleep aid, EtOH withdrawal	0.5–2 mg daily (divided doses) PO, IV	Drowsiness, dizziness, delirium, caution w/ respiratory insufficiency

Pyelonephritis treatment see page 14-7

Steroids, topical agents see page 20-4

Steroids, systemic

Drug	Description	Category / Compatibility	Indication	Dose	Adverse effects
Betamethasone (Celestone)	Anti-inflammatory – Accelerates production of surfactant	C Compatible	Fetal lung maturity	12.5 mg IM q24h × 2 doses (24–36w5dw gest)	Mat hyperglycemia, leukocytosis, fetal hypoglycemia
Dexamethasone	Anti-inflammatory	C Compatible	Fetal lung maturity	12 mg IM q12h × 2 doses (24–36w5d w gest)	Mat hyperglycemia, leukocytosis, fetal hypoglycemia
	Anti-inflammatory, rheumatologic conditions Thrombocytopenia			10 mg IV q12h	
Prednisone	Glucocorticoid analog	C Compatible	Anti-inflammatory, rheumatologic conditions, thrombocytopenia	Varies based on indication	HTN, fluid retention, euphoria, Cushing syn, hyperglycemia

Syphilis treatment see page 21-8

Tocolytics

Drug	Description	Category / Compatibility	Indication	Dose	Adverse effects
Nifedipine (Procardia)	CCB	C Compatible	Preterm labor (tocolysis)	Loading dose: 30 mg once 10–20 mg PO q6–8	HoTN, tachy, dizziness, Caution w/ magnesium
Magnesium sulfate	CCB (antagonizes procontractile effects of calcium)	A Compatible	Neuroprotection for preterm labor (prior to 32 weeks) Tocolysis (controversial)	6 g IV loading dose, then 1–2 g/h 4 g IV loading dose, then 1–2 g/h	Flushing, HA, blurry vision, drowsiness Magnesium tox: Hyporeflexia, somnolence, pulm edema, resp depression
Indomethacin (Indocin)	Prostaglandin synthetase inhib	C Compatible	Preterm labor (tocolysis)	100 mg PO loading dose, then 50 mg PO q6 × 8 doses	Oligohydramnios Premature closure of ductus arteriosus Do not administer >32 weeks in pregnancy
Terbutaline	β-adrenergic agonist	B Compatible	Preterm contractions Tachysystole ECV	0.25 mg SQ × 1 (may rpt if needed)	Tachy, nervousness, cardiac dysrhythmia. Black box warning against prolonged use b/c of mat cardiovascular effects.

Urinary Tract Infection treatment see page 14-5

Uterotonics (and see Chapter 11)

Drug	Mechanism	Indication	Dose	Adverse Effects
Oxytocin (Pitocin)	Stimulates uterine oxytocin receptors → increases uterine contractility	Postpartum hemorrhage, induction/augmentation of labor	10–80 U in 1 L crystalloid 10 U IM (if no IV access)	N/V, emesis, hyponatremia
Misoprostol (Cytotec)	Prostaglandin E₁ analog → stimulates uterine contractions	Postpartum hemorrhage; cervical ripening, 1st trimester abortion	600–1000 mcg PR, PO, or buccal 25–100 mcg q4h PV, PO, or buccal for cervical ripening	N/V, diarrhea, fever, chills, CI in women with prior hysterotomy in 3rd trimester of pregnancy
Methylergonovine (Methergine)	Ergot alkaloid → increases uterine contractility	Postpartum hemorrhage	0.2 mg IM, q2–4h up to 5 doses 0.2 mg PO q6h × 4 doses	HTN, N/V CI w/ HTN
Carboprost (Hemabate)	Prostaglandin F₂α → stimulates uterine contractions	Postpartum hemorrhage	0.25 mg IM q15–90', maximum 8 doses (2 mg) in 24 hours	N/V, diarrhea, flushing, chills, CI w/ asthma
Dinoprostone (Cervidil, Prostin E₂)	Prostaglandin E₂ → stimulates uterine contractions	Cervical ripening	10 mg in vaginal fornix for cervical ripening	N/V, diarrhea, fever, chills, HA

Figure APP-4-1 Basic Life Support, Adult Cardiac Arrest Algorithm (2015 Update)

Verify scene safety.

Victim is unresponsive.
Shout for nearby help.
Activate emergency response system
via mobile device (if appropriate).
Get AED and emergency equipment
(or send someone to do so).

Look for no breathing
or only gasping and check
pulse (simultaneously).
Is pulse **definitely** felt
within 10 seconds?

Normal breathing, has pulse

Monitor until emergency responders arrive.

No normal breathing, has pulse

Provide rescue breathing:
1 breath every 5–6 seconds, or
about 10–12 breaths/min.
• Activate emergency response
  system (if not already done)
  after 2 minutes.
• Continue rescue breathing;
  check pulse about every
  2 minutes. If no pulse, begin
  CPR (go to "**CPR**" box).
• If possible opioid overdose,
  administer naloxone if
  available per protocol.

No breathing or only gasping, no pulse

By this time in all scenarios, emergency
response system or backup is activated,
and AED and emergency equipment are
retrieved or someone is retrieving them.

CPR
Begin cycles of
30 compressions and 2 breaths.
Use AED as soon as it is available.

AED arrives.

Check rhythm.
Shockable rhythm?

Yes, shockable

Give 1 shock. Resume CPR
immediately for about 2 minutes
(until prompted by AED to allow
rhythm check).
Continue until ALS providers take
over or victim starts to move.

No, nonshockable

Resume CPR immediately for
about 2 minutes (until prompted
by AED to allow rhythm check).
Continue until ALS providers take
over or victim starts to move.

(From *Circulation*. 2010;122:S685.)

Figure APP-4-2 ACLS Adult Cardiac Arrest Algorithm (2015)

(From *Circulation*. 2015;132(suppl 2):S444.)

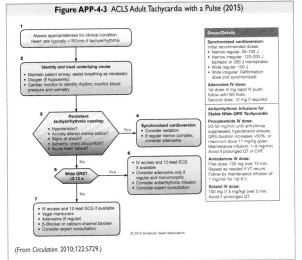

Figure APP-4-3 ACLS Adult Tachycardia with a Pulse (2015)

1
Assess appropriateness for clinical condition
Heart rate typically ≥150/min if tachyarrhythmia

2
Identify and treat underlying cause
- Maintain patent airway; assist breathing as necessary
- Oxygen (if hypoxemic)
- Cardiac monitor to identify rhythm; monitor blood pressure and oximetry

3
Persistent tachyarrhythmia causing:
- Hypotension?
- Acutely altered mental status?
- Signs of shock?
- Ischemic chest discomfort?
- Acute heart failure?

4 — Yes →
Synchronized cardioversion
- Consider sedation
- If regular narrow complex, consider adenosine

No ↓

5
Wide QRS? ≥0.12 s — Yes →

6
- IV access and 12-lead ECG if available
- Consider adenosine only if regular and monomorphic
- Consider antiarrhythmic infusion
- Consider expert consultation

No ↓

7
- IV access and 12-lead ECG if available
- Vagal maneuvers
- Adenosine (if regular)
- β-Blocker or calcium channel blocker
- Consider expert consultation

Doses/Details

Synchronized cardioversion:
Initial recommended doses:
- Narrow regular: 50–100 J
- Narrow irregular: 120–200 J biphasic or 200 J monophasic
- Wide regular: 100 J
- Wide irregular: Defibrillation dose (not synchronized)

Adenosine IV dose:
1st dose: 6 mg rapid IV push; follow with NS flush.
Second dose: 12 mg if required.

Antiarrhythmic Infusions for Stable Wide-QRS Tachycardia

Procainamide IV dose:
20–50 mg/min until arrhythmia suppressed, hypotension ensues, QRS duration increases >50%, or maximum dose 17 mg/kg given.
Maintenance infusion: 1–4 mg/min. Avoid if prolonged QT or CHF.

Amiodarone IV dose:
First dose: 150 mg over 10 min. Repeat as needed if VT recurs. Follow by maintenance infusion of 1 mg/min for 1st 6 h.

Sotalol IV dose:
100 mg (1.5 mg/kg) over 5 min. Avoid if prolonged QT.

© 2015 American Heart Association

(From *Circulation*. 2010;122:S729.)

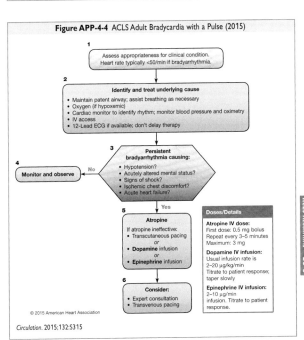

Figure APP-4-4 ACLS Adult Bradycardia with a Pulse (2015)

1
Assess appropriateness for clinical condition.
Heart rate typically <50/min if bradyarrhythmia.

2
Identify and treat underlying cause
- Maintain patent airway; assist breathing as necessary
- Oxygen (if hypoxemic)
- Cardiac monitor to identify rhythm; monitor blood pressure and oximetry
- IV access
- 12-Lead ECG if available; don't delay therapy

3
Persistent bradyarrhythmia causing:
- Hypotension?
- Acutely altered mental status?
- Signs of shock?
- Ischemic chest discomfort?
- Acute heart failure?

4 ← No
Monitor and observe

Yes ↓

5
Atropine
If atropine ineffective:
- Transcutaneous pacing
  or
- **Dopamine** infusion
  or
- **Epinephrine** infusion

6
Consider:
- Expert consultation
- Transvenous pacing

Doses/Details

Atropine IV dose:
First dose: 0.5 mg bolus
Repeat every 3–5 minutes
Maximum: 3 mg

Dopamine IV infusion:
Usual infusion rate is 2–20 μg/kg/min
Titrate to patient response; taper slowly

Epinephrine IV infusion:
2–10 μg/min
infusion. Titrate to patient response.

© 2015 American Heart Association

Circulation. 2015;132:S315

Figure APP-4-5 ACLS Opioid-associated Emergency Management (2015)

Assess and activate.
Check for unresponsiveness and call for nearby help. Send someone to call 9-1-1 and get AED and naloxone. Observe for breathing vs no breathing or only gasping.

Begin CPR.
If victim is unresponsive with no breathing or only gasping, begin CPR. If alone, perform CPR for about 2 minutes before leaving to phone 9-1-1 and get naloxone and AED.

Administer naloxone.
Give naloxone as soon as it is available. 2 mg intranasal or 0.4 mg intramuscular. May repeat after 4 minutes.

Does the person respond?
At any time, does the person move purposefully, breathe regularly, moan, or otherwise respond?

Yes →

Stimulate and reassess.
Continue to check responsiveness and breathing until advanced help arrives. If the person stops responding, begin CPR and repeat naloxone.

No ↓

Continue CPR and use AED as soon as it is available.
Continue until the person responds or until advanced help arrives.

(From *Circulation*. 2010;122:S685.)

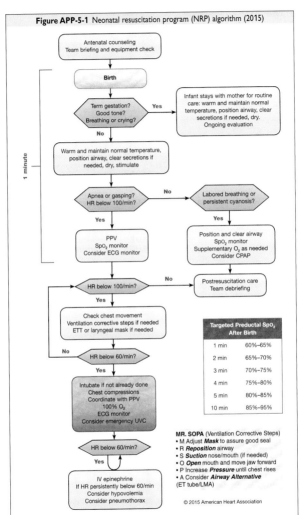

Figure APP-5-1 Neonatal resuscitation program (NRP) algorithm (2015)

Antenatal counseling
Team briefing and equipment check

Birth

Term gestation?
Good tone?
Breathing or crying? — **Yes** → Infant stays with mother for routine care: warm and maintain normal temperature, position airway, clear secretions if needed, dry. Ongoing evaluation

No

Warm and maintain normal temperature, position airway, clear secretions if needed, dry, stimulate

Apnea or gasping?
HR below 100/min? — **No** → Labored breathing or persistent cyanosis?

Yes   **Yes**

PPV
SpO_2 monitor
Consider ECG monitor

Position and clear airway
SpO_2 monitor
Supplementary O_2 as needed
Consider CPAP

HR below 100/min? — **No** → Postresuscitation care
Team debriefing

Check chest movement
Ventilation corrective steps if needed
ETT or laryngeal mask if needed

No

HR below 60/min?

Yes

Intubate if not already done
Chest compressions
Coordinate with PPV
100% O_2
ECG monitor
Consider emergency UVC

HR below 60/min?

Yes

IV epinephrine
If HR persistently below 60/min
Consider hypovolemia
Consider pneumothorax

1 minute

Targeted Preductal SpO_2 After Birth	
1 min	60%–65%
2 min	65%–70%
3 min	70%–75%
4 min	75%–80%
5 min	80%–85%
10 min	85%–95%

MR. SOPA (Ventilation Corrective Steps)
• M Adjust *Mask* to assure good seal
• R *Reposition* airway
• S *Suction* nose/mouth (if needed)
• O *Open* mouth and move jaw forward
• P Increase *Pressure* until chest rises
• A Consider *Airway Alternative*
(ET tube/LMA)

© 2015 American Heart Association

(From Wyckoff MH, Aziz K, Escobedo MB, et al. *Circulation*. 2015;132(suppl 2):S543. And published at *Pediatrics* 2015;136(suppl 2):S196. Available online at: pediatrics.aappublications.org/content/136/Supplement_2/S196)

A

17-OHP	17-hydroxyprogesterone
AA	African American
AAP	American Academy of Pediatrics
Ab(s)	antibody(ies)
AB	abortion
ABC	airway-breathing-circulation
ABG	arterial blood gas
abx	antibiotics
AC	abdominal circumference
ACEI	angiotensin-converting enzyme inhibitor
ACh	acetylcholine
aCL	anticardiolipin antibody
ACLS	Advanced Cardiac Life Support
ACOG	American College of OB/GYN
ACS	acute coronary syndrome/ American Cancer Society
ACTH	adrenocorticotropic hormone
ADH	antidiuretic hormone
AE	adverse effects
AED	antiepileptic drug
AEDF	absent end-diastolic flow
AF	amniotic fluid
AFC	antral follicle count
AFE	amniotic fluid embolism
AFI	amniotic fluid index
AFLP	acute fatty liver of pregnancy
AFP	alpha-fetoprotein
AFV	amniotic fluid volume
AG	anion gap
Ag	antigen
AH	Assisted Hatching
AI	active ingredient
AIDS	acquired immunodeficiency syndrome
AIHA	autoimmune hemolytic anemia
AIN	anal intraepithelial neoplasia
AIS	adenocarcinoma in situ/ androgen insensitivity syndrome
AKI	acute kidney injury
ALT	Alanine AminoTransferase
AMA	advanced maternal age
AMH	anti-Müllerian hormone
AML	acute myeloid leukemia
Amp	amplitude/ampicillin
AMS	altered mental status
Amy	amylase
ANA	antinuclear antibody
AP	angina pectoris/ anteroposterior
aPa/APLA	antiphospholipid antibodies
APRN	advanced practice registered nurse
APS	APLA syndrome
aPTT	activated partial thromboplastin time
AR	absolute risk
ARB	angiotensin receptor blocker
ARDS	acute respiratory distress syndrome
ARF	acute renal failure
ARR	AR reduction
ART	antiretroviral therapy/assisted reproductive technology
AS	aortic stenosis
ASA	American Society of Anesthesiologists/aspirin
ASCAs	antisaccharomyces cerevisiae antibodies
ASCCP	American Society for Colposcopy and Cervical Pathology
ASD	atrial septal defect
ASIS	anterior–superior iliac spine
ASRM	American Society for Reproductive Medicine
AST	Aspartate Aminotransferase
AT-III	antithrombin III
ATD	antithyroid drug
ATFP	arcus tendineus fasciae pelvis
ATN	acute tubular necrosis
AUA	American Urological Association
AUB	abnormal uterine bleeding
AUGS	American urogynecologic society
AVA	aortic valve area
AVF	arteriovenous fistula
avg	average
AVM	arteriovenous malformation
AVSDs	atrioventricular septal defects
a/w	associated with
Azithro	azithromycin
AZT	zidovudine

B

BASE	brief abuse screen for the elderly
BAV	bicuspid aortic valve
BB	beta blocker
BBT	basal body temperature
BC	bulbus cordis
BCC	basal cell carcinoma
BCLS	basic cardiac life support
BE	base excess
BEP	bleomycin/etoposide/cisplatin
bhCG	beta-hCG
BiAsp	biphasic insulin aspart
BID	twice daily
BMD	bone mineral density
BMI	body mass index
BMT	bone marrow transplant
BMZ	betamethasone
BPD	biparietal diameter
BPH	benign prostatic hyperplasia
BPP	biophysical profile
BPS	bladder pain syndrome
BSA	body surface area
BSO	bilateral salpingo-oophorectomy

BTL	bilateral tubal ligation
BUN	blood urea nitrogen
BV	bacterial vaginosis
C	
C	Caucasian
Ca	calcium
CA	cancer
CAD	coronary artery disease
CAH	congenital adrenal hyperplasia
CAIS	complete androgen insensitivity
CAP	community-acquired pneumonia
CARPREG	Cardiac Disease in Pregnancy Score
c/b	complicated by
CBC	complete blood count
CCAM	congenital cystic adenomatoid malformation
CCB	calcium channel blocker
CD	cesarean delivery/Crohns disease
CDC	Centers for Disease Control and Prevention
CDH	congenital diaphragmatic hernia
CEE	conjugated equine estrogen
CF	cystic fibrosis
CFU	colony-forming units
CGH	comparative genomic hybridization
CHD	congenital heart disease
CHF	congestive heart failure
chorio	chorioamnionitis
CHTN	chronic hypertension
CI	confidence interval/contraindication
CIC	clean intermittent self-catheterization
CIN	cervical intraepithelial neoplasia
CIS	carcinoma in situ
CIWA-Ar	Clinical Institute Withdrawal Assessment for Alcohol, Revised
CKC	Cold Knife Conization
CKD	chronic kidney disease
CKI	creatine kinase inhibitor
CK-MB	creatine kinase-MB
CL	cervical length
CM	Certified Midwife
CMP	Comprehensive Metabolic Profile
CMV	cytomegalovirus
CNM	Certified Nurse-Midwives
CNS	Central Nervous System
CO	cardiac output
COC	combined oral contraceptive
COCP	combined oral contraceptive pills
COH	controlled ovarian hyperstimulation
Const Del	constitutional delay
COP	colloid osmotic pressure

COPD	chronic obstructive pulmonary disease
Cort	corticosteroid
COX	cyclo-oxygenase
CP	cerebral palsy
CPAM	congenital pulmonary airway malformation
CPAP	continuous positive airway pressure
CPCs	choroid plexus cysts
CPD	cephalopelvic disproportion
CPM	Certified Professional Midwives
CPP	chronic pelvic pain
CPR	cardiopulmonary resuscitation
CR	cervical ripening
CrCl	creatinine clearance
CREST	Collaborative Review of Sterilization
CRF	chronic renal failure
CRH	corticotropin-releasing hormone
CRL	crown-rump length
CRP	c-reactive protein
crypto	cryptosporidiosis
CS	cesarean section
CSII	continuous subcutaneous insulin infusion
C&S	culture & sensitivity
CSE	combined spinal–epidural
CSF	cerebrospinal fluid
CT	computed tomography
CTA	CT angiography
CTCAE	common terminology criteria for adverse events
CTD	connective tissue disease
CTEPH	chronic thromboembolic pulmonary hypertension
CTS	carpal tunnel syndrome/conflict tactics scale
CTV	CT venography
CTX	chest x-ray/contractions
CUS	compression ultrasonography
CVA	cerebrovascular accident
CVC	central venous catheter
CVD	cardiovascular disease
CVP	central venous pressure
CVS	chorionic villus sampling
CVT	cerebral venous thrombosis
CVVH	continuous venovenous hemofiltration
c/w	consistent with
D	
DBP	diastolic blood pressure
D&C	dilation and curettage
DCIS	ductal carcinoma in situ
DCM	dilated cardiomyopathy
DDx	differential diagnosis
D&E	dilation & evacuation
DEM	Direct Entry Midwives
DES	diethylstilbestrol

DEXA	dual-energy x-ray absorptiometry	**EOC**	epithelial ovarian cancer
DHEA-S	dehydroepiandrosterone sulfate	**EPDS**	Edinburgh postnatal depression scale
DHT	dihydrotestosterone	**EPT**	expedited partner therapy
DIC	disseminated intravascular coagulation	**ER**	emergency department/room
dig	digoxin	**ERCD**	elective repeat cesarean delivery
DKA	diabetic ketoacidosis	**ERCP**	endoscopic retrograde cholangiopancreatography
DMPA	depot medroxyprogesterone acetate	**ERV**	expiratory reserve volume
DMSO	dimethyl sulfoxide	**Erythro**	erythromycin
DMT	disease-modifying treatments	**ES**	elastic stockings
		ESR	erythrocyte sedimentation rate
DOAC	direct oral anticoagulant	**ESRD**	end-stage renal disease
DPG	diphosphoglycerate	**ET**	endometrial thickness/ estrogen therapy
dsDNA	double-stranded DNA		
DSM	Diagnostic and statistical manual of mental disorders	**EUA**	examination under anesthesia
		exp	expiratory
DTR	deep tendon reflex	**evid**	evidence
DV	domestic violence		
DVT	deep vein thrombosis	**F**	
dysfxn	dysfunction	**FASD**	fetal alcohol spectrum disorder
dz	disease	**FAST**	focused assessment sonography for trauma
E		**FDA**	Food and Drug Administration
EAS	external anal sphincter	**FDG**	fluorodeoxyglucose
EBL	estimated blood loss	**FEIBA**	factor eight inhibitor bypassing activity
EBRT	external beam radiation therapy		
EBV	Epstein–Barr virus	FE_{Na}	fractional excretion of sodium
EC	emergency contraception/ endometrial carcinoma	FE_{urea}	fractional excretion of urea
		FEV	forced expiratory volume
ECC	endocervical curettage	**ffDNA**	free fetal DNA
ECG	electrocardiogram	**fFN**	fetal fibronectin
ECHO	echocardiogram	**FFP**	fresh-frozen plasma
ECMO	extracorporeal membrane oxygenation	**FH**	fundal height
		FHH	familial hypocalciuric hypercalcemia
ECT	electroconvulsive therapy		
ECV	external cephalic version	**FHM**	fetal heart motion
EDD	estimated date of delivery	**FHR**	fetal heart rate
EDS	Ehlers–Danlos Syndrome	**FHRT**	FHR tracing
EE	ethinyl estradiol	**FHT**	fetal heart tones
EF	ejection fraction	**FHx**	family history
EFM	external fetal monitoring	**FIGO**	International Federation of Gynecology and Obstetrics
EFW	estimated fetal weight		
EGA	estimated gestational age		
EH	endometrial hyperplasia	**FISH**	fluorescence in situ hybridization
EIC	endometrial intraepithelial carcinoma		
		FL	femur length
EIF	echogenic intracardiac focus	**FLM**	fetal lung maturity
		FM	fetal movement
ELISA	enzyme-linked immunosorbent assay	**FMH**	fetomaternal hemorrhage
		FMP	final menstrual period
EMACO	etoposide, methotrexate, actinomycin D, cytoxan, oncovin	**FNA**	fine-needle aspiration
		FRC	functional residual capacity
		FRAX	Fracture Risk Assessment Tool
EMAEP	etoposide, methotrexate, actinomycin, and cisplatinum/carboplatin	**FSE**	fetal scalp electrode
		FSH	follicle-stimulating hormone
		FTA-ABS	fluorescent treponemal antibody absorption
EMB	endometrial biopsy	**FTT**	failure to thrive
EMBx	endometrial biopsy	**FVIII**	factor VIII
EMG	electromyography	**FVL**	factor V Leiden
EMS	emergency medical service/ endometrial stripe	**FU**	fluorouracil
		FVC	forced vital capacity

fx	fracture or function
fxn	function

G

GA	general anesthesia
G20210A	prothrombin G20210A
GABA	gamma-aminobutyric acid
GAD	glutamic acid decarboxylase
GB	gall bladder
GBS	group B *Streptococcus*
GC/CT	Neisseria gonorrhoeae/Chlamydia trachomatis
G-CSF	granulocyte colony-stimulating factor
GCT	granulosa cell tumor
GDM	gestational diabetes mellitus
GDPP	gonadotropin-dependent (central) precocious puberty
GERD	gastroesophageal reflux disease
GFR	glomerular filtration rate
GGT	γ-glutamyl transpeptidase
GH	growth hormone
GHTN	gestational hypertension
GLT	glucose loading test
GNR	Gram negative rods
GnRH	gonadotropin-releasing hormone
G6PD	glucose-6-phosphate dehydrogenase
GS	gestational sac
GTN	gestational trophoblastic neoplasia
GTT	glucose tolerance test
GU	genitourinary
GVHD	graft-versus-host disease
GYN/ONC	gynecologic oncology

H

H	Hispanic
HA	headache/hemolytic anemia
HAART	highly active antiretroviral therapy
HAP	hospital-acquired pneumonia
HAV	hepatitis A virus
HbA	hemoglobin A
HbA1c	hemoglobin A1c
HBcAg	hepatitis B core antigen
HbEP	hemoglobin electrophoresis
HbF	hemoglobin F
HbS	hemoglobin S
HbSC	Hemoglobin SC
HbSS	Hemoglobin SS
HBV	hepatitis B virus
HDFN	hemolytic disease of the fetus and newborn
HC	head circumference
HCAP	healthcare-associated pneumonia
hCG	human chorionic gonadotropin
HCV	hepatitis C virus
HCT	hematocrit
HDL	high-density lipoprotein

HDR	high-dose rate
HDS	hemodynamically stable
HDV	hepatitis D virus
HEAA	hydroxyethoxyacetic acid
HEG	hyperemesis gravidarum
HELLP	Hemolysis, Elevated Liver enzymes, Low Platelets
HepBIg	hepatitis B immune globulin
HER	human epidermal growth factor receptor
HEV	hepatitis E virus
H/H	hemoglobin and hematocrit
HIDA	hepatobiliary iminodiacetic acid
HIFU	high-intensity focused ultrasound
HIT	heparin-induced thrombocytopenia
HIV	human immunodeficiency virus
HK	hypokinesis
HL	humerus length
HLA	human leukocyte antigen
HLHS	hypoplastic left heart syndrome
HMB	heavy menstrual bleeding
hMG	human menopausal gonadotropin
H&P	history and physical exam
HNPCC	hereditary nonpolyposis colorectal cancer
HPI	history of present illness
HoNa	hyponatremia
HoTN	hypotension
HPA	hypothalamic–pituitary–adrenal
hPL	human placental lactogen
HPO	hypothalamic–pituitary–ovarian
HPV	human papilloma virus
HQOL	health-related QOL
HRT	hormone replacement therapy
HSDD	hypoactive sexual desire disorder
HSG	hysterosalpingogram
HSM	hepatosplenomegaly
HSV	herpes simplex virus
HT	hormone therapy
HTLV	human T-cell lymphotropic virus
HTN	hypertension
HUS	hemolytic uremic syndrome
hyperaldo	hyperaldosteronism
hyperK	hyperkalemia
HyperNa	hypernatremia
hyperphos	hyperphosphatemia
HypoCa	hypocalcemia
hypoK	hypokalemia
hypophos	hypophosphatemia

I

IAS	internal anal sphincter
IBD	inflammatory bowel disease
IBS	irritable bowel syndrome

IC	inspiratory capacity/interstitial cystitis	LARC	long acting reversible contraception
ICH	intracerebral hemorrhage	LBP	low back pain
ICP	intrahepatic cholestasis of pregnancy	LBW	lean body weight/low birth weight
ICSI	intracytoplasmic sperm injection	LCIS	lobular carcinoma in situ
ICU	intensive care unit	LCHAD	long-chain 3-hydroxyacyl-CoA dehydrogenase
I&D	incision & drainage	L&D	labor and delivery
IDSM	Isotope dilution mass spectrometry	LDH	lactate dehydrogenase
IEA	inferior epigastric artery	LDL	low-density lipoprotein
IFN	interferon	LDR	low-dose rate
IGF	insulin-like growth factor	LDUH	low-dose UFH
IMRT	intensity-modulated radiation therapy	LE	lower extremity
incl	includes/including	LEEP	loop electrosurgical excision procedure
INH	isoniazid	Levo	levofloxacin
innomin	innominate	LFT	liver function tests
INR	international normalized ratio	LGA	large for gestational age
intravag	intravaginal	LH	luteinizing hormone
I&O	input/output	LMP	last menstrual period
IOL	induction of labor	LMWH	low–molecular-weight heparin
IOM	Institute of Medicine	LND	lymph node dissection
IP	infundibulopelvic/ intraperitoneal	LNG IUD	levonorgestrel-releasing intrauterine device
IPCD	intermittent pneumatic compression devices	LNG-IUS	levonorgestrel intrauterine system
IPV	intimate partner violence	LOF	leakage of fluid
IR	immediate release	LP	low pressure/lumbar puncture
IRV	inspiratory reserve volume	LPP	leak point pressure
ISD	intrinsic sphincteric deficiency	LPS	lipopolysaccharides
ITP	immune thrombocytopenia purpura	LPV	localized provoked vulvodynia
		L/S	lecithin/sphingomyelin
IUD	intrauterine device	LSC	laparoscopic
IUFD	intrauterine fetal demise	LUNA	laparoscopic uterosacral nerve ablation
IUGR	intrauterine growth restriction	LVEF	left ventricular ejection fraction
IUI	intrauterine insemination	LVSI	lymphovascular space involvement
IUP	intrauterine pregnancy		
IUPC	intrauterine pressure catheter		
IUS	intrauterine system	**M**	
IV	intravenous	MAC	methotrexate, actinomycin D, cytoxan
IVC	inferior vena cava	MAOI	monoamine oxidase inhibitor
IVDU	intravenous drug use	MAP	mean arterial pressure
IVF	in vitro fertilization	MCA	middle cerebral artery
IVH	intraventricular hemorrhage	MCC	menstrual cycle cessation
IVIG	intravenous immunoglobulin	MCV	mean corpuscular volume
IVP	intravenous pyelogram	MDCT	multidetector CT
		MDD	major depressive disorder
		MDI	metered dose inhaler/multiple daily injection
J			
JVD	jugular venous distension	MDPA	medroxyprogesterone acetate
JVP	jugular venous pressure	MDR	multidrug resistant
		MDS	myelodysplastic syndrome
K		MEC	Medical Eligibility Criteria/ meconium
K-B	Kleihauer–Betke		
KOH	potassium hydroxide	MEN	multiple endocrine neoplasia
KUB	kidneys, ureters, bladder	MESA	microsurgical epididymal sperm aspiration
		MI	myocardial infarction
L		MIBG	metaiodobenzylguanidine
LA	left atrium/lupus anticoagulant	MIF	Müllerian inhibitory factor
LAD	lymphadenopathy	MIS	Müllerian inhibiting substance
LAIV	live attenuated influenza vaccine	Mitoc	mitochondrial

MIVF	maintenance intravenous fluid	**NPV**	negative predictive value
MFM	maternal fetal medicine	**NNRTI**	nonnucleoside reverse transcriptase inhibitor
MMK	Marshall–Marchetti–Krantz		
MMMT	malignant mixed müllerian tumor (uterine carcinosarcoma)	**NNT**	number needed to treat
		NOAC	non-vitamin K oral anticoagulant
MMP	matrix metalloproteinase	**NPH**	neutral protamine Hagedorn
MMR	measles, mumps, rubella	**NRFHT**	nonreassuring fetal heart tracing
MOA	mechanism of action	**NS**	normal saline
MoM	multiple of the median	**NSAID**	nonsteroidal antiinflammatory drug
MPA	medroxyprogesterone acetate		
MR	mental retardation/mitral regurgitation	**NST**	nonstress test
		NSAIDs	nonsteroidal anti-inflammatory drugs
MRA	magnetic resonance angiography		
		NSTEMI	non-ST segment elevation MI
MRAT	melanoma risk assessment tool	**NT**	neural tube
		NT	nuchal translucency
MRgFUS	Magnetic Resonance-Guided Focused Ultrasound	**NTD**	neural tube defect
		N/V	nausea and vomiting
MRKH	Mayer–Rokitansky–Kuster–Hauser	**NVP**	negative predictive value
MRSA	methicillin-resistant *Staph aureus*	**NYHA**	New York Heart Association
MRV	magnetic resonance venography	**O**	
		OAB	overactive bladder
MS	mitral stenosis	**OASIS**	obstetric anal sphincter injury
MSAFP	maternal serum AFP	**OB**	obstetrics
MSD	mean sac diameter	**OC**	obstetric conjugate
MSH	melanocyte-stimulating hormone	**OCP**	oral contraceptive pill
		OD	optical density
MSK	musculoskeletal	**OEIS**	omphalocele-exstrophy-imperforate anus-spinal defects
MSM	Men Who Have Sex With Men		
MSSA	methicillin-sensitive *Staphylococcus aureus*		
		OGTT	oral glucose tolerance test
MTC	medullary thyroid cancer	**OHSS**	ovarian hyperstimulation syndrome
MTX	methotrexate		
MUCP	maximal urethral closure pressure	**OHVIRA**	obstructed hemivagina and ipsilateral renal anomaly
MUGA	multigated acquisition		
MUI	mixed urinary incontinence	**OI**	opportunistic infection
MV	mitral valve	**O&P**	ova and parasite
MVI	multivitamin	**OPK**	Ovulation Prediction Kit
MVP	maximum vertical pocket	**OR**	odds ratio/operating room
MVU	Montevideo Units	**OSA**	obstructive sleep apnea
		OTC	over-the-counter
N		**P**	
NAAT	nucleic acid amplification test	**PA**	posterior–anterior/pulmonary artery
NAIT	neonatal alloimmune thrombocytopenia		
		PA	primitive atrium
NB	nasal bone	**PAC**	pulmonary artery catheter
NCAH	nonclassical congenital adrenal hyperplasia	**PAIS**	partial/incomplete AIS
		PAH	pulmonary arterial hypertension
NCI	National Cancer Institute		
NE	norepinephrine	**pANCAs**	perinuclear antineutrophil cytoplasmic antibodies
NEC	necrotizing enterocolitis		
NETA	norethindrone acetate	**PARP**	poly ADP ribose polymerase
NGT	nasogastric tube	**PAP**	pulmonary artery pressure
NICHD	National Institute of Child Health and Human Development	**PAPP-A**	pregnancy-associated plasma protein A
		PCA	patient-controlled analgesia
NICU	neonatal intensive care unit	**PCEA**	patient-controlled epidural analgesia
NIH	National Institute of Health		
NIHF	nonimmune hydrops fetalis	**PCI**	percutaneous coronary intervention
nml	normal		

PCKD	polycystic kidney disease
PCN	penicillin
PCOS	polycystic ovary syndrome
PCP	primary care physician
PCr	plasma creatinine
PCR	polymerase chain reaction
PCWP	pulmonary capillary wedge pressure
PD	primary dysmenorrhea
PDA	patent ductus arteriosus
PDPH	postdural puncture headache
PE	pulmonary embolism
PEC	preeclampsia
PEFR	peak expiratory flow rate
PEG	polyethylene glycol
PET	positron emission tomography
PFT	pulmonary function test
PG	phosphatidylglycerol/prostaglandins
PGD	preimplantation genetic diagnosis
PGE2	prostaglandin E2
PGF	prostaglandin F
PGS	preimplantation genetic screening
pheo	pheochromocytoma
PHQ	Patient Health Questionnaire
pHTN	pulmonary hypertension
PHV	peak height velocity
PI	protease inhibitor
PID	pelvic inflammatory disease
PIERS	Preeclampsia Integrated Estimate of Risk
PlGF	placental growth factor
PIH	pregnancy induced hypertension
PJP	*Pneumocystis jirovecii pneumonia*
PLAP	placental alkaline phosphatase
PLT	platelets
PMB	postmenopausal bleeding
PMDD	premenstrual dysphoric disorder
PMFT	pelvic floor muscle training
PMH	past medical history
PMI	point of maximal impulse
PMN	polymorphonuclear lymphocytes
PMNC	polymorphonuclear cell
PMP	postmenopausal
PNC	prenatal care
PMS	premenstrual syndrome
PNa	plasma sodium
PNA	pneumonia
PNV	prenatal vitamin
POC	products of conception
POI	premature ovarian insufficiency
POP	progestin-only pill/pelvic organ prolapse
POP-Q	pelvic organ prolapse quantification
PORTEC	postoperative radiation therapy in endometrial cancer
PP	postpartum

PPD	purified protein derivative
PPE	palmar plantar erythrodysesthesia
PPH	postpartum hemorrhage
PPI	proton pump inhibitor
PPROM	preterm premature rupture of membranes
PPV	positive predictive value
ppx	prophylaxis
PR	per rectum/pulmonary regurgitation
PRAMS	Pregnancy Risk Assessment Monitoring System
PRBC	packed red blood cells
PRES	posterior reversible encephalopathy syndrome
PRL	prolactin
progest	progestin
PROM	premature rupture of membranes
PSI	pneumonia severity index
PSH	past surgical history
PSV	peak systolic velocity
PT	prothrombin time
ptb/PTB	preterm birth
pt	patient
PTD	preterm delivery
PTEN	Phosphatase and tensin homolog
PTH	parathyroid hormone
PTHrP	parathyroid hormone–related protein
PTL	preterm labor
PTSD	post-traumatic stress disorder
PTU	propylthiouracil
PTX	pneumothorax
PUBS	periumbilical blood sampling
PUPPP	Pruritic Urticarial Papules and Plaques of Pregnancy
PUVA	psoralen and ultraviolet A
PV	per vagina/primitive ventricle
PVA	polyvinyl alcohol
PVD	peripheral vascular disease
PVR	postvoid residual/pulmonary vascular resistance
pyelo	pyelonephritis

Q	
QD	daily
QHS	at night
QOL	quality of life

R	
RA	right atrium
RAI	radioactive iodine
RAIR	rectoanal inhibitory reflex
RAIU	radioactive iodine uptake
Rb	retinoblastoma
RBBB	right bundle branch block
RBC	red blood cell
RCRI	revised cardiac risk index
RCT	randomized control trial

RCVS	reversible cerebral vasoconstriction syndromes	**SLE**	systemic lupus erythematosus
		SMA	spinal muscular atrophy
		SMX	sulfamethoxazole
RDS	respiratory distress syndrome	**SNM**	sacral nerve modulation
RDW	red cell distribution width	**SNRIs**	serotonin and norepinephrine reuptake inhibitors
REDF	reversed end-diastolic flow		
retic	reticulocyte	**SOB**	shortness of breath
RF(s)	risk factor(s)	**sPEC**	severe preeclampsia
RhD	Rhesus D	**SPEP**	serum protein electrophoresis
RI	reticulocyte index	**Spont**	spontaneous
RIBA	recombinant immunoblot assay	**SQ**	subcutaneous
		SS	sliding scale
RFA	radiofrequency thermal ablation	**SSA/SSB**	Anti-Sjögren's-syndrome-related antigen A and B
RLS	restless leg syndrome		
RN	registered nurse	**SSI**	surgical site infection
RNA	ribonucleic acid	**SSRI**	selective serotonin reuptake inhibitor
ROA	right occiput anterior		
ROM	rupture of membranes	**Std**	standard
RPL	recurrent pregnancy loss/retroperitoneal lymphadenectomy	**STD**	sexually transmitted disease
		STEMI	ST segment elevation MI
		STI	sexually transmitted infection/disease
RPR	rapid plasma reagin		
RR	relative risk	**SUI**	stress urinary incontinence
RRMS	relapsing remitting multiple sclerosis	**SUFU**	Society of Urodynamics, Female Pelvic Medicine, & Urogenital Reconstruction
RRT	renal replacement therapy		
RSV	respiratory syncytial virus	**SV**	stroke volume
RT	radiation therapy	**SVD**	spontaneous vaginal delivery
RUSB	right upper sternal border	**SVR**	systemic vascular resistance
RUQ	right upper quadrant	**SVT**	supraventricular tachycardia
RV	residual volume/right ventricle		
rx/rxn	reaction	**T**	
		T	testosterone
S		**TA**	transabdominal
SAB	spontaneous abortion	**TAH**	total abdominal hysterectomy
SAH	subarachnoid hemorrhage	**T-ACE**	Tolerance, Annoyed, Cut down, Eye opener
SARS	severe acute respiratory syndrome		
		TB	tuberculosis
SBE	subacute bacterial endocarditis	**TBG**	thyroxine-binding globulin
		TBW	total body water
SBO	small bowel obstruction	**TC**	transcervical
SBP	systolic blood pressure	**T&C**	type and crossmatch
SCAD	spontaneous coronary artery dissection	**TCA**	tricyclic antidepressant
		TDF	testis determining factor
SCC	squamous cell carcinoma	**TDaP**	tetanus, diphtheria, acellular pertussis
SCD	sequential compression device		
SCID	severe combined immunodeficiency disease	**TDx-FLM**	fetal lung maturity test
		T2DM	Type II diabetes mellitus
SD	secondary dysmenorrhea	**TE**	tracheoesophageal
S/D	systolic/diastolic	**TENS**	transcutaneous electrical nerve stimulation
SDP	single deepest pocket		
SE profile	side-effect profile	**TESE**	testicular sperm extraction
SERM	selective estrogen receptor modulators	**TG**	triglycerides
		thal	thalassemia
SF	severe features	**TIA**	transient ischemic attack
sFlt	soluble fms-like tyrosine kinase-1 (= sVEGFR-1)	**TIBC**	total iron-binding capacity
		TFT	thyroid function test(s)
		THC	tetrahydrocannabinol/marijuana
SGA	small for gestational age		
SIDS	sudden infant death syndrome	**TLC**	total lung capacity
Signif	significant	**TLH**	total laparoscopic hysterectomy
SIRS	systemic inflammatory response syndrome		
		TMJ	temporomandibular joint
SIS	saline infusion sonography sonohysterography	**TMP**	trimethoprim
		TNF	tumor necrosis factor
SL	sublingual	**TNM**	tumor, node, metastasis

TOA	tuboovarian abscess
TOCO	tocodynamometer
TOLAC	trial of labor after prior cesarean
TOT	transobturator tape
tPA	tissue plasminogen activator
TPN	total parenteral nutrition
TPO	thyroid peroxidase
TR	tricuspid regurgitation
TRAb	TSH receptor antibody
TRALI	transfusion-related lung injury
T&S	type and screen
TSH	thyroid stimulating hormone
TSH-R	TSH receptor
TSI	TSH-stimulating immunoglobulin
TST	tuberculin skin test
TTE	transthoracic echocardiography
TTP–HUS	thrombotic thrombocytopenic purpura–hemolytic uremic syndrome
TTTS	twin-to-twin transfusion syndrome
TX/tx	treatment
TXA	tranexamic acid
TVL	total vaginal length
TVT	tension-free vaginal tape
TVUS	transvaginal ultrasound

U	
UA	urinary albumin
UAE	uterine artery embolization
UC	ulcerative colitis
UCr	urine creatinine
UCx	uterine contractions
uE3	unconjugated estriol
UFH	unfractionated heparin
ULN	upper limit of normal
UNa	urine sodium
uncirc	uncircumcised
UOP	urine output
UPEP	urine protein electrophoresis
UPSC	uterine papillary serous carcinoma
URI	upper respiratory infection
Uro	urology
US	ultrasound/ultrasonography

USPSTF	U.S. Preventive Services Task Force
UTI	urinary tract infection
UUI	urge urinary incontinence

V	
VAIN	vaginal intraepithelial neoplasia
Vanco	vancomycin
VAP	ventilation-associated pneumonia
VB	vaginal birth/vaginal bleeding
VBAC	vaginal birth after cesarean
VBP	vinblastine, bleomycin, carboplatin
VCAM	vascular cell adhesion molecule
VDRL	venereal disease research laboratory
VEGF	vascular endothelial growth factor
VIN	vulvar epithelial neoplasia/ vulvar intraepithelial neoplasia
VMSx	vasomotor symptoms
vol	volume
VS	vital signs
VSx	vasomotor symptoms
VSD	ventriculoseptal defect
VT	tidal volume
VTE	venous thromboembolism
VVF	vesicovaginal fistula
vWD	von Willebrand disease
vWF	von Willebrand factor
Vz/vac	vaccine
VZV	varicella zoster virus

W	
WGA	weeks gestational age
WHI	Women's health initiative
WHO	World Health Organization
w/	with
w/o	without
wnl	within normal limits
WWE	women with epilepsy

X	
XR	extended release/x-ray
XRT	radiation therapy/radiotherapy

Note: Page number followed by f and t indicates figure and table respectively.

A

Abdominal compartment syndrome, post-laparoscopic, 3-11
Abdominal pain, IBS symptoms and, 15-5t
Abdominal radiograph (KUB), 14-7
Abdominal wall, cutaneous nerve entrapment/myofascial pain, 5-13
Abnormal uterine bleeding (AUB), 5-8
Abortion. *See also* Spontaneous abortion
  medical, 5-18, 5-18t
  medical, contraindicated, 5-19t
  surgical, 5-19
Abscess, neuraxial anesthesia and, 4-4t
Absence seizures, 18-3
AC (fetal abdominal circumference), 9-8
Acarbose, 17-8t
Accelerations, fetal heart rate, 10-8, 10-8t, 10-10f
Accidental bowel leakage (ABL), 7-9
ACEI (angiotensin-converting enzyme inhibitor), 12-5, 12-14t
ACE inhibitors, 12-4t
Acetaminophen
  endomyometritis, 11-18
  intraamniotic infection, 11-17
  migraine, 18-2t, 18-3t
  postoperative pain management, 4-7
  pyelonephritis, 14-7
Acetowhite changes, 1-9
Achondroplasia, 9-12
Acidemia, 10-14, 13-3
Aclovate (Alclometasone dipropionate), 20-4t
ACOG (American Congress/College of OB/GYN), 13-6, 21-5
Acral lentiginous melanoma, 1-14
Acromegaly, 17-13f, 17-17
ACTH (adrenocorticotrophin)-stimulation test, 6-12
ACTH (adrenocorticotropic hormone), 17-10t, 17-11f, 17-12, 17-16
Actinomycin D, 22-16t, 25-6t
Acupuncture, 4-6t, 5-14
Acute coronary syndrome (ACS), 12-10
Acute fatty liver of pregnancy (AFLP), 12-7t, 12-8t, 15-11, 15-11t
Acute hemolytic reaction, 16-16t
Acute hypernatremia, 14-9
Acute interstitial nephritis (AIN), 14-1t
Acute kidney injury (AKI), 14-1, 14-1t
Acute pancreatitis, 15-1, 15-3t
Acute pelvic pain, 2-2, 2-2t
Acute renal failure, 3-8, 12-9
Acute tubular necrosis (ATN), 14-1t
Acute urinary retention, 3-10
Acyclovir, 21-11t
Addison disease, 17-10t, 17-11

AdenoCa (adenocarcinoma), 22-2, 22-11
Adenocarcinoma in situ (AIS), 6-7t
Adenomyoma, 5-5
Adenomyosis, 5-5
Adenosarcoma, uterine, 22-6
Adenosquamous carcinoma, 22-2, 22-11
Adjustment disorder, 19-4
Adnexal masses, 5-19, 5-21f
Adnexal torsion, 2-7–2-8
Adrenal cortex, 17-10
Adrenal disorders, 17-10
Adrenal hyperplasia
  congenital, 6-4, 6-11, 17-13f
  late-onset, amenorrhea and, 6-7t
Adrenal insufficiency, 17-11
  perioperative management, 3-3
Adrenal medulla, 17-10
Adrenal tumors, 17-11f, 17-13f
Adrenarche, 6-1
  premature, 6-2t
Adrenocorticotrophin (ACTH)-stimulation test, 6-12
Adriamycin (Doxorubicin), 25-5t
AEDs (antiepileptic drugs), 18-4t, 18-5t, 19-7t
AFC (antral follicle count), 8-2
AFE (amniotic fluid embolism), 10-14, 11-15, 13-5, 13-8, 14-2t
Affiliated obstetrical providers, 10-16
AFI (amniotic fluid index), 9-8, 10-1, 12-5
AFLP (Acute Fatty Liver of Pregnancy), 12-7t, 12-8t, 15-11, 15-11t
AFP (alpha-fetoprotein)
  adnexal masses and, 5-20t
  aneuploidy screening and, 9-12, 9-12t
  embryonal carcinoma and, 22-9
  germ cell tumors and, 22-9
AGC (atypical glandular cells), 1-8, 1-9t
AI/AR (Aortic Insufficiency/ Aortic Regurgitation), pregnancy and, 12-12t, 12-14t
AIDS, 21-1. *See also* HIV
Air/CO$_2$ embolization, 3-11, 3-12
AIS (adenocarcinoma in situ), 1-9
Albumin 5% or 25% solution, 14-9t
Albumin excretion rate, stages of, 14-4
Albuterol, 14-9
Alclometasone dipropionate (Aclovate), 20-4t
Alcohol abuse, 19-1, 19-2t. *See also* EtOH
  withdrawal, seizures and, 18-3
Aldomet (Alphamethyldopa), 25-4t
Alendronate (Fosamax), 25-12t
Alesse, 25-11t
Alkalemia, 13-3
Allergens/allergies
  anaphylaxis and, 13-7
  blood transfusions and, 16-17t
  perioperative review of, 3-1

Alloimmunization, 16-13
  in pregnancy, 16-14f
Alopecia, 22-18
Alpha-fetoprotein (AFP), 5-20t, 9-12, 22-9t
Alphamethyldopa (Aldomet), 25-4t
Alpha-thalassemia, 9-13, 16-3
Alprazolam, 19-6t
Altered mental status (AMS), 3-8.
  See also Mental status
Amcinonide (Amcort, Cyclocort), 20-4t
Amcort (Amcinonide), 20-4t
Amenorrhea, 6-6, 6-7t, 6-8, 6-9f
American Society of Anesthesiologists'
  (ASA) physical status
  classification system, 3-1t
AMH (anti-Müllerian hormone), 8-1, 8-2
Amine odor test, 5-1t
Aminoglycosides, 21-11t
5-Aminosalicylic acid (5-ASA), 15-7t
Amitriptyline, 5-14, 5-15, 7-8, 18-3t
Amlodipine, 12-4t
Amniocentesis, 9-13, 10-2, 11-8, 24-5
Amnionicity, 11-4
Amniotic band syndrome, 9-11
Amniotic fluid embolism (AFE), 11-15
Amniotic fluid index (AFI), 9-8
Amniotic fluid leakage, PPROM and, 11-7
Amniotic fluid volume, 9-8
Amniotomy, 10-7
Amoxicillin, 11-7t, 14-5t, 25-1t
Amoxicillin–clavulanate, 14-6t, 14-7t
Amphetamines, 6-8, 19-2t
Ampicillin
  characteristics/indications, 25-1t
  intraamniotic infection, 11-17t
  PPROM, 11-7t
  pyelonephritis, 14-7t
  UTIs, 14-6t
Amsel clinical criteria for bacterial
  vaginosis, 5-1t
Analgesia
  inhalational, 4-7
  medications, 25-8t
  nonpharmacologic, 4-6
  parenteral, 4-1, 4-2t
Anal incontinence, 7-9
Anal manometry, 7-10
Anal sphincter, artificial, 7-10
Anal sphincteroplasty, overlapping, 7-10
Anaphylaxis, 13-7
Anatomy. *See also* Surgery
  avascular pelvic planes, 23-4f
  blood supply of pelvic organs and
    external genitalia, 23-2f
  bony pelvis, 23-1f
  colon blood supply, 23-5f
  fetal circulation, 23-6f
  internal organs, posterior view, 23-1f
  pelvic arterial blood supply, 23-3f
  pelvis, 9-4
  upper abdominal blood supply, 23-5f

ureter course and relationship to
    vulnerable sites, 23-2f
  urogenital triangle and pelvic floor, 23-6f
Ancef (cefazolin), 25-1t
Androgen excess, 6-11
Androgen insensitivity syndrome, 6-9
Androgens, 6-7t, 17-10, 22-9t, 22-10
Android pelvis, 9-5, 9-5f, 9-5t
Anemia
  initial approach to, 16-2f
  perioperative optimization of, 3-2
  PMS or PMDD vs., 5-13
  in pregnancy, 16-1
Anesthesia, 4-1
  general, 4-6
  local, 4-5
  neuraxial, 4-2
Aneuploidy, 9-8, 9-11, 9-12
Angina, unstable, 12-10
Angiotensin receptor blocker (ARB),
    11-1, 12-4t, 12-5
Anion gap, diabetic ketoacidosis and,
    17-3t
Anorectal cytomegalovirus, 21-6
Antabuse (Disulfiram), 25-9t
Anterior colporrhaphy, 7-3
Anterior compartment defect surgery,
    7-3
Anterior pelvic organ prolapse, 7-1
Anterior pelvis, 9-4
Anterior pituitary, 17-16
Anthropoid pelvis, 9-5, 9-5f, 9-5t
Antiandrogens, 6-12
Antiangiogenesis agents, 22-17
Antibiotics
  Bartholin duct abscess, 5-3
  characteristics of specific types,
    25-1t
  endomyometritis, 11-18
  GBS disease, 10-3, 10-3f
  IBD, 15-7t
  intraamniotic infection, 11-17,
    11-17t
  ob-gyn surgery prophylaxis, 3-7t
  pneumonia, 13-4
  preoperative, 3-3
  sepsis, 3-9
  surgical abortion, 5-19
Anticardiolipin antibodies, 16-12t
Anticholinergics, 7-5, 7-6, 7-6t, 7-7
Anticoagulants, 25-4t
Anticoagulation
  duration, 16-9t
  perioperative stopping, 3-2
  recurrent pregnancy loss and, 8-4
  reversal, 16-11
  thrombophilia in pregnancy and
    postpartum, 16-11t
Anticonvulsants, steroid levels and, 18-5
Antiemetics, 25-8t
Antiepileptic drugs (AEDs), 18-4t,
    18-5t, 19-7t
Antifibrinolytics, 11-10
Anti-HBc/anti-HBs, 15-8, 15-8t

Antihypertensives, 25-4t
Anti-Müllerian hormone (AMH), 8-1, 8-2
Antimuscarinics, 7-6t, 7-7
Antiphospholipid antibodies, 8-4
Antiphospholipid antibody syndrome (APS), 16-12, 16-12t, 16-13t
Antiprogestins, 5-4
Antipsychotics, 6-6, 19-7t
Anti-RhD immunoglobulin, 16-13, 16-14t
Antithyroid drugs (ATDs), 17-9
Anti-β2 glycoprotein-I Ab, 16-12t
Antral follicle count, 8-1
Anxiety disorders, 19-4
Aortic disease, 12-12t, 12-14t
Aortic regurgitation (AR), 12-13
Aortic stenosis (AS), 12-12t, 12-13, 12-13t, 12-14t
AP (anteroposterior) diameter of pelvis, 9-4, 9-5t
ApexiCon (Diflorasone diacetate), 20-4t
Apical pelvic organ prolapse, 7-1
Apidra (Glulisine), 17-3t
Apocrine miliaria, 20-5
Appendiceal abscess, 2-7
Appendicitis, 2-2t, 15-3
APRN (advanced practice registered nurse), 10-16t
AR (aortic regurgitation), 12-13
ARB (angiotensin receptor blocker), 11-1
Arcuate uterus, 8-6f
ARDS (acute respiratory distress syndrome), 8-12, 14-6
Aromatase inhibitors, 5-4, 5-7, 6-3, 22-17
Arrest of labor in 1st stage, definition of, 10-4
Arrhythmias, 12-2
Arterial blood gas (ABG) analysis, 13-3, 13-3t, 16-8
AS (aortic stenosis), 12-12t, 12-13, 12-13t, 12-14t
ASA. See Aspirin
ASCUS (atypical cells of undetermined significance), 1-8, 1-9t
Asherman syndrome, 6-7t, 6-8
Aspart (NovoLog), 17-3t
Aspirin (ASA)
    acute coronary syndrome, 12-10
    characteristics/indications, 25-8t
    IBD, 15-7t
    migraine, 18-2t, 18-3t
    valvular heart disease, 12-14t
ASRM (American Society for Reproductive Medicine) endometriosis criteria, 5-6
Assisted hatching (AH), 8-10
Assisted reproductive technology (ART), 8-9, 8-11, 11-4
Association, congenital anomalies and, 9-9

Asthma, 4-1, 13-6, 13-7t
ASVDs (atrial and ventricular septal defects), 9-11
Asymptomatic bacteriuria, 14-4
Asystole, 26-2f
Atenolol, 12-4t
AT-III (antithrombin III), 16-10t
Atonic seizures, 18-3
Atopic eruption of pregnancy, 20-2t
Atorvastatin, 12-10
Atorvastatin (Lipitor), 1-10t
Atrial septal defect (ASD), 9-10
Atrioventricular (AV) block, 14-10
Atypical hyperplasia of breast, 1-6
Autoimmune diseases or disorders
    anemia, 16-3
    dermatologic manifestations, 20-7
    Hashimoto thyroiditis, 17-8
    hypergonadotropic hypogonadism, 6-5
Autologous blood donation, 16-16t
Avastin, 25-5t
Aygestin (norethindrone acetate), 2-10t
Azathioprine, 15-7t
Azithromycin, 2-13, 21-11t, 25-2t
Aztreonam, 14-6t

B
Bacterial infections
    blood transfusions and, 16-17t
    pneumonia, 13-4t
Bacterial vaginosis (BV), 5-1t
Bacteriuria, asymptomatic, 14-4, 14-5t
Bactrim, 25-2t
Bactrim BID, 21-11t
Balloon catheter, 10-7
Bandl's ring, 4-6
Barrier contraception, 1-17t
Bartholin duct cyst or abscess, 2-2t, 5-2
Bartholin gland cyst, 20-6t, 24-2, 24-3f, 24-5
Bartholin's gland carcinoma, 22-12, 22-13
Basal body temperature, 17-1f
Basal cell carcinoma, 1-13, 22-13
    vulvar, 22-12
BAV (bicuspid aortic valve), 12-12t, 12-14t
Bayley–Pinneau tables, 6-5
Bazedoxifene, 5-18t
Beckwith–Wiedemann syndrome, 9-11
Behçet disease, 20-7
Bell's palsy, 18-8
Bendroflumethiazide, 12-4t
Benign or nonprogressive pubertal variants, 6-2t
Benzathine, 21-11t
Benzodiazepines, 5-13, 19-6t
Betamethasone, 25-10t
Betamethasone dipropionate (Diprolene), 20-4t
Betamethasone valerate (Beta-Val, Valisone), 20-4t
Beta-mimetics, 11-8t
Beta-thalassemia, 16-3

β-Blockers
  acute coronary syndrome, 12-10
  chronic hypertension, 12-4t
  cocaine-induced hypertension and, 19-3t
  epinephrine contraindications and, 4-1
  peripartum cardiomyopathy, 12-14t
  valvular heart disease, 12-14t
β-lactam, 3-7
Bevacizumab, 22-3t, 22-17, 25-5t
BiAsp 70/30 (BIAsp 30), 17-3t
Bicarbonate, serum, 17-3
  diabetic ketoacidosis and, 17-3t, 17-4
Bicornuate uterus, 8-5f, 8-6t, 8-7, 11-16
Biguanides, 17-8t
Bile acid sequestrants, 1-11t
Binge drinking, 19-1
Bioidentical hormones, compounded, 5-18t
Biofeedback, 5-15
Biomarkers
  adnexal masses, 5-20
  bone turnover, 1-13
Biophysical fetal profile, 10-1
Bioprosthetic heart valves, 12-14
Biopsy, endometrial, 24-5
Bipolar disorder, 19-5
BIRADS (Breast Imaging Reporting and Data System) score, 1-4t
Birth defects, UTI medications and, 14-5t
Bisacodyl (Dulcolax), 9-7t
Bisacodyl suppository, 9-7t
Bishop score, 10-6t
Bisphosphonates, 1-13, 6-3, 14-10, 25-12t
Black powder burn, 5-6
Bladder
  dysfunction, neural tube defects and, 9-10
  exstrophy, 9-11
  injuries, 3-10
  innervation of, 7-1t
  overactive, 7-4, 7-5
  prolapse into vagina, 7-1
Bladder diary, 7-8
Bladder diverticulum, ovarian cyst vs., 2-7
Bleeding. See also Abnormal uterine bleeding; Hemorrhage; Postpartum hemorrhage
  post-laparoscopic, 3-11
Bleomycin, 25-5t
α-Blockers for overflow incontinence, 7-7
Blood loss with delivery, 16-1
Blood pressure (BP), hypertension and, 12-3t
Blood products for hemorrhage and critical care, 16-15t
Blood supply
  pelvic arteries, 23-3f
  pelvic arteries, surgical considerations, 23-3t

pelvic organs and external genitalia, 23-2f
Blood transfusion
  complications, 16-17t
  massive transfusion, 16-17, 16-18t
  postpartum hemorrhage, 11-10
Blood type testing, preoperative, 3-3
Blood volume, pregnancy, 12-2
Blueberry muffin rash, 21-3
Blunt trauma, 2-11
B-Lynch compression sutures, for postpartum hemorrhage, 11-10, 11-11f
Body mass index (BMI), 9-3t, 17-6t
Bone age, precocious puberty and, 6-3
Bone marrow toxicity, 25-7
Borders of standard pelvic fields, EBRT and, 22-18
Boric acid, for vaginitis, 5-2t
Botulinum toxin type A (Botox) injection, 7-6, 7-9
Bowel dysfunction, neural tube defects and, 9-10
Bowel obstruction, 3-10
Bowel preparation, preoperative, 3-3
Bowen's disease, 1-14
BPD (biparietal diameter), in fetal ultrasound, 9-8
BPH (benign prostatic hyperplasia), 7-7
Brachial plexus nerve, gynecologic surgery and, 3-5t
Brachytherapy, 22-18
  anatomic points for, 22-19
Bradycardia
  fetal heart rate, 10-8t
  with a pulse, Adult Algorithm, 26-3f
BRAT diet, 9-5
BRCA mutation, 1-6, 5-20, 22-7
Breast cancer, 1-5
Breast cysts, 1-5t
Breast development, 6-1f, 6-1t
Breast disease, benign, 1-4f
Breastfeeding
  contraception and, 10-15
  HIV/AIDS in women and, 21-2
  influenza, 13-6
  nutrition and, 9-3
  postoperative pain management and, 4-7
Breast stimulation, induction of labor and, 10-7
Breathing, nonpharmacologic analgesia and, 4-6t
Breech extraction, 4-2, 4-6
Breech presentation, 10-4, 11-16t
Brenner/transitional cell carcinoma, 22-7
Brenner tumors, 5-20
Breslow staging, for melanoma, 22-13t
Brief Sexual Symptom checklist, 5-15
Bromocriptine, 6-8
Brucellosis, 9-4
BSO (bilateral salpingo-oophorectomy), 5-7, 5-14
Bupivacaine, 4-1t, 4-4t, 4-7

Buprenorphine (Butrans), 19-3t, 25-9t
Bupropion (Wellbutrin), 25-9t
Burns, 2-11
Butoconazole, 5-2t
BV (bacterial vaginosis), 5-1t
Bypass incontinence, 7-7

C
CA-125, 5-20, 5-20t, 22-5
Cabergoline, 6-8, 8-12
Caffeine, 9-4
CAGE/CAGE-AID, 19-1t
Calcitonin, 1-13, 25-12t
Calcium, 1-13, 9-4t, 17-4
Calcium-based nephrolithiasis, 14-7
Calcium carbonate, 5-13
Calcium channel blockers (CCBs),
    11-8t, 12-4t, 12-14t
Calcium chloride, 14-9
Calcium gluconate, 14-9
Calcium supplements, 5-17
Caldwell & Moloy classification, 9-5
Canavan disease, 9-13
Cancer. See also specific types
    host–tumor interactions and, 22-17f
    screening, 1-3
Candesartan, 12-4t
Candida albicans, 5-1t
Candida glabrata, 5-1t, 5-2t
Candidiasis, 5-1t
CAP (community-acquired pneumonia),
    13-4
Captopril, 12-4t
Carbamazepine, 18-4t, 19-7t
Carbohydrates, in pregnancy, 9-4t
Carboplatin, 22-18, 25-5t
Carboplatinum, 22-17
Carboprost (Hemabate), 25-6t
Carcinosarcoma
    ovarian, 22-7
    uterine, 22-6
Cardiac arrest, BLS Healthcare Provider
    Adult Algorithm, 26-1f
Cardiac enzymes, 12-10
Cardiac output (CO), postpartum
    changes, 12-2
Cardiogenic pulmonary edema, 13-5
Cardiopulmonary arrest, maternal,
    trauma and, 2-11
Cardiovascular (CV) system
    embryologic development, 9-9t
    local anesthesia toxicity and, 4-1
    pregnancy and, 9-3
Cardiovascular disease (CVD)
    perioperative optimization of, 3-1t
    preeclampsia and, 12-9
    in pregnancy, 12-1, 12-1t
Carpal tunnel syndrome (CTS), 9-6
Carpenter and Coustan scale, 17-6t
CARPREG (maternal cardiac risk
    classification), 12-1, 12-1t
cART (combination antiretroviral
    therapy), 21-2
Case control studies, 1-21t
Case series, 1-21t

Catastrophic antiphospholipid antibody
    syndrome, 16-13
CCBs (calcium channel blockers), 11-8t,
    12-4t, 12-14t
CDC's Advisory Committee on
    Immunization Practices, 13-6
CEE (conjugated equine estrogen), 5-8,
    25-13t
Cefaclor, 14-6t
Cefazolin, 3-7t, 11-17t, 25-1t
Cefdinir, 14-6t
Cefepime, 14-7t
Cefotaxime, 14-7t
Cefotetan, 2-9t, 11-17t, 14-7t
Cefoxitin, 2-9t, 11-17t
Cefpodoxime, 14-6t
Cefpodoxime proxetil, 14-6t
Ceftriaxone, 2-9t, 2-13, 14-6t, 14-7t,
    25-2t
Celestone (Betamethasone), 25-10t
Cell cycle and checkpoints, 22-17f
Cell-free fetal DNA, 9-13
Central nervous system (CNS), 4-1, 7-1
Cephalexin, 14-5t, 25-3t
Cephalic presentation, 10-4, 10-4f,
    11-16t
Cephalosporin, 2-9t, 3-7t
Cerebral aneurysm rupture, 18-7
Cerebral palsy (CP), 10-14
Cerebral venous thrombosis, 18-7,
    18-7f
Cervical assessment, spontaneous labor
    and delivery and, 10-4
Cervical atresia, Müllerian anomalies
    and, 8-7
Cervical cancer
    annual diagnoses and deaths, 1-20t
    characteristics, 22-2
    fertility preserving surgeries for,
        8-11
    HIV/AIDS in women and, 21-1
    in pregnancy, 22-3
    radiation therapy, 22-19t
    screening, 1-7
    staging and management, 22-3t
Cervical cerclage, 11-6, 24-9
Cervical change, labor and, 10-4
Cervical Cytology Screening
    Guidelines, 1-7
Cervical cytomegalovirus, 21-6
Cervical dysplasia, 21-6
Cervical insufficiency, short cervix and,
    11-5
Cervical length (CL), 9-8, 11-8
Cervical ripening (CR), 10-7
Cervidil (Dinoprostone), 10-7, 25-6t
Cesarean delivery/section (CD, C/S)
    general anesthesia and, 4-6
    induction of labor and, 10-7
    intraamniotic infection and, 11-17
    local anesthetics and, 4-5
    neuraxial anesthesia and, 4-2, 4-4t
    postoperative pain management,
        4-7t
    procedure, 24-8

Cetrorelix, 5-4
CFTR gene, male factor infertility and, 8-8
Chancre, syphilitic, 21-7
Chancroid, 21-9, 21-10t
Chasteberry, 5-13
Chemotherapy
  cervical cancer, 22-2, 22-3t
  epithelial ovarian cancer, 22-7
  germ cell tumors, 22-9, 22-11t
  gynecologic cancers, 22-17
  medications, 25-5t
  molar pregnancy, 22-15
  tumor biology and, 22-16
  types, 22-17
Chickenpox, 21-3
Chlamydia, 5-14
Chlamydia trachomatis, 2-9, 21-10t
Chloasma, 20-1t
Chloride, diabetic ketoacidosis, 17-4
2-Chloroprocaine, 4-1t
Chloroprocaine, 4-4t
Chlorthalidone, 12-4t
Cholecystitis, 15-1, 15-2t
Choledocholithiasis with ascending cholangitis, 15-2t
Cholelithiasis, 15-1, 15-2t
Cholesterol screening and treatment, 1-10t
Cholestyramine, 1-11t
Chorioamnionicity, 11-4
Chorioamnionitis, 11-17
Choriocarcinoma, 5-20t
  gestational, 22-15
  nongestational, 22-9, 22-9t
Chorionicity, 11-4
Chorionic villus sampling (CVS), 9-12, 9-14
Chorioretinitis, 21-2, 21-4
Choroid plexus cysts (CPC), 9-10
Chromopertubation, 8-1
Chromosomal microarray, 9-14
Chromosome abnormalities
  male factor infertility and, 8-8, 8-9
  routine prenatal testing, 9-1
Chronic adrenal insufficiency, 17-12
Chronic fatigue syndrome, 5-13
Chronic hypernatremia, 14-9
Chronic hypertension (CHTN), 12-3t
  definition, 11-1
  gestational complications of, 12-3t
  medications, 12-4t
  with superimposed preeclampsia, 11-1, 11-2, 12-6t, 12-7t
Chronic kidney disease (CKD), 14-3, 14-4t
Chronic pancreatitis, 15-2
Chronic pelvic pain, 5-13
Chronic renal failure (CRF), 14-3
Chrousos syndrome, 17-13f
Chung staging for melanoma, 22-13t
Cimetidine, 7-8
CIN (cervical intraepithelial neoplasia), 1-9, 22-2

Ciprofloxacin
  chancroid, 21-11t
  characteristics/indications, 25-2t
  ob-gyn surgery prophylaxis, 3-7t
  pyelonephritis, 14-7t
  UTIs, 14-6t
Cisplatin, 22-3t, 22-17, 22-18, 25-5t
Citalopram (Celexa), 19-6t, 25-9t
CL (cervical length), 9-8, 11-8
Clamps, surgical, 24-12, 24-12f
Clark staging for melanoma, 22-13t
Classic congenital adrenal hyperplasia, 6-11
Clear cell adenocarcinoma, 22-11
Clear cell carcinoma, 22-2, 22-4
Clear cell cystadenocarcinoma, 22-7
Clindamycin
  characteristics/indications, 25-1t
  endomyometritis, 11-18
  lactational mastitis, 10-16
  ob-gyn surgery prophylaxis, 3-7t
  PID, 2-9t
  vaginitis, 5-2t
Clinical breast exam, 1-6t
Clinical pelvimetry, 9-4
Clinical trials, phases of, 1-20
Clitoromegaly, 6-9t
Cloacal exstrophy, 9-11
Clobetasol propionate (Temovate), 20-4t
Clomiphene citrate (Clomid), 8-9, 25-12t
Clomiphene citrate challenge test (CCCT), 8-1
Clomipramine (TCA), 5-13
Clonazepam, 19-6t
Clotrimazole, 5-2t
Clubfoot (talipes equinovarus), 9-12
Cluster headache, 18-1, 18-1t
CM (Certified Midwife), 10-16t
CMV negative blood products, 16-16t
CNM (Certified Nurse-Midwife), 10-16t
Coagulation factor inhibitors, 16-12
Coagulation factors, pregnancy changes in, 15-1
Coagulation system, 16-1
Coagulopathies, 4-3, 11-10, 16-10, 16-11
Cocaine, 4-1, 19-3t
COCPs (continuous oral contraceptive pills), 5-5, 5-8, 5-9
"Coffee bean" pattern, 5-20
Cohort studies, 1-21
Colace (docusate sodium), 9-7t
Colestipol, 1-11t
Colloid IV solution, 14-8t
Colon blood supply, 23-5f
Colonoscopy, 7-9
Colorectal cancer screening, 1-3
Colpocleisis
  complete, 7-3
  partial, 7-8
Colporrhaphy, anterior, 7-3
Colposcopy, 1-8, 1-9

Combined hormonal contraception (CHCs), 1-17, 1-17t, 1-18t
Combined oral contraceptives (COCs), 2-10t, 5-11, 5-13
Combined spinal–epidural (CSE) neuraxial anesthesia, 4-3
Combipatch (17β-Estradiol + norethindrone acetate), 25-13t
Compazine (Prochlorperazine), 25-8t
Complete androgen insensitivity syndrome (CAIS), 6-9, 6-9t, 6-10, 6-11
Complete breech, 10-4, 10-4f, 11-16t
Complete hydatidiform mole, 22-14, 22-14t
Complete placenta previa, 11-13
Complete testicular feminization, 6-9
Complete uterine inversion, 11-15
Complex endometrial hyperplasia with/ without atypia, 22-4, 22-4t
Compounded bioidentical hormones, 5-18t
Computed tomography (CT)
    chronic kidney disease, 14-4
    common indications, 2-1
    epithelial ovarian cancer, 22-7
    germ cell tumors, 22-9
    nephrolithiasis, 14-7
    preeclampsia, 11-1
    sex cord-stromal tumors, 22-10
    surgical site infections, 3-7
    Urogram, 14-3
Condoms, male/female, 1-17t
Condyloma lata, 21-7
Condylomata acuminata, 21-7
Condylomata lata, 21-7
Congenital adrenal hyperplasia (CAH), 6-2t, 6-11, 17-13f
Congenital anomalies, 9-9
Congenital diaphragmatic hernia (CDH), 9-11
Congenital heart disease (CHD), 9-8
Congenital pulmonary airway malformation (CPAM), 9-11
Congenital syphilis, 21-8
Congenital Zika syndrome, 21-5
Conization, cold knife (CKC), 22-3, 22-3t, 24-6
Conotruncal anomalies, hypoplastic left heart syndrome and, 9-11
Constipation
    differential diagnosis of IBS symptoms and, 15-5t
    irritable bowel syndrome with, 15-4t
    medications, 9-7t
    medications causing, 7-9
    postpartum, 10-15
    severe, pelvic pain and, 2-2t
Consultation, preoperative, 3-1
Continuous subcutaneous insulin infusion (CSII), 17-2, 17-3
Continuous urinary incontinence, 7-4
Contraception
    depression and psychiatric disease, 1-16
    medications, 25-10t
    postpartum, 10-15
Contraceptive patch, 1-17
Contraceptives, oral. See COCPs; Combined oral contraceptives; OCPs
Contraction stress test, 10-1
Contrast agents, 2-2
Contrast computed tomography (CT), 2-1
Convulsions, 12-9
Copper IUD, 1-17
Copper T IUD (ParaGard), 1-16t, 1-18, 1-19t, 25-10t
    insertion, 24-1
Cord prolapse, induction of labor and, 10-7
Cordran (Flurandrenolide), 20-4t
Coronary artery disease (CAD), 4-1, 12-10
Corticosteroids (Cort), 3-9, 15-7t, 20-4t
Cortisol deficiency, 6-11
Cortisol production disorders, 17-10t
Cortizone-10 (Hydrocortisone butyrate), 20-4t
Cotton swab test, 5-14, 5-15
Cough stress test, 7-4
Counseling
    long-term, preeclampsia, 12-9
    preconception, pulmonary hypertension, 12-11
    psychological, 6-12
Couvelaire uterus, 11-13
CPM (Certified Professional Midwife), 10-16t
Crab louse, 21-10
Craniopharyngioma, 6-7t
Critical care, blood products for, 16-15t
Crohns disease (CD), 15-5, 15-6t, 20-6
Cryoprecipitate blood products, 16-15t
Cryotherapy, 21-9
Crystalloid IV solution, 14-8t
    postpartum hemorrhage, 11-10
C/S. See Cesarean delivery/section
CSE (combined spinal–epidural) neuraxial anesthesia, 4-3
CT. See Computed tomography
CTA (CT angiography), 16-8
Cushing disease, 17-10t
Cushing syndrome
    amenorrhea and, 6-7t
    congenital adrenal hyperplasia and, 6-12
    cortisol production and, 17-10, 17-10t, 17-11f
    hyperandrogenism and, 17-13f
Cutivate (Fluticasone propionate), 20-4t
CVS (chorionic villus sampling), 9-12, 9-14
Cyclocort (Amcinonide), 20-4t
Cyclophosphamide (Cytoxan), 22-18, 25-6t
Cyclosporine A, 7-9
CYP11B1 mutation, 6-12

CYP21A2, 6-12
CYP21 mutation, 6-12
Cystadenomas, 2-7, 5-20
Cystectomy
  adnexal masses, 5-21
  adnexal torsion, 2-8
  interstitial cystitis, 7-9
  ovarian cysts, 2-7
Cystic fibrosis (CF) screening, 9-13
Cystitis
  interstitial, 7-8
  pelvic pain and, 2-2t
Cystocele, 7-1
Cystoplasty, 7-9
Cystourethroscopy, 7-5
Cysts
  bone, 17-15
  ovarian, 17-13f
  vaginal and perineal, 20-6t
Cytochrome P-450, 15-1
Cytomegalovirus (CMV), 16-17t,
    21-2, 21-4
Cytotec, 10-7, 11-10t, 25-6t

D
D&C (dilatation and curettage)
  abnormal uterine bleeding and, 5-9
  endometrial cancer, 22-5
  postmenopausal bleeding and, 5-10
  procedure, 24-5
  surgical abortion, 5-19
D&E (dilation & evacuation), 5-19
Danazol, 5-7, 6-6
Darifenacin ER (Enablex), 7-6t
Davydov neovagina, 8-7
DCIS (ductal carcinoma in situ), 1-7
Decelerations, fetal heart rate, 10-8,
    10-8t, 10-10f
Deep incisional SSI, 3-7
Defecation physiology and mechanisms,
    7-1
Deformation, definition, 9-9
Delayed acute hemolytic reaction,
    16-16t
Delayed puberty, 6-4, 6-5f
Delivery
  diabetes and, 17-6, 17-7
  herpes simplex virus and, 21-4
  multiple gestation, 11-5
  operative vaginal, 10-12, 10-12f
  spontaneous labor and, 10-4, 10-4f,
    10-4t
  twin, neuraxial anesthesia and, 4-2
  valvular heart disease and, 12-14
DEM (Direct Entry Midwife), 10-16t
11-Deoxycorticosterone, 6-12
Depo-Provera, 1-17t
Depot medroxyprogesterone acetate,
    5-11, 5-14, 5-18t
Depression, 1-16, 9-2, 19-3
Dermatologic changes in pregnancy,
    20-1t
Dermatologic conditions
  apocrine miliaria, 20-5
  gynecological cysts and, 20-6t

hidradenitis suppurativa, 20-5
lichen planus, 20-3
lichen sclerosus, 20-2
lichen simplex chronicus, 20-3
manifestations of systemic disease,
    20-6
psoriasis, 20-4
topical corticosteroids for, 20-4t
Dermatop (Prednicarbate), 20-4t
Dermoid tumors, 2-7
Descent, in labor, 10-5
Desensitization, female sexual
    dysfunction, 5-16
Desonide (DesOwen, Desonate), 20-4t
Desoximetasone (Topicort), 20-4t
Detemir (Levemir), 17-3t
Detrol/Detrol LA (Tolterodine), 7-6t
Developmental field defect, definition,
    9-9
DEXA (dual-energy x-ray
    absorptiometry), 1-13
  BMD (bone marrow density), 5-16
Dexamethasone, 22-16t, 25-10t
Dextrose 5% solution, 14-8t
DHEA, 6-12, 22-9t
Diabetes mellitus (DM). See also
    Gestational diabetes mellitus;
    Pregestational diabetes
    mellitus
  amenorrhea and, 6-7t
  epinephrine contraindications and,
    4-1
  medications, 25-7t
  menopause and, 5-17
  perioperative management, 3-2t
  pregestational, congenital anomalies
    and, 9-9
  in pregnancy, 17-5
  type 1 (T1DM), 17-2, 17-2t
  type 2 (T2DM), 17-4
  White classification, 17-5t
Diabetic ketoacidosis (DKA), 17-3
Diagonal conjugate, 9-4
Dialysis, ovarian hyperstimulation
    syndrome and, 8-12
Diaphragm with spermicide, 1-17,
    1-17t
DIAPPERS mnemonic for urinary
    incontinence, 7-4
Diarrhea, 9-8t, 15-4t, 15-5t
Diazepam, 19-6
DIC (disseminated intravascular
    coagulation), 12-9, 16-11
Dichorionic diamniotic twins, 11-4f
Dichorionic twins, 11-5
Diclofenac, 18-2t
Dicloxacillin, 10-16
Dietary adjustments, chronic kidney
    disease, 14-4
Dietary supplements, 5-13
Diflorasone diacetate (ApexiCon),
    20-4t
Diflorasone diacetate (Florone), 20-4t
Digitalis toxicity, 14-9
Digoxin, 12-14t

Dihydroergotamine, 18-2t, 18-3t
Dilaudid. *See* Hydromorphone
Diltiazem Extended release, 12-4t
Dilutional anemia of pregnancy, 16-1t
Dinoprostone (Cervidil, Prostin E₂),
    10-7, 25-6t
Diphenoxylate–atropine (Lomotil), 9-8t
Diprolene (Betamethasone
    dipropionate), 20-4t
Direct oral anticoagulant (DOAC), 16-9
Discectomy, 4-3
Discordance, multiple gestation, 11-5
Disruption, definition, 9-9
Disulfiram (Antabuse), 25-9t
Ditropan (Oxybutynin IR), 7-6t
Ditropan XL (Oxybutynin ER), 7-6t
Diuretics, 12-15t
Diverticular abscess, 2-7
Diverticulitis, 2-2t
Dizygosity, 11-4
DKA (diabetic ketoacidosis), 17-3
DMPA (depot medroxyprogesterone
    acetate), 1-17, 5-9
DMSO (dimethyl sulfoxide), 7-8
Docetaxel (Taxotere), 22-17, 25-5t
Docusate sodium (Colace), 9-7t
Domestic abuse or violence, 1-2, 1-15,
    5-13, 9-2
Donor twin, twin–twin transfusion
    syndrome and, 11-5
Donovan bodies, 21-11t
Donovanosis, 21-10t
Dopamine agonists, 6-8
Dopamine antagonists, 18-2t
Doppler ultrasound, 2-1
Doulas, 10-16
Dovetail sign, 7-9
Doxorubicin (Adriamycin, Doxil), 25-5t
Doxycycline
    characteristics/indications, 25-3t
    early pregnancy failure, 2-7t
    genital ulcers, 21-11t
    ob-gyn surgery prophylaxis, 3-7t
    PID, 2-9t
    surgical abortion, 5-19
    syphilis, 21-8t
Doxylamine, 9-5
Doxylamine succinate, 25-8t
Drug reaction
    fixed, dermatologic manifestations
        of, 20-7
    hyperandrogenism and, 17-13f
Drug use (abuse)
    screening tools, 19-1t
    seizures and, 18-3
Dulcolax (bisacodyl), 9-7t
Duodenal atresia, 9-8
DV. *See* Domestic abuse or violence
DVT (deep vein thrombosis), 16-7f,
    16-7t
    characteristics, 16-6
    perioperative, 3-7, 3-8t
Dysautonomia, familial, 9-13
Dysgerminomas, 5-20t, 22-8, 22-9t
Dyslipidemia, 5-17

Dysmenorrhea, 2-2t, 5-11, 5-12f
Dyspareunia, 5-15, 7-3
Dysplasia, definition, 9-9
Dysthymia, 19-3

E
E2 (cyclin) embryonal carcinoma, 22-9
Early congenital syphilis, 21-8
Early term, definition, 9-1
ECG (electrocardiogram) changes
    hypokalemia, and, 14-9
    in pregnancy, 12-2
Echocardiography, 16-8
Echogenic bowel, 9-11
Eclampsia
    definition, 11-1, 18-5
    headache and, 18-1t
    management and treatment, 12-8t
    pregnancy-related hypertension and,
        12-6, 12-7t
Ectopic pregnancy, 2-2t, 2-3, 2-7
EDD (expected due date), 9-1, 9-1t
Edema, lower extremity, 9-6
Edinburgh postnatal depression scale
    (EPDS), 19-4
EE (ethinyl estradiol)/norethindrone,
    2-10t
EFW (estimated fetal weight), 9-1, 9-8
Elder abuse, 1-15
Elderly patients, perioperative
    optimization of, 3-3
Elective repeat cesarean delivery
    (ERCD), 10-13, 10-13t
Electrical injuries, 2-11
Electrocoagulation, 5-5
Electroconvulsive therapy (ECT), 19-4,
    19-5, 19-6
Electrolyte imbalances, seizures and,
    18-3
Electrolytes, distending, 3-11
Electromyography, 7-10
Ella (Ulipristal), 1-18
Elocon (Mometasone furoate), 20-4t
EMACO (etoposide, methotrexate,
    actinomycin D, cytoxan,
    oncovin), 22-16t
EMAEP (etoposide, methotrexate, act D,
    carboplatin), 22-16t
Embolectomy, 16-9, 16-9t
Embolism, 16-9
Embryo cryopreservation, 8-10
Embryologic development by organ
    system, 9-9t
Embryonal carcinoma, 5-20t, 22-9
Emergency contraception (EC), 1-18,
    1-18t
Emtricitabine, 2-13
Enablex (Darifenacin ER), 7-6t
Enalapril, 12-4t
Endoanal ultrasound (US), 7-9
Endocarditis prophylaxis, 12-14
Endocervical curettage, 1-9
Endocrine changes during pregnancy,
    9-3
Endodermal sinus tumor, 5-20t, 22-8,
    22-9t

Endometrial ablation, 5-5, 5-9, 24-6
Endometrial adenocarcinoma, 22-4, 22-7
Endometrial biopsy, 24-5
Endometrial cancer, 1-20t, 8-11, 22-5t
Endometrial curettage, 2-4
Endometrial hyperplasia (EH), 22-4, 22-4t, 22-19t
Endometrial stromal sarcoma, 22-6
Endometrioid carcinoma, 22-2
Endometriomas, 2-7, 5-20
Endometriosis, 5-5, 5-13, 5-14, 8-1t
Endomyometritis, 11-18
Enema, 9-7t
Engagement, in labor, 10-5
Enhanced recovery after surgery (ERAS), 3-5
Enoxaparin (Lovenox), 25-4t
Enteric gram-negative rods, 2-9
Enterococcus, surgical site infections and, 3-6
Environmental teratogens, 9-9
Enzymes, pregnancy changes in, 15-1
Ependymoma, 4-3
Epidemiology terms, 1-20t
Epidermoid cyst, 20-6t
Epidermolysis bullosa, 1-14
Epidural block, 4-3, 4-3f, 4-5f
Epilepsy, 18-3, 18-4t, 18-5t
Epinephrine, 4-1
Epithelial endometrial cancer types, 22-5t
Epithelial neoplasm (tumors), 2-7, 22-4
Epithelial ovarian cancer (EOC), 22-7
Eprosartan, 12-4t
ERCD (elective repeat cesarean delivery), 10-13, 10-13t
Ergotamine, 18-3t
Eros Therapy, 5-16
Ertapenem, 11-17t
Erythema multiforme, 20-7
Erythematous papule, 21-9
Erythromycin, 11-7t, 21-11t, 25-2t
Escherichia coli, 3-6
ESRD (end-stage renal disease), 14-3
Essure (hysteroscopic sterilization), 1-17
Estimated fetal weight (EFW), 9-1, 9-8
17β-Estradiol (Climara, Estrace), 25-13t
Estradiol-17β vaginal cream, 5-17t
Estradiol-17β vaginal ring, 5-17t
Estradiol vaginal tablet, 5-17t
Estrogen
    acute uterine bleeding, 2-10t
    endometriosis, 5-7
    female sexual dysfunction, 5-16
    GD-independent precocious puberty, 6-3
    lipids and, 1-11
    osteoporosis, 1-13
    ovulation and, 17-1, 17-1f
    urinary incontinence, 7-5
    vaginal, menopause and, 5-17
    vulvar pain, 5-15
Estrogen therapy (ET), 5-17
Ethnicity, screening diabetes in pregnancy and, 17-6t

Ethosuximide, 18-4t
EtOH (ethanol). See also Alcohol abuse
    routine prenatal visit question, 9-2
    screening tools, 19-1t
Etonogestrel implant (Implanon/ Nexplanon), 1-16t
    abnormal uterine bleeding, 5-9
    insertion, 1-17, 24-1, 24-2f
    primary dysmenorrhea, 5-11
Etoposide, 22-17, 25-5t
Euprolide, 8-12
Exercise
    anxiety disorders, 19-4
    cholesterol management, 1-11t
    chronic pelvic pain, 5-14
    in pregnancy, 9-3
    weight-bearing, 1-13
Expanding tumors, 22-16
Expulsion, in labor, 10-5
Extended field EBRT, 22-18, 22-19t
Extended radical hysterectomy, 22-1
Extension, in labor, 10-5
External anal sphincter (EAS), 7-1
External beam radiation (EBRT), 22-18, 22-19t
External cephalic version (ECV), 11-16
External rotation, in labor, 10-5
External urethral sphincter, 7-1t
Extraperitoneal insufflation, laparoscopy and, 3-10
Extraurethral incontinence, 7-7
Extravascular anemia, 23-1t
Ezetimibe, 1-11t

F
Facial bladder neck slings, 7-7
Factor V Leiden (FVL), 16-10t
Factor VIII (blood product), 16-16t
Factor Xa inhibitors, 16-9t
Fallopian tubes, tubal factor infertility and, 8-3
False pelvis, 9-4
Familial hypocalciuric hypercalemia (FHH), 17-15
Fat necrosis, 1-5t
Febrile nonhemolytic reaction, 16-16t
Fecal incontinence, 7-9
Fecundity, 8-1
Female bony pelvis, 23-1f
Female mortality causes, 1-20t. See also Maternal mortality
Female orgasmic disorder, 5-15
46,XX Female pseudohermaphroditism, 6-12
Female sexual differentiation pathway, 6-10f
Female sexual dysfunction, 5-15, 5-17
Female sexual interest/arousal D/O, 5-15
Female sterilization, 1-17
Femoral nerve, gynecologic surgery and, 3-4t
Femoral neuropathy, postpartum, 18-9
Fenofibrate, 1-11t

Fentanyl (Sublimaze), 4-2t, 4-4t, 4-7t, 25-8t
Ferning, PPROM and, 11-7
Ferrous gluconate/sulfate/fumarate, 16-2t
Fertility preservation, 8-10
Ferriman–Gallwey score, 17-13, 17-14f
Fesoterodine ER (Toviaz), 7-6t
Fetal alcohol spectrum disorder (FASD), 19-2t
Fetal anatomy assessment, 9-8
Fetal assessment, trauma and, 2-11
Fetal circulation, 23-6f
Fetal cord blood gas analysis, 10-14, 10-14t
Fetal echocardiography, 9-8
Fetal growth restriction, 10-1. See also IUGR
Fetal heart rate (FHR)
    abnormal, cord blood gas analysis and, 10-14
    accelerations and decelerations, 10-10f
    decelerations, neuraxial anesthesia and, 4-4t
    intrapartum monitoring, 10-7
    monitoring, diabetic ketoacidosis and, 17-4
    routine prenatal testing, 9-2
    sample tracings, 10-9f
    tracings in labor, 10-8t
    variability, 10-11f
Fetal lie, spontaneous labor and delivery and, 10-4
Fetal lung maturity testing by amniocentesis, 10-2
Fetal meconium, 11-16
Fetal movement count, 10-1
Fetal presentation, 10-4, 10-4f
Fetal radiation exposure, 2-1t
Fetal testing, antenatal, 10-1, 10-1t
Fetal ultrasound: anatomy and echocardiography, 9-8
Fever
    neuraxial anesthesia and, 4-3t
    postoperative, 3-6, 3-6t
    postpartum, 10-15
fFN (fetal fibronectin), 11-8
FFP (fresh-frozen plasma), 16-15t
FH (fundal height), 9-1, 9-2
FHR. See Fetal heart rate
Fibrates, 1-11t
Fibroadenoma, 1-5t
Fibroids, uterine, 5-3
Fibromas, 2-7, 5-20, 22-10
Fibromyalgia, 5-13
FIGO (International Federation of Gynecology and Obstetrics)
    cervical cancer staging, 22-1t
    endometrial cancer staging, 22-5t
    gestational trophoblastic neoplasia staging, 22-15t
    modified WHO prognostic scoring for GTN adapted by, 22-16t
    ovarian cancer staging, 22-8t

uterine cancer staging, 22-6t
    vaginal cancer staging, 22-12t
    vulvar cancer staging, 22-13t
Filling cystometry, 7-5
Final menstrual period (FMP), 5-16
Fioricet, 18-3t
1st trimester, 9-2t, 9-3, 9-8, 9-12
Fixed drug reaction, 20-7
Flagyl (Metronidazole)
    characteristics/indications, 25-3t
    ob-gyn surgery prophylaxis, 3-7t
    PID, 2-9t
    sexual assault postexposure prophylaxis, 2-13
    vaginitis, 5-2t
Fleet (sodium phosphate), 9-7t
Flexion, in labor, 10-5
Florone (Diflorasone diacetate), 20-4t
Fluconazole, 5-2t
Fludrocortisone, 6-12
Fluid management, 3-9, 14-3, 14-10, 17-4
Fluid overload, 3-11
Fluids and electrolytes, for IV composition, 14-8t
FluMist, 13-6
Fluocinolone acetonide (Synalar), 20-4t
Fluocinonide (Lidex), 20-4t
Fluoxetine (Prozac), 18-3t, 19-6t, 25-9t
Flurandrenolide (Cordran), 20-4t
Fluticasone propionate (Cutivate), 20-4t
Flu vaccine, 9-3, 13-6
Foam stability index, 10-2
Folate deficiency, 16-3
Folic acid, 9-4, 9-4t
Follicle remnant, 17-1
Follicular cysts, 2-7
Follicular phase of menstruation, 17-1
Folliculitis, 20-2t
Fondaparinux, 16-9
Food warnings during pregnancy, 9-4
Forceps
    operative vaginal delivery and, 10-12, 10-12f
    surgical, 24-11, 24-11f
Fosfomycin, 14-5t, 25-3t
4 Factor prothrombin complex concentrate, 16-16t
Fox–Fordyce disease, 20-5
Fractions, of EBRT, 22-18
Fragile X permutation screening, 9-13
Frank breech, 10-4f, 11-16t
FRAX risk assessment tool, 1-13
Free T_3 (fT_3), 17-9t
Free T_4 (fT_4) or free T_4 index (FTI), 17-9t
"Fried egg" cellular appearance, 22-8
FSH (follicle-stimulating hormone)
    deficiency, panhypopituitarism and, 17-16
    delayed puberty and, 6-5
    menstrual cycle and, 6-1
    ovulation and, 17-1, 17-1f
    testing, infertility and, 8-1
Full term, definition, 9-1

Functional (transient) hypogonadotropic hypogonadism, 6-6
Functional hypothalamic amenorrhea, 6-8
Fundal height (FH), 9-1, 9-2
Fungi, pneumonia and, 13-4t
Furosemide, 14-10

G

Gabapentin, 5-15, 5-16, 18-4t
GAD (generalized anxiety disorder), 19-4
Gadolinium, 2-2
Galactorrhea, 1-5, 17-16
Ganirelix, 5-4
Gardnerella vaginalis, 2-9, 5-1t
Gartner duct cyst, 20-6t
Gastroenteritis, 2-2t
Gastrointestinal (GI) system
    anomalies, 9-11
    changes in pregnancy, 9-3, 15-1
    chemotherapy and, 22-18
    embryologic development, 9-9t
    laparoscopic injuries, 3-11
Gastroschisis, 9-11
GBS (group B *Streptococcus*), 3-6, 9-3, 10-3, 10-3f
GDM (gestational diabetes mellitus), 9-2, 17-5
Gelnique (Oxybutynin patch), 7-6t
Gemcitabine, 22-17
Gemcitabine (Gemzar), 25-5t
Gender identity disorders, 6-11, 6-12
General anesthesia, 4-6
Generalized seizures, 18-3
Genetic amniocentesis, 9-13
Genetic screening, 9-12
Genetic syndromes. See Chromosome abnormalities
Genitalia
    ambiguous, 6-11, 6-12
    external, blood supply to, 23-2f
Genital ulcers, 21-10t
Genital warts, 21-6, 21-7
Genitofemoral nerve, gynecologic surgery and, 3-4t
Genitopelvic pain/penetration D/O, 5-15
Genitourinary (GU) tract, 8-7, 9-9t, 22-18
    anomalies, 9-11
    fistulas, 7-8
Gentamicin
    characteristics/indications, 25-1t
    endomyometritis, 11-18
    intraamniotic infection, 11-17t
    ob-gyn surgery prophylaxis, 3-7t
    PID, 2-9t
    UTIs, 14-6t
Germ cell tumors
    characteristics, 2-7, 22-8
    markers, 22-9t
    ovarian, serum biomarkers in, 5-20t
    treatment, 22-11t

Gestational age (GA)
    1st trimester ultrasound and, 9-8
    prenatal care and, 9-2t
    vacuum delivery and, 10-12
Gestational diabetes mellitus (GDM)
    characteristics, 17-7
    management in pregnancy, 17-6
    multiple gestation and, 11-5
    screening, 9-2, 17-5, 17-6
Gestational hypertension (GHTN), 11-1, 12-3t, 12-6t, 12-7t, 12-9t
Gestational hypertensive disorders, 11-1
Gestational thrombocytopenia, 16-5
Gestational trophoblastic neoplasia (GTN), 22-14, 22-14f, 22-14t
    FIGO staging, 22-15t
    treatment regimens, 22-16t
GFR (glomerular filtration rate), 14-1, 14-3, 14-4
Gigantism, 17-17
Glargine (Lantus), 17-3t, 25-7t
Glasgow criteria, 1-14
Glucocorticoids, 6-12
Glucose, plasma, 17-3, 17-3t, 17-7t.
    See also Oral glucose tolerance test
α-Glucosidase inhibitors, 17-8t
Glulisine (Apidra), 17-3t
Glyburide, 17-7t
Glycemic control in pregnancy, 17-6t
GnRH (gonadotropin-releasing hormone), 6-1
GnRH (gonadotropin-releasing hormone) agonists
    abnormal uterine bleeding, 5-9
    adenomyosis, 5-5
    endometriosis, 5-7
    leiomyoma, 5-4
    pelvic congestion syndrome, 5-14
    PMS or PMDD, 5-13
GnRH (gonadotropin-releasing hormone) analogs, 5-7
GnRH (gonadotropin-releasing hormone) antagonists, 5-4
Goiter, 17-10f
GoLytely – electrolytes (polyethylene glycol), 9-7t
Gompertzian tumor, 22-16
Gonadarche, 6-1
Gonadotropin-dependent (central) precocious puberty (GDPP), 6-3, 6-4f
Gonadotropin-independent (peripheral) precocious puberty, 6-3, 6-4f
Gonadotropins (Follistim, Fertinex, Gonal-f), 8-9, 25-12t
Gonorrhea, 5-14
Grand multipara, 9-1
Granuloma inguinale, 21-10t
Granulosa cell tumor (GCT), 22-10
Graves disease, 17-9, 17-10f
Gravidity, 9-1
"Ground glass" appearance, 5-20
Group B *Streptococcus* (GBS), 3-6, 9-3, 10-3, 10-3f

Growth hormone (GH), 6-6, 17-16
Growth restriction. See Fetal growth restriction; IUGR
GTT (glucose tolerance test), 9-1
Gynecoid pelvis, 9-5, 9-5f, 9-5t
Gynecologic surgery, common nerve injury in, 3-4t
Gynecomastia, 6-9t

H
Haemophilus ducreyi, 21-9, 21-10t
Haemophilus influenzae, 2-9
HAIR-AN syndrome, 17-13f
Halcinonide (Halog), 20-4t
Halobetasol propionate (Ultravate), 20-4t
Halogenated anesthetics, 4-6, 11-15
Haloperidol, 19-6, 19-7t
HAP (hospital-acquired pneumonia), 13-4
Hashimoto thyroiditis, 17-8
HbA1c, 17-6t
HBcAg, 15-8, 15-8t
HBeAg, 15-8, 15-8t
HbEP (hemoglobin electrophoresis), 9-13
HBsAg, 15-8, 15-8t
HC (head circumference), 9-8
β-hCG (human chorionic gonadotropin), 5-20t, 9-12, 9-12t
hCG (human chorionic gonadotropin), 8-12, 17-2, 22-9, 22-9t
Headache (HA)
  approach to, by history, 18-1f
  characteristics, 18-1
  postdural puncture, 4-4t
  postpartum, 10-15
Head entrapment, 4-6
Head presentation, 10-4
Heart failure, 12-15
Heart sounds, 12-2
HELLP syndrome, 12-7t, 12-8t, 15-10, 15-11t, 16-3t. See also Preeclampsia
Hemabate, 11-10t
Hematologic changes of pregnancy, 9-3, 16-1
Hematoma, epidural, 4-4t
Hematuria, 14-3
Hemivaginas, obstructed, 8-7
Hemodynamic profile, pregnancy and, 12-2
Hemoglobin, diagnostic amniocentesis and, 9-14
Hemoglobinopathies, 9-13, 16-3
Hemolytic anemia, 16-3
Hemophilias, 16-12
Hemorrhage. See also Postpartum hemorrhage
  blood products for, 16-15t
  liver, pregnancy-related hypertension and, 12-9
  post-hysteroscopic, 3-12
  risk, neuraxial anesthesia and, 4-2
  subarachnoid, 18-1t, 18-7

Hemorrhoidal branch of pudendal nerve, 7-1
Hemorrhoids, 7-9, 9-7
Henderson–Patterson bodies, 21-9
Heparin, 7-8, 12-14t, 25-4t
Heparin-induced thrombocytopenia (HIT), 16-5, 16-6t
Hepatitis, viral, 15-7
Hepatitis A virus (HBA), 15-8
  vaccine, 15-9
Hepatitis B virus (HBV), 15-8
  blood transfusions and, 16-17t
  in pregnancy, 21-5
  vaccine, 15-9
Hepatitis C virus (HCV), 15-8
  blood transfusions and, 16-17t
  diagnosis by serology, 15-9t
  in pregnancy, 21-5
Hepatitis D virus (HCD), 15-9
Hepatitis E virus (HCE), 15-9
Herbal medications, 5-13
Hernia
  pelvic pain and, 2-2t
  Trocar site, 3-11
Herpes gestationis, 20-1t
Herpes simplex virus (HSV), 21-1, 21-2, 21-4, 21-10t
Herpes simplex virus, chancroid, 2-2t
Hetastarch, 14-9t
Hextend, 14-9t
Hidradenitis suppurativa, 20-5
High-intensity focused ultrasound (HIFU), 5-4, 5-5
Hirsutism, 17-13, 17-14f
HIV. See also AIDS
  blood transfusions and, 16-17t
  postexposure prophylaxis (PEP), 2-12–2-13
  in women, 21-1
Hormonal regulation, 17-1
  menstrual cycle, 17-1f
Hormone replacement therapy (HRT), 5-16, 6-11, 25-13t
Hormone therapy (HT), 5-17, 5-17t, 5-18t, 22-11t
Horn, rudimentary, 8-7
hPL (human placental lactogen), 17-2
HPO (hypothalamic–pituitary–ovarian) axis, 6-1
HSD3B2 mutation, 6-12
HSIL (high-grade squamous intraepithelial lesion), 1-8
HSM (hepatosplenomegaly), cytomegalovirus and, 21-4
HTN. See Hypertension
Humalog (Lispro), 17-3t
Humalog Mix 75/25 (Lispro 75/25), 17-3t
Human papilloma virus (HPV), 1-8, 2-13, 21-6
Humulin 70/30 (70% NPH/30% regular), 17-3t
Humulin L (Insulin zinc), 17-3t
Humulin N (Isophane insulin), 17-3t

Humulin R, 17-3t
Humulin U (Insulin zinc extended), 17-3t
Hurley staging, for hidradenitis suppurativa, 20-5
Hyaline membrane disease, 10-2
Hydatidiform moles, complete or partial, 22-14, 22-14t
Hydralazine, 11-1, 12-4t, 12-5t, 12-15t, 25-4t
Hydrocephalus, 9-10, 21-2
Hydrochlorothiazide, 12-4t
Hydrocodone (Vicodin), 25-9t
Hydrocortisone, 6-12, 14-10, 15-7t, 20-4t
Hydrocortisone butyrate (Locoid, Cortizone-10), 20-4t
Hydrocortisone probutate (Pandel), 20-4t
Hydrocortisone valerate (Westcort), 20-4t
Hydromorphone (Dilaudid), 4-4t, 4-7t, 25-8t
Hydrops fetalis, 11-2, 21-3
Hydrosalpinx, 2-1, 2-7
21-Hydroxylase deficiency, 6-12
11β-Hydroxylase deficiency, 6-12
17-Hydroxypregnenolone, 6-12
17-Hydroxyprogesterone (17-OHP), 6-12
3β-Hydroxysteroid dehydrogenase deficiency, 6-12
Hydroxyzine, 7-8
Hymen, imperforate, 6-8
Hyoscyamine sulfate, 9-8t
Hyperandrogenism, 6-12, 17-12, 17-13f
Hypercalcemia, 14-10, 17-15
  PTH-related, 17-14
Hyperchloremia, 14-10
Hyperemesis gravidarum (HEG), 9-6
Hyperglycemia, 17-4
Hypergonadotropic hypogonadism, 6-5, 8-8
Hyperkalemia (hyperK), 6-11, 14-9
Hypermagnesemia, 14-10
Hypernatremia, 14-9
Hyperosmolar hyperglycemic state, 17-4
Hyperphosphatemia, 14-10
Hyperprolactinemia, 6-5f, 6-8, 17-13f, 17-16
Hypertension (HTN), 5-17, 12-3t, 17-6t. See also Chronic hypertension
Hypertensive crisis, 12-5
Hypertensive disorders, 12-1
Hypertensive emergency, 12-5
Hypertensive urgency, 12-5
Hyperthyroidism, 3-3, 4-1, 17-9, 17-9t, 17-10f
Hypnosis, 4-6t
Hypocalcemia, 14-10, 17-15
Hypochloremia, 14-10
Hypogastric nerves (T11–L2), 7-1t

Hypogonadotropic hypogonadism, 6-4, 6-5
Hypokalemia, 14-9
Hypomagnesemia, 14-10
Hyponatremia (hypoNA), 10-7, 14-10
Hypoparathyroidism, 17-15
2° Hypoparathyroidism, 17-15
Hypoperfusion, 3-8
Hypophosphatemia, 14-10
Hypoplasia, 8-5f
Hypoplastic left heart syndrome (HLHS), 9-10
Hypospadias, 6-9t
Hypotension (HoTN), 4-3t
Hypothalamic amenorrhea, 6-7t
Hypothyroidism, 3-3, 17-8, 17-9t
Hypovolemia, 4-3
Hypoxia, 3-8, 10-14
Hysterectomy
  abnormal uterine bleeding, 5-9
  acute uterine bleeding, 2-10t
  adenomyosis, 5-5
  cervical cancer, 22-3t
  chronic pelvic pain, 5-14
  endometriosis, 5-7
  gestational trophoblastic neoplasia, 22-16t
  pelvic congestion syndrome, 5-14
  total abdominal, procedure, 24-7
  types of, 22-1
  uterine fibroids, 5-4
  vaginal procedure, 24-8
Hysterosalpingogram (HSG), 8-1
Hysteroscopic myomectomy, 5-4
Hysteroscopic sterilization (Essure), 1-17
Hysteroscopic tubal ligation, 24-7
Hysteroscopy
  acute uterine bleeding, 2-10t
  Asherman syndrome, 6-8
  complications, 3-11
  infertility testing, 8-1
  leiomyoma, 5-4
  operative procedure, 24-6
  postmenopausal bleeding, 5-10

I
Ibandronate (Boniva), 25-12t
Ibuprofen (Advil, Motrin), 11-18, 18-2t, 18-3t, 25-8t
IC/BPS (interstitial cystitis/bladder pain syndrome), 7-8
ICSI (intracytoplasmic sperm injection), 8-9
Ifosfamide, 22-18, 25-6t
IgE (immunoglobulin E), 13-7
IgG (immunoglobulin G), 21-3
IgM (immunoglobulin M), 21-3
Iliac veins, internal, embolization of, 5-14
Iliococcygeal suspension, 7-3
Iliohypogastric nerve, 3-4t, 5-13
Ilioinguinal nerve, 3-4t, 5-13
Imaging, 2-1, 2-1t. See also specific types

Imipenem–cilastatin, 14-6t
Imipramine (Tofranil), 7-6t
Immature (malignant) teratoma, 5-20t,
    22-8, 22-9t
Immune hydrops, 11-2
Immunotherapy, 22-17
Imodium (loperamide), 9-8t
Impetigo herpetiformis, 20-1t
Inadequate blockade, neuraxial
    anesthesia and, 4-4t
Incision cellulitis, 3-7
Incision selection, preoperative, 3-3
Incomplete androgen insensitivity
    syndrome (CAIS), 6-9t
Incomplete breech, 10-4f
Incomplete uterine inversion, 11-15
Incontinence
    anal, 7-9
    bypass, 7-7
    overflow, 7-7
    screening, 1-2
    urinary, 7-4
Incontinence pessary, 7-5
Indapamide, 12-4t
Indigo carmine amniotic infusion, 11-7
Indomethacin (Indocin), 11-8t, 25-7t
Induction of labor (IOL)
    Bishop score, 10-6t
    cervical ripening and, 10-7
    characteristics/indications, 10-6
    complications, 10-7
    median hours in labor, 10-5t
Infection. See also Sexually-transmitted
    infections/disease
    Bartholin duct abscess, 5-2
    congenital anomalies and, 9-9
    diagnostic amniocentesis, 9-13
    HIV/AIDS in women, 21-1
    post-hysteroscopic, 3-12
    soft tissue, neuraxial anesthesia and,
        4-3
    TORCH, 21-2
    Zika, 21-4
Infertile androgen abnormality/
    insensitivity syndromes, 6-9t
Infertility
    causes, 8-1t
    congenital adrenal hyperplasia and,
        6-12
    evaluation, 8-1
    medications, 25-12t
    tubal factor, 8-3
Infiltrating ductal breast cancer, 1-7
Infiltrating lobular breast cancer, 1-7
Inflammatory bowel disease (IBD), 15-5,
    15-6t, 15-7t
Inflammatory breast cancer, 1-7
Influenza in pregnancy, 13-6, 21-5
Influenza vaccine, 13-5, 13-6
Informed consent, 3-1
INH (isoniazid), 21-6
Inhibin, 22-9t
Inhibin A, 9-12, 9-12t
Inotropes, 12-15t
Institute of Medicine (IOM), 9-3t

Insulin
    diabetic ketoacidosis, 17-4
    forms, 25-7t
    hyperkalemia, 14-9
    management during labor, 17-7
    management in pregnancy, 17-7f
    types and pharmacodynamics,
        17-3t
Insulin resistance, 6-12
Insulin zinc (Lente, Humulin L, Novolin L),
    17-3t
Insulin zinc extended (Ultralente,
    Humulin U), 17-3t
Integrated genetic screening, 9-13
Interferon gamma release assay, 21-6
Intermediate-acting insulin, 17-3t
Internal anal sphincter (IAS), 7-1
Internal rotation, in labor, 10-5
Interspinous diameter of pelvis, 9-4
Interstitial brachytherapy, 22-18
Interstitial cystitis, 7-8
Interval sterilization, 1-17
Intimate partner violence, 1-15
Intimate terrorism, 1-15
Intraamniotic infection, 11-17
Intracavitary brachytherapy, 22-19
Intracranial calcifications, 21-2
Intracranial pressure, 4-3
Intracytoplasmic sperm injection (ICSI),
    8-10
Intrahepatic cholestasis of pregnancy
    (ICP), 15-9
Intrapartum fetal monitoring, 10-7
Intrapartum hemodynamic changes,
    12-2
Intrauterine devices (IUDs), insertion,
    24-1
Intrauterine growth restriction (IUGR),
    9-1, 9-8, 11-3
Intrauterine insemination (IUI), 8-9
Intravascular anemia, 23-1t
Invasive mole, 22-14, 22-15t
Iodine-based contrast, 2-2
Iodine deficiency, 17-8
Iodine uptake, 17-9t, 17-10f
Irbesartan, 12-4t
Iron, 9-4t, 16-2t
Iron deficiency anemia, 16-1t, 16-2t
Irradiated blood products, 16-16t
Irritable bowel syndrome (IBS), 5-13,
    15-4, 15-4t, 15-5t
Irving method for postpartum tubal
    ligation, 24-9
Isolated precocious puberty, 6-3
Isophane insulin (NPH, Humulin N,
    Novolin N), 17-3t, 25-7t
IUFD (intrauterine fetal demise), 11-5
IUGR (intrauterine growth restriction),
    9-1, 9-8, 11-3
IUP (intrauterine pregnancy), 5-17
IVF (in vitro fertilization)
    assisted reproduction, 8-10
    IV fluid composition for, 14-8t
    Müllerian anomalies and, 8-7
    sperm aspiration and, 8-9

Jarisch–Herxheimer reaction, 21-8
JNC 8 hypertension classification, 12-3t

K

Kallmann syndrome, 6-6
Kayexalate (sodium polystyrene
    sulfonate), 14-9
Keflex (Cephalexin), 25-3t
Kegel exercises, 7-5
Kenalog (Triamcinolone acetonide),
    20-4t
Ketones, serum, 17-3, 17-3t
Klebsiella granulomatis, 21-10t
Kleihauer–Betke (KB) test, 11-13,
    16-14
Klinefelter syndrome, 8-8
KUB (kidneys, ureters, bladder)
    abdominal radiograph, 14-7

L

Labetalol, 11-1, 12-4t, 12-5t, 25-4t
Labioscrotal fusion, partial, 6-9t
Labor
    diabetes and, 17-7
    maternal hemodynamic changes,
        12-2t
    neuraxial anesthesia and, 4-4t
    pain, 4-1, 4-2t
    spontaneous, 10-4, 10-5f, 10-5t
    support, nonpharmacologic analgesia
        and, 4-6t
    valvular heart disease and, 12-14
Labor curve, 10-4
Lactated Ringer's solution, 14-8t
Lactational amenorrhea, 1-18
Lactational mastitis, 10-16
LactMed (pharmaceuticals & lactation
    database), 10-16
Lactulose, 9-7t
LAD (lymphadenopathy), 21-11t
LAIV (live attenuated influenza vaccine),
    13-6
Lamellar body count, 10-2
Lamotrigine, 18-4t, 19-7t
Lantus (Glargine), 17-3t, 25-7t
Laparoscopy
    chronic pelvic pain, 5-14
    complications, 3-10
    detorsion, 2-8
    endometriosis, 5-6, 5-7
    infertility testing, 8-1
    operative procedure, 24-7
    ovarian cysts, 2-7
Laparotomy, 2-7, 11-15
Large bowel obstruction, 3-10
Late congenital syphilis, 21-8
Latency antibiotics, 11-7, 11-7t
Latent syphilis, 21-7
Lateral–femoral cutaneous nerve,
    gynecologic surgery and, 3-4t
Lateral femoral cutaneous neuropathy,
    postpartum, 18-9
Lateral pelvis, 9-4
Late term, definition, 9-1

Latzko procedure, 7-8
Laxatives, 9-7t
LCIS (lobular carcinoma in situ), 1-7
LDH (lactate dehydrogenase), 5-20t,
    22-8, 22-9t
Le Fort colpocleisis, 7-4
Leg cramps, pregnancy and, 9-7
Leiomyoma, 2-2t, 5-3
Leiomyomata, 2-7
Leiomyosarcoma, 22-6
Lente (Insulin zinc), 17-3t
Lentigo maligna melanoma, 1-14
Leopold maneuver, 11-16
Letrozole (Femara), 5-4, 8-9, 25-12t
Leucovorin, 21-3
Leukocytes, 16-1
Leukoreduced blood products, 16-16t
Leuprolide, 5-4, 5-13
Leuprolide acetate, 5-7
Levator ani complex, 7-1
Levemir (Detemir), 17-3t
Levetiracetam, 18-4t
Levofloxacin, 2-9t, 14-6t, 14-7t
Levonorgestrel (emergency
    contraception), 1-18, 1-18t
Levonorgestrel-releasing intrauterine
    system (LNG-IUD, IUS)
    abnormal uterine bleeding, 5-9
    contraception, 1-16t, 1-17
    endometriosis, 5-7
    insertion, 24-1
    leiomyoma, 5-4
    primary dysmenorrhea, 5-11
LH (luteinizing hormone)
    deficiency, panhypopituitarism and,
        17-16
    delayed puberty and, 6-5
    menstrual cycle and, 6-1
    ovulation and, 17-1, 17-1f
    testing, infertility and, 8-1
Lice, pubic, 21-10
Lichen planus, 20-3
Lichen sclerosus, 20-2
Lichen simplex chronicus, 20-3
Lidex (Fluocinonide), 20-4t
Lidocaine, 4-1, 4-4t, 4-7, 5-15, 7-8
Linea terminalis, 9-4
Lipids and cholesterol, 1-10f, 1-10t.
    See also Dyslipidemia
Lisinopril, 12-4t
Lispro (Humalog), 17-3t, 25-7t
Lispro 75/25 (Humalog Mix 75/25),
    17-3t
Listeriosis, 9-4
Lithium, 19-7t, 25-9t
Liver failure, 12-9, 15-11
Liver hemorrhage, 12-9
LMWH (low–molecular-weight
    heparin), 12-14t, 16-9, 16-9t
LNG-IUD. *See* Levonorgestrel-releasing
    intrauterine system
Local anesthesia toxicity, 4-1, 4-4t
Local anesthetics, 4-1t, 4-5, 4-5f, 5-15
Locoid (Hydrocortisone butyrate),
    20-4t

Loestrin, 25-11t
Lomefloxacin, 14-6t
Lomotil (diphenoxylate–atropine), 9-8t
Long-acting reversible contraception (LARC), 1-16t
Long-chain L-3 hydroxyacyl-CoA dehydrogenase deficiency (LCHAD), 15-11
Longitudinal vaginal septum, 8-6
Loop electrosurgical excision procedure (LEEP), 24-4, 24-4f
Loperamide (Imodium), 9-8t
Lorazepam (Ativan), 19-6, 19-6t, 25-10t
Losartan, 12-4t
Lovastatin, 1-10t–1-11t
Lovenox (Enoxaparin), 4-3, 25-4t
Low back pain, 9-6
Lower-extremity edema or varicosities, 9-6
Low-lying placenta, 11-13
LP (lumbar puncture) shunt, 4-3
LPP (leak point pressure), 7-5
L/S (lecithin/sphingomyelin) ratio, 10-2
LSIL (low-grade squamous intraepithelial lesion), 1-8, 1-9t
Lugol iodine, 1-9
Lung volumes and capacities, 13-1f
Lupus anticoagulant, 16-12t
Lupus erythematosus, systemic (SLE), 9-9
Luteal phase of menstruation, 17-1
Lymphogranuloma venereum, 21-10t. See also Chlamydia trachomatis
Lynch syndrome, 5-20, 22-7

M

M3 muscarinic receptor, 7-1t
Macroadenoma, 17-16
Macrobid (Nitrofurantoin), 14-6t, 25-2t
Macrocytic anemia, 16-3
Macrosomia, 9-8
Magnesium, 17-4, 18-6t
Magnesium citrate, 9-7t
Magnesium hydroxide (MOM), 9-7t
Magnesium sulfate
    antihypertensive effects, 25-4t
    digitalis toxicity, 14-9
    preeclampsia, 11-1, 12-9t
    preterm delivery and, 11-8t
    tocolytic effects, 25-7t
    uterine inversion, 11-15
Magnetic resonance-guided focused ultrasound (MRgFUS), 5-4
Magnetic resonance imaging (MRI)
    acute kidney injury, 14-3
    breast cancer, 1-6t
    chronic kidney disease, 14-4
    common indications, 2-1
    endometriosis, 5-6
    epithelial ovarian cancer, 22-7
    leiomyoma, 5-4
    preeclampsia, 11-1
Male circumcision, 24-10
Male factor infertility, 8-8
Male pseudohermaphroditism, 6-9, 6-10

Male sexual differentiation pathway, 6-10f
Malformation, definition, 9-9
Malignancy. See also Cancer
    ovarian cyst vs., 2-7
Malodorous lochia/discharge, postpartum, 10-15
Malpresentation, 11-16
Mammography/mammogram, 1-4t, 1-6t
MAOIs (monoamine oxidase inhibitors), 4-1
Marijuana, 6-7t, 9-2, 19-2t
Marsupialization
    Bartholin gland cyst, 5-3, 20-7t, 24-3f, 24-5
    Gartner duct cyst, 20-7t
Martius flap, 7-8
"Mask of Pregnancy," 20-1t
Massage, 4-6t, 5-14
Massive transfusion, 16-17, 16-18t
Mastalgia, 1-5t
Mastitis, 1-5t
    lactational, 10-16
Maternal Mental Health Safety Bundle, 19-4
Maternal mortality. See also Female mortality causes
    preeclampsia and, 12-10t
    tuberculosis, 21-5–21-6
Maternal serum alpha-fetoprotein (MSAFP), 9-11
Maternal serum aneuploidy screening, 9-12
Mature teratoma, 22-9
MCA (middle cerebral artery) Doppler, 21-3
McDonald cervical cerclage, 11-6, 24-10
McIndoe neovagina, 8-7
MCPAP for Moms Toolkit, Massachusetts, 19-4
MDD (major depressive disorder), 19-3
Mechanical heart valves, 12-14
Meconium aspiration syndrome, 10-2, 11-17
Meconium-stained amniotic fluid, 11-16
Medications, perioperative review of, 3-1
Medroxyprogesterone (Depo-Provera), 25-10t
Medroxyprogesterone (MPA), 5-8, 5-9
Medroxyprogesterone acetate (MDPA, Prempro), 5-14, 5-18t, 6-7, 25-13t
Megaloblastic anemia, 16-3
Megestrol acetate, 5-9
Meigs–Wertheim hysterectomy, 22-1
Melanoma
    Clark, Breslow, and Chung staging for, 22-13t
    screening, 1-14
    vaginal, 22-11
    vulvar, 22-12, 22-13
Membrane stripping, 10-7
Menarche, 6-1, 17-1
Meningitis, amenorrhea and, 6-7t

Meningocele, 9-10
Meningomyelocele, 9-10
Menopause, 5-16, 17-1
Menstrual cycle, 17-1, 17-1f
Mental status. See also Altered mental status
    diabetic ketoacidosis and, 17-3t
Meperidine, 4-2t, 4-7
Mepivacaine, 4-6
Meralgia paresthetica, 18-8
6-Mercaptopurine, 15-7t
Mercury consumption. See Methylmercury
MESA (microsurgical epididymal sperm aspiration), 8-9
Mesalamine, 15-7t
Mesenchymal tumors (sarcomas), uterine, 22-4
Mesh augmentation and mesh kit procedures, 7-4
Mesna, 22-18
Metabolic acidosis
    acute kidney injury and, 14-3
    arterial blood gas analysis, 13-3
    fetal cord blood gas analysis, 10-14
    predicted changes for, 13-3t
Metabolic alkalosis, 13-3, 13-3t
Metabolic syndrome, 6-12
Metamucil (psyllium), 9-7t
Metastatic tumors, ovarian, 22-7
Metformin (Glucophage), 17-8t, 25-7t
Methadone, 19-3t, 25-9t
Methamphetamines in pregnancy, 19-2t
Methotrexate (MTX)
    characteristics/indications, 25-6t
    ectopic pregnancy, 2-4, 2-4t
    gestational trophoblastic neoplasia, 22-16t
    IBD, 15-5, 15-7t
    medical abortion, 5-19t
Methyldopa, 12-4t
Methylergonovine (Methergine), 11-9, 11-10t, 25-6t
Methylmercury, 9-4. See also Mercury consumption
Methylprednisolone, 15-7t
Metoclopramide (Reglan), 9-5, 25-8t
Metronidazole (Flagyl)
    characteristics/indications, 25-3t
    ob-gyn surgery prophylaxis, 3-7t
    PID, 2-9t
    sexual assault postexposure prophylaxis, 2-13
    vaginitis, 5-2t
MIA (Multivariate Index Assay), 5-20, 5-20t
Miconazole, 5-2t
Microadenoma, 17-16
Microangiopathic anemia, 16-3t
Microcephaly, 21-4
Microcytic anemia, 16-2
Micronor (Norethindrone), 5-14, 25-11t
Micturition, physiology and mechanisms of, 7-1t

Middle cerebral artery Doppler velocimetry, 10-2
Midline block, during EBRT, 22-18
Midurethral slings, 7-6
Midwives, education and accreditation, 10-16t
Mifepristone, 5-4, 5-18, 5-18t
Migraine, 18-1, 18-1t, 18-2, 18-2t
Mild androgen insensitivity syndrome, 6-11
Mineralocorticoids, 6-12
Mineral oil enema, 9-7t
Minislings (single-incision slings), 7-7
Minor antigens (Ag), 16-14
Mirabegron (Myrbetriq), 7-6t
Miralax (polyethylene glycol), 9-7t
Mirena IUD, 5-5
Mirena IUS, 1-16t, 25-10t. See also Levonorgestrel-releasing intrauterine system
Mirror syndrome, 11-2
Miscarriage
    recurrent pregnancy loss and, 8-4
    spontaneous, 2-1, 2-5
Misoprostol, 5-18, 5-18t, 11-9
Misoprostol (Cytotec, PGE₁), 10-7, 11-10t, 25-6t
Mitral regurgitation (MR), 12-12t, 12-13, 12-13t
Mitral stenosis (MS), 12-12t, 12-13, 12-13t
Mixed germ cell tumor, 22-8, 22-9t
Mixed urinary incontinence (MUI), 7-4
Modified Pomeroy postpartum tubal ligation, 24-9
Modified radical hysterectomy, 22-1
Molar pregnancy, 22-14, 22-14f
Molluscum contagiosum, 21-9
Mometasone furoate (Elocon), 20-4t
Monochorionic diamniotic twins, 11-4f, 11-5
Monochorionic monoamniotic twins, 11-5
Monodermal teratomas, 22-9
Monozygosity, 11-4
Mood disorders, 5-13
Morphine, 4-2t, 4-4t, 4-7t, 12-10, 25-9t
Mortality causes, female, 1-20t
Mosaicism, 1-9
Motor vehicle collisions, 2-11
Moxifloxacin, 2-9t
MPA (medroxyprogesterone), 5-8, 5-9
MRgFUS (magnetic resonance-guided focused ultrasound), 22-1
MRI (magnetic resonance imaging). See Magnetic resonance imaging
MRKH (Mayer–Rokitansky–Kuster–Hauser), 8-6
MRSA (methicillin-resistant Staphylococcus aureus), 10-16
MTX. See Methotrexate
Mucinous adenocarcinoma, 22-2
Mucinous epithelial ovarian cancer, 22-7
Mucinous epithelial uterine tumors, 22-3

Müllerian anomalies, 8-4, 8-5f, 9-11
Multidrug-resistant infection, 13-4
Multiparous, definition, 9-1
Multiple daily injection (MDI) therapy, 17-2
Multiple gestation, 11-4, 11-4f
Multiple sclerosis, 18-8
Musculoskeletal anomalies, 9-12
Myoclonic seizures, 18-3
Myofascial pain syndrome, 5-14
Myomas, 5-3
Myomectomy, 5-4
Myrbetriq (Mirabegron), 7-6t

N
Nafarelin acetate, 5-7
Nalbuphine, 4-2t
Naloxone, 19-3t, 26-4f
Naproxen, 18-2t, 18-3t
Narcotics, 5-11
Nasal bone, 9-12
Nausea and vomiting of pregnancy (NVP), 9-5
Necrotizing fasciitis, 3-7
Neisseria gonorrhoeae, 2-9
Neonatal alloimmune thrombocytopenia (NAIT), 16-15
Neonatal resuscitation program (NRP) algorithm, 27-1f
Nephrolithiasis, 2-2t, 14-7
Nephrolithotomy, percutaneous, 14-8
Nerve sheath tumors, 2-7
Neural tubes
    defects, 9-1, 9-10
    embryologic development, 9-9t
Neuraxial anesthesia, 4-2–4-4
Neuropathies in pregnancy, 18-8
Neurosyphilis, 21-8
Neurotoxicity, chemotherapy and, 22-18
Newborn respiratory distress, 10-2
Nexplanon (Etonogestrel implant) insertion, 24-1, 24-2f
Niacin, 1-11t
Nicardipine, 11-1
Nicotinic acid, 1-11t
Nicotinic cholinergic receptor, 7-1t
Nifedipine
    antihypertensive effects, 25-4t
    chronic hypertension, 12-4t
    hypertensive crisis, 12-5t
    migraine, 18-3t
    preeclampsia, 11-1
    preterm delivery and, 11-8t
    primary dysmenorrhea, 5-11
    tocolytic effects, 25-7t
Nipple discharge, 1-5, 17-16
Nitrates, 12-10
Nitrendipine, 12-4t
Nitric oxide (N₂O), 4-6
    inhalational, 4-7
Nitrofurantoin (Macrobid), 14-6t, 25-2t
Nitrofurantoin monohydrate, 14-5t

Nitroglycerine, 4-6, 11-15, 12-5t, 12-15t
Nitroprusside, 11-1
Nivolumab, 22-17
Noncalcium-based nephrolithiasis, 14-7
Nonclassical congenital adrenal hyperplasia (NCAH), 6-11
Noncontrast computed tomography (CT), 2-1
Nonelectrolyte fluids, distending, 3-11
Nongestational choriocarcinoma, 22-9, 22-9t
Nonimmune hydrops, 11-2
Nonimmune hydrops fetalis (NIHF), 9-10
Nonmegaloblastic anemia, 16-3
Nonstress test (NST), 10-1, 11-13
Non-vitamin K oral anticoagulant (NOAC), 16-9, 16-9t
Norethindrone (Micronor), 5-14, 25-11t
Norethindrone acetate, 5-7, 5-9, 25-13t
Normocytic anemia, 16-3
Nortriptyline, 19-6t
Novolin L (Insulin zinc), 17-3t
Novolin N (Isophane insulin), 17-3t, 25-7t
Novolin R, 17-3t, 25-7t
NovoLog (Aspart), 17-3t
NPH (Isophane insulin), 17-3t
NSAIDs (nonsteroidal anti-inflammatories)
    abnormal uterine bleeding, 5-9
    adenomyosis, 5-5
    characteristics/indications, 25-8t
    chronic pelvic pain, 5-14
    endometriosis, 5-7, 5-14
    lactational mastitis, 10-16
    leiomyoma, 5-4
    postoperative pain management, 4-7
    preterm delivery and, 11-8t
    primary dysmenorrhea, 5-11
NSTEMI (non-ST segment elevation MI), 12-10
NT (nuchal translucency), 9-1, 9-12
NTD (neural tube defect), 9-1, 9-10
Nuchal translucency (NT), 9-12
Nuclear medicine, 2-2
Nugent score, 5-1
Nutrients in pregnancy, 9-4
Nutrition
    in pregnancy, 9-3
    total parenteral nutrition, 15-12, 15-12t
Nuva-Ring (Ethinyl estradiol/etonogestrel vaginal ring), 25-11t
NYHA (New York Heart Association), 12-1t
Nystatin, 5-2t

O
OAB (overactive bladder), 7-4, 7-5
Obesity, 1-11, 3-3, 6-12, 9-3
Obstetric anal sphincter injury (OASIS), 7-9

Obstetric conjugate (OC), 9-4
Obstetric laceration repair, 24-10
Obturator nerve, 3-4t
Obturator neuropathies, postpartum, 18-9
OCPs (oral contraceptive pills)
    characteristics/indications, 25-11t
    continuous, abnormal uterine bleeding, 5-8, 5-9
    contraception, 1-17
    endometriosis, 5-7, 5-14
    leiomyoma, 5-4
    primary amenorrhea and, 6-6
    uterine/vaginal obstruction, 8-7
OCs. See Obstetric conjugate
OEIS complex (Omphalocele, Exstrophy of the bladder, Imperfect anus, Spinal defects), 9-11
Ofloxacin, 2-9t, 14-6t
Olaparib, 22-17
Olaprib, 25-5t
O'Leary uterine artery ligation sutures, 11-10, 11-11f
Oligohydramnios, 11-5
Oliguria, perioperative, 3-9
Omphalocele, 9-11
Ondansetron (Zofran), 9-5, 25-8t
Oophorectomy, 2-7, 5-7, 5-13, 5-21, 24-7
Operative hysteroscopy, 24-6
Operative laparoscopy, 24-7
Operative reports, perioperative evaluation of, 3-1
Operative vaginal delivery, 10-12, 10-12f
    complications, 10-13
Opioids
    characteristics/indications, 25-8t
    combination of local anesthetic and, 4-4
    labor pain, 4-1
    Life-Threatening Emergency (Adult) Algorithm, 26-4f
    as neuraxial anesthetic, 4-4t
    postoperative pain management, 4-7
    in pregnancy, 19-3t
Oral glucose tolerance test (OGTT), 17-5, 17-6t
Organ space, 3-7
Orgasmic headache, 18-1
Oropharyngeal cytomegalovirus, 21-6
Orthocyclen, 25-11t
Ortho Evra Patch (Norelgestromin/ ethinyl estradiol transdermal system), 25-11t
Ortho Tri-Cyclen, 25-11t
Osmotic laxative, 9-7t
Osteogenesis imperfecta, 9-12
Osteoporosis, 1-12, 5-16, 5-17
    medications, 25-12t
O'Sullivan scale, modified, 17-6t
Ovarian cancer
    annual diagnoses and deaths, 1-20t
    epithelial, 22-7

fertility preserving surgeries for, 8-11
    FIGO staging for, 22-8t
    germ cell tumors, 22-8, 22-11t
    sex cord-stromal tumors, 22-10
Ovarian cysts, 2-2t, 2-7, 17-13f
Ovarian hyperstimulation syndrome (OHSS), 8-11
Ovarian torsion, 2-2t, 5-21
Ovarian transposition surgery, 8-10
Ovarian tumors, 2-2t, 17-13f
Ovarian veins, embolization of, 5-14
Ovaries, preservation procedure, 24-8
Overactive bladder (OAB), 7-4, 7-5
Overflow incontinence, 7-4, 7-7
Ovral, 25-11t
Ovulation, 17-1
Ovulation disorders, 8-11
Ovulation induction, 8-3, 8-9, 8-11
Oxybutynin ER (Ditropan XL), 7-6t
Oxybutynin IR (Ditropan), 7-6t
Oxybutynin patch (Gelnique), 7-6t
Oxycodone (Roxicodone, Percocet), 25-9t
Oxytocin (Pitocin), 10-7, 11-9, 11-10t, 25-6t

P
Paclitaxel (Taxol), 22-3t, 22-17, 22-18, 25-5t
Paget disease
    breast, 1-7
    vulva, 22-12, 22-13
Pain
    abdominal, 15-5t
    abnormal wall, 5-13
    acute pelvic, 2-2, 2-2t
    Bartholin duct cyst or abscess, 5-2
    chronic pelvic, 5-13
    differential diagnosis of IBS symptoms and, 15-5t
    genitopelvic, 5-15
    IC/BPS, 7-8
    low back, 9-6
    pelvic, 5-14
    postoperative, 4-7
    postpartum, 10-15
    round ligament, 9-6
    shoulder, 3-11
    upper abdominal, 15-3t
    vulvar, 5-14
PAIS (partial/incomplete androgen insensitivity syndrome), 6-10, 6-11
PALM-COEIN classification, 5-8
Palmer's point, 3-11
Pancreatitis, 15-1, 15-3t
Pandel (Hydrocortisone probutate), 20-4t
Panhypopituitarism, 17-16
Panic disorder, 19-4
PAPP-A (pregnancy-associated plasma protein A), 9-12
Pap smear, 1-8, 1-8t, 5-1
Paracervical blocks, 4-5f

ParaGard (Copper T IUD), 1-16t, 1-18, 1-19t, 25-10t
  insertion, 24-1
Parametrial boost, after EBRT, 22-18, 22-19t
Parathyroid disorders, 17-14
Paratubal cysts, 2-7
Parenteral analgesia, 4-1–4-2, 4-2t
Parietal pain, 2-5
Parity, 9-1
Parkland method for postpartum tubal ligation, 24-9
Paroxetine, 5-16, 19-6t
PARP inhibitors, 22-17
Partial-Birth Abortion Ban Act (2003), 5-18
Partial exenteration hysterectomy, 22-1
Partial/focal seizures, 18-3
Partial hydatidiform moles, 22-14, 22-14t
Parvovirus, 21-3
Parvovirus B19, 21-2
Patient-controlled analgesia (PCA), 4-2t, 4-7t
Pazopanib, 22-17
PCEA (patient-controlled epidural analgesia), 4-7t
PCOS (polycystic ovarian syndrome), 6-7t, 8-2, 17-6t, 17-13t
PCR (polymerase chain reaction), 8-9
PDPH (postdural puncture headache) risk, 4-3
PEA (pulseless electrical activity), 26-2f
Peak expiratory flow rate (PEFR), 13-1
Peak height velocity (PHV), 6-1, 6-1t
PEGylated liposomal doxorubicin, 22-17
Pelvic congestion syndrome, 5-14
Pelvic floor, urogenital triangle and, 23-6f
Pelvic floor muscle training (PMFT), 7-5
Pelvic floor physical therapy, 5-14, 5-15, 5-16
Pelvic fractures, 2-11
Pelvic inflammatory disease (PID), 2-2t, 2-8, 8-3
Pelvic kidney, 2-7
Pelvic organ prolapse (POP), 7-1, 7-3
Pelvic organ prolapse quantification (POP-Q), 7-2, 7-2f
Pelvic pain, acute, 2-2, 2-2t
Pelvic Pain Assessment, 5-14
Pelvic plexus efferents (S2–4), 7-1t
Pelvimetry, 9-4
Pelvis
  anatomy, 9-4
  arterial blood supply, 23-3f
  arterial blood supply surgical considerations, 23-3t
  avascular planes, surgical considerations, 23-4f
  bony anatomy, 23-1f
  shapes, 9-5f
  shapes, Caldwell & Moloy classification, 9-5

Pemphigoid gestationis, 20-1t
Penetrating trauma, 2-11
Penicillins (PCNs), 10-16, 21-8t, 21-11t, 25-3t
Penile cytomegalovirus, 21-6
Pentosan polysulfate, 7-8
Pentosan polysulfate sodium, 5-14
Percutaneous nephrolithotomy, 14-8
Perimenopause, 5-13, 5-16
Perinatal death, 12-10t
Perineal cysts, 20-6t
Perineal sensation, anal incontinence and, 7-9
Perioperative oliguria, 3-9
Perioperative patient management, 3-1
Peripartum cardiomyopathy, 12-15, 12-15t
Peripartum onset of major depressive disorder, 19-3
Peripheral precocity, 6-2t
Peritoneal inclusion cysts, 2-7
Periviable, definition, 9-1
Permanent hypogonadotropic (secondary) hypogonadism, 6-6
Permethrin, 21-10
Peroneal nerve, gynecologic surgery and, 3-4t
Peroneal neuropathy, postpartum, 18-9
Persistent depressive disorder, 19-3
Personality disorders, 5-13
Pessaries, 7-5, 7-6
PG measurement, 10-2
pH
  arterial, diabetic ketoacidosis and, 17-3, 17-3t
  PPROM and, 11-7
  vaginal, 5-15
Pharmacotherapy
  anxiety disorders, 19-4
  bipolar disorder, 19-5
  depression, 19-4
  psychosis, 19-5
  schizophrenia, 19-6
Phenobarbital, 18-4t
Phenothiazine, 4-1
Phenytoin, 18-4t
Pheochromocytoma, 17-12
Phobias, 19-5
Phosphate, 17-4
PHQ-9 (depression screening questionnaire), 19-4
Phthirus pubis, 21-10
Phyllodes tumor, 1-7
Physical activity, 19-5. See also Exercise
Physical inactivity, 17-6t
Physical therapy (PT), 5-14
Pica, 9-4
PID (pelvic inflammatory disease), 2-2t, 2-8, 8-3
PIERS (Preeclampsia Integrated Estimate of Risk), 18-5
Piperacillin, 11-17t
Piperacillin/tazobactam, 25-2t
Pitocin (Oxytocin), 10-7, 11-9, 11-10t, 25-6t

Pituitary, amenorrhea and, 6-7t
Pituitary adenomas, 6-8
Pituitary disorders, 17-16
Piver–Rutledge–Smith classification (1974), 22-1
Placenta accreta, 11-14
Placenta increta, 11-14
Placental abruption, 2-11, 11-12, 12-3t, 12-9t
Placental location, fetal ultrasound of, 9-8
Placental site trophoblastic disease, 22-15
Placental site trophoblastic tumor, 22-14
Placenta percreta, 11-14
Placenta previa, 11-13
Plan B (emergency contraception), 1-18, 1-18t
Planned vaginal breech delivery, 11-16
Plasma IV solution, 14-8t
Plasma volume, 16-1
Platelets, 16-15t
Platinum, 22-17
Platypelloid pelvis, 9-5, 9-5f, 9-5t
Pneumonia (PNA), 13-4
Polycystic kidney disease, 14-4
Polycystic ovary syndrome (PCOS), 6-7t, 8-2, 17-6t, 17-13f
Polyembryoma, 22-9, 22-9t
Polyethylene glycol (Miralax, GoLytely – electrolytes), 9-7t
Polyhydramnios, 11-5, 11-9
Polymorphic eruption of pregnancy, 20-1t
Pontine micturition center, 7-1
Positioning, preoperative, 3-3
Positive predictive value (PPV), 1-20t
Postcolporrhaphy, 7-3
Posterior compartment defect surgery, 7-3
Posterior pelvic organ prolapse, 7-1
Posterior pelvis, 9-4
Posterior pituitary, 17-16
Postmenopausal bleeding, 5-10
Postoperative fever, 3-6, 3-6t
Postoperative ileus, 3-5
Postoperative pain management, 4-7
Postpartum blues, 19-4
Postpartum care, 10-15, 17-7
Postpartum cerebral angiopathy, 18-6
Postpartum compression neuropathies, 18-9
Postpartum depression, 19-3
Postpartum hemodynamic changes, 12-2
Postpartum hemorrhage (PPH), 11-9, 11-10, 11-12t. See also Uterine atony
Postpartum hypertension, 12-9
Postpartum hypoparathyroidism, 17-15
Postpartum visit, 10-15
Post term, definition, 9-1
Potassium, 17-4
Potassium sensitivity test, 7-8
Pox virus, 21-9

PPROM (preterm premature rupture of membranes), 11-6
Prader orchidometer, 8-8
Pravastatin, 1-10t–1-11t
pRBCs, 16-15t
Precocious puberty, 6-2, 6-2t, 6-4f
Prednicarbate (Dermatop), 20-4t
Prednisone, 6-12, 15-7t, 25-10t
Preeclampsia (PEC). See also HELLP syndrome
    definition, 11-1
    headache and, 18-1t
    management and treatment, 12-7t, 12-9, 12-9t
    medications, 25-4t
    pregnancy outcomes, 12-9t
    severe, management algorithm, 12-8f
    superimposed on chronic hypertension, 11-1
    with and without severe features, 12-6t
Pregestational diabetes mellitus, 9-9, 17-6, 17-6t
Pregnancy. See also Ectopic pregnancy; under Prenatal
    cardiovascular changes in, 12-2
    clinical pelvimetry, 9-4, 9-5f, 9-5t
    early failure, 2-5–2-7
    ECG changes in, 12-2
    fetal ultrasound, 9-8
    hypertension related to, 12-6t, 12-7, 12-7t, 12-8f, 12-9t
    Müllerian anomalies and, 8-6t, 8-7
    recurrent loss, 8-4
Pregnancy Risk Assessment Monitoring System (PRAMS), 1-16
Pregnancy termination
    medical, 5-18, 5-18t
    medical contraindications, 5-19t
    surgical, 5-19
Pregnancy test, 3-3, 5-14
Pregnenolone, 6-12
Preimplantation genetic testing, diagnosis, screening, 8-11
Premarin, 2-10t, 25-13t
Premature menopause, 5-16
Premature ovarian insufficiency (POI), 8-2
Premenstrual dysphoric disorder (PMDD), 5-12
Premenstrual syndrome (PMS), 5-12
Premixed insulin, 17-3t
Prenatal complaints, common, 9-5
Prenatal testing, routine, 9-1–9-13
Prenatal visits, routine, 9-1, 9-1t, 9-2t
PRES (posterior reversible encephalopathy syndrome), 18-6
Presacral neurectomy, 5-7
Prescription drug abuse, 19-1
Pressure-flow study, 7-5
Preterm deliveries, 12-3t, 12-9t
Preterm labor (PTL), 11-8
Preterm premature rupture of membranes (PPROM), 8-6, 11-6

Previable, definition, 9-1
Primary amenorrhea, 6-6, 6-10
Primary dysmenorrhea (PD), 5-11
Primary headache, 18-1
Primary hypercortisolism, 17-10t
Primary hyperparathyroidism, 17-14
Primary hypocortisolism, 17-10t
Primary hypogonadism, 6-5, 8-8
Primary hypothyroidism, 17-8, 17-10f
Primary ovarian insufficiency, 6-6, 6-7
Primary progressive multiple sclerosis, 18-8
Primigravida, definition, 9-1
Primiparous, definition, 9-1
PR muscle, defecation and, 7-1
Probenecid, 2-9t
Procardia, 25-4t. See also Nifedipine
Prochlorperazine (Compazine), 25-8t
Progesterone
    abnormal uterine bleeding, 5-9
    challenge test, 6-7
    endometriosis, 5-7
    as hormone of pregnancy, 17-2
    ovulation and, 17-1f
    serum, ectopic pregnancy, 2-4
    therapy (PT), 5-17
Progesterone IUD, 5-17t
Progestin-only contraception, 1-17t, 1-18t
Progestins
    abnormal uterine bleeding, 5-9
    acute uterine bleeding, 2-10t
    adenomyosis, 5-5
    endometriosis, 5-7
    high-dose, primary amenorrhea and, 6-6
    hormone therapy, 5-18t
    lipids and, 1-11
    pelvic congestion syndrome, 5-14
    primary dysmenorrhea, 5-11
Progressive central precocious puberty, 6-2t
Progressive relapsing multiple sclerosis, 18-8
Prolactin (PRL), 6-5, 6-5f, 8-1
Proliferative phase of ovulation, 17-1f
PROM (premature rupture of membranes), 11-6
Promethazine, 9-5
Promethazine HCl (Phenergan), 25-8t
Propranolol, 18-3t
Prostaglandin F$_{2\alpha}$, 11-10t
Prostaglandins, 11-9
Prosthetic valves, 12-14, 12-14t
Protein, in pregnancy, 9-4t
Protein C/S, 16-10t
Proteins, pregnancy changes in, 15-1
Proteinuria, 11-1, 14-1
Prothrombin G20210A mutation, 16-10t
Provera (Medroxyprogesterone), 2-10t. See also Medroxyprogesterone
Prurigo gestationis, 20-2t
Pruritic urticarial papules and plaques of pregnancy (PUPPP), 20-1t

Pruritus, 4-4t, 21-10
Pseudohypoparathyroidism, 17-15
Pseudoincontinence, 7-9
PSI (pneumonia severity index), 13-4
Psoriasis, 20-4
Psychiatric disease screening, 1-16
Psychiatric medications, 19-6t, 25-9t
Psychosis, 19-5
Psychotherapy, 5-14, 19-4, 19-5
Psyllium (Metamucil), 9-7t
PTH (parathyroid hormone), 1-13, 17-14
PTH-related hypercalcemia, 17-14
PTHrP (parathyroid hormone–related protein), 17-14
Pubarche, 6-1
Puberty
    characteristics, 6-1
    delayed, 6-4, 6-5f
    GD-dependent precocious, 6-3
    GD-independent precocious, 6-3
    isolated precocious, 6-3
    precocious, 6-2, 6-2t
Pubic hair, 6-1f, 6-1t
Pubic lice, 21-10
Pudendal block, 4-5f
Pudendal nerve, 3-4t, 7-1, 7-1t
Pudendal nerve block, 24-10
Pulmonary angiography, 16-8
Pulmonary disease, 3-1t
Pulmonary edema, 12-2, 12-9, 13-5
Pulmonary embolism (PE)
    characteristics, 16-6
    diagnostic evaluation, 16-7, 16-8t
    perioperative, 3-7, 3-8t
    pretest probability scoring of, 16-8t
Pulmonary function testing, 13-1, 13-1f, 13-2f
Pulmonary hypertension, 12-11, 12-11t
Pulmonary insufficiency, 14-7
Pulmonary system embryologic development, 9-9t
Punctuation, 1-9
Pustular psoriasis of pregnancy, 20-1t
PVR (postvoid residual resistance), 7-4
Pyelonephritis, 2-2t, 14-6
Pyrimethamine, 21-3

Q
qSOFA (quick SOFA) score, 3-8
Q-tip test, 7-4
Quad screen, 9-1, 9-12
Querleu–Morrow classification of radical hysterectomy, 22-1t
Quickening (1st fetal movement), 9-2

R
Radiation therapy (RT)
    cervical cancer, 22-2, 22-3t
    endometrial cancer, 22-6
    germ cell tumors, 22-9, 22-11t
    gynecologic cancers, 22-19t
    types, 22-18
Radical hysterectomy, 22-1, 22-1t, 22-3t
Radical trachelectomy, 22-3

Radical vaginectomy, 22-11
Radiofrequency ablation, 5-5
Radiography (XR), 2-1, 2-11
Radiologic pelvimetry, 9-5
RAI (radioactive iodine), 17-10
RAIR (rectoanal inhibitory reflex), 7-1
Raloxifene, 1-13, 25-12t
Raltegravir, 2-13
Randomized control trial (RCT), 1-21t
Rash, syphilitic, 21-7
RBC mass (red blood cell mass), 16-1
RCT (randomized control trial), 1-21t
Recipient twin, twin–twin transfusion
    syndrome and, 11-5
Recombinant factor VII, 11-10
Rectal prolapse repair, 7-10
Rectocele, 7-1
Rectovaginal fistula, 7-9
Rectum, prolapse into vagina, 7-1
Recurrent pregnancy loss (RPL), 8-3
Recurrent UTI, 14-4
Red top tube test, 16-17
5α-Reductase androgen abnormality/
    insensitivity syndromes, 6-9t
Referrals, for depression, 19-4
Referred pain, 2-5
Reglan, 6-6. See also Metoclopramide
Reifenstein androgen abnormality/
    insensitivity syndromes, 6-9t
Relapsing-remitting (RR) multiple
    sclerosis, 18-8
Relaxation exercises, 5-16
Relaxin, 17-2
Remifentanil, 4-2t
Renal agenesis, 9-11
Renal changes during pregnancy, 9-3
Renal failure, acute, 12-9
Renal replacement therapy (RRT), 14-3
Renewing tumors, 22-16
Reproductive organs, 23-1f, 23-2f
Reprotox (online schizophrenia
    resource), 19-6
Respiratory acidosis, 10-14, 13-3,
    13-3t
Respiratory alkalosis, 13-3, 13-3t
Respiratory changes in pregnancy, 9-3,
    13-2, 21-5
Respiratory distress syndrome (RDS),
    10-2
Restitution, in labor, 10-5
Retained placenta, 4-6, 11-10
Retroplacental clot, 11-13
Retropubic colposuspension, 7-6
Reversible cerebral vasoconstriction
    syndromes (RCVS), 18-1,
    18-1t
Revised Cardiac Risk Index (RCRI),
    3-1t, 3-2t
RFA (ultrasound-guided radiofrequency
    thermal ablation), 5-4
Rh alloimmunization, 16-13
Rho(D) Ig (immunoglobulin), 5-19
Rhythm method, 1-18
RIPE combination, for TB, 21-6

Risedronate (Actonel), 25-12t
Risk factors (RFs), perioperative
    evaluation of, 3-1
Risperidone, 19-6
RMI (Risk of Malignancy Index), 5-20,
    5-20t
Rocephin (Ceftriaxone), 25-2t
Rod fusion, 4-3
ROMA (Risk of Ovarian Malignancy),
    5-20, 5-20t
Rome III and Rome IV IBS diagnostic
    criteria, 15-4t
Ropivacaine, 4-1t, 4-4t
Rosuvastatin (Crestor), 1-10t
Rotational flaps, 8-7
Round ligament pain, 9-6
Rubella, 21-2, 21-3

S
Sacral nerve modulation (SNM), 7-6,
    7-9, 7-10
Sacrocolpoperineopexy, 7-3
Sacrocolpopexy, 7-3
Sacrospinous ligament fixation, 7-3
Saddle block, 4-5f
SAH (subarachnoid hemorrhage),
    18-1t, 18-7
Salpingectomy, 2-5, 8-3
Salpingostomy, 2-5
Salt wasting, 6-12
Sanctura (Trospium chloride), 7-6t
Sanctura XR (Trospium ER), 7-6t
Sarcoidosis, 6-7t
Sarcoma botryoides, 22-11
Schizophrenia, 19-6
Scissors, surgical, 24-11, 24-11f
Sclerotherapy, 5-14
Screening. See also Testing
    breast cancer, 1-7t
    cervical cancer, 1-7, 1-9t
    cholesterol, 1-10t
    colorectal cancer, 1-3
    cystic fibrosis, 9-13
    depression and psychiatric disease,
        1-16
    genetic, 9-12
    gestational diabetes mellitus, 9-2,
        17-5, 17-6t
    incontinence, 1-2
    skin cancer, 1-3, 1-13
    substance abuse, 19-1t
    Tay–Sachs, 9-13
SDP (single deepest pocket), fetal
    ultrasound, 9-8
Seasonale, Seasonique, 25-11t
Sebaceous gland cyst, 20-6t
2nd trimester, 9-2t, 9-3, 9-8, 9-12, 9-12t
Secondary amenorrhea, 6-6
Secondary carcinomas, vaginal cancer
    and, 22-11
Secondary dysmenorrhea (SD), 5-11
Secondary headache, 18-1
Secondary hypercortisolism, 17-10t
Secondary hyperparathyroidism in renal
    disease, 17-15

Secondary hypocortisolism, 17-10t
Secondary hypogonadism, 6-6, 8-8
Secondary hypothyroidism, 17-8
Secondary progressive multiple sclerosis, 18-8
Secretory epithelial uterine tumors, 22-3
Secretory phase of ovulation, 17-1f
Sedatives, 19-3t
Sedlis criteria for cervical cancer, 22-3t
Seizure disorders, 18-3
Seizures, 11-1
Self-breast exam, 1-6t
Semen analysis, 8-8, 8-8t
Semirigid ureteroscopy, 14-8
Senna, 9-7t
Sepsis, 3-8
Septate uterus, 8-6f, 8-6t, 8-7
Septic shock, 3-8
Sequence, definition, 9-9
Sequential genetic screening, 9-13
SERMs (selective estrogen receptor modulators), 1-13, 25-12t
Serologic testing, for syphilis, 21-8
Serous epithelial ovarian cancer, 22-7
Sertoli–Leydig cell tumors, 22-10
Sertraline, 19-6t
Sertraline (Zoloft), 25-9f
Sex-cord stromal tumors, 22-10
Sex therapy, 5-16
Sexual assault, 2-12–2-13
Sexual Assault Nurse Examiner (SANE), 2-12
Sexual differentiation pathways, 6-10f
Sexual intercourse, induction of labor and, 10-7
Sexually-transmitted infections/disease (STIs)
  HIV/AIDS in women, 21-1
  HPV, 21-6
  screening, 1-2
  sexual assault postexposure prophylaxis, 2-12–2-13
  syphilis, 21-7
  Zika, 21-4
Sexual response cycle, 5-15
SGA (small for gestational age), 12-3t, 12-9t
Sheehan syndrome, 6-7t, 6-8, 17-10t
Shirodkar cervical cerclage, 11-6, 24-10
Shock wave lithotripsy, 14-8
Short-acting insulin, 17-3t
Short cervix, 11-5, 11-6f
Short stature, congenital adrenal hyperplasia and, 6-12
Shoulder breech, 10-4
Shoulder dystocia, 4-2
Shoulder pain, post-laparoscopic, 3-11
Sickle cell anemia, 16-3t
Sickle cell disease and variants, 16-4
Sideroblastic anemia, 16-2t
SIG E CAPS (Sleep, Interest, Guilt, Energy, Concentration, Appetite, Psychomotor, Suicide), 19-3

Sigmoidoscopy, flexible, 7-9
Sildenafil, 5-16
Simple endometrial hyperplasia with/ without atypia, 22-4, 22-4t
Simple extrafascial hysterectomy, 22-1
Simple seizures, 18-3
Simvastatin, 1-10t–1-11t
Single-incision slings (minislings), 7-7
Sinusoidal pattern, fetal heart rate, 10-8, 10-8t, 10-9f
SIS (saline infusion sonography/ sonohysterography)
  abnormal uterine bleeding, 5-8
  infertility testing, 8-1
  leiomyoma, 5-4
  postmenopausal bleeding, 5-10
  recurrent pregnancy loss and, 8-4
Skene duct cyst, 20-6t
Skin. See also Dermatologic changes in pregnancy; Dermatologic conditions
  cancer screening, 1-3, 1-13
  preoperative preparation of, 3-6
  reactions, chemotherapy and, 22-18
Sleep disturbance, 19-4, 19-5
SMA (spinal muscular atrophy), 9-12
Small bowel obstruction, 2-2t, 3-10
Small cell carcinoma, 22-2
Smoking, 9-2, 17-9. See also Tobacco
Smoking cessation, 5-17, 19-2
SNRIs (serotonin and norepinephrine reuptake inhibitors), 5-16, 19-6t
Soapsuds enema, 9-7t
Social anxiety, 19-4
Sodium bicarbonate, 14-3, 14-9
Sodium chloride (NaCl) 7.5% solution, 14-8t
Sodium chloride (NaCl) 9% solution, 14-8t
Sodium ferric gluconate, 16-2t
Sodium phosphate (Fleet), 9-7t
Sodium polystyrene sulfonate (Kayexalate), 14-9
SOFA score, 3-8
Soft markers, in fetal anatomy assessment, 9-8
Solifenacin (Vesicare), 7-6t
Sonohysterography (saline infusion sonogram). See SIS
Sorbitol, 9-7t
Speculum exam, chronic pelvic pain and, 5-14
Sperm cryopreservation, 8-10
Spherocytosis, hereditary, 16-3t
Spina bifida, 9-10
Spinal headache (postdural puncture), 4-4t
Spinal neuraxial block, 4-3
Spiramycin, 21-3
Spirometry, 13-1
Spontaneous abortion (SAB) or miscarriage, 2-2t, 2-5
Spontaneous labor and delivery, 10-4, 10-5t

Squamous cell carcinoma (SCC), 1-14, 22-2, 22-11, 22-12
Squamous epithelial uterine tumors, 22-3
SSRIs (selective serotonin reuptake inhibitors), 5-13, 5-16, 19-6t
Staphylococcus aureus, 3-6
Static tumors, 22-16
Statins, 1-11t
STEMI (ST segment elevation MI), 12-10
Steroid cell tumors, 22-10
Steroids, 18-2t, 18-5, 25-10t. *See also* Corticosteroids
Stevens–Johnson syndrome, 20-7
Stillbirth, 21-3
Stones. *See* Cholecystitis; Cholelithiasis
Stool diary, 7-9
Strassman metroplasty, 8-7
Streptococcus agalactiae, 2-9
Stress urinary incontinence (SUI), 7-4, 7-6
Stroke, 5-20, 18-6
Stromal tumors, 2-7
Struma ovarii (ovarian dermoid), 17-10f
Subacute bacterial endocarditis (SBE), 3-3
Subarachnoid hemorrhage (SAH), 18-1t, 18-7
Subclinical hypothyroidism, 17-8, 17-9, 17-10f
Subdermal Implant (Etonogestrel implant), 25-11t
Substance abuse, 9-2, 19-1, 19-1t medications, 25-9t
Substance use disorder, 19-1
Sufentanil, 4-4t, 4-7, 4-7t
Sulbactam, 11-17t
Sulfadiazine, 21-3
Sulfasalazine, 15-7t
Sulfonylureas (glyburide, glipizide, glimepiride), 17-7t, 25-7t
Sumatriptan, 18-2t, 18-3t
Superficial incisional SSI, 3-7
Suppository, for constipation, 9-7t
Surfactant/albumin ratio, 10-2
Surgery
    avascular pelvic planes and, 23-4t
    common gynecologic, 24-5
    common instruments for, 24-11
    common obstetric, 24-8
    enhanced recovery after, 3-5
    epithelial ovarian cancer, 22-7
    germ cell tumors, 22-9
    gynecologic, common nerve injury in, 3-4t
    hyperthyroidism, 17-10
    pelvic arterial blood supply and, 23-3t
    postoperative fever, 3-6, 3-6t
    postoperative ileus, 3-5
    wound classification, 3-6t
Surgical site infections (SSIs), 3-6
    preoperative antibiotics and, 3-3

Swyer syndrome, 6-6, 6-7t
Synalar (Fluocinolone acetonide), 20-4t
Syndromes, definition, 9-9
Syphilis, 6-7t, 21-2, 21-7, 21-9, 21-10t
Syphilitic meningitis, 21-8

T
T_3 resin uptake (T_3RU), 17-9t
T6–L1 nerve root block with local anesthetic, 4-7t
T-ACE, 19-1t
Tachyarrhythmias, 9-11
Tachycardia with a pulse, Adult Algorithm, 26-3f
Tachypnea, 10-2
Tachysystole, 10-7
Talipes equinovarus (clubfoot), 9-12
Tamoxifen, 6-3
Tamponade, intracavitary, 2-10t
Tampon test, 11-7
Tanner stages (staging), 6-1f, 6-1t, 6-2
Tap-water enema, 9-7t
Taxane, 22-17
Taxotere (docetaxel), 22-17, 25-5t
Tay–Sachs screening, 9-13
Tazobactam, 11-17t
TE (thromboembolism), 5-17t
Tegaserod (Zelnorm), 9-7t
Temovate (Clobetasol propionate), 20-4t
Tenaculum site for nerve blocks, 4-5f
Tenofovir, 2-13
TENS (transcutaneous electrical nerve stimulation), 4-6t
Tension-free vaginal tape, retropubic sling (TVT), 7-6
Tension-type headache, 18-1
Teratogens, 9-9, 19-2t
Teratoma, 5-20, 6-7t
Terbutaline, 11-8t, 11-15, 25-7t
Terconazole, 5-2t
TERIS (online schizophrenia resource), 19-6
Tertiary syphilis, 21-8
TESE (testicular sperm extraction), 8-9
Testing. *See also* Screening
    preoperative, 3-1
    by RCRI factors, 3-2t
Testosterone, 5-16, 5-18t, 22-9t, 22-10
Tetanus/diphtheria/pertussis (Tdap), 2-13
Tetracycline, 21-8t
Thalassemias, 9-13, 16-2t, 16-3
Thecomas, 22-10
Thelarche, 6-1
    premature, 6-2t
Therapeutic amniocentesis, 9-14
Thiazide diuretic, 12-4t
Thiazolidinediones (pioglitazone, rosiglitazone), 25-7t
Thimerosal, 13-6
3rd trimester, 9-2t, 9-3, 12-2t
Thoracic anomalies, 9-11

Thrombocytopenia
  approach to, 16-5f
  characteristics, 16-4, 16-4t
  management, 16-5t
  neonatal alloimmune, 16-15
  neuraxial anesthesia and, 4-3
  perioperative optimization, 3-2
Thrombolysis, 16-9, 16-9t
Thrombophilia evaluation, 16-10, 16-10f, 16-10t
Thrombosis
  cerebral venous, 18-1f, 18-1t, 18-7
  deep vein, 5-3, 8-4
  splenic vein, 15-2
  venous sinus, 18-1
Thyroid disease perioperative management, 3-3
Thyroid disorders, 5-13, 17-10f
Thyroid function tests, 17-9t
Thyroiditis, 17-9, 17-10f
Thyroid-stimulating hormone (TSH), 5-13, 8-2, 17-9t
Thyroid storm, 17-9, 17-10
Thyrotoxicosis factitia, 17-10f
Thyroxine-binding globulin (TBG), 17-9t
TIBC (total iron-binding capacity), 16-2t
Tibial nerve stimulation, percutaneous, 7-10
Tibolone, 5-18t
Ticarcillin/clavulanate, 14-6t
Tinidazole, 5-2t
Tioconazole, 5-2t
TMP/SMX (trimethoprim/ sulfamethoxazole), 10-16, 14-5t, 14-7t, 25-2t
TNM (tumor, lymph node, metastasis) staging, 1-7t
TOA (tuboovarian abscess), 2-2t, 2-7
Tobacco, 9-2, 19-2t. See also Smoking
Tocolytics, 11-8t, 25-7t
Tofranil (Imipramine), 7-6t
TOLAC (trial of labor after prior cesarean), 10-13, 10-13t
Tolterodine (Detrol/Detrol LA), 7-6t
Tonic–clonic seizures, 18-3
Topicort (Desoximetasone), 20-4t
Topotecan (Hycamtin), 22-17, 25-5t
TORCH infections, 21-2
TOT (transobturator sling), 7-7
Total abdominal hysterectomy, 24-7
Total alkaline phosphatase, 15-1
Total parenteral nutrition (TPN), 15-12, 15-12t
Total spinal blockade, 4-4t
Total T₄ (T₄), 17-9t
Total triiodothyronine (T₃), 17-9t
Touch, nonpharmacologic analgesia and, 4-6t
Toviaz (Fesoterodine ER), 7-6t
Toxic adenomas, 17-9
Toxicity
  bone marrow, 22-17
  digitalis, 14-9
  local anesthesia, 4-1, 4-4t
Toxoplasmosis, 9-4, 21-2

TPAL system, 9-1
TPN (total parenteral nutrition), 15-12
Tranexamic acid, 2-10t, 5-8, 11-10
Tranquilizers, 6-7t, 19-3t
Transabdominal ultrasound (US), 2-1
Transfusion associated circulatory overload (TACO), 16-17t
Transfusion-related acute lung injury (TRALI), 16-17t
Transient (functional) hypogonadotropic hypogonadism, 6-6
Transient tachypnea of the newborn, 10-2
Transobturator sling (TOT), 7-7
Transvaginal ultrasound (TVUS)
  abnormal uterine bleeding, 5-8
  adenomyosis, 5-5
  adnexal masses, 5-20
  common indications, 2-1
  endometriosis, 5-6
  infertility testing, 8-1
  postmenopausal bleeding, 5-10
Transverse diameter of pelvis, 9-4, 9-5t
Transverse vaginal septum, 6-7t, 6-8, 8-6
Transversus abdominis plane block, 4-7t
Trauma, 2-11, 2-12f, 5-14
Treponema pallidum, 21-7, 21-10t
Triamcinolone acetonide (Kenalog, Triderm), 20-4t
Trichomonas, 5-1t, 5-14
Tricyclic antidepressants (TCA), 4-1, 5-15, 19-6t
Triderm (Triamcinolone acetonide), 20-4t
Trimethoprim, 14-6t
Triple screen, 9-1, 9-12
Triptan–NSAID combination, 18-2t
Trisomy 13/18, 9-10
Trisomy 21 (T21), 9-8, 9-11
Trocar site hernia, 3-11
Troponin, 12-10
Trospium chloride (Sanctura), 7-6t
Trospium ER (Sanctura XR), 7-6t
True pelvis, 9-4
Truvada, 2-13
TSH (thyroid-stimulating hormone), 5-13, 8-2, 17-9t
TST (tuberculin skin test), 21-6, 21-6t
Tubal diseases, 8-1t
Tubal factor infertility, 8-3
Tubal ligation, 4-2, 4-7, 8-3, 24-7, 24-9
Tuberculin skin test (TST), 21-6, 21-6t
Tuberculosis (TB), 6-7t, 21-5
Turner (XO) syndrome, 6-5, 6-7t, 9-10
TVT (tension-free vaginal tape, retropubic sling), 7-6
Twin delivery, 4-2
Twin–twin transfusion syndrome (TTTS), 11-5

U
UAE (uterine artery embolization)
  acute uterine bleeding, 2-10t
  adenomyosis, 5-5
Uchida method for postpartum tubal ligation, 24-9

UFH (unfractionated heparin), 16-9, 16-9t
Ugly duckling sign, 1-14
Ulcerative colitis (UC), 15-5, 15-6t
Ulipristal (Ella), 1-18
Ultralente (Insulin zinc extended), 17-3t
Ultrasound (US)
    common indications, 2-1
    early pregnancy, 2-2
    early pregnancy failure, 2-6
    ectopic pregnancy, 2-4
    redating EDD with, 9-1t
Ultrasound-guided radiofrequency thermal ablation (RFA), 5-4
Ultravate (Halobetasol propionate), 20-4t
Umbilical artery Doppler velocimetry, 10-1
Umbilical cord
    blood gas analysis, 10-6, 10-14, 10-14t
    fetal ultrasound, 9-8
    prolapse, induction of labor and, 10-7
Unconjugated estriol (UE3), 9-12, 9-12t
Unfractionated heparin (UFH), 16-9, 16-9t
Unicornuate uterus, 8-5f, 8-6t, 8-7
Upper abdominal blood supply, 23-5f
Upper abdominal pain, differential diagnosis of, 15-3t
UPSC (uterine papillary serous carcinoma), 22-4
Ureter, 23-2f
Ureteral diverticulum, 2-7
Ureteric injuries, 3-10
Ureterovaginal fistulae, 7-8
Urethra, innervation of, 7-1t
Urethral plugs, 7-5, 7-6
Urethral pressure profile, 7-5
Urethral sphincter, 7-1t
Urge urinary incontinence (UUI), 7-4, 7-5, 7-6t
Urinary diversion, 7-9
Urinary dysfunction, 5-17
Urinary incontinence, 7-4, 25-10t
Urinary retention, postpartum, 10-15
Urinary system changes in pregnancy
    acute kidney injury, 14-1
    chronic kidney disease, 14-3
    fluids and electrolytes, 14-8
    nephrolithiasis, 14-7
    pyelonephritis, 14-6
    urinary tract infections, 14-4
Urinary tract infections (UTIs), 14-4, 14-5t
Urinary tract injury, 3-11
Urodynamic testing, 7-5
Uroflowmetry, 7-5
Urogenital atrophy, 5-17
Urogenital fistulae, 7-7
Urogenital triangle, 23-6f
US. See Ultrasound

Uterine artery embolization, 5-9
Uterine atony, 11-10t, 11-11f
Uterine bleeding, 2-9, 5-8
Uterine cancer, 22-4, 22-4t, 22-5t, 22-6t
Uterine compression sutures, 11-11f
Uterine didelphys, 8-4, 8-5f, 8-6t, 8-7
Uterine fibroids, 5-3
Uterine inversion, 11-15
    general anesthesia and, 4-6
    postpartum hemorrhage and, 11-10
Uterine massage, 11-11f
Uterine obstruction, 8-7
Uterine perforation, 3-12
Uterine prolapse, 7-1
Uterine sarcomas, 22-6
Uterine septum, 8-7
Uterine tetany, 10-7
Uterosacral ligament suspension, 7-3
Uterosacral nerve ablation, 5-7
Uterotonics, 25-6t

V
Vaccines/vaccinations
    hepatitis A and B, 15-9
    hepatitis B, 21-5
    HPV, 21-7
    influenza, 9-3, 21-5
    pneumococcal, 13-5
    recommendations and types, 1-19f
    routine prenatal visit, 9-3
    varicella, 21-3
VACTERL (Vertebral anomalies, Anal atresia, Cardiac defects, TE fistula, Renal defects, Limb defects), 9-11
Vacuum, operative vaginal delivery and, 10-12, 10-12f
Vagina, 3 levels of support of, 7-2
Vaginal agenis/MRKH, 8-6
Vaginal atresia, 8-6
Vaginal birth after cesarean (VBAC), 10-13, 10-13t
Vaginal bleeding. See Postpartum hemorrhage
Vaginal cancer, 1-20t, 22-11, 22-12t, 22-19t
Vaginal cuff cellulitis, 3-7
Vaginal cysts, 20-6t
Vaginal cytomegalovirus, 21-6
Vaginal flora, 2-9
Vaginal hysterectomy, 24-8
Vaginal mesh types and procedures, 7-4
Vaginal obstruction, 8-7
Vaginal pH, 5-15
Vaginal ring, 1-17, 5-17t, 25-11t
Vaginismus, 5-15
VAIN (vaginal intraepithelial neoplasia), 22-11
Valacyclovir, 21-11t
Valisone (Betamethasone valerate), 20-4t
Valproate, 19-7t
Valproic acid, 18-4t
Valsalva maneuver, 7-2

Valsartan, 12-4t
Valvular heart disease, 12-12t
Vancomycin, 25-3t
VAP (ventilation-associated pneumonia), 13-4
Variability, fetal heart rate, 10-8, 10-8t
Varicella virus (VZV), 21-2, 21-3
Varicosities, 9-6
Vasa previa, 11-14
Vascular injury, laparoscopy and, 3-11
Vascular thrombosis, 16-12t
Vasomotor menopausal symptoms (VMsx), 5-16
Vasopressors, 3-9
VBAC (vaginal birth after cesarean), 10-13
VBP (vinblastine, bleomycin, carboplatin), 22-16t
Vecchietti procedure, 8-7
Venlafaxine, 5-16, 19-6t
Venous thromboembolic disease, 16-6, 16-7f, 16-9
Ventricular fibrillation (VF), 26-2f
Ventriculomegaly, 9-10, 21-4
Verapamil, 18-3t
Verrucous carcinoma, 1-14
  vulvar, 22-12, 22-13
Vesicare (Solifenacin), 7-6t
Vestibulectomy, 5-15
VF (ventricular fibrillation), 26-2f
Viability, prenatal testing of, 9-1
VIN (vulvar epithelial neoplasia/vulvar intraepithelial neoplasia), 22-12
Viral hepatitis, 15-7
Viral infections, 13-4t
Virchow's triad, 16-6
Visceral pain, 2-4
Vitamin A, 9-4
Vitamin B6 (pyridoxine), 5-13, 9-5, 25-8t
Vitamin B$_{12}$ deficiency, 16-3
Vitamin D supplements, 1-13, 5-17, 9-4
Vitex agnus-castus (chasteberry), 5-13
Voiding cystogram, 14-4
Voiding diary, 7-8
von Willebrand disease (vWD), 16-11
VT (tidal volume), 26-2f
VTE (venous thromboembolism), 3-7, 3-8t, 16-6, 16-9t
Vulvar cancer, 1-20t, 22-12, 22-13t, 22-19t
Vulvar carcinoma, 22-12
Vulvar cytomegalovirus, 21-6
Vulvar pain, 5-14
Vulvar sarcoma, 22-12, 22-13
Vulvar varicosities, 9-6
Vulvodynia, 5-14
Vulvovaginitis, 5-1
VVF (vesicovaginal fistula) repair, 7-8

W

Warfarin (Coumadin), 12-14t, 16-9, 16-9t, 25-4t
Water immersion, nonpharmacologic analgesia and, 4-6t
Water injections, sterile, nonpharmacologic analgesia and, 4-6t
Weapons, sexual assault reporting and, 2-13
Weight gain during pregnancy by BMI, 9-3t
Wells DVT score, 16-7t, 16-8t
Well-Woman (Annual) Exam, 1-1, 1-1t, 1-2, 1-3t
Wertheim's hysterectomy, 22-1
Westcort (Hydrocortisone valerate), 20-4t
Wet prep
  chronic pelvic pain, 5-14
  vulvar pain, 5-15
Whirlpool sign, 2-8
White classification of diabetes mellitus, 17-5t
Whole blood, 16-16t
Williams' vulvovaginoplasty, 8-7
Withdrawal method, 1-17
Women's health epidemiology and research, 1-20t
Women's Health Initiative (WHI), 5-17
Word catheter, 24-2, 24-3f
World Health Organization (WHO), 12-1t, 18-5, 22-16t
Wound infiltration, 4-7t
Wright–Giemsa stain, 21-11t

X

Xeroderma pigmentosum, 1-14
XR (radiography), 2-1. See also Radiography

Y

Yeast culture, 5-15
Yolk sac tumor, 22-8, 22-9t
Yuzpe method, 1-18

Z

ZAHARA I (maternal cardiac risk classification), 12-1
Zelnorm (tegaserod), 9-7t
Zika, 21-4
Zithromax, 25-2t
Zofran (Ondansetron), 9-5, 25-8t
Zolpidem (Ambien), 25-9t
Zona fasciculata, 17-10
Zona glomerulosa, 17-10
Zona reticularis, 17-10
Zoster, 21-3
Zosyn (Piperacillin/tazobactam), 25-2t
Zygosity, 11-4